Board Review Series

Emergency Medicine

Board Review Series

Emergency Medicine

Latha Stead, M.D.
Resident, Department of Emergency Medicine
Jacobi-Montefiore Emergency Medicine Residency Program
Bronx, New York

Reviewers:

Stephen H. Thomas, M.D., F.A.C.E.P.
Director, Undergraduate Medical Education
Associate Director, Prehospital Medicine
Department of Emergency Medicine,
Harvard Medical School
Attending Physician,
Massachusetts General Hospital
Boston, Massachusetts

Barbara A. McIntosh, M.D., F.A.C.E.P.
Attending Physician,
Queens Hospital Center
Attending Physician, St. John's Hospital,
Catholic Medical Center
Former Associate Medical Director,
New York City Emergency Medical Services
Queens, New York

Steven Nazario, M.D.
Assistant Professor of Emergency Medicine
Albert Einstein College of Medicine
Attending Physician,
Jacobi Medical Center
Bronx, New York

Barbara G. Lock, M.D.
Resident, Department of Emergency Medicine
Jacobi-Montefiore Emergency Medicine Residency Program
Bronx, New York

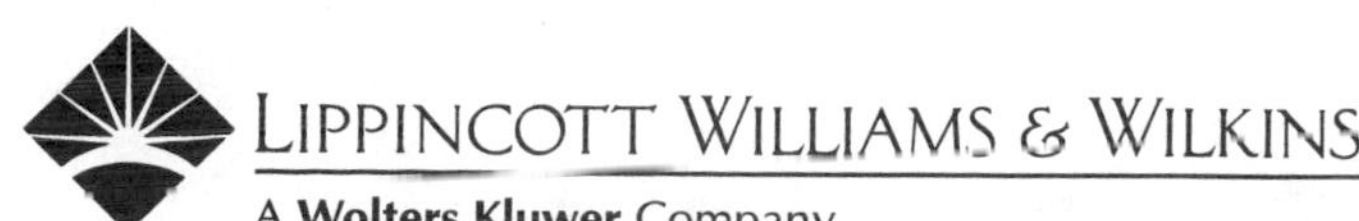

LIPPINCOTT WILLIAMS & WILKINS
A **Wolters Kluwer** Company
Philadelphia • Baltimore • New York • London
Buenos Aires • Hong Kong • Sydney • Tokyo

Editor: Elizabeth Nieginski
Editorial Director: Julie Scardiglia
Development Editors: Emilie Linkins
Marketing Manager: Kelley Ray
Managing Editor: Marette Smith

351 West Camden Street
Baltimore, Maryland 21201-2436 USA

530 Walnut Street
Philadelphia, Pennsylvania 19106 USA

Printed in the United States of America

Library of Congress Cataloging-in-Publication Data
ISBN#0-683-30617-0

To purchase additional copies of this book call our customer service department at **(800) 638-3030** or fax orders to **(301) 824-7390.** International customers should call **(301) 714-2324.**

00 01 02
1 2 3 4 5 6 7 8 9

Dedication

To my parents, Ganti & Prabha, my beloved husband Matt, my brother Murali & baby Thor . . .

you are my inspiration and the reason I accomplish anything in life

With special thanks to my teachers,

Herbert S. Chase Jr., M.D.
Clinical Associate Professor of Medicine
College of Physicians & Surgeons
Columbia University, New York, New York

Martin J. Davis, D.D.S.
Dean of Student Affairs
School of Dental & Oral Surgery
Columbia University, New York, New York

Jay H. Lefkowitch, M.D.
Clinical Professor of Pathology
College of Physicians & Surgeons
Columbia University, New York, New York

Amalia C. Kelly, M.D.
Clinical Associate Professor of Obstetrics & Gynecology
College of Physicians & Surgeons
Columbia University, New York, New York

. . .for making my dream of becoming a doctor happen

Foreword

Emergency medicine developed as a specialty in its own right during the last quarter of the 20th century. When this new medical discipline first appeared it raised some questions, particularly within mainstream academic medicine. This was largely because the new field was aimed not at "knowing more and more about less and less"—which had been the longstanding tradition of specialization and subspecialization in American medicine—but was targeted at breadth rather than depth of knowledge. Indeed, the problem of defining this new discipline was determining along what tissue plane (i.e., how deeply into the body of medical knowledge) to dissect to free the broad slice of the specialty's core content. The solution presented itself, quite naturally, as a contextual one, determined by the temporal profile of the patient's presentation. Emergency medicine has become a broad-based, time-delimited specialty.

The format of *BRS Emergency Medicine* is entirely congruent with these two dimensions of the discipline. First, the concise outline format combined with liberal use of figures and tables provides ready access to clinically useful diagnostic and therapeutic information. It is conducive to rapid scanning at the bedside. Second, each of the 20 chapters offers a summary of clinical presentations, diagnostic strategies, treatment options, and appropriate disposition for common emergency department problems. With a review test at the end of each chapter and a comprehensive exam at the end of the text, the book contains over 400 USMLE-style questions and answers. This format reflects a fundamental understanding of the need for information to be integrated into some larger conceptual framework if it is to be retained in memory. The chapters can be read as an overview, which might be undertaken at a pace of roughly one chapter following each of the 20 or so shifts a clinical clerk is likely to work during an average one-month emergency department rotation. Along with each chapter, the review questions can then be worked to test the mastery of the material. At the end of the book, taking the comprehensive examination will provide the student with an overall review.

This text was authored by an emergency medicine resident during her training. It contains substantial contributions from her many colleagues in the residency program, and reflects a great deal of careful content editing undertaken by several members of the faculty. Medical students emerging from their preclinical years should find this book enormously helpful in optimizing the educational value of an emergency medicine clerkship.

E. John Gallagher, MD
Professor & University Chair
Department of Emergency Medicine
Albert Einstein College of Medicine
April 2, 2000

Contents

Preface

BRS Emergency Medicine provides a quick review of the major topics in emergency medicine. It is meant to help to prepare the third and fourth year medical student for the USMLE Steps 2 and 3 and the emergency medicine clerkship examinations. It is useful not only for exam review, but also as a quick reference for medical students and residents rotating in the emergency department.

The text is presented in the tight outline format of *BRS,* which makes review of core concepts quick and easy. The book is divided into 20 chapters which cover emergencies by system. Each chapter ends with a review test consisting of USMLE-style study questions to test the student's knowledge of the information covered in that chapter. The comprehensive examination at the end of the text is designed to test knowledge across systems, as emergencies rarely present within a single system. Clinical vignettes describing how an actual patient might present to the emergency department are emphasized. This question format reflects the style of the USMLE Steps 2 and 3 and the emergency medicine clerkship examinations.

As a first and second year medical student, I owned every *BRS* title available at the time, and relied on them to get me through clerkship examinations and the USMLE Step 1. When I entered the third year of medical school, however, I found there were very few clinical *BRS* titles, and was pleased to author this book as part of the expansion of the *BRS* series to include more clinical titles. I hope this book will be as useful as the other titles in the *BRS* series. I welcome any comments or suggestions for future editions, and wish you fun and luck in your emergency medicine experience.

Latha Stead

Acknowledgments

My sincere thanks to the entire staff at Lippincott Williams & Wilkins. Elizabeth Nieginski introduced me to the world of publishing and has been a great source of inspiration and encouragement throughout this project. Her cheerful e-mails kept me going during the times when I thought I didn't have what it took to write a useful review book. My editing and production teams, Julie Scardiglia, Lisa Bolger, Emilie Linkins, Elizabeth Durand, Karla Schroeder, and Marette Smith, worked hard to maintain stylistic consistency of the manuscript, while Wayne Heim expertly created the artwork.

Special thanks to all my contributors and reviewers. Certain people deserve special mention:

Dr. Anthony Ciociari, for compiling the comprehensive examination.

Dr. John Gallagher, for his support and encouragement.

Dr. Barbara Lock, my friend and colleague, for her critical review of and substantial contribution to several chapters. She selflessly dedicated her precious free time to making this book up to date.

Dr. Stephen Thomas for going above and beyond his role as reviewer to make this work as accurate as possible. As my preceptor in medical school, he sold me on the idea of emergency medicine. An inspiring teacher and a fabulous role model, he has urged me to excel along every step of the way.

Contributors

Katherine J. Chou, M.D.,
Assistant Professor of Pediatrics
Albert Einstein College of Medicine
Assistant Director of Pediatric Emergency Services
Jacobi Medical Center
Bronx, New York

Anthony Ciorciari, M.D.
Assistant Professor of Emergency Medicine
Albert Einstein College of Medicine
Attending Physician, Jacobi Medical Center
Bronx, New York

Elaine Dennis, M.D., M.B.A.
Resident, Department of Emergency Medicine
Jacobi-Montefiore Emergency Medicine Residency Program
Bronx, New York

Eddys Disla, M.D.
Chief, Division of Rheumatology
Department of Medicine
Cabrini Medical Center
New York, New York

Marie Doulaverakis, D.D.S.
Resident, Department of Orthodontics
Columbia University School of Dental & Oral Surgery
New York, New York

Shashi D. Ganti, M.D., F.A.A.O.
Ophthalmologist, Private Practice
Palo Alto, California

Michelle Garcia, M.D.
Resident, Department of Emergency Medicine
Mount Sinai/Elmhurst Emergency Medicine Residency Program
New York, New York

William A. Gluckman, D.O., EMT-P
Associate Medical Director, University Emergency Medical Service
Instructor of Surgery
University of Medicine and Dentistry New Jersey
Newark, New Jersey

Peter W. Greenwald, M.D.
Resident, Department of Emergency Medicine
Jacobi-Montefiore Emergency Medicine Residency Program
Bronx, New York

Peter Gruber, M.D., F.A.C.E.P.
Trauma Coordinator
Jacobi-Montefiore Emergency Medicine Residency Program
Assistant Professor of Emergency Medicine
Albert Einstein College of Medicine
Bronx, New York

Glenn R. Hornstein, M.D., F.A.A.P
Resident, Department of Emergency Medicine
Jacobi-Montefiore Emergency Medicine Residency Program
Bronx, New York

Siu-Fai Li, M.D.
Assistant Professor of
Emergency Medicine
Albert Einstein College of Medicine
Attending Physician,
Jacobi Medical Center
Bronx, New York

Barbara G. Lock, M.D.
Resident, Department of Emergency
Medicine
Jacobi-Montefiore Emergency Medicine
Residency Program
Bronx, New York

Heather Long, M.D.
Resident, Department of
Emergency Medicine
Jacobi-Montefiore Emergency Medicine
Residency Program
Bronx, New York

Frank Lovaglio, M.D.
Instructor of Emergency Medicine
Albert Einstein College of Medicine
Attending Physician,
Jacobi Medical Center
Bronx, New York

Charles M. Martinez, M.D.
Assistant Professor of
Emergency Medicine
Albert Einstein College of Medicine
Attending Physician,
Jacobi Medical Center
Bronx, New York
Police Surgeon,
New York City Department of Police

Eliza Ng, M.D.
Resident, Department of Obstetrics
& Gynecology
Jacobi Medical Center
Bronx, New York

Victor Pazos, M.D.
Cardiology Fellow, Dept. of Medicine
Mt. Sinai Medical Center
Miami, Florida

Michael Rohman, M.D., F.A.C.S., F.A.A.S.T., F.S.T.S,
Professor of Surgery
New York Medical College
Attending Trauma Surgeon
Jacobi Medical Center
Bronx, NY

Nirav N. Shah, M.D.
Chief Resident, Department of
Emergency Medicine
Long Island Jewish Medical Center
New Hyde Park, New York

Chandra Sharma, M.D.
Chief, Division of Neurology
Department of Medicine
Cabrini Medical Center
New York, New York

Nathaniel Tindel, M.D.
Attending Spine Surgeon
Dept. of Orthopedics
Jacobi Medical Center
Bronx, NY

Son-Yih Tu, M.D.
Instructor of Emergency Medicine
Attending Physician,
St. Luke's Roosevelt Medical Center
New York, New York

Johnny J. Vazquez, M.D.
Resident, Department of
Emergency Medicine
Lincoln Medical and Mental
Health Center
Bronx, New York

Smeeta Verma, M.D.
Director, Undergraduate
Medical Education
Assistant Professor of
Emergency Medicine
Albert Einstein College of Medicine
Attending Physician,
Jacobi Medical Center
Bronx, New York

1

Resuscitation, Basic Life Support, and Advanced Cardiac Life Support

I. Airway

—**Airway, breathing, and circulation** are the three components of the **ABCs,** the first issues that must be addressed in any patient encounter.

—Patency of the airway is checked by clinical presentation. If the patient can cough or speak, the airway is at least partially patent.

—Some of the more common causes of airway obstruction include:

—**foreign bodies** (especially in children)

—**edema** (as with anaphylaxis)

—a **lax tongue** falling back into the pharynx in an obtunded patient.

—The presence of **stridor** (high-pitched, upper airway, inspiratory sounds) usually indicates some degree of obstruction.

—If the airway is obstructed, opening the airway is attempted, as outlined in section IV.

—If the Basic Life Support (BLS) techniques fail, more definitive airway management must be undertaken.

A. Indications for intubation

1. Failure to maintain a patent airway

—Burn injury to airway and penetrating neck trauma may result in failure to maintain a patent airway.

2. Failure to protect the airway

—Aspiration, status epilepticus, drug overdose, severe head injury (GCS <9), or central nervous system (CNS) lesions may result in failure to protect the airway.

—Suggestive clues include inability to handle secretions and absence of gag and swallow reflexes.

3. **Hypoxia refractory to oxygenation via face mask**

B. **Types of intubation**

1. **Blind nasotracheal intubation**

—The diameter of the tube must be **0.5–1.0 mm** smaller than the corresponding endotracheal tube size (see I B 2). In children, the size of the tube can be estimated to be the size of the child's fifth digit.

—The depth of the tube (from the external nares to 5 ± 2 cm above the carina) should be 26 cm in women and 28 cm in men.

a. **Indications** include inability to open mouth (secondary to severe oral trauma or trismus), a short, thick neck, and inability to move the neck.

b. **Contraindications** include **apnea, head trauma** (e.g., basilar skull or central facial fracture), **CSF rhinorrhea,** an expanding neck hematoma, an uncooperative patient, choanal atresia, known bleeding diathesis, and an anticipated need for thrombolytic therapy

c. **Complications** include epistaxis, nasal septum or turbinate trauma, airway obstruction from bleeding, sinusitis (long-term), and retropharyngeal lacerations (rare).

—violation of cranial vault by blind nasotracheal intubation in cases of trauma

2. **Endotracheal intubation**

—is the method most commonly used.

—is the mainstay of difficult intubations.

—requires direct visualization of the airway (Figure 1-1).

—The **diameter of the tube** should be **6.5–8.0 mm in women** and **8.0–8.5 mm in men.** In **children,** the size of the tube is calculated as follows: **(age in years/4) + 4** mm.

—The depth of the tube (distance from lips to 5 ± 2 cm above the carina) should be 21 cm in women and 23 cm in men. In children, the depth is calculated as follows: (age in years/2) + 12 cm.

a. **Methods for checking endotracheal tube (ETT) placement**

(1) Direct visualization of the tube passing through the vocal cords (see Figure 1-1)

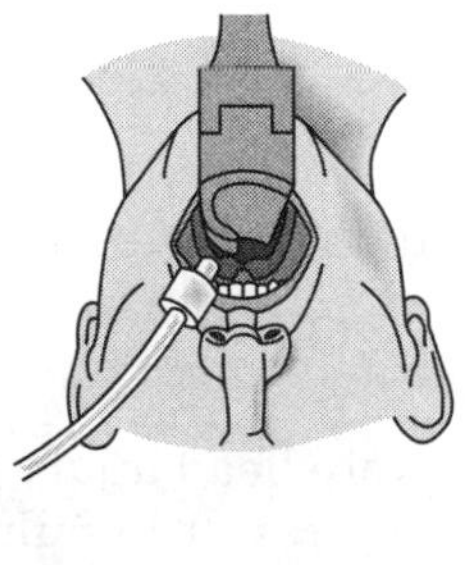

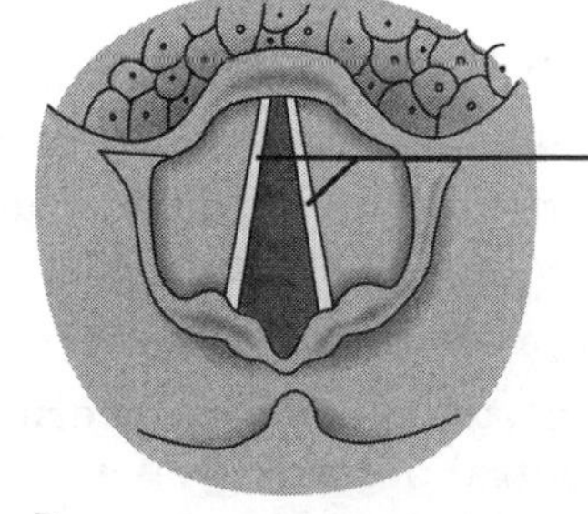

Figure 1-1. (*A*) Endotracheal intubation. (*B*) Note direct visualization of the V-shaped vocal cords. (Adapted from LifeART. Copyright 1998, Lippincott Williams & Wilkins. All rights reserved.)

(2) Pulmonary and gastric auscultation
(3) Condensation in ETT
(4) Aspiration technique
—Easy aspiration suggests tube is positioned in the trachea.
—Difficult aspiration suggests tube is positioned in the esophagus.
(5) Resistance to bagging (suggests esophageal intubation)
(6) Chest radiograph: tip of ETT should be aligned with T3 vertebra
(7) End-tidal carbon dioxide detector

b. **Contraindications** include
—massive orofacial trauma
—hemorrhage and severe trismus

c. **Complications** include
—vocal cord damage secondary to laryngospasm (can be prevented by anesthetizing vocal cords before procedure)
—subglottic stenosis
—esophageal or right main-stem bronchus intubation
—dental trauma
—cervical spine injury

3. **Rapid sequence intubation (RSI)**

—is a technique in which sedation and neuromuscular blockade are used virtually simultaneously without positive pressure ventilation in between.

—fastest method to obtain a **definitive airway**

—low complication rate

a. **Indications** include inability of patient to cooperate with awake intubation, altered mental status, seizure activity, trismus of oral muscles, severe trauma, and increased intracranial pressure (ICP).

b. Potential **complications** include **vomiting** and subsequent **aspiration,** because in emergent settings one must assume the patient has a full stomach.

c. The **procedure** involves

—**preparation** of all equipment (e.g., checking ETT balloon, suction, bag valve mask device, and pulse oximetry).

—**preoxygenation** (5 minutes of 100% oxygen by non-rebreather mask).

—**pretreatment** (Tables 1-1 and 1-2).

(1) For patients with increased ICP, use lidocaine or fentanyl.
(2) For preventing succinylcholine-associated muscle fasciculations, use a "priming" dose (0.01 mg/kg) of a competitive neuromuscular blocking agent such as atracurium, rocuronium, pancuronium, or vecuronium.
(3) For children use atropine 0.01–0.02 mg/kg IV to prevent the paradoxical bradycardia associated with succinylcholine to which children are especially susceptible.

—**sedation** with thiopental, methohexital, etomidate, midazolam, diazepam, fentanyl, or ketamine

Table 1-1. Induction Agents used in Rapid Sequence Intubation

Induction Agent	IV Dose	Onset of Action	Duration of Action	Indications	Contraindications
Thiopental	3.0–5.0 mg/kg	< 1 min	5–10 min	↑ ICP	Hypotension, asthma, cardiogenic shock, pulmonary edema
Methohexital	1.0–3.0 mg/kg	< 1 min	5–10 min	↑ ICP	Seizures, hypotension, asthma
Etomidate	0.3 mg/kg	< 1 min	5 min	↑ ICP, CAD	Age < 10 years, pregnant/ lactating, myoclonic epilepsy, severe hepatic disease
Fentanyl	3–15 μg/kg	2–4 min	45 min	↑ ICP	Hypotension
Midazolam	0.5–1.0 mg/kg	< 1 min	6–15 min	↑ ICP	Hypotension
Diazepam	0.04–0.3 mg/kg (children); 5–10 mg (adults)	1–2 min	2–4 h	↑ ICP	Hypotension
Ketamine	1.0–1.5 mg/kg	1 min	10–20 min	Status asthmaticus	Head trauma, ↑ ICP
Propofol	1.5–3.0 mg/kg	< 1 min	5–10 min	↑ ICP	Hypotension, severe CAD

CAD = coronary artery disease; *ICP* = increased intracranial pressure.

—**paralysis** with a **noncompetitive** neuromuscular blocking agent (e.g., succinylcholine) (see Table 1-2).

4. **Cricothyrotomy**

—is a surgical airway through the cricothyroid membrane

—provides a definitive airway

—is an invasive technique

a. **Indications** include

—massive trauma to the nose and mouth

—uncontrollable oral hemorrhage

—inhalation injury resulting in massive nasal and oral edema

—inability to control the airway with other methods

b. **Contraindications** include

—laryngeal injury

—patient age under 10 years (because the cricothyroid membrane in children is too small) [Figure 1-2]

Table 1-2. Neuromuscular Blocking Agents Used in Rapid Sequence Intubation

Depolarizing Agent	IV Push Dose	Onset of Action	Duration of Action	Continuous IV Infusion Rate
Noncompetitive				
Succinylcholine	1.0–1.5 mg/kg (can use 3–4 mg IM in children if no IV access)	30 sec	3–5 min	0.5–1.0 mg/min
Competitive				
Atracurium	0.5 mg/kg	2–5 min	20–45 min	0.4–0.8 mg/kg/h
Rocuronium	0.8 mg/kg	1–2 min	30–45 min	0.6–0.72 mg/kg/h
Pancuronium	0.1 mg/kg	3–5 min	80–100 min	0.02–0.1 mg/kg/h
Vecuronium	0.1 mg/kg	2–3 min	20–40 min	0.1 mg/kg/h

IM = intramuscular; *IV* = intravenous.

—ability to intubate safely by other methods

—In children under 10 years of age, a needle cricothyrotomy with percutaneous transtracheal ventilation is preferred.

c. **Complications** include excessive hemorrhage, aspiration, prolonged hypoxic state (because of time this technique requires), trauma to vocal cords and thyroid, esophageal perforation, subcutaneous emphysema, and altered phonation.

II. Breathing

—Once the airway is secured, attention is directed to breathing.

A. Oxygen delivery devices

—Any patient in respiratory distress or with potential for hypoxia should receive supplemental oxygen, with the goal of keeping oxygen saturation above 96%.

—Table 1-3 summarizes the methods used to deliver oxygen.

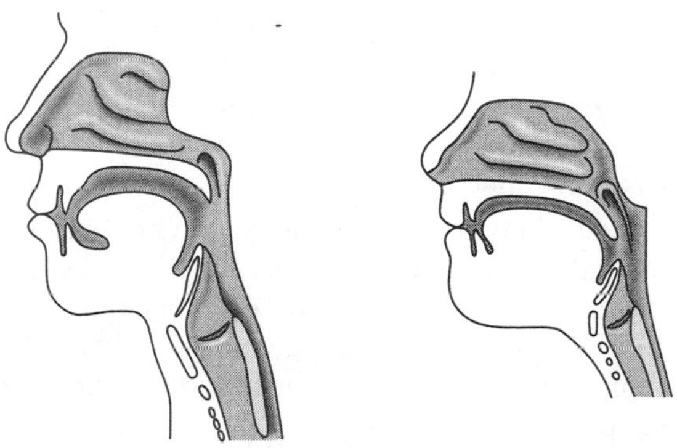

Figure 1-2. Airway anatomy. Note the differences between the adult (*A*) and pediatric (*B*) airways. (Adapted from LifeART. Copyright 1998, Lippincott Williams & Wilkins. All rights reserved.)

Table 1-3. Oxygen Delivery Devices

Delivery Devices	Oxygen Concentration (%)	Flow Rate (L)	Indications
Nasal cannula	25–45	1–6	Conscious, spontaneously breathing patient; not appropriate for arrest setting
Venturi mask	40–60	4–10	Conscious spontaneously breathing patient; not appropriate for arrest setting
Non-rebreather mask	80–95	8–12	Conscious, spontaneously breathing patient; not appropriate for arrest setting
Bag–valve–mask device	100	12–15	Apneic, nonintubated patients

B. Mechanical ventilation

—In intubated patients, the work of breathing may be assisted by ventilators.

1. Ventilators have several **modes** (Table 1-4).
2. Certain ventilator **settings** are manually preset, such as respiratory rate (RR), tidal volume (TV), percent of oxygen content of inspired gas (FIO_2), and positive end-expiratory pressure (PEEP).
   a. **RR** is set at 8–12 breaths/min in patients with normal lungs. A rate of 5–6 breaths/min may be used for patients with obstructive lung disease to facilitate permissive hypercapnia. For patients in whom hyperventilation is desired (e.g., head trauma, cerebral edema), RR may be set as high as 18–20 breaths/min.
   b. The **TV** is set at 5–15 ml/kg in patients with normal lungs. The aim is to adjust TV to keep peak airway pressures < 35 mm Hg; however, too low a TV may result in hypoxia and atelectasis.
   c. **FIO_2** is set at 0.2–1.0 in patients with normal lungs. The initial setting is 0.5. The aim is to set the lowest FIO_2 that will produce an oxygen saturation > 90% and a partial pressure of oxygen (PO_2) > 60 mm Hg. Increase the FIO_2 setting in patients with fever, hypercarbia, acidemia, and blood dyscrasias in whom the oxygen saturation is inherently compromised.
   d. **PEEP** is used when an acceptable oxygen saturation (i.e., > 90%) is not achievable with a desirable FIO_2 (i.e., < 0.5). Start with 5 cm H_2O and increase at 15-minute intervals by 3 cm H_2O until desired parameters are reached. PEEP improves oxygenation by keeping the alveoli patent during expiration and narrows the alveolar-arterial oxygen difference.
3. **Monitoring.** Patients on mechanical ventilation

   —should be monitored to ensure that optimal ventilation and perfusion conditions are maintained, especially when the patient is totally paralyzed and cannot breathe spontaneously.

Table 1-4. Ventilator Modes

Ventilator Mode	Description	Advantages and Indications	Disadvantages
CMV	Ventilator delivers a preset volume regardless of patient effort; spontaneous breaths not allowed (patient cannot breathe between mechanical breaths)	Useful for apneic, paralyzed, comatose, and acute overdose patients and those being deliberately hyperventilated (e.g., ↑ ICP)	Respiratory alkalosis may result, requires neuromuscular paralysis and sedation, difficult to wean
AC	Ventilator responds to patient's spontaneous effort, ensuring adequate tidal volume; if no patient effort, then cycles at preset rate.	Good initial choice of ventilator mode in conscious patients	Allows patients to spontaneously (self) hyperventilate
IMV	Equivalent to CMV + spontaneous breathing; ventilator does not assist patient but allows spontaneous breathing while delivering a predetermined number of tidal volumes	Requires less sedation than CMV or AC and no neuromuscular paralysis, good for muscle conditioning, less tendency for patient to self-hyperventilate	Breath stacking
SIMV	Equivalent to AC + spontaneous breathing; similar to IMV, but synchronized to patient's breathing; mechanical breath either coincides with a spontaneous breath or falls between spontaneous breaths	Prevents breath stacking, facilitates weaning, useful for obstructive airway disease	Requires intact respiratory effort
PS	Maintains airway at a constant preset inspiratory pressure until patient's inspiratory flow falls below 25% of peak level	Lowest peak airway pressure of all modes, requires less patient work, facilitates weaning, useful for restrictive airway disease	Requires spontaneously breathing patient, not good for patients with fluctuating respiratory effort or pulmonary compliance

AC = assist control; *CMV* = controlled mechanical ventilation; *IMV* = intermittent mandatory ventilation; *PS* = pressure support; *SIMV* = synchronized intermittent mandatory ventilation.

—should be placed on a cardiac monitor to check blood pressure, pulse, and oxygen saturation. It may also be desirable to monitor cardiac output, pulmonary capillary wedge pressure, and central venous pressure by means of a Swan-Ganz catheter. Bilateral breath sounds should be confirmed periodically in order not to miss a pneumothorax.

—An **arterial blood gas (ABG)** should be obtained 15 minutes after the initial ventilator settings are made and after each change in the ventilator settings to assess partial pressure of carbon dioxide (PCO_2).

a. In most patients, a PCO_2 of 40 mm Hg is desirable.

b. In patients who are being deliberately hyperventilated, Pco_2 is targeted to 28–30 mm Hg.

c. In patients with chronic carbon dioxide retention, Pco_2 is targeted to 50 mm Hg.

4. **Adverse effects**

a. **Barotrauma** can result from high pressures, which can lead to

—pneumothorax (tension pneumothorax is the most common complication)

—pulmonary interstitial emphysema

—subcutaneous emphysema

—pneumomediastinum

—pneumoperitoneum

—air embolism

b. **Decreased cardiac output** can result from decreased venous return to the right side of the heart secondary to increased intrathoracic pressure. Decreased cardiac output often is associated with PEEP > 15 cm H_2O and can lead to

—increased ischemia of the gastric mucosa and secondary bleeding

—decreased renal blood flow, leading to renal insufficiency and decreased urinary output

—decreased hepatic flow, leading to increased hepatic vessel resistance

c. **Oxygen toxicity** can result in **retrolental fibroplasia** and is associated with high Fio_2 settings.

d. **Pneumonia** is associated with nonsterile technique and poor humidification of the ventilation system. The most common infectious organisms are gram-negative enteric bacteria.

e. **Ulceration, stenosis,** or **necrosis** of the nasopharynx and oropharynx also may occur.

III. Circulation

—is focused on after the airway and breathing have been addressed.

—is addressed by monitoring vital signs, establishing IV access, controlling hemorrhage, and providing chest compressions as necessary.

A. Vital signs (i.e., pulse and blood pressure)

—The pulse is a quick, noninvasive way of determining gross circulatory status.

1. A palpable **radial** pulse denotes an approximate systolic blood pressure (SBP) of **80 mm Hg.**
2. A palpable **femoral** pulse denotes an approximate SBP of **70 mm Hg.**
3. A palpable **carotid** pulse denotes an approximate SBP of **60 mm Hg.**

B. Capillary refill time

—is another quick, easy gauge of perfusion.

—is the time it takes for color to return to a blanched nail bed.

—normal capillary refill time is 2–3 seconds, with 5 seconds considered abnormally delayed.

C. IV access

1. Peripheral access

—is often faster than central line placement.

—affords excellent access for volume replacement when done with two **large-bore needles (14- to 16-gauge)** in the **antecubital** or **upper arm veins.**

—In **infants and small children** [i.e., < 11 kg (24 lb)], a **22- to 24-gauge** needle should be used.

—In **older children,** an **18- to 22-gauge** needle may be more appropriate.

2. Central access

—may be obtained via different veins.

—Each approach has its own advantages and disadvantages (Table 1-5).

3. Intraosseous (IO) access

—is used in **children** when IV access is difficult to obtain.

—is attempted via the **anteromedial aspect of the tibia** or the **distal femur.**

—The marrow of the bone drains into the central venous system, and may provide faster access.

—Virtually **all drugs that can be given IV can also be given IO.**

D. Chest compressions

1. Closed compressions (see IV B 2)

Table 1-5. Comparison of Different Approaches for Central Venous Access

Central Venous Access	Advantages	Disadvantages
Subclavian	Left preferred over right for transcutaneous pacing, low infection rate, most comfortable for patient	Least safe during a code, highest risk of pneumothorax (2%), interference with CPR, contraindicated in the presence of clavicular fracture
Internal jugular	Less risk of pneumothorax compared to subclavian, easier access during CPR compared to subclavian, right preferred over left due to anatomy, fastest circulation time	Increased risk of carotid artery puncture, least comfortable for patient
Femoral	Safest in acute situations (trauma, code), no risk of pneumothorax, easiest access during a code	Highest incidence of infection, increased risk of thrombosis, slowest circulation time

CPR = cardiopulmonary resuscitation.

2. Open compressions

—are done **after thoracotomy** in cases of penetrating trauma to the chest.

—are most successful if done **within 20 minutes of cardiac arrest.**

IV. Basic Life Support (BLS)

A. Foreign body airway obstruction

1. Conscious victim

a. Determine obstructed airway.

—Shout "Can you cough?" and "Can you speak?"

—Look for the **universal distress signal** (i.e., a hand wrapped around the throat). Inability to make vocal sounds or the presence of stridor also usually signals an obstructed airway.

b. Activate the emergency medical system (EMS).

c. Clear the airway.

(1) In adults and children, use the **Heimlich maneuver.**

—Stand behind the victim with your fists two fingerbreadths below the xiphoid process.

—Deliver upward abdominal thrusts until the airway is cleared (i.e., foreign body is expelled) or the victim becomes unconscious.

(2) In **infants,** use an alternative method consisting of **back blows and chest thrusts,** because the force of the Heimlich maneuver may result in rupture of abdominal organs.

—With the infant placed prone over the rescuer's forearm, deliver five forceful back blows between the infant's shoulder blades using the heel of the hand.

—Next, while carefully supporting the head and neck, turn the infant to a supine position with the head lower than the trunk and deliver five quick downward chest thrusts with 2–3 fingers of one hand one fingerbreadth below the nipple line.

—Continue alternating back blows with chest thrusts until the foreign body is expelled or the victim becomes unconscious.

2. Unconscious victim

a. Determine unresponsiveness.

—Shout "Are you okay?"

b. Activate the EMS.

c. Open the airway.

—Use the head tilt-chin lift method (Figure 1-3*A*) unless C-spine injury is suspected.

—If C-spine injury is suspected, use the modified jaw thrust maneuver (Figure 1-3*B*).

d. Determine breathlessness.

—Observe the chest (i.e., look, listen, and feel for breathing) for 5 seconds.

e. Ventilate.

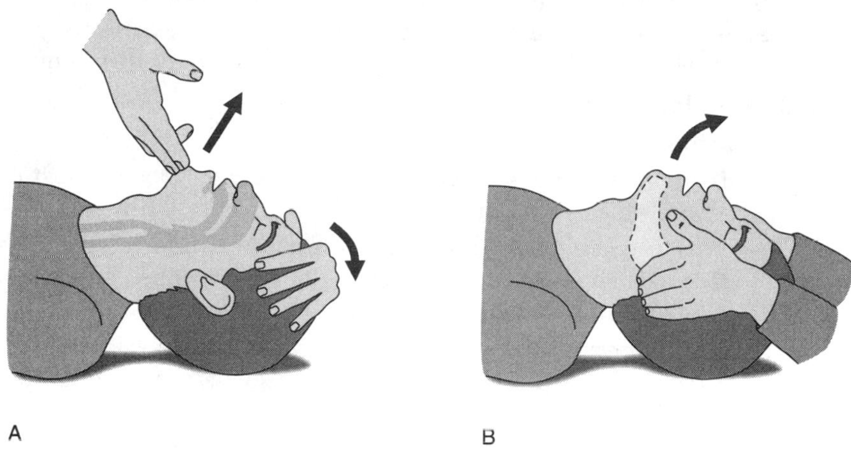

Figure 1-3. Head positioning techniques for opening the airway. (*A*) Head tilt-chin lift technique to open airway.(*B*) Jaw thrust technique to open airway. This technique is used when C-spine injury is suspected. (Adapted from LifeART Emergency Medicine Professional Collection. Copyright 1998, Lippincott Williams & Wilkins. All rights reserved.)

—Maintain an open airway, seal the mouth, and pinch the nose. If using a bag-valve-mask device, place the mask over the nose and mouth.

—Give two full breaths (or squeezes).

—If ventilation is unsuccessful, reposition the head and repeat the procedure.

—If ventilation still is unsuccessful, it is likely that the airway is obstructed.

f. Clear the airway.

—Use the **Heimlich maneuver** for adults and children [see IV A 1 c (1)].

—Use alternating **back blows** and **chest thrusts** for infants [see IV A 1 c (2)].

g. Check for foreign bodies.

—Open the mouth with the head tilt-chin lift or cross-finger technique.

—Do a finger sweep to locate the foreign body.

h. Ventilate.

—Repeat the ventilation sequence (see IV A 2 e) until airway is clear (rescue breathing).

—This ventilation sequence should be repeated once every 5 seconds in adults and once every 3 seconds in children.

—The major adverse effect associated with rescue breathing is **gastric distention,** especially in children. To minimize this risk, rescue breathing is performed with slow breaths given over 1.0–1.5 seconds, of volume just sufficient to cause the chest to rise.

B. Cardiopulmonary resuscitation (CPR)

1. Determine pulselessness.

—Locate the carotid artery and feel for a pulse (5 seconds).

—If the victim has no pulse, circulation must be provided in addition to breathing.

—In children, locating a pulse may be difficult. However, because **cardiac arrest in children usually is secondary to respiratory arrest,** a child who is not breathing probably also has circulatory compromise.

2. **Begin closed chest compressions.**
   a. **Adults**
      —If there is no pulse, locate the landmark for closed chest compressions, which is 2–3 fingerbreadths above the xiphoid process.
      —With the heel of one hand on the sternum and the heel of the other hand on top of the first hand, give chest compressions that are **1.5–2.0 inches deep,** at the rate of **80–100/min.**
      —In **one-person CPR,** the ratio of chest compressions to breaths is **15:2.** In **two-person CPR,** the ratio of chest compressions to breaths is **5:1.**
      —Take 5 seconds to check for pulse after the first minute, and then check every few minutes.
   b. **Children and infants**
      —Using 2–3 fingers of one hand, compressions are given one fingerbreadth below the nipple line at a depth of **0.5–1.0 inch,** at a rate of **at least 100/min.**
      —The ratio of chest compressions to breaths is **5:1.**
3. **Activate the EMS**
   a. **Adults**
      —Immediately activate the EMS.
   b. **Children**
      —Perform 1 minute of rescue breathing before activating the EMS system, because pediatric cardiac arrest is primarily respiratory in origin.

V. Cardiopulmonary Arrest and Advanced Cardiac Life Support (ACLS)

—ACLS picks up where BLS leaves off (i.e., at CPR).

—Figure 1-4 is the universal **ACLS algorithm** devised by the American Heart Association.

A. Ventricular tachycardia (VT) [Figure 1-5] and ventricular fibrillation (VF) [Figure 1-6]

—Check for VT/VF on the monitor.

1. For treatment of VT with a pulse, see V E 1.
2. For treatment of VT without a pulse, treat like VF, as outlined below (Figure 1-7).
   a. **Defibrillate (shock) three times.**
      —Defibrillate at 200 J, 300 J, and 360 J in adults. In children, defibrillate at 2 J/kg, then at 4 J/kg, and again at 4 J/kg.
      —Check the rhythm after each shock before proceeding to the next one.
   b. **Check for VT/VF.**
      —If VT/VF is persistent, continue CPR, oxygenate, and obtain IV access.

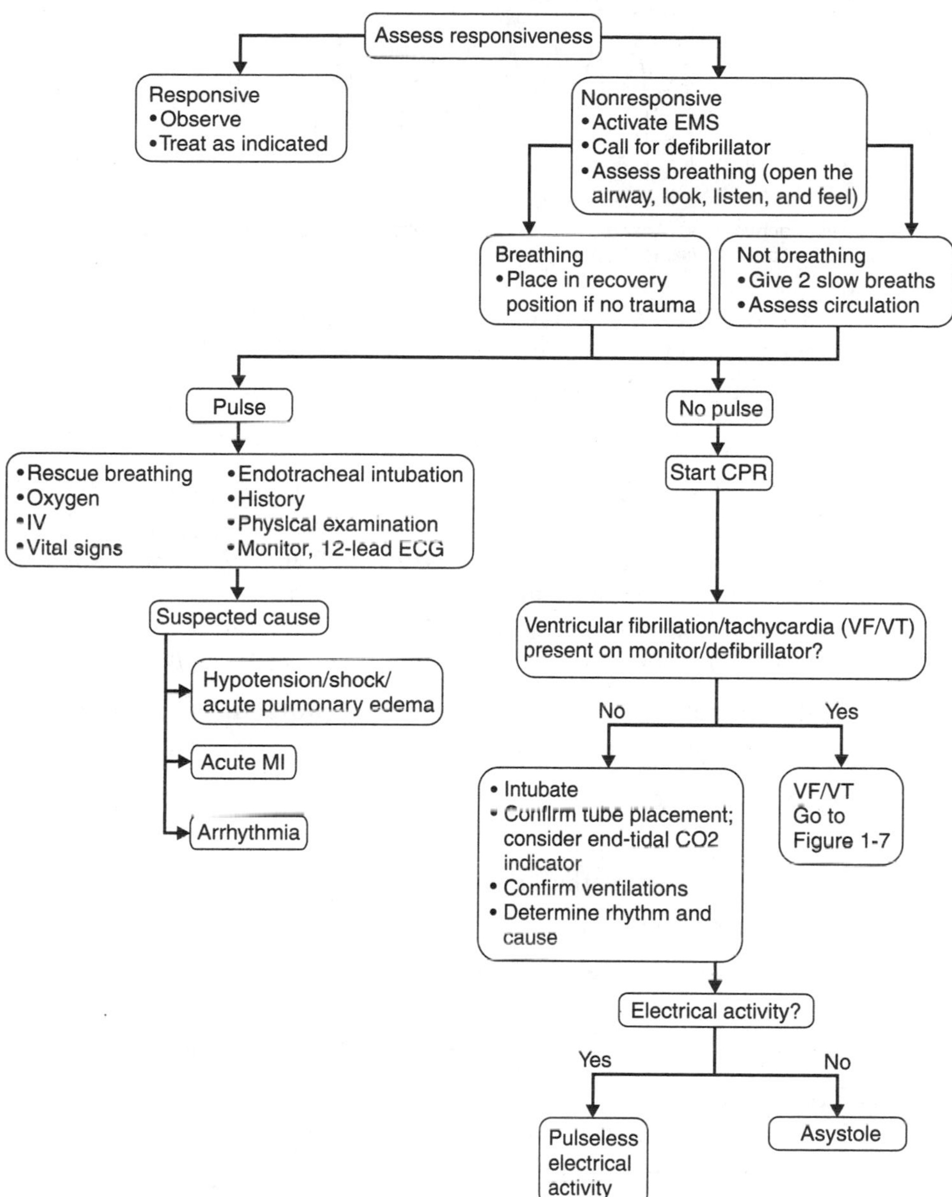

Figure 1-4. Universal advanced cardiac life support (ACLS) algorithm. *ABCs* = airway, breathing, circulation; *CPR* = cardiopulmonary resuscitation; *ECG* = electrocardiogram; *EMS* = emergency medical services; *IV* = intravenous. (Reproduced with permission. *Advanced Cardiac Life Support,* 1997. Copyright American Heart Association.)

c. **Deliver another shock** at the intensity last used, followed by administration of **epinephrine.**

—Give **adults** 1 mg of epinephrine IV push, and repeat every 3–5 minutes until a pulse is established.

—Give **children** 0.01 mg/kg IV push of epinephrine, and repeat every 3–5 minutes at a dose of 0.1 mg/kg.

d. Administer the following **medication sequence** if VT/VF persists.

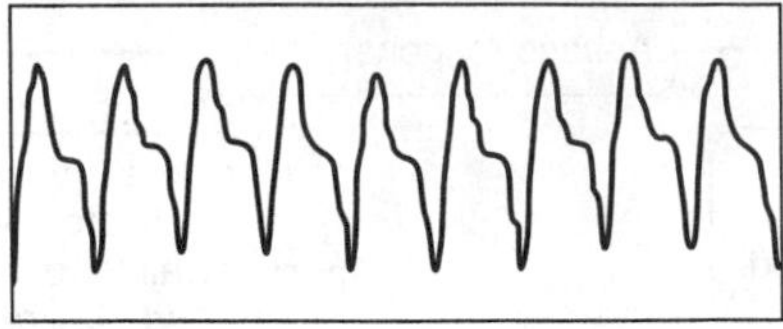

Figure 1-5. Ventricular tachycardia. (Adapted from LifeART Emergency Medicine Professional Collection. Copyright 1998, Lippincott Williams & Wilkins. All rights reserved.)

Defibrillate at 360 J (adults) or 4 J/kg (children) and check the rhythm on the monitor **after each dose of medication.**

—Administer **lidocaine** 1.0–1.5 mg/kg IV push. (Note: a single dose of 1.5 mg/kg lidocaine is acceptable for cardiac arrest). Repeat in 3–5 minutes to a maximum dose of 3 mg/kg.

—Administer **bretylium** 5 mg/kg IV push. Repeat once at 10 mg/kg IV push.

—Administer **magnesium sulfate** 1–2 mg IV for suspected hypomagnesemic states and torsades de pointes.

—Administer **procainamide** for persistent refractory VF. Administer 30 mg/min to a maximum total dose of 17 mg/kg.

B. Pulseless electrical activity (PEA) [electromechanical dissociation]

1. **Causes** of PEA can be summarized by the acronym, MATCH^{4}ED.

—**M:** massive myocardial infarction

—**A:** acidosis

—**T:** tension pneumothorax

—**C:** cardiac tamponade

—**H^4:** hypovolemia, hypoxia, hypothermia, hypokalemia

—**E:** embolism

—**D:** drug overdose (e.g., tricyclics, β-blockers, calcium channel blockers)

2. **Treatment**

a. Intubate the patient and obtain IV access.

b. Treat any underlying conditions.

c. Administer **epinephrine.**

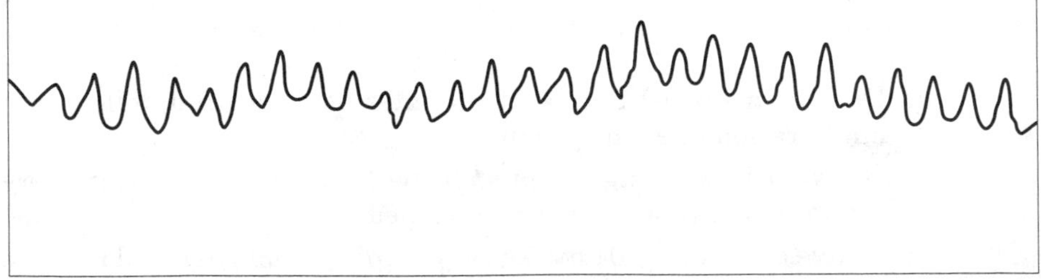

Figure 1-6. Ventricular fibrillation.

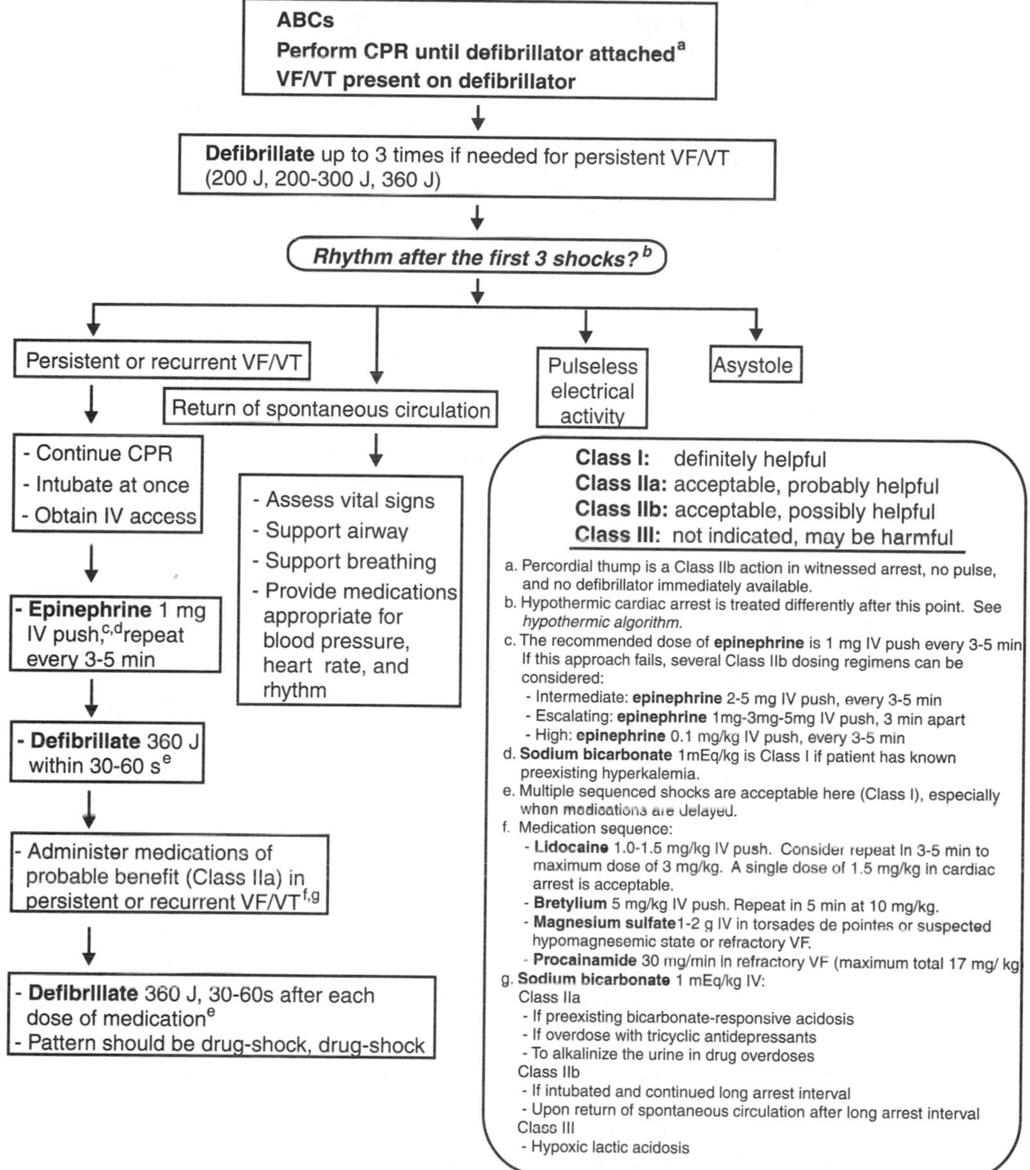

Figure 1-7. Algorithm for treatment of ventricular fibrillation/pulseless ventricular tachycardia (VF/VT). *ABCs* = airway, breathing, circulation; *CPR* = cardiopulmonary resuscitation; *IV* = intravenous; *PEA* = pulseless electrical activity. (Reproduced with permission. *Advanced Cardiac Life Support,* 1997. Copyright American Heart Association.)

—Give adults 1 mg IV push, and repeat every 3–5 minutes.

—Give children 0.01 mg/kg IV push, and repeat every 3–5 minutes. Remember that subsequent doses are given at 0.1 mg/kg.

d. If **bradycardia** is present, administer **atropine.**

—Give adults 1 mg IV, and repeat every 3–5 minutes up to a maximum dose of 0.04 mg/kg.

—Give children 0.02 mg/kg, and repeat only once. Note that the minimum dose of atropine is 0.1 mg, regardless of the weight of the child, because too small a dose of atropine is associated with paroxysmal slowing of the heart.

C. Asystole

—If the monitor shows asystole ("flatline"), confirm this in another lead. Then:

1. Intubate and obtain IV access.
2. If asystole is confirmed, consider immediate **transcutaneous pacing.**
3. Administer **epinephrine.**
   —Give adults 1 mg IV push, and repeat every 3–5 minutes.
   —Give children 0.01 mg/kg IV push, and repeat every 3–5 minutes. Remember that subsequent doses are given at 0.1 mg/kg.
4. If symptomatic **bradycardia** is present, administer **atropine.**
   —Give adults 1 mg IV, and repeat up to a maximum dose of 0.04 mg/kg.
   —Give children 0.02 mg/kg IV (minimum dose=0.1 mg), and repeat up to a maximum dose of 0.04 mg/kg.
5. If asystole persists, consider termination of efforts.

D. Paroxysmal supraventricular tachycardia (PSVT) [adults]

—Treatment of PSVT is aimed at interrupting the cycle of impulses traveling to the ventricles to return them to the atrioventricular (AV) node and prevent them from terminating prematurely.

1. Vagal maneuver

—is the treatment of choice.

—slows conduction via the AV node by increasing parasympathetic tone.

—One of the most common vagal maneuvers is the **carotid sinus massage,** which is performed by applying firm pressure over the carotid sinus for 5–10 seconds. It is contraindicated in patients with carotid bruits. **Simultaneous bilateral carotid sinus massage should never be attempted.**

—Other vagal maneuvers include ice water immersion of the face and performing a Valsalva maneuver.

2. Pharmacotherapy

—consists of **adenosine and verapamil.**

a. Adenosine

—is used first because of its fewer side effects and short half-life.

—is administered via **rapid** IV push followed by a saline flush.

—is given up to three consecutive times at doses of 6 mg, 12 mg, and 12–18 mg at intervals of 1–2 minutes.

b. Verapamil

—is administered intravenously over 2 minutes in doses of 5 mg (adults) or 075–0.15 mg/kg (children > 2 years of age).

—Adverse effects include hypotension, which can be managed with 1.5–4.0 mg/kg (adults) or 10–20 mg/kg (children) IV calcium chloride.

c. Other **antiarrhythmics**

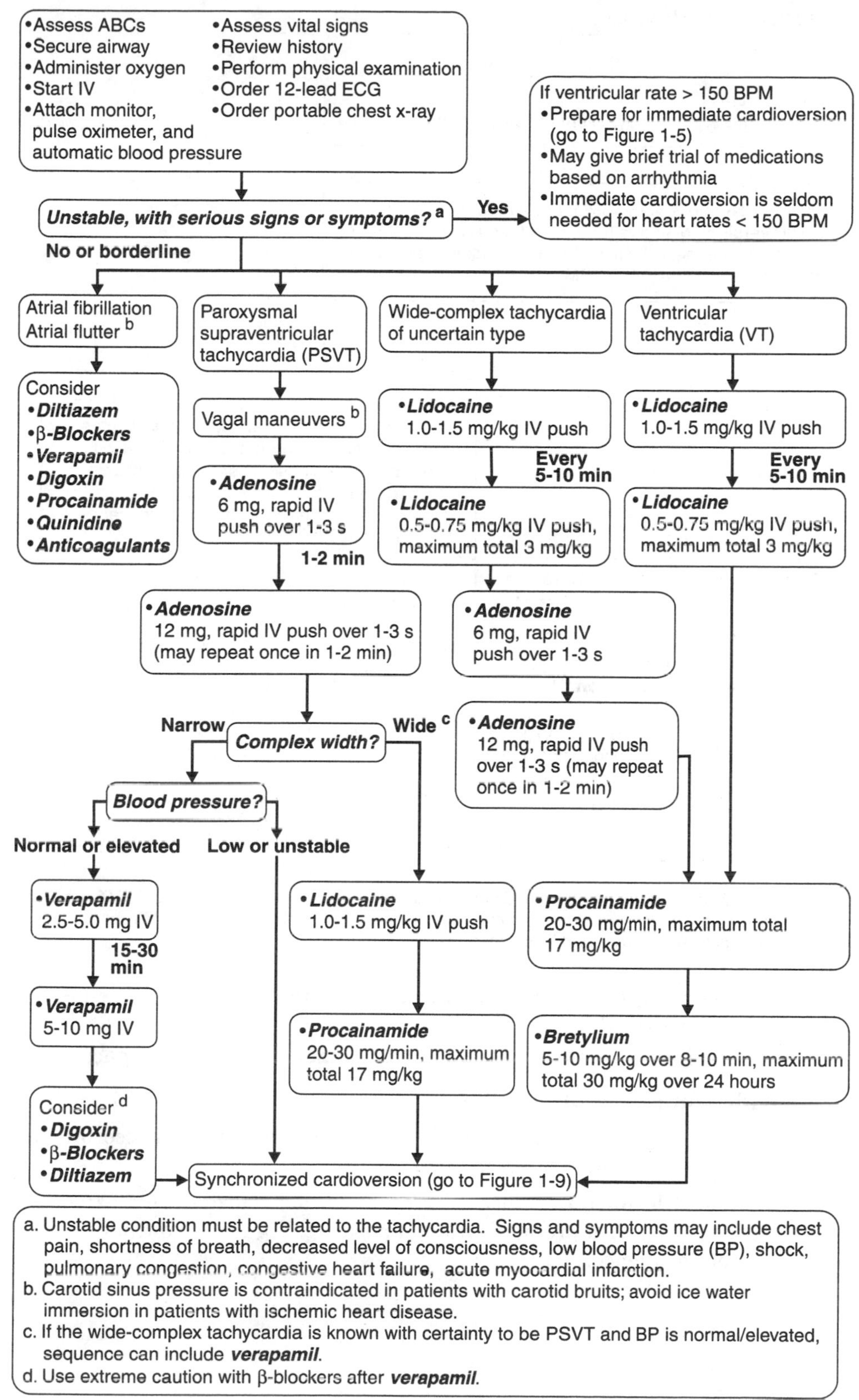

Figure 1-8. Algorithm for treatment of tachycardia. *ABCs* = airway, breathing, circulation; *BPM* = beats per minute; *ECG* = electrocardiogram; *IV* = intravenous. (Reproduced with permission. *Advanced Cardiac Life Support,* 1997. Copyright American Heart Association.)

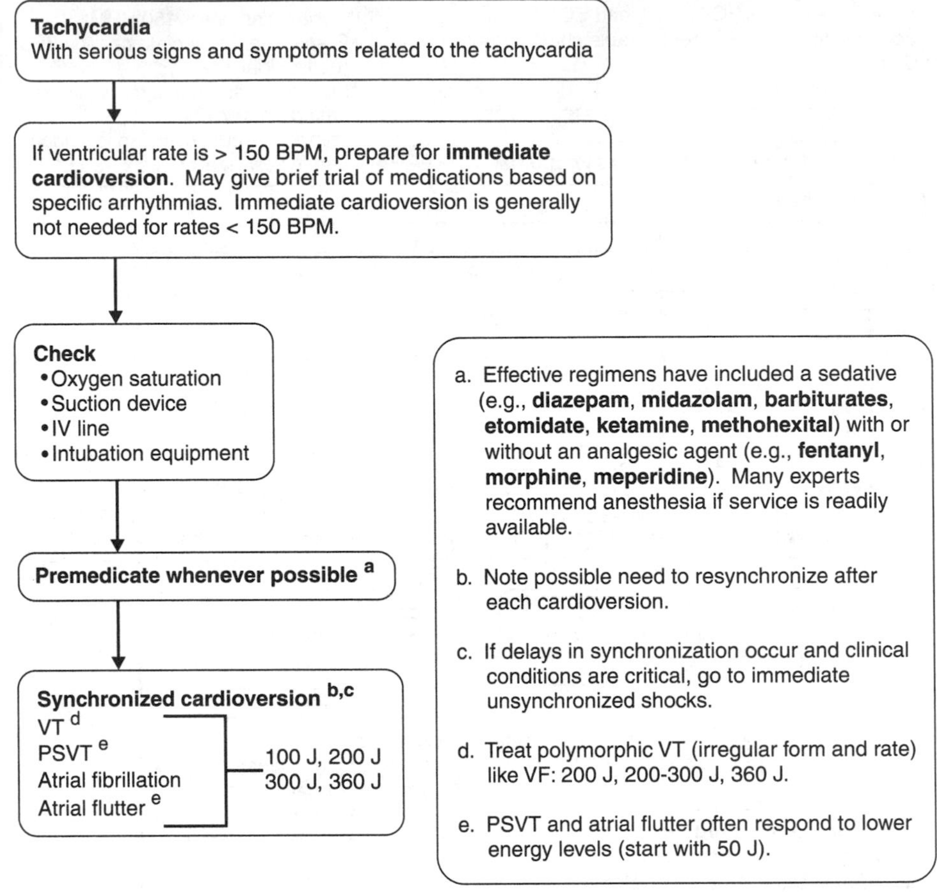

Figure 1-9. Electrical cardioversion algorithm. *BPM* = beats per minute; *IV* = intravenous; *PSVT* = paroxysmal supraventricular tachycardia; *VT* = ventricular tachycardia. (Reproduced with permission. *Advanced Cardiac Life Support,* 1997. Copyright American Heart Association.)

—are used if narrow-complex PSVT persists despite adenosine and verapamil.

—include digoxin, β-blockers, **diltiazem,** or overdrive pacing.

E. Wide-complex tachycardia

1. **Stable patients** (includes VT with a pulse) are treated according to the algorithm shown in Figure 1-8.
2. **Unstable patients** with wide-complex tachycardia are treated by cardioversion with premedication, if possible. Figure 1-9 outlines the treatment sequence.

Study Questions

1. A young woman is walking home from work when she passes out on the sidewalk. A crowd of people forms, some of whom attempt to arouse her by talking to her, but she does not respond. A man from the crowd states that he has training in cardiopulmonary resuscitation (CPR) and steps forward to help. Which of the following should be his first step in the management of this patient?

(A) Call for help and then determine whether the patient is breathing and has a pulse
(B) Begin chest compressions and breathing at a rate of 15:2, while waiting for help
(C) Administer 5 back blows followed by 5 quick downward chest thrusts to see if the patient might spontaneously recover
(D) Recruit another person and begin two-person CPR, alternating compressions and breaths at a rate of 15:2

2. A patient in the coronary care unit is found unconscious. The monitor reveals the rhythm strip below. The crash cart is in the room. Which of the following is the most appropriate first step in the management of this patient?

(A) Administer 0.5 mg of epinephrine intravenous (IV) and check for a pulse
(B) Defibrillate at 200 J and check for pulse
(C) Begin chest compressions at a rate of 80–100/min
(D) Make sure the IV line, oxygen, and monitor are in place
(E) Lift the patient to a standing position and perform a Heimlich maneuver

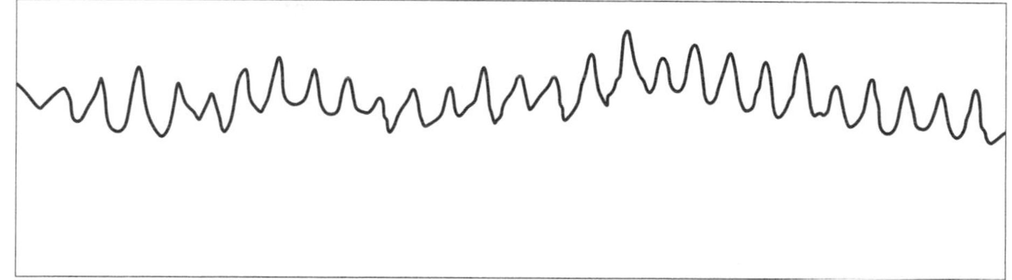

3. Which of the following is true regarding central venous access via the femoral vein?

(A) There is risk of pneumothorax
(B) There is no risk of thrombosis
(C) There is a high incidence of infection
(D) There is great difficulty obtaining access
(E) There is fastest circulation time

4. A 52-year-old woman experienced cardiac arrest 5 minutes ago. She has a 2-L O_2 nasal cannula and an intravenous (IV) line in place. The electrocardiogram (ECG) shows fine ventricular fibrillation (VF). Femoral, brachial, and carotid pulses are absent. Cardiopulmonary resuscitation (CPR) is being performed by other members of the on-call team. As the code leader, which of the following should be your first step in the management of this patient?

(A) Confirm pulselessness while preparing for immediate defibrillation
(B) Administer 1 mg IV push of epinephrine, then defibrillate
(C) Administer 50 mEq IV bolus of sodium bicarbonate, then defibrillate
(D) Administer both the epinephrine (1 mg IV push) and sodium bicarbonate (50 mEq IV bolus), then defibrillate
(E) Administer 1.0 mg of atropine IV and check for a pulse

5. A 47-year-old man is brought to the emergency department by ambulance. The cardiac monitor demonstrates electrical activity, but no pulse is obtainable. As the treatable etiologies of pulseless electrical activity (PEA) are being considered, intravenous (IV) access is confirmed. Which of the following medications should be administered to the patient first?

(A) Calcium chloride, 5 ml of 10% solution IV bolus
(B) Epinephrine, 1 mg IV push
(C) Isoproterenol, 4 mg/min IV infusion
(D) Sodium bicarbonate, 1 mEq/kg IV
(E) Atropine, 1 mg IV push

6. Which of the following statements regarding endotracheal intubation is true?

(A) It allows adjunctive ventilatory equipment to be used more effectively
(B) It increases the risk of aspiration of gastric contents
(C) It is the immediate priority in ventricular fibrillation (VF)
(D) If done properly, it may result in one lung being inflated
(E) There are few situations in which it is the method of choice

7. A 72-year-old man has been in ventricular fibrillation (VF) for several minutes. The VF is refractory to defibrillation and epinephrine. Which of the following is the correct regimen for the administration of lidocaine?

(A) Lidocaine, 1.0–1.5 mg/kg IV push followed by defibrillation; repeat if necessary in 3–5 minutes to a maximum dose of 3 mg/kg
(B) Lidocaine, 1.0–1.5 mg/kg IV push followed by a pulse check; repeat if necessary in 3–5 minutes to a maximum dose of 3 mg/kg
(C) Lidocaine, 1.0–1.5 mg/kg IV push followed by defibrillation; repeat if necessary in 3–5 minutes at double the dose to a maximum dose of 3 mg/kg
(D) Lidocaine, 1.0–1.5 mg/kg IV push followed by a pulse check; repeat if necessary in 3–5 minutes at double the dose to a maximum dose of 3 mg/kg.
(E) Lidocaine 1.0–1.5 mg/kg IV push followed by defibrillation; repeat if necessary in 3–5 minutes at one half the dose to a maximum does of 3 mg/kg.

8. Which of the following rapid sequence intubation (RSI) induction agents cannot be used in head trauma?

(A) Thiopental
(B) Methohexital
(C) Ketamine
(D) Etomidate
(E) Midazolam

9. Although succinylcholine is the choice depolarizing neuromuscular blocking agent in rapid sequence intubation (RSI), it should be avoided in which of the following situations?

(A) Narrow-angle glaucoma
(B) Cataracts
(C) Altered mental status
(D) Hypokalemia
(E) Hypernatremia

Directions: The response options for Items 10–13 are the same. You will be required to select one answer for each item in the set.

Questions 10–13

Match each drug listed below with the correct description.
(A) Epinephrine
(B) Procainamide
(C) Atropine
(D) Magnesium

10. The first drug used in the treatment of ventricular fibrillation

11. Drug of choice for torsades de pointes

12. Drug of choice for symptomatic bradycardia

13. Drug used for persistent refractory ventricular fibrillation

Directions: The response options for Items 14–16 are the same. Each item will state the number of options to choose. Choose exactly this number.

Questions 14–16

Match each statement below with the appropriate drugs.
(A) Adenosine
(B) Lidocaine
(C) Thiopental
(D) Verapamil
(E) Etomidate
(F) Epinephrine
(G) Diltiazem
(H) Midazolam
(I) Propranolol
(J) Bretylium

14. Induction agents used for patients with head trauma (select 3 drugs)

15. Drugs used in the treatment of paroxysmal supraventricular tachycardia (select 4 drugs)

16. Drugs used in the treatment of ventricular fibrillation (select 3 drugs)

Answers and Explanations

1–A. Because the man does not have training in advanced cardiac life support (ACLS) and does not have access to a defibrillator, basic life support (BLS) techniques must be used. The role of BLS is to sustain the victim until further help arrives. Upon arriving at the scene of an unconscious victim, the first step is to call for help (i.e., ambulance, paramedics, 911). Then the patient's situation (e.g., responsiveness, breathing, pulse) should be assessed. Cardiopulmonary resuscitation (CPR), which is the combination of chest compressions and breaths, should not be started unless the patient is not breathing and does not have a pulse. If a pulse is present, rescue breathing alone may be sufficient. Immediately beginning chest compressions bypasses the initial evaluation of the patient. Administering back blows is inappropriate because back blows are used in infants, not adults. Recruiting another person to help with 2-person CPR alternating compressions and breaths at a rate of 15:2 not only bypasses the initial evaluation, but states the wrong compression:breath rate. The rate of compressions to breaths in two-person CPR is 5:1, not 15:2. Lifting the patient to a standing position is inappropriate because the patient may have sustained cervical spine trauma which could worsen with improper movement.

2–B. The EKG shows ventricular fibrillation (VF). As delineated in the American Heart Association's advanced cardiac life support (ACLS) algorithm, the first step after establishing VF in a patient is to defibrillate, which can immediately restore sinus rhythm. The initial intensity is 200 J, followed by 260 J and then 360 J, if unsuccessful. Checking for the intravenous (IV) line, supplemental oxygen, and cardiac monitor should only be done after defibrillation. Also, because the patient is in the coronary care unit, he probably already has IV access, and he may or may not be intubated. A monitor is obviously in place. Chest compressions are inappropriate before the initial three shocks (defibrillation) are administered. The administration of epinephrine occurs if VF persists after defibrillation and if the IV line, oxygen, and cardiac monitor as necessary are in place. Atropine is administered for bradycardia or asystole. It is not part of the standard algorithm for VF.

3–C. Femoral vein cannulation carries no risk of pneumothorax due to its distance from the lungs. Femoral vein cannulation carries with it the highest risk of thrombosis and infection. Central venous access via the femoral vein often is easier than any of the other approaches, especially in a code situation. Circulation time via femoral vein access is slowest when compared to other approaches.

4–A. The first priority in the treatment of ventricular fibrillation is immediate defibrillation, because this measure on its own can restore sinus rhythm. Medications are administered only after three consecutive shocks are delivered and fail to restore sinus rhythm. After that, the medication sequence is epinephrine, lidocaine, and bretylium. Sodium bicarbonate is not routinely used for the treatment of VF. Atropine is given for bradycardia.

5–B. Pulseless electrical activity includes electromechanical dissociation, idioventricular rhythms, ventricular escape rhythms, and brady-asystolic rhythms. Once PEA is established, the airway should be secured with intubation. Then IV access is obtained, and blood flow is assessed with Doppler ultrasound, end-tidal CO_2, echocardiography, or an arterial line. At this point, causes of PEA are considered so that any treatable causes can be addressed immediately (see V B 1). The first drug administered after this point is epinephrine 1 mg IV push.

6–A. Endotracheal intubation in place allows adjunctive ventilatory equipment, such as the bag-valve-mask device, to be used more effectively with less effort on the part of the rescuer. Endotracheal intubation decreases, not increases, the risk of aspiration. The immediate priority in ventricular fibrillation (VF) is defibrillation, not endotracheal intubation. If done improperly, endotracheal intubation may result in only a single lung being inflated. It is the method of choice for most situations.

7–A. The correct dose of lidocaine when given IV push is 1.0–1.5 mg/kg. Repeat dose is the same dose given after a 3- to 5-minute interval. Treatment of VF with lidocaine is followed by defibrillation, not a pulse check (see universal algorithm, Fig. 1–4). The dose of lidocaine when given via the endotracheal tube is 2–4 mg/kg.

8–C. Ketamine is contraindicated in the setting of head trauma, as it increases intracranial pressure (ICP). Thiopental, methohexital, etomidate, and midazolam are all safe for use in patients with increased ICP.

9–A. Succinylcholine (SCh) is associated with a number of side effects, including hyperkalemia, malignant hyperthermia, prolonged apnea, histamine release, and muscle fasciculations. Muscle fasciculations in turn result in an increase in intragastric and intraocular pressure (IOP). The rise in IOP would exacerbate the already elevated IOP in narrow-angle glaucoma and is therefore contraindicated in this situation. However, complications from muscle fasciculations can be overcome by the administration of a prefasciculating dose of a competitive neuromuscular blocker such as vecuronium. The presence of cataracts or hypernatremia does not influence SCh use. Altered mental status is one of the indications for using RSI and SCh. Hyperkalemia would be a contraindication to SCh use, but hypokalemia is not. See Table 1-2.

10–A. The treatment of ventricular fibrillation can be summarized by the following mnemonic: Shock, shock, shock, everybody shock, little shock, big shock, mama shock, papa shock.

Shock, shock, shock: defibrillate x 3: at 200 J, 300 J, and 360 J in adults and at 2 J/kg, 4J/kg, and 4 J/kg in children

Everybody shock: **Epinephrine** 1 mg/kg IV
Little shock: **Lidocaine** 1.0–1.5 mg/kg IV
Big shock: **Bretylium** 5 mg/kg IV, can repeat once at 10 mg/kg

Mama shock: **Magnesium** 1–2 g IV
Papa shock: **Procainamide** 20–30 mg/min (max. dose is 17 mg/kg)

11–D. Magnesium sulfate is the drug of choice for the treatment of torsades de pointes. The optimum dosage has not been established. Generally, treatment begins with 1–2 g IV push, watching for hypotension. Dosages of up to 10 g have been used. Torsades de pointes is a type of polymorphic ventricular tachycardia characterized by a ventricular rate greater than 200/min and a spiraling of the QRS complexes. It often is the result of underlying electrolyte imbalances such as hypomagnesemia.

12–C. Atropine is the drug of choice for symptomatic bradycardia and brady-asystolic cardiac arrest. The dose for symptomatic bradycardia is 0.5–1.0 mg, which may be repeated at 5-minute intervals. Consider a pacemaker for patients who require prolonged atropine or with recurrent episodes of bradycardia. The dose for brady-asystolic cardiac arrest (asystole) is 1 mg IV repeated every 3–5 minutes as needed. The maximum dose of atropine in both settings is 0.04 mg/kg. Note that the minimum dose of atropine is 0.1 mg regardless of the patient's weight, because a smaller dose can actually produce paroxysmal bradycardia.

13–B. As per the American Heart Association, procainamide is used for persistent ventricular fibrillation that is refractory to epinephrine, lidocaine, and bretylium. The dose is 20–30 mg/min until the arrhythmia is suppressed. This rate may not produce an effective dose fast enough, but a rate faster than this produces profound hypotension. Therefore, the drug is not widely used in code situations. Treatment with procainamide must be stopped when the QRS complex is widened by 50% or more, or the PR or QT interval is lengthened by 50% or more. Heart block and cardiac arrest are potential complications. Procainamide is relatively contraindicated in the presence of hypokalemia and hypomagnesemia because it can potentiate ventricular arrhythmias in these situations.

14–C, E, F. See Table 1-1 for a listing of common induction agents. Thiopental, etomidate, and midazolam are good for patients with head injury because they do not increase the intracranial pressure (ICP). Fentanyl and diazepam also are good choices. Ketamine, on the other hand, is contraindicated in this setting because it does raise ICP.

15–A, D, G, I. Adenosine is the first drug of choice (after vagal maneuvers) for the treatment of non-wide-complex (narrow-complex) PSVT. The dose is 6 mg rapid IV push followed by a saline flush, because the half-life of the drug is only 10 seconds. Repeat doses of 12 mg and 12–18 mg are given at 1- to 2-minute intervals. Patients should be warned about a possible distressing but fleeting chest pain and flushing as the drug goes in. Because of the short half-life of the drug, the PSVT may recur, and one may consider verapamil or diltiazem, which are longer-acting. Verapamil and diltiazem block slow calcium channels, resulting in potent negative inotropic (verapamil) and negative chronotropic (verapamil and diltiazem) activity. These effects are useful in terminating supraventricular tachycardias that re-enter via the AV node (the most common type). Verapamil and diltiazem are indicated in the treatment of PSVT that does not require cardioversion (i.e., patient is hemodynamically stable). The dose of verapamil is 1.5–5 mg slow IV push, which may be repeated in 15–30 minutes. The dose of diltiazem is 0.25 mg/kg slow IV push. Watch for hypotension with these drugs. Adenosine, verapamil, and diltiazem are considered first-line therapies for PSVT. If these fail, then many other therapies are acceptable if judged to be clinically useful. These include β-blockers (such as propranolol), digoxin, sedation, overdrive pacing, and electrical cardioversion.

16–B, F, J. See explanation for Question 10.

2

Cardiovascular Emergencies

I. Acute Chest Pain

A. Overview

1. **Causes**
   - a. **Life-threatening** causes include **myocardial infarction (MI)** (see II), **esophageal rupture** (see Chapter 4), **aortic dissection** (see IV), **cardiac tamponade** (see VI), **pulmonary embolism** (see Chapter 3), and **pneumothorax** (see Chapter 3).
   - b. Other causes include pneumonia, musculoskeletal pain, malignancy, peptic ulcer disease, cholecystitis, pancreatitis, herpes zoster, and anxiety.
   - c. It is imperative to determine which causes are life-threatening and which ones afford the luxury of an elective work-up.
2. **Risk factors** may help to focus on the causes of chest pain that are more likely in a particular patient. Remember to **evaluate all patients thoroughly,** even if they do not fall into a classic risk group.
   - a. Risk factors for **coronary artery disease (CAD)** include male gender, age > 40 years, smoking, hypertension, hypercholesterolemia, diabetes mellitus, and family history (particularly of MI/CAD under 50 years of age).
   - b. Risk factors for **thromboembolic disease** include previous history of thromboembolic disease; estrogen use; trauma to legs or pelvis; immobilization; long plane, train, or car trips; and hypercoagulable states [e.g., pregnancy, cancer, congestive heart failure (CHF)].
   - c. Risk factors for **aortic aneurysms** include hypertension (most significant factor), atherosclerosis, Marfan's syndrome, pregnancy, and valvular aortic stenosis.

B. Physical examination.

When assessing chest pain it is important to determine the P-Q-R-S-T.

1. **P = provoking or palliative factors**
   —Pain may be related to **movement** (positional), **eating** (prandial), **exertion** (exertional), or **emotional** factors.

—Pain that increases with inspiration is termed **pleuritic,** meaning that the cause is likely pulmonary.

—Factors that alleviate pain [e.g., rest, nitroglycerin (NTG), position change, antacids] also must be considered.

2. **Q = quality**

—The description or quality of the pain (e.g., **sharp, stabbing, crushing, aching**) can provide important clues for arriving at the diagnosis.

—**For example,** the pain of MI often is described as a squeezing tightness, whereas the pain of aortic dissection is sharp and tearing.

3. **R = radiation**

—Pain may radiate to the **arm, back, shoulder,** or **retrosternal area.**

—The site to which the pain radiates (or does not radiate) also helps to determine the diagnosis.

—**For example,** the pain of aortic dissection classically radiates to the interscapular area.

4. **S = severity**

—Because outward expression of pain may vary across cultures, it is important to determine the severity of the pain **as the patient experiences it.**

—Ask the patient to rate his or her pain on a **scale** of 1 to 10. Figure 2-1 depicts a pain scale that is not hindered by language.

—Also determine if the severity was **maximal at onset,** or if it **gradually became worse.**

5. **T = timing** (duration)

—The duration of pain **varies based on the cause. For example,** the pain of unstable angina lasts 1 to 10 minutes, whereas the pain of MI lasts 30 minutes to 3 hours.

—**Fleeting pain lasting 1 to 2 seconds usually is not cardiac in origin.**

II. Myocardial Infarction

A. Clinical presentation

1. Symptoms

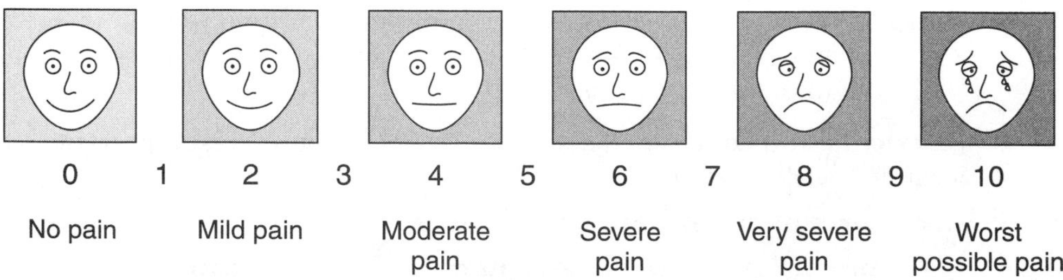

Figure 2-1. A pain scale used for rating severity of pain.

—Pain generally is **intense,** described as **crushing** or **squeezing** pressure. It is **retrosternal** and often radiates down the left arm, neck, and sometimes the jaw.

—The patient usually is **diaphoretic** and **pale,** with **cool, moist skin.**

—Many patients clutch their chests or report **indigestion.**

—The picture is that of a person who appears **acutely ill,** with **fear, anxiety,** and **an impending sense of doom.**

—Additional symptoms include weakness, confusion, hiccuping (due to diaphragmatic irritation), nausea, vomiting, and shortness of breath.

2. Physical examination

—Heart sounds S_1 and S_2 may be **muffled** due to global hypokinesis.

—An S_3 **gallop** (always pathologic) may be heard as the left ventricle fails. It may be necessary to place the patient in the left lateral decubitus position to fully appreciate a gallop.

—An S_4 sound also may be heard, representing either a **noncompliant LV secondary to ischemia** or a **benign sound** (common in the elderly).

—The **heart rate** may be slow, normal, or fast.

—The **blood pressure (BP)** may be low, normal, or high.

—**Fine rales** in the lung bases may or may not be present.

—Presence of **jugular venous distention (JVD)** suggests a **right ventricular (posterior) infarct,** often accompanied by **cyanotic, edematous extremities** and **clear lungs,** signifying RV dysfunction.

B. Diagnostic tests

1. Chest radiograph

—is usually **normal.**

—may show enlargement of the left ventricle if there was prior left ventricular dysfunction.

—Previously existing cardiomyopathy may show up as cardiomegaly, and wet lungs from CHF may reveal haziness.

—**There are no radiographic findings pathognomonic for unstable angina or MI.**

2. Electrocardiogram (ECG)

a. Transmural (Q wave) MI

—Presence of ST elevations with subsequent development of **pathologic Q waves** is diagnostic for Q wave MI.

—Pathologic Q waves have a width of 0.04 seconds or more, and an amplitude $\geq$ 25% of the R wave in that lead.

—Because Q waves may take up to 72 hours to develop, a person presenting with MI may have a perfectly normal ECG. Therefore, it is **imperative not to rule out MI based solely on the ECG.**

—The MI can be classified based on the location of the Q waves.

(1) Inferior (diaphragmatic) MI: Q waves in II, III, aVF

(2) High lateral MI: Q waves in I, aVL
(3) Anteroseptal MI: Q waves in V_1 through V_3
(4) Anterolateral MI: Q waves in V_4 through V_6
(5) Localized anterior MI: Q waves in V_2 through V_4
(6) Anterior (massive) MI: Q waves in V_1 through V_6, I, aVL
(7) Right ventricular MI: Q waves in V4R and V5R (R = right ventricular lead)
(8) Posterior wall MI: large R in both V1 and V2, and Q in V6

b. Non–Q wave MI

—involves the **subendocardial zone of the left ventricle.**

—does not exhibit any abnormal Q waves or ST elevations on the ECG.

—exhibits marked **ST segment depression** of 1 mm or more, resulting in either horizontal or down-sloping ST segments in all precordial leads.

—Often there are no obvious or diagnostic ECG changes. In such cases, **CK-MB elevation** must be present to make the diagnosis of non–Q wave MI. Otherwise, the diagnosis of unstable angina must be made.

3. Cardiac enzymes

—serve as a useful adjunct in the diagnosis of MI, especially when the presentation of chest pain may appear benign. (Remember that up to 4% of MIs have an atypical presentation, often seen in the elderly).

—One "negative" set of cardiac enzymes **cannot be used to rule out MI in the emergency department.**

—Damaged myocardial cells release enzymes that can be used as markers for cardiac injury. Table 2-1 summarizes the time course of the different enzymes.

a. The earliest marker is **myoglobin,** which is also released from skeletal muscle, making it a less specific marker for myocardial injury in the setting of skeletal muscle injury (e.g., trauma, postoperative period).

b. Troponin, the most recently identified cardiac marker, is extremely **specific** and **sensitive** for cardiac muscle, making it ideal for detecting cardiac injury in the setting of skeletal muscle trauma, microinfarcts, and MIs that are several days old.

c. The most widely used markers are **creatinine kinase (CK)** and **lactate dehydrogenase (LD).**

(1) **CK** exists as

Table 2-1. Cardiac Enzyme Markers

Enzyme	Rise (hours post-CP)	Peak (hours)	Return to baseline (days)
Myoglobin	1–2	4–6	1
Troponin	3–6	12–24	7–10
CK-MB	4–6	12–36	3–4
LD	12	24–48	10–14

CK-MB = creatinine kinase-MB; *CP* = chest pain; *LD* = lactate dehydrogenase.

—**CK–MM** from muscle.
—**CK–BB** from the brain.
—**CK–MB** from the heart.

(2) **LD** exists as
—**LD_1** (cardiac) and **LD_2** (RBCs). An **LD_1:LD_2 ratio** > 1.0 is indicative of MI.
—**LD_3** (pulmonary).
—**LD_4** (liver) and **LD_5** (striated muscle).

C. Treatment

1. Medical therapy

a. **IV-O_2 monitor** is the basic treatment for any patient with chest pain.

b. **NTG** (Table 2-2)
—is useful in the rapid relief of **angina.**

Table 2-2. Primary Drugs Used for Treatment of Mycardial Infarction (MI) and Unstable Angina

Drug	Actions	Recommended Dose
Aspirin (ASA)	↓ Cardiac mortality (at least 20%) Antiplatelet activity	160–325 mg po (preferably chewed for faster onset)
Nitroglycerin (NTG)	Vasodilator, ↓ cardiac mortality (20%–30%)	0.4 mg sublingually repeated every 2–5 minutes up to 3 times; if no relief, use 5–10 mg/min IV at 2- to 5-minute intervals to a maximum of 100 mg/min
β_1-Blockers (metoprolol, atenolol)	↓ Preload, ↓ cardiac mortality blocks catecholamine drive	cardioselective (β_1) blockers: metoprolol: 5–15 mg IV over 5 min atenolol: 5–10 mg IV over 5 min
Magnesium	↓ Incidence of arrhythmia	1–2 g over IV 10–20 minutes followed by continuous infusion of 1–2 g/h
Morphine sulfate	↓ Preload blocks catecholamine drive	2 mg IV bolus every 5 minutes titrated to effect
Thrombolytics (streptokinase, urokinase, anistreplase, alteplase, retaplase)	Open occluded arteries, salvage ischemic myocardium, ↓ mortality and morbidity of MI	streptokinase: 1.5 IU IV over 60 min urokinase: 2 million U IV, then 1 million U over 60 min anistreplase: 30 U IV over 2–5 min (concurrent heparinization not necessary) alteplase: 15 mg IV bolus, then 75 mg/kg (max. 50 mg) IV over 30 min then 0.5 mg/kg (max. 35 mg) IV over 60 min retaplase: two 10 mg IV boluses given over 2 min, 30 min apart
Heparin	Anticoagulation, prevent progression of coronary artery and mural thrombosis	80 U/kg IV bolus followed by 18 U/kg/h infusion

IV = intravenous; *MI* = myocardial infarction

—can be administered by mouth, by nasal spray, transdermally, sublingually, and intravenously.

(1) **Side effects** include headache and flushing. These can be used to gauge NTG therapy.

—If there is no pain relief, and flushing and/or headache do not occur, increase the dose of NTG.

—If these symptoms do occur but are not accompanied by pain relief, consider the possibility that the pain is not one that can be relieved by NTG (i.e., the pain may not be cardiac in origin, or may not be caused by esophageal spasm).

(2) **Contraindications**

—NTG is not indicated for RV infarcts. Hypoperfusion is secondary to RV dysfunction, in which forward cardiac output is not sufficient to preload the LV. The treatment for RV infarcts is aimed at increasing RV output (and, subsequently, LV output) using Starling's law and increasing RV preload with volume expansion. NTG, which decreases preload, would decrease RV output and could potentially extend the infarct by producing hypotension, including in the coronary bed.

c. **Aspirin** (see Table 2-2)

(1) An **absolute contraindication** is allergy to aspirin.

(2) **Relative contraindications** include gastrointestinal (GI) bleeding and presence of a bleeding diathesis.

d. **β-Blockers** (see Table 2-2)

—are also useful in angina prophylaxis.

—β_1-selective agents such as **metoprolol** are preferred.

—In the setting of MI, the goal is to administer β-blockers **within 8 hours,** targeting a heart rate between **60 and 90 beats/min.**

(1) **Absolute contraindications** include

—heart rate < 60 beats/min.

—systolic BP (sBP) < 100 mm Hg.

—second- or third-degree heart block.

—moderate to severe left ventricle dysfunction.

—severe chronic obstructive pulmonary disease (COPD).

—signs of peripheral hypoperfusion.

—congestive heart failure (CHF).

(2) **Relative contraindications** include

—concurrent use of calcium channel blockers.

—brittle diabetes (difficult to control).

—first-degree heart block.

—severe peripheral vascular disease.

—asthma.

e. **Magnesium** (see Table 2-2)

—deficiency has been shown to produce cardiac arrhythmias [particularly torsades de pointes and ventricular fibrillation (VF)], results in secondary hypokalemia (which causes arrhythmias), and also may predispose to digitalis intoxication.

f. Morphine (see Table 2-2)

—is underused in the treatment of angina.

—serves to alleviate **pain and anxiety;** a relaxed patient is more cooperative and has less myocardial oxygen demand than an anxious patient.

—If it becomes necessary to reverse the effects of morphine (i.e., in the setting of respiratory depression), use 0.4–2.0 mg/kg of **naloxone.**

g. Thrombolytics (see Table 2-2)

—available in the United States include **streptokinase, urokinase, anisoylated plasminogen streptokinase activator complex (APSAC, anistreplase), alteplase, and retaplase.** The latter two are recombinant human tissue plasminogen activators.

—should be administered within 30 minutes of entering the emergency department.

—Note that thrombolytics are used in the treatment of MI, but **not for unstable angina.**

(1) The two most common and serious **complications** include hemorrhagic stroke and bleeding requiring transfusion.

(2) Indications include

—acute MI by ECG criteria of > 0.1 mV ST segment elevation in at least two contiguous leads, or new left bundle branch block.

—absence of cardiogenic shock.

—ability to administer the agent quickly after onset of symptoms.

(a) < 6 hours: most beneficial

(b) 6–12 hours: less useful, but still provides important benefits

(c) 12 hours: diminishing benefits, may still be useful in selected patients

(3) Absolute contraindications include

—active internal bleeding.

—suspected aortic dissection.

—recent head trauma or known intracranial neoplasm or aneurysm.

—history of cerebrovascular accident (CVA) within last 6 months.

—known traumatic CPR (i.e., rib fractures resulting from CPR).

—pregnancy.

—persistent hypertension (systolic BP > 180 mm Hg, diastolic BP > 110 mm Hg) after medical treatment.

(4) Relative contraindications include

—major surgery or trauma < 2 weeks ago.

—hypertension (systolic BP > 180 mm Hg, diastolic BP > 110 mm Hg on at least two separate readings) before medical treatment.

—history of chronic severe hypertension with or without drug therapy.

—active peptic ulcer disease.

—history of ischemic or embolic CVA.

—known bleeding diathesis or current use of anticoagulants [prothrombin time (PT) > 15 seconds].

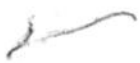

—prolonged (> 10 minutes) cardiopulmonary resuscitation (CPR).

—hemorrhagic ophthalmic conditions and diabetic hemorrhagic retinopathy.

—advanced liver and kidney disease.

—infectious endocarditis.

—exposure to streptokinase/APSAC within the past 6 months, if these agents are to be used again currently.

h. **Heparin** (see Table 2-2)

—is a **mandatory adjunct to tissue plasminogen activator,** and also is used concurrently with other thrombolytic therapy.

—can also be used on its own as therapy for angina, but is a third-line medication, after aspirin and NTG.

i. **Calcium channel blockers, lidocaine,** and **angiotensin-converting enzyme (ACE) inhibitors**

—are **not currently recommended** for treatment of acute MI in the emergency department.

j. **Volume expansion**

—is used for treatment of right ventricle infarct to increase preload and cardiac output.

k. **Arterial vasodilators**

—are used if left and right ventricle infarct are present.

l. GP IIb-IIIa receptor inhibitors

—used for non Q wave MI

—see Section III D 3

2. **Surgical therapy**

a. **Percutaneous coronary transluminal angioplasty (PTCA)**

—is a procedure in which coronary vessel flow is restored by physically breaking up the occluding clot or thrombus.

—is indicated for patients in whom thrombolysis is contraindicated.

—Patient requires prior cardiac catheterization to localize thrombus.

—Patient is concurrently anticoagulated with heparin.

(1) **Relative contraindications** include arterial dissection, and long or eccentric-shaped lesions that are technically difficult to lyse.

(2) **Complications** of PTCA include arterial dissection, MI, and sudden death. Overall mortality is approximately 20%.

(3) Due to above complications and high restenosis rate, PTCA is generally reserved for patients with single or double vessel disease, patients with discrete proximal lesions, and patients who either refuse surgery or are poor surgical candidates.

b. **Coronary artery bypass grafting (CABG)**

—is a highly successful procedure in which diseased coronary arteries are bypassed with grafts from either the saphenous vein, the internal mammary artery, or both.

—is indicated for patients with triple vessel disease and in whom medical management of angina fails.

—As with PTCA, patient requires prior cardiac catheterization to delineate lesions.

III. Unstable Angina

A. Definition. Unstable angina is new-onset angina, angina at rest, or angina that is worsening in terms of longer duration or increasing frequency or severity.

B. Clinical presentation

—same as for myocardial infarction (see II A)

C. Diagnostic tests

—same as for myocardial infarction (see II B)

D. Treatment

1. Unstable angina often is a warning sign of impending MI and therefore should be treated aggressively. Many of the therapies are the same as for MI:
   - **a.** Oxygen by nasal cannula or face mask to keep oxygen saturation >95%
   - **b.** Aspirin (ASA)
   - **c.** Nitroglycerin (NTG)
   - **d.** β-Blockers
   - **e.** PTCA
   - **f.** CABG
2. Some of the therapies for unstable angina differ from those used for MI:
   - **a. Thrombolytics** are **contraindicated** in the treatment of unstable angina.
   - **b. Enoxaparin** is a low-molecular-weight heparin recently approved for the treatment of unstable angina. The recommended dosage is 1 mg/kg subcutaneously every 12 hours. It is usually given with 100–325 mg of aspirin orally for at least 2 days or until the patient is clinically stable.
   - **c. GP IIb-IIIa receptor inhibitors** prevent clot formation by blocking the activation of glycoprotein IIa-IIIb receptor and cross-linking of adjacent platelets by fibrinogen. This is the final common pathway in platelet aggregation, and inhibition at this point results in more than 90% blockage of platelet activity. GP IIb-IIIa receptor inhibitors are indicated for the treatment of both unstable angina and non–Q wave MI, but not for Q wave MI. Therapy with these drugs may serve as a bridge to further therapy such as PTCA or CABG, or may be used in patients who are managed medically. Three drugs in this class are currently approved in the United States:
     - **(1) Abciximab:** 0.25 mg/kg bolus, then .125 μg/kg/min (maximum dose=10 μg/min) intravenous infusion for 12 hours.
     - **(2) Eptifibatide:** 180 μg/kg bolus, then 2 μg/kg/min IV infusion for 72 hours.

(3) **Tirofiban:** 0.4 μg/kg/min for 30 minutes, then 0.1 μg/kg/min for 12–108 hours. Used concurrently with heparin.

E. Disposition

—Patients with unstable angina should be admitted to the telemetry or coronary care unit.

IV. Thoracic Aneurysms and Aortic Dissection

—Although ruptured thoracic aneurysm and aortic dissection may seem to be very similar clinical entities, it is essential to remember that they have entirely different pathophysiologies and **distinct clinical presentations.**

A. Definitions

—An **aneurysm** is a **ballooning defect in the vessel wall.** Aneurysms often are **chronic,** and may or may not rupture.

—A **dissection** is a **tear of the arterial intima.** Traumatic thoracic dissections often are associated with **deceleration injuries**.

B. Clinical presentation

1. Symptoms

—**Thoracic aneurysms** usually present with poorly defined chest pain, especially if the aneurysm is expanding rapidly. Once the aneurysm has expanded to the point that the pressure on the weakened vessel wall is too great, the aneurysm will rupture.

—**Aortic dissection** usually presents with hypertension (which may be the precipitant of the intimal tear), acute onset of pain described as "tearing," and radiation to the interscapular area. The associated symptoms that develop depend on which section(s) of aorta are occluded as the intimal canal (false lumen) expands and compresses the true lumen. As a result, the patient may complain of **hoarseness** (caused by compression of the recurrent laryngeal nerve), **chest pain** (caused by compression of the coronary ostia), or **back or extremity pain** (caused by compromise of distal flow to the kidneys or limbs). A proximal dissection may propagate back to the aortic root and pericardium, producing aortic insufficiency and cardiac tamponade, both of which are ominous signs.

2. Physical examination

a. Physical examination findings of **thoracic aneurysm** are minimal, because they tend to be asymptomatic. If rupture occurs, an acute increase in pain and hypertension will be noted, by which point it has become a surgical emergency.

b. Physical examination findings suggestive of **aortic dissection** include

—acute **neurologic symptoms** (syncope, coma, convulsions, hemiplegia).

—**absent or diminished pulses.**

—**arterial ischemia to the leg.**

—a new **aortic regurgitation murmur,** which characteristically radiates down the right sternal border rather than the left.

—a **palpable thrust** in the right second or third intercostal spaces.

—a **pulsating sternoclavicular joint** secondary to swelling at the base of the aorta.

C. Diagnostic tests

1. Chest radiograph may demonstrate

—a **widened mediastinum.**

—**abnormal aortic contour.**

—a **"calcium sign,"** which reflects separation of intimal calcification from the adventitial surface.

—With traumatic rupture of the aorta, one may note

—tracheal deviation to the right.

—obliteration of space between pulmonary artery and aorta.

—esophageal (or NGT) deviation to the right.

—depression of left main stem bronchus.

—widened paratracheal stripe.

—widened paraspinal interfaces.

—presence of pleural or apical cap.

—left hemothorax.

—fractures of 1st or 2nd rib.

—fracture of scapula.

2. Contrast computed tomography (CT) is best for diagnosis.

3. Magnetic resonance angiography (MRA) also may be necessary.

4. Transesophageal echocardiography (TEE) and **aortography** also are useful tests.

D. Treatment

1. Medical therapy

a. Sodium nitroprusside

—is used to control BP.

—is titrated to a sBP of 100–120 mm Hg.

—Starting infusion dose is 5 μg/kg/min for adults, to a maximum of 20 μg/kg/min, or 1 μg/kg/min for children, to a maximum of 4 μg/kg/min.

—Note: cyanide toxicity is a potential complication. Prevent by wrapping solution bag and tubing in opaque material (e.g., aluminum foil).

b. β-Blockers

—are used to control the pulse.

Boluses of **propranolol** (1.5 mg IV every 2–4 hours) should be administered until the target pulse rate of 60/min is obtained.

—Alternative drugs include **esmolol,** which has a short half-life and is easier to titrate, and **labetalol,** which is both an α- and a β-blocker.

c. **Opiate analgesia**

—can be used as a supplement to control BP and pulse.

—**Morphine,** 5–10 mg IV, is given in 2-mg increments.

2. **Surgery**

—is the definitive treatment for proximal thoracic dissections and any ruptured aneurysm.

—If such a situation is suspected, it is imperative that the patient go to the operating room as soon as possible.

V. Acute Pericarditis

—is inflammation of the pericardium.

A. **Causes** include

—**viral infection** (coxsackievirus, echovirus)

—**bacterial infection** (*Staphylococcus aureus, Streptococcus pneumoniae,* β-hemolytic streptococci, *Mycobacterium tuberculosis*)

—**fungal infection** (*Histoplasma capsulatum*)

—**autoimmune diseases** [systemic lupus erythematosus (SLE), rheumatoid arthritis]

—**malignancy,** especially tumors of the breast and lung

—**trauma**

—**idiopathic**

—**MI** (Dressler's syndrome)

—**uremia**

B. **Clinical presentation**

1. **Symptoms**

a. The **pain** of pericarditis

—is typically described as **"sharp"** or **"stabbing"**

—has a **gradual onset**

—is worse when the patient is supine, and is alleviated by sitting up and leaning forward; thus, it is **pleuritic** and **positional**

—is often referred to the neck, back, and left shoulder, particularly to the left trapezial ridge

—is distinguished from anginal pain in that it is **not relieved by NTG**

b. The patient also presents with **fever**

2. **Physical examination**

a. The most important physical finding is a **pericardial friction rub,** pathognomonic for pericarditis. The pericardial friction rub

—is a scratchy, low-pitched sound best heard with the diaphragm of the stethoscope over the left sternal border, with the patient sitting up and leaning forward.

—is intermittent.

b. Examination also reveals a **resting tachycardia, dysphagia, dyspnea on inspiration, paradoxical pulse,** and **Kussmaul's sign** (inspiratory neck vein distention).

C. Diagnostic tests

1. Echocardiography

—is the diagnostic **test of choice** for detecting a pericardial effusion associated with pericarditis.

—may reveal a **thickening of the pericardial wall.**

2. Chest radiograph

—demonstrates an enlarged cardiac silhouette (Figure 2-2) only if there is a large pericardial effusion. Otherwise, it is normal.

3. ECG changes include

—PR segment depression followed by **ST segment elevation** in all leads except aVR, where there is reciprocal depression.

—overall **low-voltage QRS complexes** and **T wave flattening** (Figure 2-3).

D. Treatment

—consists of **nonsteroidal anti-inflammatory agents (NSAIDs),** such as **ibuprofen** (400–600 mg four times daily) and **indomethacin** (25–50 mg four times daily).

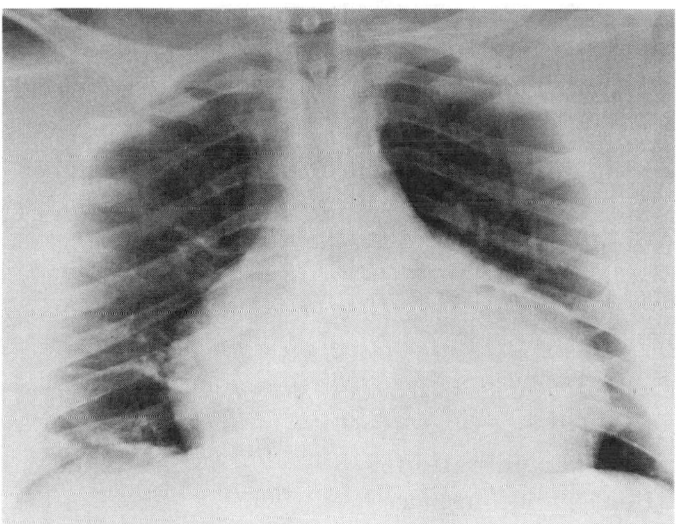

Figure 2-2. Chest radiograph demonstrating an enlarged cardiac silhouette. (Reprinted with permission from Daffner RH: *Clinical Radiology: The Essentials,* 2nd ed. Philadelphia, Lippincott Williams & Wilkins, 1999.)

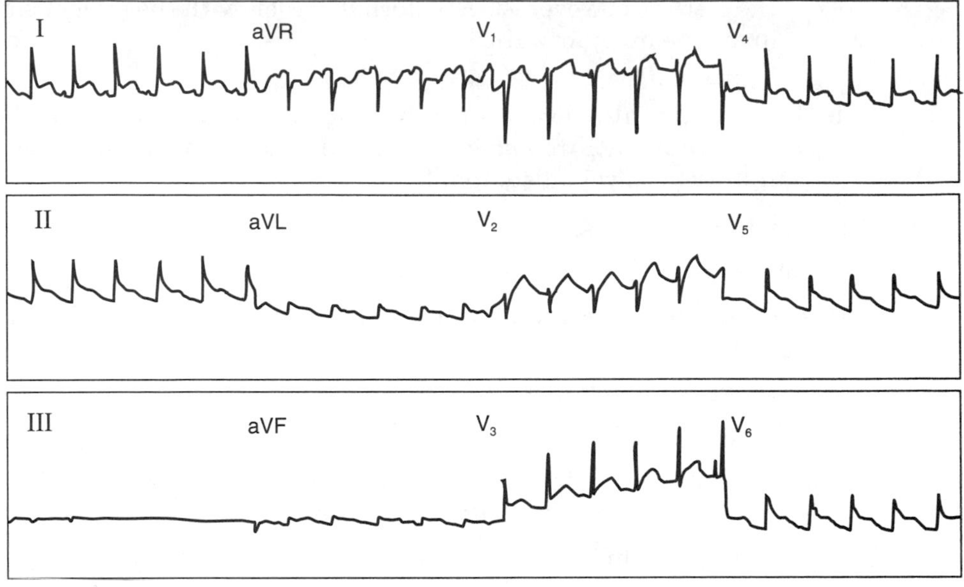

Figure 2-3. Electrocardiogram (ECG) of pericarditis demonstrating low-voltage QRS complexes and T wave flattening. (Adapted with permission from Chung EK: *Pocket Guide to ECG Diagnosis.* Cambridge, MA, Blackwell Science Publishers, 1996, p 473.)

—Additionally, the underlying cause for the pericarditis must be sought and treated.

VI. Cardiac Tamponade

A. **Pathophysiology.** Results from rapid accumulation of fluid in the pericardial space. The excess pericardial fluid prevents the atria and ventricles from filling adequately during diastole, which decreases the volume of blood available during systole, producing hemodynamic compromise.

B. **Causes**

1. **Penetrating trauma to the chest** is the most common preceding event.
2. Cardiac tamponade may result as a **complication of pericarditis** of any cause.

C. **Clinical presentation**

1. **Symptoms** include
   —acute dyspnea.
   —tachycardia.
2. **Physical examination**
   a. **Beck's triad** includes
      —**hypotension** secondary to decreased systemic arterial pressure.
      —**distended neck veins** secondary to increased venous pressure.
      —**muffled heart sounds**.

b. **Pulsus paradoxus** is an exaggerated waxing and waning of the pulse due to inspiratory decrease in arterial pressure of > 10 mm Hg.

D. **Diagnostic tests**

1. **Chest radiograph** usually demonstrates an enlarged cardiac silhouette. The lung fields usually are clear.
2. **ECG** may demonstrate low QRS voltage, T wave flattening (see Figure 2-3), and **electrical alternans** (Figure 2-4).

E. **Treatment**

—**Pericardiocentesis** is the definitive treatment for cardiac tamponade.

VII. Congestive Heart Failure

A. **Overview**

1. **Causes** (Table 2-3)

—The most common cause of right heart failure (RHF) is left heart failure (LHF).

2. **Risk factors** include

—tachyarrhythmias, such as atrial fibrillation.

—increased sodium load.

—acute myocardial ischemia or infarction.

—noncompliance with medications.

—ingestion of drugs that impair myocardial function.

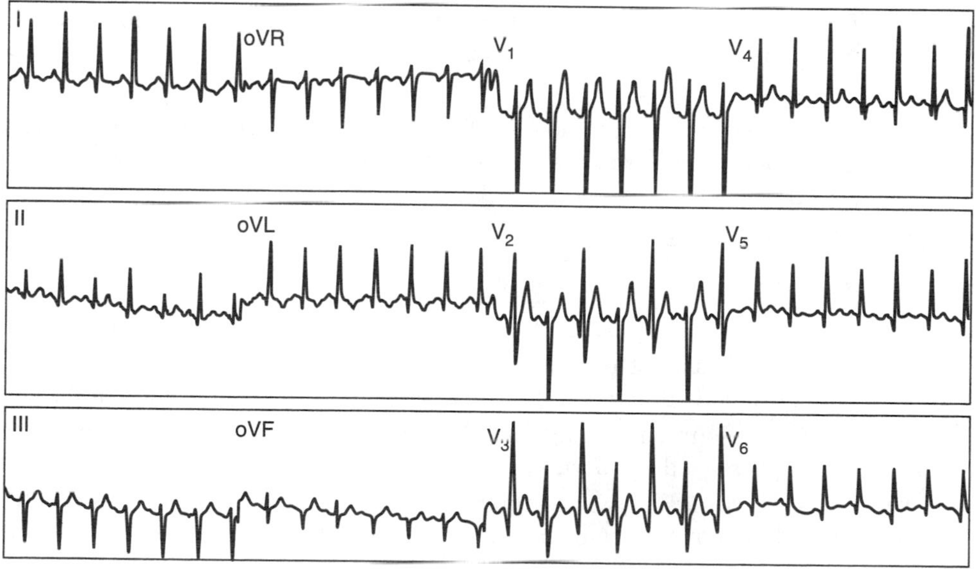

Figure 2-4. Electrocardiogram (ECG) of cardiac tamponade demonstrating electrical alternans. Note the alteration of the QRS complex in every other beat. (Adapted with permission from Chung EK: *Pocket Guide to ECG Diagnosis*. Cambridge, MA, Blackwell Science Publishers, 1996, p 379)

Table 2-3. Features of Left and Right Heart Failure

	Causes	Symptoms	Physical Findings	Chest X-ray Findings
LHF	Left-sided MI and bacterial endocarditis, valvular HD (AS, AR, MR), systemic hypertension, ↑ pulmonary venous pressure	Pulmonary congestion, dyspnea on exertion, orthopnea, paroxysmal nocturnal dyspnea, nocturia, cough, fatigue and weakness, white or pinkish frothy sputum (if pulmonary edema)	Tachycardia, tachypnea, diaphoresis, S_3 gallop, pulmonary rales and wheezes, Cheyne-Stokes respiration	Prominent pulmonary vasculature, cardiomegaly, Kerley B lines
RHF	LHF, right-sided MI and bacterial endocarditis, valvular HD (MS, IHSS), pulmonary hypertension, ↑ systemic pressure	Right upper quadrant pain (secondary to distention of hepatic capsule)	JVD, hepatomegaly, hepatojugular reflex, peripheral edema, ascites, cyanosis, hypo- or hypertension	Widened SVC, pleural effusion

AR = aortic regurgitation; *AS* = aortic stenosis; *HD* = heart disease; *IHSS* = idiopathic hypertrophic subaortic stenosis; *JVD* = jugular venous distention; *LHF* = left heart failure; *MI* = myocardial infarction; *MR* = mitral regurgitation; *MS* = mitral stenosis; *RHF* = right heart failure; *SVC* = superior vena cava.

—physical overexertion.

B. Clinical presentation

1. **Symptoms** of LHF result from increased pulmonary venous pressure, whereas symptoms of RHF result from increased systemic pressure (see Table 2-3).
2. **Physical examination** (see Table 2-3). CHF often presents as **acute pulmonary edema,** a situation with the risk of impending respiratory failure.

C. Diagnostic tests

1. **Chest radiograph** findings

   —depend on the amount of **pulmonary congestion** present.

   a. At pressures of 15 mm Hg, vascular markings are limited to the upper lung fields due to lesser resistance compared to the lower lung fields.

   b. As pressures reach 20 mm Hg, interstitial edema develops as a result of increased left atrial pressure.

      —markings at the periphery of lower lung fields, known as **Kerley B lines** are present, in cases of **interlobular edema.**

      —vary in cases of LHF and RHF (see Table 2-3).

      —detect enlarged cardiac silhouette and peribronchial cuffing in late CHF.

2. **ECG** findings

—may demonstrate changes suggestive of MI or ischemia as an acute cause of CHF.

—may reveal **ventricular hypertrophy** (tall R waves in precordial leads) and **atrial hypertrophy** (tall, upright P waves) in cases of chronic failure.

—may note an arrhythmia, which may be the cause for the CHF.

—Although all of these signs may be seen in CHF, none of them is diagnostic for CHF.

D. Treatment

1. Be prepared to **intubate** if necessary.
2. Use **IV-O_2-monitor,** as for any patient with a cardiac emergency.
3. Give **NTG** 0.4 mg sublingually to alleviate pain, if patient is not hypotensive. If the patient does not respond, switch to a drip of 5 μg/min.
4. Administer a potent diuretic to reduce the pulmonary edema.

—Preferred diuretics are **furosemide** (40–80 mg IV) and **bumetanide** (1–2 mg IV).

—Do not forget to **monitor serum electrolytes,** especially potassium.

5. Give morphine sulfate for analgesia if patient is not hypotensive.
6. For patients with **hypotension** (systolic BP < 90 mm Hg)

—the choice inotropic agent is **dobutamine,** which has the advantage of increasing cardiac output without increasing peripheral vascular resistance. It is administered as a 5–10 μg/kg/min drip.

—**Dopamine** (1–10 μg/kg/min) also may be used for inotropic support, especially if the patient is hypotensive.

a. At low doses (1–5 μg/kg/min), dopamine promotes diuresis.
b. At higher doses (5–10 μg/kg/min), dopamine increases BP.

—A third drug used for inotropic support is **amrinone,** a phosphodiesterase inhibitor. It is used at doses of 10–15 μg/kg/min, titrated to hemodynamic profile for severe CHF refractory to diuretics, vasodilators, and conventional inotropic agents.

7. For patients presenting with **hypertension** also, consider **sodium nitroprusside** in an IV drip titrated to BP: 5 μg/kg/min in adults, to a maximum of 20 μg/kg/min, or 1 μg/kg/min in children, to a maximum of 4 μg/kg/min.

VIII. Hypertensive Emergencies

A. Definition: hypertensive emergency versus hypertensive urgency (Table 2-4)

B. Clinical presentation

1. **Symptoms**

Table 2-4. Hypertensive Emergency Versus Hypertensive Urgency

	End-Organ Damage	Blood Pressure	Treatment Schedule
Hypertensive emergency	Yes (brain, heart, kidney)	>130 mm Hg *or* presence of end organ damage	30–60 minutes, gradually
Hypertensive urgency	No	>115 mm Hg (diastolic)	24–48 hours, gradually

a. Central nervous system (CNS) symptoms may include **headache, nausea, vomiting, vertigo, tinnitus, aphasia, lethargy,** or **coma.**

b. In a patient with cardiovascular damage, **chest pain, dyspnea, orthopnea, cough,** and **right upper quadrant pain** (from passive hepatic congestion) may be noted.

c. Renal end-organ damage may present as **anuria, oliguria, mental status changes, weight loss,** and **weakness.**

2. **Physical examination**

—should focus on systems that may have end-organ damage.

a. Beginning with the CNS, do a thorough **neurologic examination,** looking for diplopia, hemiparesis, and seizures.

b. **Funduscopic examination** may reveal arteriovenous nicking, hemorrhages, or exudates, but it is the finding of **papilledema** that is diagnostic for hypertensive encephalopathy.

c. Check the **BP** in both arms, paying attention to peripheral pulses. Perform **orthostatic BP testing** (if the patient can tolerate it) to rule out dehydration.

d. **Cardiac examination** may reveal cardiomegaly with a prominent left ventricular impulse. S_3 and S_4 sounds also may be heard.

e. **Chest auscultation** may demonstrate basilar rales.

f. Other findings may include JVD, cyanosis, hepatojugular reflex, and dependent edema.

C. **Differential diagnosis**

1. **Pheochromocytoma**

—is distinguished by **episodic** hypertension, often accompanied by diarrhea and flushing.

—is treated with **phentolamine,** an α_1-blocker.

2. **Abrupt cessation of clonidine or β-blockers**

—May precipitate withdrawal and severe rebound hypertension.

—Treat immediate crisis with **nitroprusside,** then resume regimen, with gradual tapered decrease.

3. **Tyramine crisis**

—Patients on monoamine oxidase inhibitors who ingest foods high in tyramine (aged cheese, Chianti wine, pickled herring) can have a severe hypertensive crisis.

—Treat with **phentolamine.**

4. **Ingestion of sympathomimetics**

—such as amphetamines, cocaine, phencyclidine (PCP), lysergic acid diethylamide (LSD), "cold medicines" (which often contain α_1-blockers), and "diet pills" may result in severe hypertension, usually associated with agitation and delirium.

—**Sodium nitroprusside** can be used to control symptoms, as can β-blockers and phentolamine.

D. Diagnostic tests

1. **Chest radiograph** may reveal pulmonary edema and cardiomegaly.
2. **ECG** may show evidence of myocardial ischemia, CHF, or left ventricular hypertrophy (LVH).

E. Treatment

1. Initially, all patients are put on **IV-O_2-monitor.**
2. The **goal** of therapy is to lower the BP to a **sBP** of **140–160 mm Hg** and a **diastolic BP (dBP)** of **90–110 mm Hg.** However, the BP must be brought down **gradually** to prevent cerebral edema, because a 25% reduction in mean arterial pressure (MAP; 2/3 dBP + 1/3 sBP) is the lower limit of cerebral autoregulation.
3. **Pharmacologic agents**

a. **Sodium nitroprusside**

—is the **drug of choice** for **all hypertensive crises, except preeclampsia** and **eclampsia.**

—An infusion of 5 μg/kg/min (in D_5W) is given and titrated to desired BP.

b. **Labetalol**

—is administered in boluses of 20 mg IV (or 1–2 mg/kg IV).

—may be given as an infusion (in D_5W) at 2 mg/min.

—is stopped once the desired BP is reached.

—The α-blocking activity of labetalol on smooth muscle decreases the BP, and its β-blocking effect prevents reflex tachycardia.

—**β-Blockers should not be used in patients with COPD, CHF, and heart block.**

c. **Nimodipine**

—is used in cases of **acute subarachnoid hemorrhage** in patients with good neurologic status, because it decreases the associated vasospasm.

—The recommended dosage is 60 mg orally every 4 hours for 21 days.

—Side effects include hypotension (dose-related), edema, and headache.

d. **NTG (IV or sublingual)**

—is used for cases of **angina** to control pain; the nitroprusside lowers the BP. **NTG, morphine,** and **furosemide** (20–40 mg IV) may be added to the nitroprusside regimen in cases of **pulmonary edema.**

e. **Magnesium sulfate** and **hydralazine**

—are the optimal treatment for hypertensive emergencies in pregnancy (i.e., **preeclampsia** and **eclampsia**) [see Chapter 16].

f. **Benzodiazepines,** usually given for sedation, also help lower the BP, and are the choice agents for hypertension associated with cocaine, PCP, and other sympathomimetic overdose.

IX. Endocarditis

A. Overview

1. **Causes** are summarized in Table 2-5.
2. **Risk factors** include
   - —intravenous drug abuse (IVDA)
   - —rheumatic or congenital heart disease
   - —prosthetic heart valve(s)
   - —intracardiac pacemaker
   - —mitral valve prolapse, pulmonic stenosis, and other valvular lesions
   - —history of endocarditis
3. Complications for **infectious endocarditis** include
   - —**CHF** (the most frequent complication)
   - —**neurologic complications,** including CVAs, meningoencephalitis, and cranial or peripheral nerve lesions secondary to emboli from the infected valves

B. Clinical presentation

1. **Symptoms** include
   - —**CHF, pulmonary edema,** or both
   - —**chest pain** (may or may not be present)
   - —**fever, chills, tachycardia, joint pains,** and **anorexia**
   - —The patient appears **acutely ill,** and also may report **fatigue, nausea,** and **vomiting.**

Table 2-5. Etiologies of Infectious Endocarditis

Organism	Incidence
Streptococcus viridans	30–40%
Other streptococci (*bovis, epidermidis*)	15–25%
Enterococci	5–15%
Staphylococci	20–35%
Pseudomonas, serratia, hemophilus, fungi	Rare, usually restricted to intravenous drug abusers and immunocompromised patients

2. **Physical examination.** Findings for subacute (versus acute) **bacterial endocarditis** include:

—**petechiae,** especially in the mouth, in the conjunctivae, and above the clavicles.

—**Osler nodes,** which are painful nodules of the palmar surface of the fingertips.

—**splinter hemorrhages** under the nails.

—**Roth spots,** which are retinal hemorrhages with a pale central halo.

—**Janeway lesions,** which are red macules found predominantly on the palms and soles, but which also may be present on the flanks and extremities.

—Cardiac examination almost always reveals a **murmur,** which may be of new onset or increased intensity. The characteristics of the murmur depend on the valve affected (Table 2-6).

Table 2-6. Classification of Heart Murmurs

Valve Defect	Characteristics of Murmur	Location of Murmur
Mitral stenosis	Low-pitched, rumbling, mid-diastolic murmur with presystolic crescendo localized to the apex; accentuating precordial thrust of RV; loud opening S_1 snap	Best heard in left third to fourth interspace
Mitral insufficiency	Harsh, medium-pitched, pansystolic murmur; accentuated precordial thrust of LV; systolic thrill; S_3 often present; ↑ P_2	At apex with radiation to left axilla and base
Aortic stenosis	High-pitched, blowing, diamond-shaped, systolic murmur; ↓ A_2; accentuated precordial thrust at the apex; systolic thrill; narrowed pulse pressure	Right second to third interspace
Aortic insufficiency	Harsh, decrescendo, blowing, diastolic murmur; ↑ A_2; S_3 heard over the apex; widened pulse pressure; "pistol shot" femorals; "water hammer" pulse; capillary pulsations	Heard over left sternal border
Tricuspid stenosis	Medium-pitched, pansystolic murmur; accentuated precordial thrust of RV, diastolic thrill at left sternal border; opening snap of TV at right sternal border	Left lower sternal margin
Tricuspid insufficiency	Low-pitched, presystolic or mid-diastolic, rumbling murmur; prominent jugular pulses	Left sternal border in fifth interspace

LV = left ventricle; *RV* = right ventricle; *TV* = tricuspid valve.

C. Diagnostic tests

1. Three sets of **blood cultures,** preferably taken from different sites, are used to make the diagnosis.
   —In 90% of cases of endocarditis, the first culture set yields a positive result.
   —Three negative sets are used to rule out endocarditis. The presence of sustained (versus transient) bacteremia as seen in endocarditis is crucial to the diagnosis.
2. **Two-dimensional echocardiography and transesophageal echocardiography (TEE)**
   —can detect blood flow patterns and the presence of vegetations, making them useful diagnostic adjuncts.
3. **Chest radiograph** may show
   —signs of **pulmonary edema,** with a heart size smaller than that expected for the degree of edema.
   —straightening of the left sternal border in cases of mitral stenosis, due to left atrial enlargement.
4. **ECG**
   —is **not confirmatory** because the changes also are seen in many other conditions.
   —**Aortic stenosis** shows depressed T waves in lead I and the precordial leads.
   —Signs of left atrial hypertrophy (LAH) [tall, upright P waves] and right ventricular hypertrophy (RVH) [tall R waves in V_4 through V_6] are seen with **mitral stenosis.**
   —**Mitral regurgitation** presents with LVH and left axis deviation.

D. Treatment

1. Most patients with endocarditis are very sick and require **hospital admission**.
2. **Antibiotics**
   a. **Empiric treatment for native valves** is nafcillin or oxacillin 50 mg/kg intravenously every 6 hours plus gentamicin 1.0 mg/kg intravenously every 8 hours.
   b. **Empiric treatment for prosthetic valves** is vancomycin 15 mg/kg every 12 hours plus gentamicin 1.0 mg/kg intravenously every 8 hours plus rifampin 600 mg by mouth every 24 hours.
   c. **Antibiotic prophylaxis** as per the 1997 American Heart Association guidelines is indicated for:
      —patients with predisposing factors (see VIII A).
      —dental extractions and implants
      —periodontal procedures
      —endodontic procedures
      —tonsillectomy
      —rigid bronchoscopy
      —sclerotherapy for esophageal varices

—endoscopic retrograde cholangiography (ERCP)
—biliary tract surgery
—prostate surgery
—cystoscopy
—urethral dilation

(1) **Prophylaxis for dental or minor GI or GU procedures in patients without prior history of endocarditis and able to tolerate:**
  (a) ampicillin, 50 mg/kg (maximum dose=2g)
  (b) If the patient is penicillin-allergic, then administer clindamycin 20 mg/kg, or azithromycin 15 mg/kg or clarithromycin 15 mg/kg, or cephalexin 50 mg/kg or cefadroxil 50 mg/kg. Administration of each of these is by mouth one hour before the procedure. Can be given IV 30 minutes before procedure if patient cannot tolerate the medication by mouth.

(2) **Prophylaxis for major GI or GU procedures in patients without prior history of endocarditis:**
  (a) **Amoxicillin** 50 mg/kg (maximum dose=2 g) is administered orally, **or ampicillin** 50 mg/kg IM/IV 30 minutes before procedure.
  (b) If the patient is penicillin-allergic, then use vancomycin 20 mg/kg IV (maximum dose is 20 mg) over 1–2 hours. Infusion to be completed 30 minutes before procedure.

(3) **Prophylaxis for patients with prior history of endocarditis.**
  (a) Use ampicillin 50 mg/kg IM/IV + gentamicin 1.5 mg/kg IV within 30 minutes of starting procedure and then ampicillin 1 g IM/IV or amoxicillin 1 g by mouth 6 hours later.
  (b) If the patient is penicillin-allergic, then use vancomycin 20 mg/kg IV over 1–2 hours + gentamicin 1.5 mg/kg IV. Infusion to be completed 30 minutes before procedure.

d. **NTG, furosemide,** and **morphine** are used for pulmonary edema.

e. IV **diltiazem** is used for atrial fibrillation.

f. **Heparin** therapy is used for suspected embolization.

3. Relative indications for **surgical management** of endocarditis include
—prosthetic valve endocarditis.
—unsuccessful treatment with antibiotics.
—repeated major emboli.
—sepsis despite medical treatment.
—aortic/mitral valve incompetence with impending heart failure.
—myocardial (valve ring) abscess.

X. CARDIAC ARRHYTHMIAS

A. Atrial fibrillation

1. Overview

a. **Definition.** Atrial fibrillation is a fast, chaotic rhythm that originates in the atrium and results in a rapid and irregular ventricular response.

b. **Risk factors**
—age
—diabetes mellitus
—heart disease (all types, including rheumatic heart disease, Wolff-Parkinson-White syndrome, atrial septal defect, and congestive heart failure)
—hypertension
—acute alcohol intoxication (holiday heart)
—thyrotoxicosis (see Chapter 12 IV)
—pericarditis
—pulmonary embolism
—chronic obstructive pulmonary disease (COPD)
—drugs (particularly digoxin and quinidine)

2. **Clinical features**

a. **Symptoms** may include
—palpitation
—fatigue
—dizziness
—chest pain

b. **Physical examination findings** may include
—tachycardia
—irregularly irregular cardiac rhythm
—hypotension

3. **Diagnostic tests**

a. **ECG** to look for
—no discernible p waves
—rapid ventricular rate (120–200 bpm)

b. **Echocardiogram** to look for valvular heart disease and atrial hypertrophy

c. **Thyroid function tests** to look for hyperthyroidism

4. **Treatment**

a. If **hemodynamically unstable** (patient has chest pain, dyspnea, or ventricular rate > 140): **synchronized cardioversion** (See Figure 1-5).

b. If **hemodynamically stable,** attempt to control rate by administering:
—**diltiazem** 0.25 mg/kg IV or
—**verapamil** 0.1–0.2 mg/kg IV
—**labetalol** 20 mg IV over 2 minutes, can repeat every 10 minutes up to maximum dose of 300 mg total (adults). Pediatric dose not well established.
—**metoprolol** 5 mg IV, can be repeated at 5-minute intervals and titrated to blood pressure (adults). Pediatric dose not well established.

—**digoxin** 10–15 μg/kg IV loading dose (much slower onset)

—note that calcium channel blockers and digoxin are **contraindicated** in patients with Wolff-Parkinson-White syndrome (see X C).

—**chemical cardioversion** may be achieved with **isobutalide** 0.01 mg/kg over 10 minutes, which may be repeated once. This is usually done under conscious sedation.

c. **Once rate is controlled, administer:**

—diltiazem 10 mg/hr **infusion** (or other rate controlling medication drip) titrated to heart rate

—**anticoagulation with heparin** to prevent intra-atrial thrombi. Loading dose is 80 U/kg IV bolus followed by 18 U/kg maintenance drip. Aim to keep activated partial thromboplastin time (APTT) between 60 and 85 seconds or 1.5–2.0 times the patient's normal value. If long-term anticoagulation is needed, warfarin is added to keep the international normalized ratio (INR) between 2 and 3.

5. **Disposition**

a. Patients with new onset or symptomatic atrial fibrillation are admitted for further work-up and optimization of anticoagulation.

b. Patients with chronic or asymptomatic atrial fibrillation may be discharged with outpatient follow-up.

B. **Atrial Flutter**

1. **Overview**

—is a rhythm produced by a re-entry circuit in the atria

—is less stable than atrial fibrillation due to rapid ventricular rate

2. **Clinical features** are the same as for atrial fibrillation (see X A).

3. **Diagnostic tests**

a. ECG to look for (Figure 2-5)

—**sawtooth shaped p waves,** best seen in leads II, III, and AVF

—usually regular PR interval

—atrial rate is 220–350 bpm

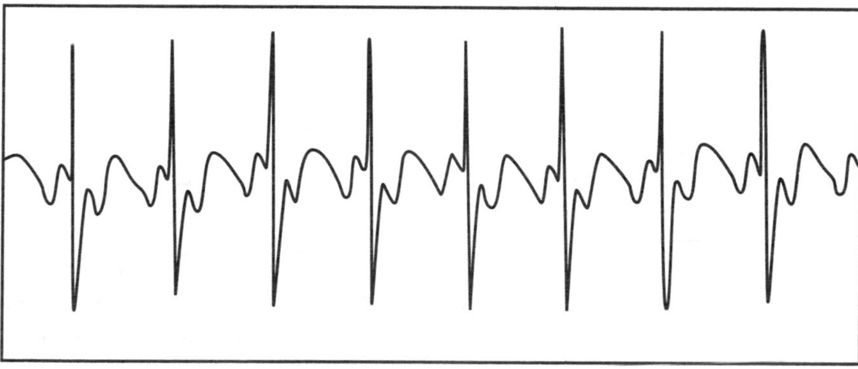

Figure 2-5. Atrial flutter. (Adapted from LifeART Emergency Medicine Professional Collection. Copyright 1998, Lippincott Williams & Wilkins. All rights reserved.)

b. Echocardiogram to look for valvular lesions and wall motion abnormalities

4. **Treatment**

a. If hemodynamically **unstable** (patient has chest pain, dyspnea, or ventricular rate > 140): synchronized cardioversion (see Figure 1-5).

b. If hemodynamically **stable,** attempt to convert to sinus rhythm

—vagal maneuvers to slow heart rate

—quinidine:

—adults: 200 mg IV. Maximum infusion rate is 10 μg/minute.

—children: not recommended. 2–10 mg/kg IV every 3–6 hours as needed

—procainamide:

—children: 3–6 mg/kg over 5 minutes to a maximum of 100 mg. Infusion (drip) dose is 20–80 μg/kg/minute.

—adults: 15–18 mg/kg over 5 minutes to a maximum of 1500 mg. Infusion (drip) dose is 1–5 mg/min.

—may also consider diltiazem, verapamil, β-blockers and digoxin as for atrial fibrillation above

c. **Anticoagulation not necessary**

5. **Disposition.** Patients should be admitted for further work-up.

C. **Wolff-Parkinson-White Syndrome**

1. **Overview.** Wolff-Parkinson-White syndrome is a congenital disorder where cardiac impulses from the sinus node are conducted via bypass tracts (accessory pathways) to the ventricle. In the absence of ectopic tachyarrhythmias, it is a benign asymptomatic syndrome.

2. **Diagnostic tests**

a. ECG to look for

—short PR interval

—long QRS interval

—presence of delta wave (Figure 2-6)

—Other ECG findings

—atrial fibrillation in Wolff-Parkinson-White syndrome will present as broad, bizarre QRS complexes

—QS or Q waves in II, III, and AVF (mimics inferior wall MI)

b. Echocardiogram to establish presence of accessory pathways, especially when diagnosis of Wolff-Parkinson-White syndrome not established (rarely done in the ED).

3. **Treatment**

a. Quinidine and procainamide are the drugs of choice for converting SVT and atrial fibrillation in Wolff-Parkinson-White syndrome.

b. Adenosine may be used for acute treatment of reciprocating tachycardia with normal QRS complexes

c. Verapamil, diltiazem and digoxin are contraindicated in the presence of Wolff-Parkinson-White syndrome.

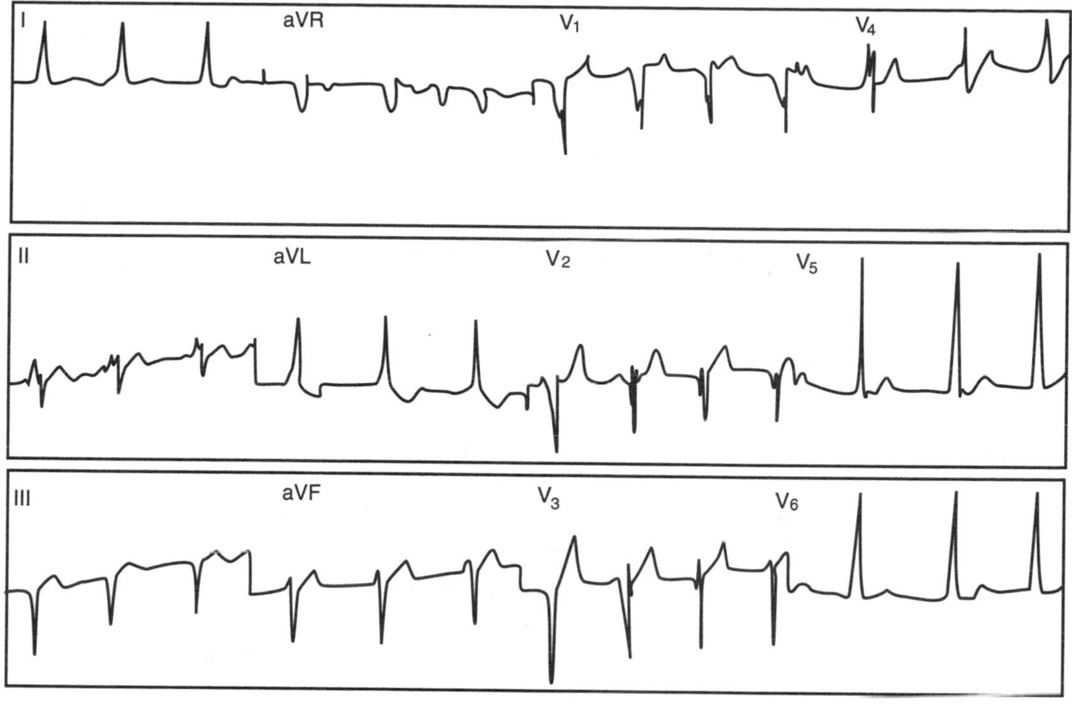

Figure 2-6. Wolff-Parkinson-White syndrome. Note slurred QRS complex (delta wave). (Adapted from LifeART Emergency Medicine Professional Collection. Copyright 1998, Lippincott Williams & Wilkins. All rights reserved.)

4. **Disposition**
   a. Patients whose arrhythmia has been well controlled and who are asymptomatic after a period of observation may be discharged home with outpatient follow-up.
   b. Patients with chest pain, dyspnea or an unstable rhythm should be admitted for further work-up.

D. Heart blocks

1. **First degree block** (Figure 2-7)
   —PR interval >.20 seconds
   —All p waves followed by a QRS complex
   —Atrial rate is equal to ventricular rate
2. **Second degree heart block** (Figure 2-8)
   a. **Type I (Wenckebach)**
      —Progressive prolongation of PR interval followed by one or more nonconducted beats at regular intervals
      —Block usually occurs at the level of the atrioventricular node (AVN)
      —QRS complexes are normal
      —Usually associated with increased parasympathetic tone
      —Atrial rate is faster than the ventricular rate
   b. **Type II (Mobitz)**
      —Constant PR interval, one beat is dropped at fixed interval

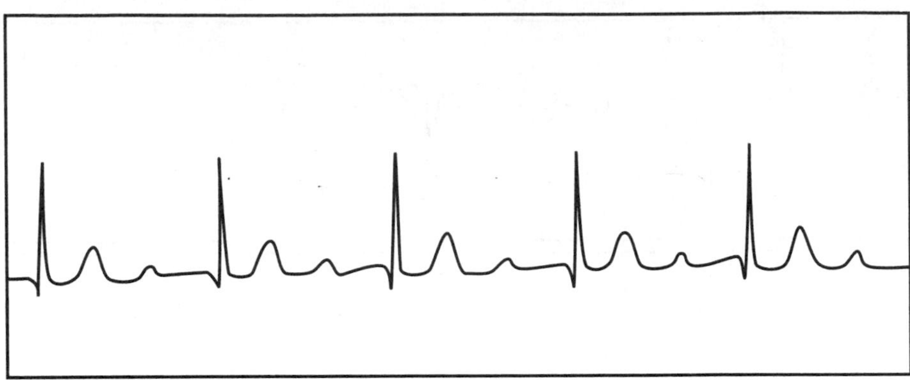

Figure 2-7. First degree heart block. Note prolonged PR interval. (Adapted from LifeART Emergency Medicine Professional Collection. Copyright 1998, Lippincott Williams & Wilkins. All rights reserved.)

—Block usually occurs at the level of the bundle branch (BB)
—QRS is wide if block is at BB and normal if at the bundle of His
—Usually associated with organic lesion in conduction pathway, particularly anteroseptal MI
—Can quickly degenerate into third degree heart block
—Poorer prognosis than type I
—Atrial rate is faster than the ventricular rate

3. **Third degree heart block** (Figure 2-9)
   —Total dissociation of atrial and ventricular rhythm
   —Normal appearing p waves
   —Pattern of p waves unrelated to pattern of QRS (varying PR and QRS intervals)
   —Block can occur at the level of the AVN with a heart rate of 40–60 bpm, which is a stable rhythm
   —Block can occur below the level of the AVN with a heart rate $<$ 40 bpm, which is an unstable rhythm
   —Atrial rate is faster than the ventricular rate
4. **Clinical features**
   a. **Symptoms** may include
      —chest pain
      —dyspnea
      —decreased level of consciousness
   b. **Physical examination findings** may include
      —hypotension
      —bradycardia
      —rales on pulmonary auscultation
5. **Treatment**
   —Usually not necessary for first degree and second degree type I blocks

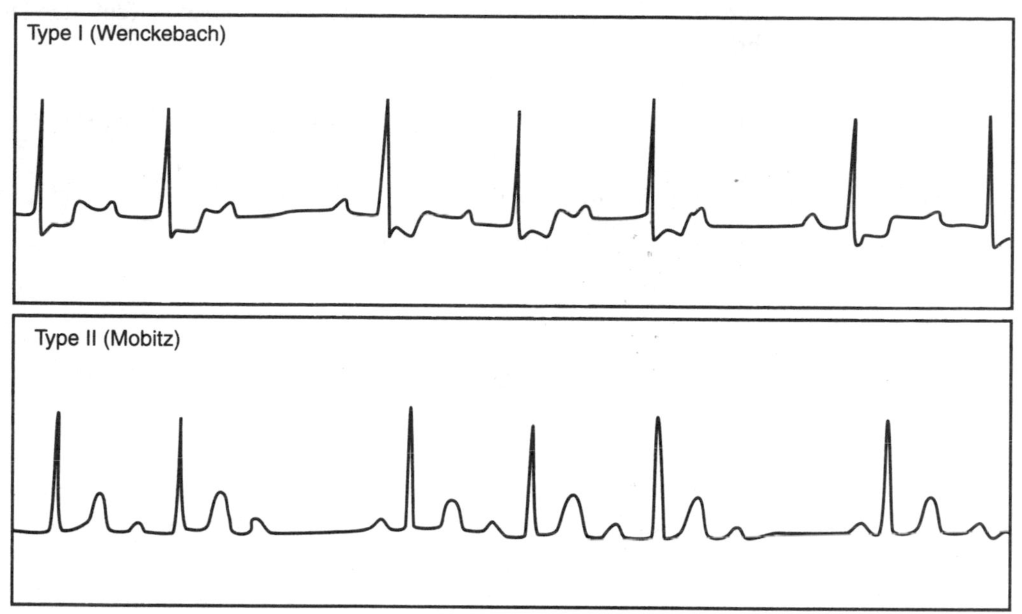

Figure 2-8. Second degree heart block. (Adapted from LifeART Emergency Medicine Professional Collection. Copyright 1998, Lippincott Williams & Wilkins. All rights reserved.)

—Often necessary for second degree type II and third degree blocks because patients are symptomatic

a. If the patient is hemodynamically **unstable** or if there is third degree block below level of AVN, then **immediate transcutaneous pacing** (bridge to transvenous pacemaker) is appropriate.

b. If the patient is hemodynamically **stable,** then manage rate and blood pressure:

—**Atropine** 0.5–1.0 mg IV repeated every 3–5 minutes (maximum dose 0.03 mg/kg)

—**Epinephrine** 1–2 μg/min intravenous infusion

—**Dopamine** 5–20 μg IV infusion

—Low dose (1–5 μg/min) has dopaminergic effect, used to increase renal output

—Medium dose (5–10 μg/min) has α and β1 effect, used to increase cardiac output.

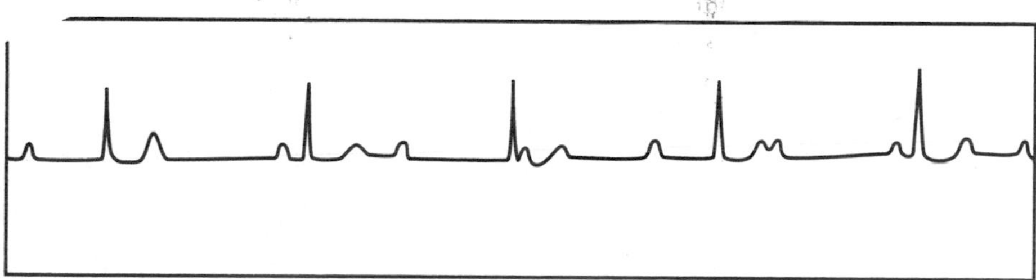

Figure 2-9. Third degree heart block. Note dissociation of atrial and ventricular rhythms. (Adapted from LifeART Emergency Medicine Professional Collection. Copyright 1998, Lippincott Williams & Wilkins. All rights reserved.)

—High dose (10–20 μg/min) has mostly α adrenergic effect, used for shock

—**Isoproterenol** 2–20 μg/min intravenous infusion

c. Lidocaine is contraindicated in the treatment of third degree block with ventricular escape beats.

E. Ventricular tachycardia and fibrillation (See Chapter 1 V A)

F. Pulseless electrical activity (See Chapter 1 V B)

G. Asystole (See Chapter 1 V C)

H. PSVT (See Chapter 1 V D)

I. Wide complex tachycardia (See Chapter 1 V E)

Review Test

1. A 73-year-old man with a history of hypertension and coronary artery disease (CAD) presents to the emergency department with acute onset of excruciating chest pain that radiates to the back. Physical examination reveals absent peripheral pulses and hoarseness. Which of the following is the most appropriate next step in the management of this patient?

(A) Obtain an electrocardiogram (ECG) to look for rhythm disturbances
(B) Decide whether the patient is a candidate for thrombolytic therapy
(C) Order a computed tomography (CT) scan of the thorax, with contrast
(D) Obtain a surgical consult immediately
(E) Observe with cardiac monitoring

2. A 26-year-old man is brought to the emergency department by ambulance after being stabbed in the chest with a dagger during a street fight. His blood pressure (BP) is 83/57 mm Hg. His heart sounds, although muffled, indicate tachycardia. Physical examination reveals distended neck veins and clear and equal breath sounds. While waiting for the results of the chest radiograph, which of the following is the first priority?

(A) Administration of epinephrine for BP support
(B) Administration of morphine to alleviate pain
(C) Preparation for emergent pericardiocentesis
(D) Administration of cardiac massage to slow the heart rate
(E) Administration of propranolol to control the tachycardia

3. A 37-year-old woman with a history of depression and suicidal tendencies is brought to the emergency department because she had two episodes of vomiting while dining in a nearby restaurant. Physical examination reveals a blood pressure (BP) of 220/170 mm Hg. The patient is agitated, acts confused, and pleads with you to let her die. Your attempts to elicit a detailed history or list of current medications are futile. Which of the following is the most appropriate next step in the management of this patient?

(A) Administer haloperidol, 1 mg intramuscularly, for the confusion, then try to contact the patient's psychiatrist.
(B) Administer lorazepam, 0.5 mg intramuscularly, to calm the patient so a detailed history can be obtained.
(C) Administer sodium nitroprusside, 10 g/kg/min intravenously, to control BP.
(D) Put the patient on one-on-one observation and call for a psychiatric consult.
(E) Physically restrain the patient so she cannot harm herself.

4. A 37-year-old man with a medical history significant for Marfan's syndrome, mitral regurgitation, and aortic insufficiency presents to the emergency department with severe chest pain that has been present for the past 4 hours. He describes the pain as sharp and tearing, and states that he feels it radiating between his shoulder blades. Ten days ago, he experienced similar symptoms that subsided after he took some painkillers. Except for this episode, he reports feeling well. Which of the following is the most likely diagnosis?

(A) Perforated gastric ulcer
(B) Aortic dissection
(C) Gastroesophageal reflux
(D) Acute myocardial infarction (MI)
(E) Acute bacterial endocarditis

5. Which of the following are contraindications to β-blocker therapy?

(A) Heart rate of 55 beats per minute
(B) Severe left ventricle (LV) dysfunction
(C) First degree heart block
(D) Severe chronic obstructive pulmonary disease (COPD)
(E) All of the above

6. Nitroglycerin (NTG) therapy is contraindicated for which of the following?

(A) Unstable angina
(B) Anterior wall myocardial infarction (MI)
(C) Inferior wall MI
(D) Right ventricular MI
(E) Lateral wall MI

7. Which of the following is the pharmacologic therapy of choice in a hypertensive emergency?

(A) Sodium nitroprusside
(B) Phentolamine
(C) Magnesium sulfate
(D) Propranolol
(E) Hydralazine

8. A 35-year-old man presents to the emergency department with pleuritic chest pain that began about 7 hours ago. He states that the pain is sharp, radiates to his left shoulder, and is alleviated by leaning forward. He reports having flu-like symptoms for the past week. He is worried that he is having a heart attack because he has a "lousy" family history. Which of the following would make acute myocardial infarction (MI) as a diagnosis in this patient most unlikely?

(A) Absence of Q waves on the electrocardiogram (ECG)
(B) Lack of response to a trial of nitroglycerin (NTG)
(C) The patient's young age
(D) Radiation of the pain to the left shoulder
(E) Positive family history

9. Which of the following drugs are used in the treatment of acute Q wave MI?

(A) Nifedipine
(B) Tirofiban
(C) Heparin
(D) Enoxaparin
(E) Eptifibatide

Directions: The response options for Items 10–13 are the same. You will be required to select one answer for each item in the set.

Questions 10–13

Match each of the physical examination findings with the correct cardiac murmur.

(A) Mitral stenosis
(B) Mitral insufficiency
(C) Aortic stenosis
(D) Aortic insufficiency
(E) Tricuspid stenosis
(F) Tricuspid insufficiency
(G) Pulmonary stenosis

10. Diastolic murmur with a loud opening snap, best heard in the fourth interspace on the left

11. Blowing, diastolic murmur with widened pulse pressure and capillary pulsations

12. Blowing, diamond-shaped, systolic murmur with narrowed pulse pressure

13. Pansystolic murmur best heard at the right sternal border

Answers and Explanations

1–D. This patient most likely has a ruptured thoracic aneurysm, a life-threatening emergency. The treatment of choice is surgical repair, which should not be delayed to obtain further diagnostic studies, such as an electrocardiogram (ECG) [choice A] or a computed tomography (CT) scan (choice C). Even with emergency surgery, operative mortality is 50%. Deciding whether the patient is a candidate for thrombolytic therapy (choice B) would be appropriate for acute myocardial infarction (MI), after initial management has been completed. Although it may appear that this patient is having an MI, the absent peripheral pulses and hoarseness are practically diagnostic for a ruptured aneurysm.

2–C. This patient most likely has cardiac tamponade. His physical examination findings include the classic triad of hypotension, distended neck veins, and muffled heart sounds, which is highly suggestive of the diagnosis. Also, cardiac tamponade is often seen after penetrating trauma to the chest. The treatment of choice is pericardiocentesis. This should be preceded by an IV fluid bolus to increase preload. Administration of morphine (choice B) would make the patient even more hypotensive, while administration of epinephrine (choice A) may worsen the tachycardia.

Cardiac massage (choice D) is *never* indicated in a patient who still has a pulse and BP. Administration of a β blocker (choice E) such as propranolol would decrease the preload and make the patient even more hypotensive.

3–C. This patient may have end-organ damage, as suggested by the confusion and vomiting. Therefore, it is imperative to control her blood pressure (BP) immediately with the administration of sodium nitroprusside. From the history that was obtained, it is possible that this patient is presenting with a hypertensive crisis secondary to coingestion of tyramine and monoamine oxidase inhibitors, in which case the treatment of choice would be phentolamine. However, because there is no way to confirm this diagnosis, administration of phentolamine is not an option. All of the other choices address the patient's psychiatric profile and not the immediate crisis; waiting to talk to the patient's psychiatrist (choice A), obtain a history (choice B), or obtain a psychiatric consult (choice C) could result in the patient's death. After the BP is under control, it would be appropriate to obtain a psychiatric follow-up. Physical restraint (choice E) may become necessary but again, it does not address the primary problem.

4–B. Marfan's syndrome is a risk factor for aortic dissection, which is the most likely diagnosis in this patient. Perforated gastric ulcer (choice A) and gastroesophageal reflux (choice C) do not typically present with intrascapular pain. Although it is possible that the patient is having acute, self-limiting myocardial infarctions (MIs) [choice D], the nature of the symptoms is not severe enough, especially considering this would be his second MI within 2 weeks. In addition, an MI is accompanied by a sense of doom, which this patient does not report. Acute bacterial endocarditis is a severe infection. If the patient had acute bacterial endocarditis (choice E) that had been left untreated for 1 week, he would be septic.

5–E. All of the choices listed are contraindications to β-blocker therapy. Second or third degree heart block is an absolute contraindication, whereas first degree heart block (choice C) is only a relative contraindication. Signs of peripheral hypoperfusion (heart rate of 55 beats per minute, severe left ventricle dysfunction, and severe chronic obstructive pulmonary disease) also are absolute contraindications to β-blocker therapy.

6–D. Nitroglycerin is contraindicated for the treatment of right ventricular (RV) infarcts because the decrease in preload would make less blood available to this area, resulting in potential extension of the infarct. The appropriate treatment for posterior wall or RV infarcts is volume expansion. (See section II C 1 b 2.)

7–A. In the absence of a specific cause for malignant hypertension, a sodium nitroprusside infusion of 0.5–10 μg/kg/min titrated to blood pressure (BP) is the pharmacologic therapy of choice. There are certain emergencies for which other drugs are more appropriate, such as phentolamine (choice B) for hypertensive crisis associated with monoamine oxidase inhibitors and magnesium sulfate and hydralazine (choices C and E) for eclampsia. Propranolol (choice D), a β-blocker with antihypertensive properties, has no role in the treatment of hypertensive emergencies.

8–B. Pain that does not respond to nitroglycerin (NTG) is unlikely to be cardiac in origin, especially in this patient. This patient is experiencing pericarditis, typified by the pleuritic but positional chest pain. Based on the patient's history of flu-like symptoms for 1 week, it is likely that this is a viral pericarditis. Lack of Q waves on the electrocardiogram (ECG) [choice A] in no way rules out myocardial infarction (MI), because non–Q wave MI occurs regularly. The patient's age (choice C), although not within the typical age range for MIs, does not rule out MI, especially in light of his family history. History of drug use, especially cocaine, should be elicited in young patients with chest pain. Radiation of the pain to the left shoulder (choice D) can be seen in acute MI and pericarditis. A positive family history (choice E) is a risk factor for MI.

9–C. Calcium channel blockers such as nifedipine (choice A) are currently contraindicated in the therapy of acute myocardial infarction (AMI) due to their substantial negative inotropic effect, which exacerbates ischemia. GP IIb-IIIa receptor inhibitors such as tirofiban and eptifibatide (choices B and E) and the low-molecular-weight heparin enoxaparin (choice D) are approved only for the treatment of unstable angina and non Q wave myocardial infarction (MI), not for acute Q wave MI. Heparin is used as an adjunct to thrombolysis in the treatment of Q wave MI.

10–A. Mitral stenosis is a diastolic murmur with a loud opening snap, best heard in the fourth interspace on the left.

11–D. Aortic insufficiency is a blowing, diastolic murmur with widened pulse pressure and capillary pulsations.

12–C. Aortic stenosis is a blowing, diamond-shaped, systolic murmur with narrowed pulse pressure.

13–E. Tricuspid stenosis is a pansystolic murmur best heard at the right sternal border.

3

Pulmonary Emergencies

I. Acute Respiratory Failure (ARF)

A. Overview

1. Definition

—is a state in which spontaneous respirations are inadequate for sustenance of life.

—requires supplemental oxygen and mechanical ventilation.

2. Causes include

—altered mental status (see Chapter 6 I).

—sepsis.

—trauma.

B. Clinical presentation

1. Symptoms

a. The patient with impending ARF generally appears to be in distress, and may be confused or obtunded.

b. Perioral or peripheral **cyanosis** and **diaphoresis** often are noted.

2. Physical examination findings may include:

—accessory respiratory muscle use.

—intercostal and subclavicular **retractions.**

—**extremes of respiratory rate** (> 30 breaths/min or < 6 breaths/min).

—**asymmetrical expansion of the chest** secondary to **splinting,** which may result from pneumothorax, rib fractures, large areas of atelectasis or pleural effusions.

—pleuritic chest pain.

C. Diagnostic tests

1. Arterial blood gas (ABG)

—allows determination of the A-a gradient (i.e., alveolar to arterial oxygen gradient) [Table 3-1]. The **normal A-a gradient = 10 mm Hg + (0.3 × patient's age).** The **formal calculation** is done as follows: $[(713)(FiO_2) - PaCO_2/.8] - PaO_2$.

—measures partial pressure of O_2 (PO_2) and partial pressure of CO_2 (PCO_2). Generally ARF is imminent when $PO_2 < 60$ mm Hg or $PCO_2 > 45$ mm Hg.

2. Pulse oximetry

—is a noninvasive way to obtain O_2 saturation.

—may be misleading. Sometimes a good pulse oximetry reading can mask a serious underlying abnormality such as carbon monoxide poisoning. Also, the presence of nail polish may produce a falsely positive result. When in doubt, do an ABG.

3. Complete blood count (CBC)

—may reveal polycythemia or leukocytosis.

a. Polycythemia may suggest a response to chronic hypoxemia.

b. Leukocytosis may suggest an infectious cause for respiratory distress.

4. Chest radiograph

—can generate differential diagnoses by classifying the radiograph as black or white.

a. A "black" or radiolucent film suggests a normal film, pulmonary embolism (PE), asthma, chronic obstructive pulmonary disease (COPD), or pneumothorax.

b. A "white" or radiopaque film suggests bacterial or aspiration pneumonia, pulmonary edema, or pleural effusion.

D. Treatment

—is twofold.

1. Manage the airway acutely with **intubation** and **mechanical ventilation,** with supplemental oxygen as necessary. Indications for intubation and mechanical ventilation include:

a. Patient having difficulty protecting the airway due to altered mental status or recurrent aspiration.

b. Acute respiratory acidosis

2. Treat the underlying cause of ARF.

Table 3-1. Mechanisms of Hypoxemia

Mechanism	A-a Gradient	Result of Supplemental Oxygen
Hypoventilation	No increase	Improved condition
Reduced FIO_2	No increase	Improved condition
$\dot{V}/\dot{Q}$ mismatch	Increase	Improved condition
Shunt	Increase	No improvement
Diffusion abnormality	Increase	No improvement

A-a = alveolar to arterial oxygen gradient; FIO_2 = fraction of inspired oxygen; $\dot{V}/\dot{Q}$ = ventilation-perfusion.

II. Pleural Effusion

A. Overview

1. Definition

—is a collection of fluid in the pleural space.

—The pleural fluid can be an exudate or a transudate (Table 3-2).

2. Causes include

—pneumonia

—pulmonary embolism

—tuberculosis

—rib fracture(s)

—CHF

—cirrhosis

—nephrotic syndrome

—glomerulonephritis

—uremia

—neoplasm(s)

—superior vena cava syndrome

—rheumatologic disease

—drug reaction

Table 3-2. Comparison of Exudates and Transudates

	Exudate	Transudate
Mechanism	Pleural membrane/vasculature damage, ↑ capillary permeability, ↓ lymphatic drainage	Abnormal formation/absorption of PF, ↑ capillary pressure, ↓ oncotic pressure
Etiologies	Infection (*Streptococcus pneumoniae, Staphylococcus aureus, Haemophilus influenzae, Mycoplasma* spp), neoplasm (lung > breast > lymphoma > others), pulmonary infarction, esophageal rupture, inflammation, trauma, pancreatitis	Congestive heart failure (usually bilateral), renal failure (usually bilateral), cirrhosis (usually right-sided)
Protein concentration	Specific gravity > 3 g/dl	Specific gravity < 3 g/dl
Protein	PF:serum ratio > 5	PF:serum ratio < 5
LDH concentration	> 200 IU/ml	< 200 IU/ml
LDH	PF:serum ratio > 6	PF:serum ratio < 6
SG	> 1.016	< 1.016

LDH = lactate dehydrogenase; *PF* = pleural fluid; *SG* = specific gravity.

B. Clinical presentation

1. **Symptoms** may include
   - —pleuritic chest pain
   - —dyspnea
   - —cough
   - —hemoptysis
2. **Physical examination findings** may include
   - —fever
   - —chills
   - —tachypnea
   - —chest wall **splinting**
   - —tracheal deviation to the contralateral side
   - —**dullness to percussion**
   - —**reduced tactile fremitus**
   - —a **friction rub**
   - —**diminished** or **absent breath sounds** over the effusion site

C. Diagnostic tests

1. **Chest x-ray**
   - —PA, lateral, and oblique views can demonstrate the location of the effusion (Figure 3-1), whether it is loculated, a mass suggestive of tumor, or edema suggestive of congestive heart failure (CHF).

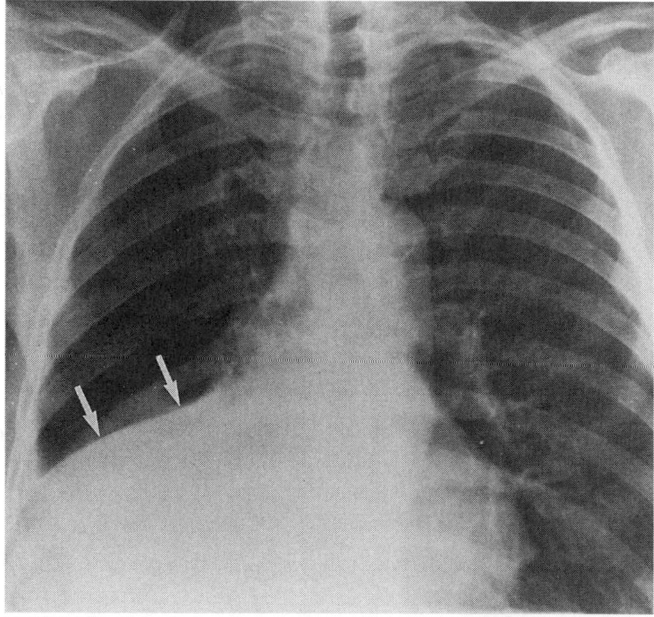

Figure 3-1. Large right pleural effusion. (Reprinted with permission from Daffner RH: *Clinical Radiology: The Essentials,* 2nd ed. Philadelphia, Lippincott Williams & Wilkins, 1999.)

—Blunted costophrenic angles indicate an effusion of at least 150 ml of pleural fluid.

2. **Pulse oximetry**

   —determines O_2 saturation.

3. **CBC** to look for **leukocytosis**

4. **Renal profile and serum lactate dehydrogenase (LDH)**

   —to compare electrolytes in serum to those in the pleural fluid, useful for determining nature of effusion.

D. Treatment

1. Management of airway, breathing, and circulation (**ABCs**) is especially important for large pleural effusions, in which the degree of respiratory and circulatory compromise may be significant.

2. **Thoracocentesis**

   —is therapeutic in large effusions.

   —is used for diagnostic purposes in small effusions.

   —The withdrawn pleural fluid is sent to the lab for cell count, pH, amylase, LDH, protein, and glucose levels.

   —Gram stain and bacterial culture are also requested.

3. **Tube thoracostomy (chest tube)**

   —is indicated when the pleural effusion is suspected to be a hemothorax or an empyema, or when esophageal perforation is present.

   —A 28–34 French tube is inserted into the fourth or fifth intercostal space at the anterior axillary line.

E. Disposition

1. Patients with small transudative effusions of known etiology who are clinically stable can be discharged home after 6 hours of observation in the emergency department (ED). A follow-up visit with the primary care physician should be scheduled for 24 to 48 hours after discharge.

2. Patients with exudative effusions usually are admitted for work-up of the cause.

3. Patients with severe respiratory compromise should be admitted to the intensive care unit (ICU), regardless of the size of the effusion.

III. Pneumothorax

—is the presence of free air in the interpleural space.

A. Overview

1. **Simple pneumothorax**

   a. **Spontaneous pneumothorax**

      —can occur without any apparent underlying cause (primary) or may be due to underlying alteration of lung architecture (secondary).

      —**Risk factors** include Marfan syndrome, mitral valve prolapse, changes in atmospheric pressure (as with aviation, scuba diving, ambient pressure changes), α_1-antitrypsin deficiency, smoking, COPD, tuberculosis (TB), lung cancer, and any process that alters lung parenchyma.

b. **Traumatic pneumothorax**

—can occur as a result of iatrogenic causes such as thoracocentesis, central line insertion, or needle biopsy, or from trauma that occurred outside of the hospital.

2. **Tension pneumothorax**

—occurs when the free air in the interpleural space is under high pressure.

B. Clinical presentation

1. Simple pneumothorax

a. **Symptoms may include**

—sudden onset pleuritic chest pain

—chest wall deformity

b. **Physical examination** findings may include

—**hyperresonance** and **decreased breath sounds on the affected side.**

—crepitus.

—retractions.

—mild tachycardia.

—normal blood pressure.

2. Tension pneumothorax

—If the clinical presentation suggests tension pneumothorax, treatment must be immediate. No diagnostic tests are necessary.

a. **Symptoms** may include

—sudden onset pleuritic chest pain

—agitation

—air hunger

b. **Physical examination** findings may include

—**Heart sounds** and breath sounds are **decreased on the affected side** due to mediastinal shift.

—Severe impairment of venous return results in pronounced tachycardia, decreased cardiac output, hypotension, and imminent shock.

—Extreme presentations demonstrate marked hemodynamic compromise, to the point of cardiac arrest.

C. Diagnostic tests

1. **Chest radiograph** is the way to make the definitive diagnosis for simple pneumothorax.

a. **A radiolucent band devoid of markings** is shown between the chest wall and the lung (Figure 3-2), which is demarcated by sharp edges running roughly parallel to each other.

b. Other findings may include:

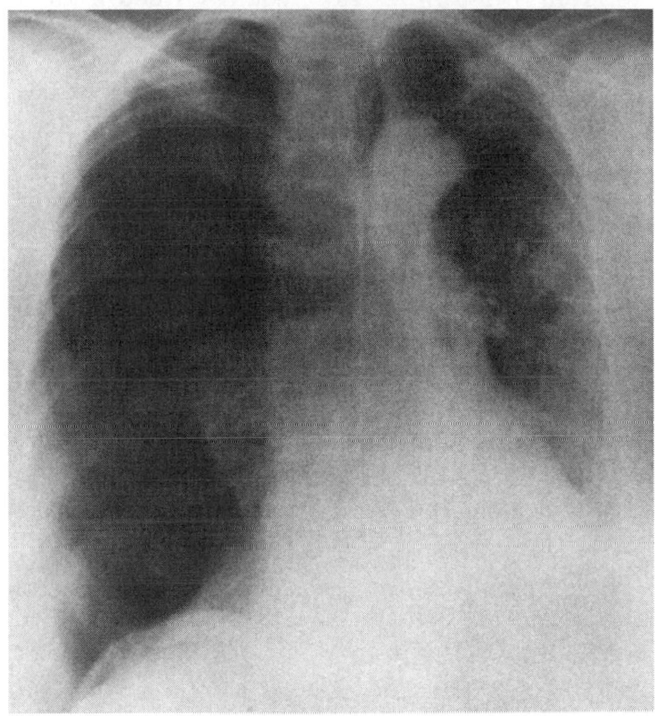

Figure 3-2. Right-sided pneumothorax. Note the lack of vascular markings. (Reprinted with permission from Harris JH, Harris WH, Novelline RA: *The Radiology of Emergency Medicine,* 3rd ed. Baltimore, Williams & Wilkins, 1993.)

—deviation of the trachea away from the affected side.

—rib fractures.

—mediastinal shift with kinked vessels.

—If unable to visualize on a plain film, an end-expiratory or left lateral decubitus film should be helpful.

—The size of the pneumothorax is estimated based on the size of the radiolucent band as a percentage of lung volume. An average interpleural distance of 2.0 cm represents a pneumothorax of approximately 20% to 25%.

2. **Pulse oximetry** to determine O_2 saturation
3. **Electrocardiogram (ECG)** of a left-sided pneumothorax

—can mimic acute myocardial infarction.

—may show right axis deviation (RAD) with Q waves in the anterior leads.

—normalizes if repeated with the patient in the erect position.

D. Treatment

1. Monitor and manage **ABCs.**
2. Administer **100% O_2** to maintain adequate oxygenation and hasten the rate of absorption of air from the pleural space back into the lungs.
3. **Remove air from the pneumothorax.**

a. **Tension pneumothorax** requires **needle decompression followed by tube thoracostomy**.
   —Insert a 14- to 16-gauge needle with plastic cannula into the second intercostal space in the midclavicular line.
   —A hissing sound will be heard as the air escapes.
   —**Tube thoracostomy** (chest tube placement) is performed following needle decompression.

b. **Spontaneous pneumothoraces** in stable patients can resolve on their own, with a 20% pneumothorax taking approximately 2 weeks to resolve. Therefore, a small pneumothorax (15%-20%) that does not show progressive enlargement over several hours on repeat chest x-ray does not require treatment. If treatment is needed, aspiration or tube thoracostomy is performed.

   (1) Aspiration
   —is done with a 16-gauge catheter placed in the second intercostal space at the midclavicular line.
   —The patient's head is elevated to a 30-degree angle.
   —A three-way stopcock is attached once the catheter is advanced. This allows air to be aspirated from one end while it prevents air from leaking back into the pleural space.
   —If more than 3 L of air is aspirated, a persistent air leak must be suspected.
   —**Contraindications** include tension pneumothorax, significant underlying lung disease, cardiopulmonary instability (e.g., imminent shock), hemothorax, pleural effusion, and bilateral pneumothorax.

   (2) Tube thoracostomy
   —A chest tube is inserted at the fourth or fifth intercostal space along the midaxillary line and is attached to a water seal with or without suction.
   —The chest tube is left in place for approximately 24 hours after reexpansion of the lung.
   —**Indications** include tension and traumatic pneumothorax, significant underlying lung disease, respiratory distress, persistent air leak, bilateral pneumothorax, presence of pleural fluid, large volume of air, and previous contralateral pneumothorax.

E. Disposition

1. Patients who are clinically stable with a small pneumothorax can be discharged home after 6 hours of observation if the repeat chest x-ray does not show increasing size.
2. All discharged patients should be instructed to follow up with their primary care physician in 24 hours and then once weekly until the pneumothorax resolves completely, to return to medical attention sooner if dyspnea occurs, and to avoid strenuous activity.
3. Patients with tension or traumatic pneumothorax should be admitted to the ICU with a follow-up chest x-ray.

IV. Pulmonary Embolism (PE)

—may present in a multitude of ways, including sudden cardiac arrest.

—There are no signs, symptoms, laboratory values, or chest x-ray or ECG findings that are diagnostic of, or consistently present with, PE.

—Diagnosis requires a high index of suspicion.

A. **Risk factors** include

—prior history of PE or deep venous thrombosis.

—recent pregnancy or surgery.

—prolonged immobilization.

—malignancy, especially peritoneal.

—hypercoagulable state.

—deficiency of antithrombin III, protein C, or protein S.

—presence of circulating lupus anticoagulant.

—use of oral contraceptives.

—obesity (i.e., > 120% ideal body weight).

—presence of a central line.

—orthopaedic trauma, especially of the long bones and pelvis.

—polycythemia and thrombocytosis.

B. Clinical presentation

1. **Symptoms** of PE include **dyspnea, pleuritic chest pain, anxiety, cough, hemoptysis, sweating,** and **syncope.**
2. **Physical examination** may reveal **tachypnea,** rales, accentuated S_2, tachycardia, fever, **diaphoresis,** S_3 or S_4 gallop, thrombophlebitis, **lower extremity edema,** and cyanosis.

C. **Diagnostic tests** (Figure 3-3)

1. **CBC**

   —Leukocytosis is often present.

   —Platelets may be reduced from their baseline level.

2. **ABG**

   —**A large A-a gradient** (> 20 mm Hg) may be suggestive of PE; however, most pulmonary pathologies cause impaired gas exchange, resulting in an increased A-a gradient.

   —A low PO_2 may be noted (**hypoxemia**); however, this finding also may be seen with asthma and pneumonia.

3. **ECG**

   —is normal in 50% of patients with PE.

   —shows $\mathbf{S_1Q_3T_3}$ (classic finding) in approximately 20% of all patients with PE.

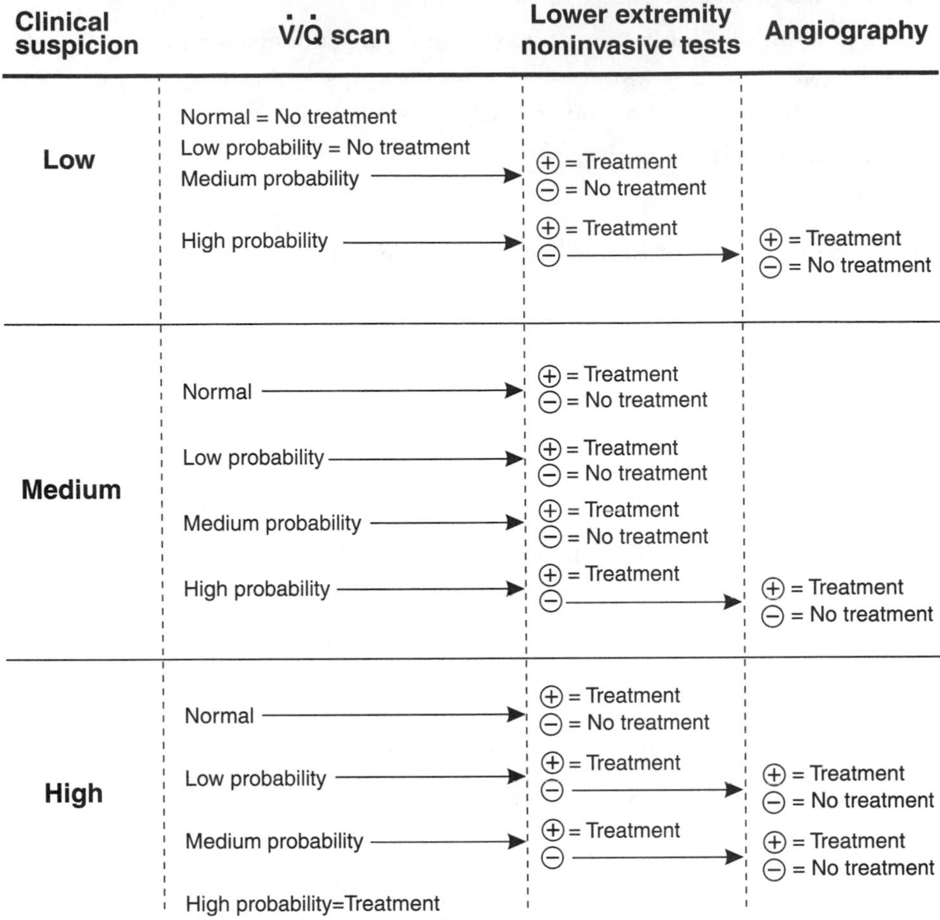

Figure 3-3. Clinical decision tree for pulmonary embolus. *LENI* = lower extremity noninvasive tests; *V̇/Q̇* = ventilation-perfusion.

—Other ECG abnormalities that may be noted include p-pulmonale (tall, peaked P wave in lead II), right axis deviation (RAD), and atrial fibrillation.

—Pulseless electrical activity (one of the causes of PE) may be noted.

4. **Chest x-ray**

—in PE usually is normal.

—may show an elevated hemidiaphragm, focal infiltrates, pleural effusion, and atelectasis.

—**Hampton's hump** (triangular wedge that protrudes off the diaphragm) and **Westermark's sign** (dilation proximal to and collapse distal to an embolus) are relatively specific to PE, but are rarely seen. If present, Westermark's sign is the first radiographic abnormality to be encountered.

5. **Ventilation-perfusion (V̇/Q̇) scan** (nuclear scintigraphic scan)

—is **done in all cases of suspected PE.**

—Eight views of the lung are obtained for each scan: ventilation and perfusion.

—When radioisotope is injected, areas of decreased perfusion or ventilation emit less signal.

—The ventilation and perfusion scans are compared to look for mismatch of signal.

—A perfusion defect that is greater than the ventilation defect is suggestive of PE.

—Normal and low probability (both considered nondiagnostic) require no treatment when clinical suspicion is low.

—If $\dot{V}/\dot{Q}$ scan is medium or high probability, additional testing [lower extremity noninvasive testing (LENIs)] is indicated.

—see Figure 3-3 for treatment algorithm.

6. **Lower extremity noninvasive testing** (LENIs)

   —measures flow patterns in the leg, used to look for deep vein thrombosis.

   —The most common tests are **impedance plethysmography** and **Doppler ultrasound.**

7. **Pulmonary angiography**

   —is the definitive test for PE.

   —The disadvantage is that it is **invasive.**

8. **Helical computed tomography (CT) scan**

   —has excellent sensitivity for PE.

   —is fast and noninvasive.

   —is not available at all institutions.

D. Treatment

—is aimed at addressing the current embolic event, preventing future recurrences, and improving long-term morbidity. Mortality from untreated PE is approximately 80%.

1. Monitor and manage **ABCs,** including supplemental $\mathbf{O_2}$ by face mask or nasal cannula.
2. Administer **morphine sulfate** at a dose of 2–10 mg intravenously (IV) over 30 minutes for pain relief.
3. **Anticoagulation therapy**

   a. Administer **heparin** 80 U/kg IV bolus, then 18 U/kg/h drip.

   —The goal is to achieve therapeutic anticoagulation [approximately 1.5–2.0 × baseline activated partial thromboplastin time (APTT)] within 48 hours.

   —Check the APTT every 6 hours.

   (1) If the APTT is subtherapeutic, increase the drip by 10%.
   (2) If the APTT is supratherapeutic but less than 100 seconds, decrease the drip by 10%.
   (3) If the APTT is greater than 100 seconds, hold the drip for 1 hour, then decrease it by 10%.

b. **Low-molecular-weight (fractionated) heparins** (LMWH)
 —offer an alternative to regular (unfractionated) heparin (Table 3-3).
 —have greater factor Xa–to–antifactor IIa activity.
 —are being used to prevent deep venous thrombosis in the setting of orthopaedic and abdominal surgery (e.g., enoxaparin).
 —are advantageous because of their once-daily subcutaneous (SC) administration and the freedom from measuring serial APTTs.

c. **Warfarin**
 —is started after 2 to 7 days of heparin to keep the international normalized ratio (INR) between 2 and 3.
 —is overlapped with heparin because warfarin takes approximately 48 hours to reach therapeutic levels.

4. **Thrombolytics** (see Chapter 2, Table 2–2, for specific thrombolytic agents and their dosages)
 —are optional in the treatment of pulmonary embolism.
 —are especially beneficial for patients with severe hemodynamic compromise, patients with exhausted cardiopulmonary reserve, or patients in whom multiple recurrences are likely.

5. **Embolectomy**
 —is reserved for massive PE that is refractory to all other medical treatment.

E. Disposition

1. Patients diagnosed with, or with suspicion of, PE are admitted for work-up and initiation of anticoagulation therapy.
2. Patients in whom PE has been ruled out and who are clinically stable may be discharged home with a follow-up appointment with the primary care physician.

Table 3-3. Comparison of Heparins

	Unfractionated Heparins	**Fractionated Heparins**
Molecular weight	15,000 daltons	4500 daltons
Route of administration	IV	SC
Half-life	90 min	24 h
Dosage for PE	80 U/kg bolus, then 18 U/kg/h drip	No bolus; 10–60 mg every day for 10–14 days
Required laboratory tests	APTT (every 6 h until therapeutic effect, then once a week)	Serial APTTs not required

APTT = activated partial thromboplastin time; *IV* = intravenous; *PE* = pulmonary embolus; *SC* = subcutaneous.

V. Pneumonia

—is an infection of the lower respiratory tract that is a leading cause of hospitalization, disability, and death.

A. Bacterial and viral pneumonia

1. Causes (Table 3-4)

2. Clinical presentation

a. Symptoms

—of **bacterial pneumonia** include fever, **shaking chills,** pleuritic chest pain, productive cough, **purulent** or **rust-colored sputum,** dyspnea, and cyanosis.

Table 3-4. Antimicrobial Therapy for Pneumonia

Type of Patient	Causative Organisms	Drug Regimen
CAP No comorbidities Outpatient treatment	*Streptococcus pneumoniae, Mycobacterium pneumoniae, Chlamydia pneumoniae, Haemophilus influenzae, Legionella* spp, *Chlamydia psitacci*	Erythromycin 500 mg PO daily × 7–10 d *or* azithromycin 500 mg PO × 1 then 250 mg PO × 4 d *or* clarithromycin 500 mg PO bid × 7–10 d
CAP + comorbidities Outpatient treatment	Same as above + oral anerobes	Azithromycin 500 mg PO × 1 then 250 mg PO × 4 d *or* clarithromycin 500 mg PO bid × 7–10 d *or* levofloxacin 500 mg PO daily × 7–10 d *or* sparfloxacin 400 mg PO × 1 then 200 mg PO × 7 d *or* grepafloxacin 600 mg PO daily × 7–10 d
CAP Admitted to regular floor	Same as CAP with comorbidities	Azithromycin 500 mg IV q 24 h + ceftriaxone 1–2 g IV q 24 h (can use any 2nd or 3rd generation IV cephalosporin)
CAP Admitted to ICU	All of the above + *Staphylococcus aureus* and *Coxiella burnetti*	Azithromycin 500 mg IV q 24 h + ceftriaxone 1–2 g IV q 24 h + vancomycin 1 g q 12 h
HIV Able to tolerate oral intake $PO_2 > 70$ mm Hg	All of the above + *Pneumocystis carinii* (PCP)	For PCP: Dapsone 100 mg PO daily × 21 d + TMP-SX 2 DS tabs PO q 8 h × 21 d
HIV unable to tolerate oral intake $PO_2 < 70$ mm Hg	All of the above + *Pneumocystis carinii* (PCP)	For PCP: TMP-SX 15 mg of TMP component/kg/d divided into q 6–8 h × 21 d + prednisone 40 mg PO bid × 5 d then 40 mg PO daily × 5 d then 20 mg PO daily × 5 d

CAP = community acquired pneumonia; *d* = days; *PO* = by mouth; *TMP-SX* = trimethoprim-sulfamethoxasole. Comorbidities – age>60, smoker, diabetes, cancer, end-stage renal disease, other comorbid disease.

—of **viral pneumonia** often are preceded by a prodrome of general malaise, headache, and myalgias. Cough usually is prominent and **nonproductive**.

b. **Physical examination**

—of **bacterial pneumonia** reveals **decreased breath sounds,** dullness to percussion, egophony, vocal fremitus, crackles, rhonchi, rales, pleural friction rub, tachycardia, and tachypnea.

—of **viral pneumonia** reveals few if any abnormalities in the lungs.

3. **Diagnostic tests**

a. **CBC**

(1) A high granulocyte count is suggestive of bacterial pneumonia.
(2) A high lymphocyte count is suggestive of viral infection.
(3) An eosinophilia is suggestive of parasitic or allergic etiology.

b. **Chest radiograph**

(1) The presence of an infiltrate is suggestive of pneumonia.
(2) The heart borders and hemidiaphragms can be used to determine the diagnosis.

—In a normal chest x-ray, both heart borders and both hemidiaphragms should be clearly visible.

—An ill-defined right heart border suggests a middle lobe consolidation, whereas a blunted left heart border suggests a left upper lobe consolidation.

—An ill-defined right hemidiaphragm suggests a right lower lobe infiltrate, whereas an obscured left hemidiaphragm suggests a left lower lobe infiltrate.

c. **ABG**

—determines the severity of illness.

d. **Blood cultures**

—are used to look for specific organisms.

e. **Gram's stain**

—of sputum is used to quickly assess the type of organism.

4. **Treatment**

a. Monitor and manage **ABCs,** including supplemental O_2.

b. Determine **antimicrobial therapy** based on the cause of the pneumonia (see Table 3-4).

5. **Disposition**

a. Compliant patients who are not in acute distress and have a community-acquired pneumonia can be treated as outpatients.

b. Hospital admission is favored when

—hypoxemia is present (i.e., $Po_2 < 60$ mm Hg).

—the patient is > 60 years old.

—comorbid disease is present [e.g., CHF, diabetes mellitus, renal insufficiency, malignancy, post-splenectomy, sickle cell anemia, human immunodeficiency virus (HIV), alcoholism, active TB].

—there is risk of aspiration due to recent head trauma, altered mental status, abdominal distention, seizures, or drug overdose.

—there are extrapulmonary complications (e.g., septic arthritis, peritonitis, abscess, meningitis, large pleural effusions).

—the patient was recently hospitalized or recent treatment failed.

—there is predominance of gram-negative bacteria on sputum stain.

—the patient is unable to tolerate oral intake.

—the patient is undomiciled or unable to care for him- or herself.

c. Patients with hypotension, decreased urinary output, or signs of imminent shock or impending respiratory failure should be admitted to the ICU.

B. Aspiration pneumonia

1. Overview

a. Definition

—inflammation of the lung parenchyma secondary to entry of foreign material into the tracheobronchial tree, producing reflex airway constriction, interstitial edema, and alveolar collapse.

—may be seen shortly after aspiration of the foreign material or up to 5 days later, depending on the volume of the aspirate and the status of the patient.

b. Pathogenesis

(1) A $\dot{V}/\dot{Q}$ mismatch is present secondary to shunting.

(2) The inflammatory reaction destroys surfactant-producing alveoli and pulmonary capillaries.

(3) This is followed by intrapulmonary mucosal hemorrhage and degeneration of bronchial epithelium. Inflammation of lung parenchyma also may occur.

c. Risk factors

—altered mental status

—paralyzed vocal cords

—impaired swallowing or coughing

—paralytic ileus

—hiatal hernia

—malfunctioning nasogastric tube

—forced feeding

—upper airway obstruction

—myopathies or neuropathies

—near drowning

d. Complications

—secondary bacterial infection (common)

—lung abscess

—adult respiratory distress syndrome (ARDS)

—death due to Mendelson's syndrome

2. Clinical presentation

a. Symptoms may include

—**dyspnea, drooling,** large amounts of blood-tinged, **frothy sputum,** and **cyanosis.**

b. **Physical examination findings** may include
—**tachypnea**
—tachycardia
—hypotension (variable)
—auscultation may reveal **wheezing,** rales, or rhonchi
—in foreign body aspiration, breath sounds over the object may be decreased or absent.

3. **Diagnostic tests**
   a. **ABG**
   —is used to look for hypoxemia and respiratory acidosis.
   —The A-a gradient will be elevated.
   b. **Chest radiograph**
   —is used to look for foreign objects.
   —may also show lobar collapse, atelectasis, and pulmonary infiltrates.

4. **Treatment**
   a. **Prevention**
   —is the best form of treatment.
   b. **Bronchoscopy** and **pulmonary toilet**
   —provide relief from obstruction.
   —are followed by investigation and elimination of the underlying cause.
   c. **Antibiotics** are used
   —if superimposed bacterial pneumonia is suspected.
   —if the patient is an immunocompromised host.

5. **Disposition**
   a. Patients without respiratory distress in whom the aspirated material has been successfully removed can be discharged home with a follow-up appointment with the primary care physician the following day.
   b. Patients with liquid aspirations and respiratory compromise are admitted to the regular ward or the ICU, depending on the severity of the situation.

VI. Noncardiogenic Pulmonary Edema (NCPE)

A. Overview

1. **Pathogenesis.** NCPE results from
   —elevated pulmonary capillary hydrostatic pressure.
   —damage to vascular endothelium by factors that disrupt pulmonary surfactant and decrease lung compliance.

2. **Causes**
   —drug overdose (e.g., opiates, aspirin)
   —near drowning
   —thermal injury

—inhalation of toxic gases
—trauma
—sepsis
—shock
—high-altitude illness
—PE
—ARDS
—pulmonary lymphatic obstruction
—aspiration of gastric contents
—eclampsia
—disseminated intravascular coagulation
—radiation pneumonitis
—postoperative or postcardioversion period

B. Clinical presentation

1. The main **symptoms** are **dyspnea** and **tachypnea**.
2. The major finding on **physical examination** is the presence of **bilateral rales.**

C. Diagnostic tests

1. **ABG**

   —is used to assess the need for mechanical ventilation.

   —Respiratory alkalosis, hypoxia, and an elevated A-a gradient are noted.

2. **Chest radiograph**

   —shows a normal-sized heart, distinguishing NCPE from cardiogenic pulmonary edema, in which cardiomegaly is usually present.

   —shows patchy alveolar infiltrates.

3. **ECG**

   —is used to rule out rhythm disturbances as a cause for the dyspnea and tachypnea.

D. Treatment

—of the underlying condition is most important.

—It is also necessary to monitor and manage **ABCs,** including supplemental O_2.

—Mechanical ventilation may become necessary.

E. Disposition

1. Most patients with NCPE should be hospitalized.
2. Patients who are intubated and those with impending respiratory failure should be admitted to the ICU.
3. Patients who do not have significant hypoxia can be discharged after 6 hours of observation.

VII. Asthma

—is characterized by hyperactive airways that result in spasm of bronchial smooth muscle, airway edema, and mucus production.

A. Overview

1. Causes

—Many environmental (extrinsic) and personal (intrinsic) factors can trigger an acute attack.

a. **Extrinsic factors** include dust-mite feces, cockroaches, ozone, cigarette smoke, gas fumes, latex, drugs (e.g., β-blockers, nonsteroidal anti-inflammatory drugs), and sulfites (food preservative).

b. **Intrinsic factors** include upper respiratory tract infection, menstrual cycle, and psychological stress.

2. Incidence

a. In childhood, boys are more commonly affected than girls.

b. In puberty, males and females are equally affected.

c. In adults, women are more commonly affected than men.

B. Clinical presentation

1. Symptoms

—The **clinical hallmark** of asthma is **wheezing,** although it may not always be present.

—Other symptoms include cough and shortness of breath.

—In status asthmaticus, the patient is fatigued, dehydrated, and in imminent respiratory failure. This stage is marked by hypoxia and acidosis.

2. Physical examination findings may include

—**pulsus paradoxus** (i.e., a drop of 10 mm Hg or more in BP during inspiration).

—inspiratory and expiratory **wheezing**

—**rales**

—**hyperresonance**

—**decreased breath sounds**

—a prolonged expiratory phase

—a silent chest (i.e., absence of breath sounds) in an ill-appearing patient may denote impending respiratory arrest.

—tachycardia

—**tachypnea**

—**use of accessory muscles** (scalenes and sternocleidomastoids)

—cyanosis also may be noted, but clubbing is rarely seen.

C. Diagnostic tests

1. Peak flowmetry

—is useful for assessing the severity of the attack.

—can be used to guide treatment decisions. Serial measurements allow assessment of ED interventions.

—should be performed in all asthma presentations.

2. **ABG**

—is not routinely useful, unless mechanical ventilation is being contemplated.

3. **Pulse oximetry**

—can be used to monitor mild to moderate hypoxemia.

4. **CBC**

—is used to look for sepsis and pneumonia.

—A high eosinophil count points to other causes of wheezing (e.g., aspergillosis, Löffler's pneumonia).

5. **Chemistry profile**

—is used to check electrolyte imbalances. Note that these also may be caused by corticosteroids, diuretics, and β agonists.

6. **Theophylline level**

—is used to rule out toxicity.

—is important because many asthma patients are chronically on theophylline, a drug with a narrow therapeutic index.

7. **Chest x-ray**

—is not routinely required.

—is obtained if diagnosis of asthma exacerbation is uncertain (i.e., possibility of pneumothorax, foreign body, pneumonia) or if this is the first presentation of the patient that is consistent with asthma.

—may show increased anteroposterior (AP) diameter, flattening of the diaphragms, and scattered atelectasis from mucus plugs.

8. **ECG**

—shows right axis deviation (RAD), clockwise rotation, and right bundle-branch block in severe asthma.

—Abnormal P waves and nonspecific ST changes also may be seen.

D. Treatment

1. Monitor and manage **ABCs,** including supplemental humidified O_2 by face mask or nasal cannula.

2. **Pharmacologic therapy**

—is aimed at binding airway receptors to prevent the cascade of airway hyperreactivity that results in release of debris by various cells, airway edema, and smooth muscle contraction.

a. **Epinephrine** (Table 3-5)

—often is given in the field and works via vasoconstriction, preventing airway edema.

b. **β_2 Agonists** (see Table 3-5)

Table 3-5. Medications Used in Asthma

Drug	Dosage	Mechanism of Action	Route of Administration	Side Effects
Epinephrine	Adults 3 mg SC Children: 0.01 mg/kg SC	Vasoconstriction Bronchodilation	SC, IV	Tachycardia
β_2 agonists	2.5 mg via nebulizer every 20 min to effect	Direct bronchial smooth muscle dilator	MDI, nebulizer, dry inhaler	Tachycardia, nausea, hypokalemia
Cortico-steroids	Prednisone: 60 mg PO Methylprednisolone: 60–125 mg IV Hydrocortisone: 200–500 mg IV	Reduced sensitivity of airways to triggers	PO, IV, MDI	Oral candidiasis
Anticholin-ergics	500 μg every 15 min up to 3 times	Binding to cholinergic receptors in airways	MDI, nebulizer	Dry mouth
Magnesium sulfate	2 g IV over 20 min	Poorly understood	IV	Toxicity: lethargy, loss of deep tendon reflexes, respiratory paralysis, cardiac arrest
Leukotriene inhibitors	Zafirlukast: 20 mg PO bid Zileuton: 600 mg PO qid	↓ smooth muscle spasm ↓ mucus production ↑ mucociliary transport ↓ vascular permeability	PO	Tachycardia, nausea
Methyl-xanthines	Theophylline Acute therapy: loading dose = 5 mg/kg; maintenance dose = 2 mg/kg q 8–12 h Chronic therapy: 50–300 mg PO bid	Poorly understood	IV, PO	Toxicity: seizures, tachycardia, hyperven-tilation, agitation, electrolyte imbalances
Heliox	2–10 L/min by face mask	↓ peak airway pressures Improved oxygenation	Face mask Nebulizer	None

IV = intravenous; *MDI* = metered dose inhaler; *PO* = by mouth; *SC* = subcutaneous.

—such as albuterol and terbutaline are the first-line drugs in the treatment of acute asthma.

—do not prevent airway inflammation, but do provide immediate relief of the symptoms via bronchodilation.

—Inhaled β_2 agonists are the preferred route for acute attacks.

c. **Anticholinergics** (see Table 3-5)

—such as ipratropium bromide are used in the treatment of moderate to severe asthma.

—act by inhibiting the airway anticholinergic receptors.

—can be coadministered with inhaled β_2 agonists in the same nebulizer.

d. **Corticosteroids** (see Table 3-5)

—are the mainstay in control of the inflammatory aspect of asthma.

—also are helpful in the acute asthma attack because they reduce sensitivity of airways to environmental triggers, allowing other medications (e.g., β_2 agonists) to function better.

e. **Magnesium sulfate** (see Table 3-5)

f. **Leukotriene inhibitors** (see Table 3-5)

—target each of the leukotriene receptors in the airway.

—Leukotrienes cause smooth muscle spasm, increased mucus production, decreased mucociliary transport, and increased vascular permeability.

—Zafirlukast and zileuton are nonspecific inhibitors that block leukotriene receptors LTC_4, LTD_4, and LTE_4.

—Montelukast specifically inhibits the receptor LTD_4.

g. **Methylxanthines**

—such as theophylline relax bronchioles via a poorly understood mechanism.

—currently are in disfavor and are not used, except in cases of severe refractory asthma or in cases in which the patient takes this medication on a chronic basis.

h. **IV hydration**

—is used to replace insensible losses.

i. **Heliox**

—is a mixture of helium and oxygen gases used via face mask or nebulizer for patients with severe asthma.

j. **Mucolytics** and **sedatives**

—are contraindicated in the treatment of asthma.

E. Disposition

1. Patients with fever, peak flowmetry values less than 40% of baseline, significant comorbidities, and failure to improve after ED treatment should be admitted to the floor.
2. Intubated patients and those with impending respiratory failure should be admitted to the ICU.
3. Most other patients can be safely discharged home with a short (3–5 days) course of oral corticosteroids. Patients who are chronically dependent on steroids should go home with a longer (10–14 days) course that is tapered down.

4. All discharged patients should follow up with the primary care physician within 2 or 3 days.
5. Counseling regarding removal of the sources of the patient's asthma exacerbations also should be provided.

VIII. Hemoptysis

A. Overview

1. Definition

—is the coughing up of blood that originates in the lower respiratory tract.

—can be defined as minor (< 250 ml/24 hr) or massive (> 250 ml/24 hr).

—Death from hemoptysis results from asphyxiation secondary to impaired gas exchange rather than blood loss.

2. Causes

a. **Life-threatening** causes include

—**fungus balls** (mycetomas).

—significant **hypoxemia.**

—significant **blood loss.**

(1) Massive hemoptysis usually results from hemorrhage from the bronchial arteries.

(2) Minor hemoptysis usually results from hemorrhage from the bronchial capillaries.

b. **Other causes include**

—bronchiectasis (most common).

—TB.

—neoplasm.

—bronchitis.

—infection (fungal, parasitic, bacterial, viral).

—pulmonary abscess.

—trauma.

—cardiogenic (CHF, mitral stenosis).

—renal (Wegener's granulomatosis, Goodpasture's syndrome).

—pulmonary arteriovenous malformation.

B. Clinical presentation

1. **Symptoms** depend on the cause of hemoptysis.
   a. Patients with TB usually report a history of **night sweats, fever,** and **weight loss.**
   b. Patients with bronchogenic carcinoma may report anorexia in addition to weight loss.
   c. Patients with pneumonia may report fever and a productive yellow or green sputum.
2. **Physical examination** also may reveal etiologic clues.
   a. **Tachypnea** suggests blood in the pulmonary cavity or underlying lung disease.

b. **Peripheral cyanosis** points to hemoglobin desaturation.
c. **Inspiratory crackles** are indicative of alveolar blood.
d. **Clubbing** is seen with bronchiectasis and bronchogenic carcinoma.
e. **Blood pressure** generally is normal, unless the degree of hemoptysis is so great as to cause hypotension.

C. Diagnostic tests

—are important to determine the origin of the bleeding.

—Hemoptysis actually may be blood from the upper airway (ear, nose, throat, pharynx, or larynx) or from the gastrointestinal tract.

1. **Chest x-ray**

   —is critical because it may reveal mycetomas, lung masses, and extravascular blood in the pulmonary cavity.

2. **Prothrombin time (PT)** and **APTT** are used to identify coagulopathies.
3. **CBC** is done to look for leukocytosis and thrombocytopenia.
4. **ABG** is done to determine the need for mechanical ventilation.
5. **Type and crossmatch of packed red blood cells**

   —is done in cases of massive blood loss in which transfusion may become necessary.

6. **Purified protein derivative (PPD) test**, anergy panel, sputum and stool for acid-fast bacilli are done to look for TB.
7. **Blood and urine cultures** (including fungal) are done to look for a causative organism if infection is present.
8. **Echocardiogram**

   —is obtained if mitral stenosis or CHF is suspected.

9. $\dot{V}/\dot{Q}$ scan, pulmonary angiography, helical CT, and lower-extremity Doppler ultrasound are options if PE is suspected.
10. Bronchoscopy and CT

    —are options if pulmonary neoplasm is suspected.

D. Treatment

1. Monitor and manage **ABCs**.

   —Supplemental O_2 is helpful in tachypneic patients.

2. Position the **bleeding lung downward** to prevent blood from seeping into the contralateral lung.
3. Use a **cough suppressant** to prevent dislodging of hemostatic clots.

   —Opiates are particularly helpful because they decrease tachypnea and relieve anxiety.

4. **Intubation** should be done if unable to clear blood from the airway.

   —It is best done with a large-diameter endotracheal tube.

   —It is preferably done in the side contralateral to the bleeding to maximize ventilation.

E. Disposition

1. Patients with massive hemoptysis, unstable vital signs, and risk of respiratory failure should be admitted to the ICU.
2. Patients with massive hemoptysis, stable vital signs, and no impending risk of respiratory failure may be admitted to a regular ward.
3. Patients with minor hemoptysis, stable vital signs and hematocrit, and no further hemoptysis after a few hours of observation in the ED can be discharged home with a follow-up appointment with the primary care physician.
4. Patients with persistent symptoms and a negative chest radiograph should be referred to an otolaryngologist for direct laryngoscopic evaluation.

IX. Tuberculosis (TB)

A. Overview

1. **Definition**
   - a. **TB** is a highly contagious infection by *Mycobacterium tuberculosis* that is spread by inhalation of infected aerosol particles. Exposure, however, does not equal disease.
   - b. **Miliary TB** is the hematogenous form of TB.
2. **Incidence**
   - a. The lifetime risk of developing TB is only 10% in an otherwise healthy host, despite much higher exposure rates.
   - b. *M. tuberculosis* is an organism that prefers ventilated, well-perfused areas; therefore, the most common sites of infection are the
     - —apical and posterior segments of the upper lobe of the lung.
     - —superior segment of the lower lobe of the lung.
     - —renal cortex.
     - —meninges.
     - —epiphyses of long bones.
     - —vertebrae.
3. **Risk factors** include
   - —urban, homeless, socioeconomically disadvantaged, and institutionalized populations.
   - —immunosuppressed individuals due to systemic illnesses [e.g., acquired immune deficiency syndrome (AIDS), diabetes, cancer, or chronic steroid use].
   - —malnourished individuals.
   - —individuals who have close contact with infected individuals.
   - —individuals who engage in intravenous drug abuse.

B. Clinical presentation

1. **Symptoms** include cough, **night sweats, hemoptysis,** fever, and weight loss.

2. **Physical examination** findings may include cervical and axillary lymphadenopathy, pleuritic chest pain, tachypnea, inspiratory crackles, hepatosplenomegaly, and clubbing.

C. **Diagnostic tests**

1. **Blood** and **fungal cultures**

—are taken to isolate the involved organism.

2. **Acid-fast bacilli stains**

—of sputum, blood, urine, and stool are used to look for *M. tuberculosis.*

—Note: other *Mycobacteria* spp, *Nocardia* spp, and other bacteria also can cause a positive acid-fast bacilli stain, so specific identification must be done.

3. **Chest radiograph** may show

—**cavitary lesions** in the upper lobes.

—mediastinal lymphadenopathy and upper lobe pleural effusion or atelectasis.

—**caseating granulomas** (old classic TB lesion), which may represent prior infection or advanced present infection.

4. **Mantoux test**

a. PPD (0.1 ml) is placed intradermally on the forearm and read 48 hours later.

b. A positive test is defined as

—≥5 mm palpable induration in HIV patients, IV drug abusers whose HIV status is unknown, close contacts of either of these groups, and patients with an abnormal chest x-ray suggestive of primary TB infection.

—≥ 10 mm palpable induration in IV drug abusers (HIV negative), institutionalized or urban populations, children under the age of 4, persons born in countries with a high incidence of TB, and persons with comorbid disease.

—≥15 mm palpable induration for all others.

c. In persons unable to mount delayed-type hypersensitivity, the Mantoux test will be falsely negative. These persons should get an anergy panel.

5. **Anergy panel**

—is done to demonstrate that the patient is anergic versus truly TB-free.

—0.1 ml of three antigens, Candida, mumps, and tetanus, are injected intradermally.

—A palpable induration of 3 mm or more at 48 hours is considered a positive test, which means the person is not anergic.

—If a person is anergic, investigation into etiology must be sought.

—**Causes** of anergy include HIV, immunosuppression, recent measles-mumps-rubella (MMR) vaccination, physiologic or psychological stress, viral infections, cancer, and sarcoidosis.

D. **Treatment**

1. Monitor and manage **ABCs,** including supplemental O_2.

Table 3-6. First-Line Bactericidal Drugs for the Treatment of Tuberculosis

Drug	Dose	Adverse Effects
Isoniazid	10 mg/kg PO/IM daily; maximum dose of 300 mg/day	Increased LFTs, hepatitis with long-term use, peripheral neuropathy
Rifampin	10–20 mg/kg PO/IV daily; maximum dose of 600 mg/day	Decreased levels of many drugs via induction of cytochrome P-450, orange discoloration of secretions, GI upset, cholestasis, thrombocytopenia, increased LFTs, hepatitis with long-term use
Pyrazinamide	15–30 mg/kg PO daily; maximum dose of 2 g/day	Hyperuricemia, arthralgias, increased LFTs
Ethambutol	15–25 mg/kg PO daily	Optic (retrobulbar) neuritis
Streptomycin	15–35 mg/kg PO daily	Ototoxicity, nephrotoxicity, hypokalemia

GI = gastrointestinal; *IM* = intramuscular; *IV* = intravenous; *LFTs* = liver function tests; *PO* = by mouth.

2. **Respiratory isolation** until the acid-fast bacilli test comes out negative three times.
3. **Pharmacologic therapy** (Table 3-6)
   a. **Prophylaxis** for household contacts and PPD converters without active disease involves **6 months of isoniazid.**
      —Alcohol diminishes the effect of isoniazid and should be avoided during the treatment period. Alcohol also increases the hepatotoxicity of isoniazid, so liver function tests should be monitored.
      —Isoniazid causes depletion of vitamin B_6, resulting in peripheral neuropathy.
      —Pyridoxine should be coadministered with isoniazid to prevent depletion of vitamin B_6.
   b. Treatment of **active TB** involves **6 months of isoniazid and rifampin**.
      —Addition of pyrazinamide is recommended for the first 2 months.
      —Note that combination capsules (isoniazid + rifampin and isoniazid + rifampin + pyrazinamide) are available and may promote patient compliance.
   c. Treatment of **multidrug-resistant TB** involves a minimum of a **four-drug regimen.**
      —The fourth drug can be ethambutol, streptomycin (ototoxic), or ofloxacin.

E. Disposition

1. Most patients with TB can be managed as outpatients as long as there are no issues of noncompliance.
2. Admission is appropriate for

—patients with acute presentations (room air hypoxia, massive hemoptysis).

—noncompliant patients.

—patients in whom the diagnosis is uncertain.

—patients who have multidrug-resistant TB.

—patients who are homeless or unable to care for themselves.

Review Test

1. A 42-year-old Wall Street executive has sudden onset of shortness of breath, weakness, and diaphoresis. He is afebrile. Physical examination reveals bibasilar rales. His electrocardiogram (ECG) is shown below. Which one of the following is the most likely diagnosis?

(A) Myocardial infarction
(B) Pulmonary embolism
(C) Spontaneous pneumothorax
(D) Acute pericarditis
(E) Ruptured aortic aneurysm

2. Which of the following patients with pulmonary embolism (PE) would benefit from embolectomy?

(A) Patient with exhausted cardiopulmonary reserve
(B) Patient with severe hemodynamic compromise
(C) Patient who is prone to multiple recurrences of pulmonary embolism
(D) Patient with a massive PE that is refractory to all medical treatment
(E) All of the above patients

3. A 64-year-old man presents with dyspnea, tachycardia, and a small amount of frothy, pinkish sputum. He is afebrile. His chest radiograph demonstrates a small pleural effusion. On tapping, the pleural fluid is found to be clear, with a specific gravity of 1.002, a lactate dehydrogenase (LDH) of 123 U/L, and a protein concentration of 2 g/dl. This patient's presentation is most consistent with which of the following conditions?

(A) Bacterial pneumonia
(B) Occult malignancy
(C) Acute pancreatitis
(D) Congestive heart failure (CHF)
(E) Tuberculosis (TB)

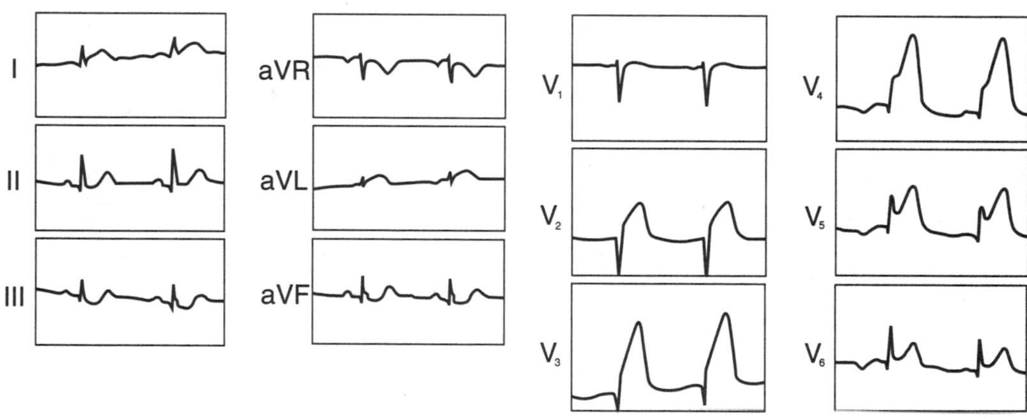

4. A 23-year-old man presents in distress with dyspnea and chest pain after a gang fight. The patient states that he was beaten and stabbed on the right side. Vital signs are as follows: blood pressure, 90/60 mm Hg; temperature, 37.7°C (100°F); respirations, 28/min; pulse, 126/min. Physical examination reveals intercostal retractions and decreased breath sounds on the right. Chest x-ray demonstrates fracture of ribs 5, 6, and 7; mediastinal shift to the left; and a pneumothorax of approximately 30%. Which of the following is the most appropriate next step in the management of this patient?

(A) Observation for 6 hours in the emergency department, then discharge home
(B) Admission to a regular ward
(C) Tube thoracostomy in the emergency department
(D) Intravenous (IV) antibiotics
(E) Hyperbaric oxygen therapy

5. Which of the following patients is at greatest risk for developing pulmonary embolism (PE)?

(A) A 22-year-old Olympic athlete with asthma
(B) A 30-year-old automobile accident victim with a broken femur
(C) A 47-year-old policeman who uses intranasal cocaine
(D) A 60-year-old dance teacher with hyperthyroidism
(E) A 33-year-old homemaker with diabetes mellitus

6. Which of the following are first-line drugs in the treatment of acute asthma?

(A) β-agonist nebulizer
(B) leukotriene inhibitor
(C) theophylline
(D) cromolyn sodium
(E) β-blocker

7. Which of the following is a non-life-threatening cause of hemoptysis?

(A) hemoptysis associated with mycetomas
(B) hemoptysis associated with severe hypoxemia
(C) hemoptysis associated with renal disease
(D) hemoptysis of 350 ml over the past 18 hours
(E) all of the above

8. Which of the following represents a positive Mantoux (PPD) test for tuberculosis (TB)?

(A) A 5-mm induration in a 27-year-old unemployed shelter resident who is human immunodeficiency virus (HIV)-positive
(B) A 9-mm induration in a 33-year-old housewife with asthma who is otherwise healthy
(C) An 8-mm induration in an 87-year-old nursing-home resident with end-stage renal disease
(D) A 6-mm induration in a 40-year-old HIV-negative male prisoner
(E) A 10-mm induration in a 22-year-old college student with no past medical history.

9. Which of the following patients is at greatest risk for aspiration pneumonia?

(A) A 42-year-old alcoholic man with a heroin overdose
(B) A 34-year-old woman with severe asthma
(C) A 72-year-old male stroke victim with an intact gag reflex
(D) A 50-year-old man with well-controlled non-insulin-dependent diabetes mellitus
(E) A 21-year-old female athlete with influenza type A.

10. Which of the following are suggestive of bacterial pneumonia?

(A) production of nonviscous white sputum
(B) bradycardia and bradypnea
(C) leukocytosis and elevated granulocyte count
(D) diffuse "whiteout" pattern on chest radiograph
(E) hemoptysis and night sweats

Answers and Explanations

1–B. The electrocardiogram (ECG) shows the classic $S_1Q_3T_3$ pattern of pulmonary embolism (PE). Remember, however, that only 10% to 20% of patients with PE will show this ECG pattern. Most patients will have either a nonspecific ST change or a normal ECG. None of the other choices (myocardial infarction, spontaneous pneumothorax, acute pericarditis, and ruptured aortic aneurysm) would present with a $S_1Q_3T_3$ pattern.

2–D. Embolectomy is reserved for massive PE that is refractory to all other medical treatment. The other choices describe patients who are at high risk, but medical therapy (versus surgical embolectomy) is still first line.

3–D. The characteristics of the pleural fluid are suggestive of a transudate. Transudates are due to defects in formation or absorption (or both) of pleural fluid. They occur in heart, liver, and kidney failure. Exudates result from damage to the pleural membrane or vasculature, or both. They are seen with infection, inflammation, and neoplasia. Bacterial pneumonia (choice A), occult malignancy (choice B), acute pancreatitis (choice C), and tuberculosis (TB) (choice E) all represent processes associated with exudates. Only congestive heart failure (CHF) is associated with a transudate. Furthermore, the patient's symptoms of dyspnea with frothy, pinkish sputum are suggestive of cardiogenic pulmonary edema.

4–C. This patient has a traumatic pneumothorax, for which the treatment is tube thoracostomy, or the insertion of a chest tube. This is done in the emergency department (ED). Observation (choice A) is appropriate only for small (< 20%) pneumothoraces in an asymptomatic patient. Admission to a regular ward (choice B) is inappropriate because this patient has a traumatic pneumothorax with rib fractures and is hypotensive. He should be admitted to the intensive care unit (ICU). Intravenous (IV) antibiotics (choice D) do not address the patient's pneumothorax, although he may need them later if he develops an infection from the wound. Hyperbaric oxygen (choice E) would only further exacerbate an existing pneumothorax.

5–B. Fractures of the long bones (especially the femur) and the pelvis are a known risk factor for pulmonary embolism (PE). Any state that predisposes to the formation of thrombi is a risk for development of PE. Neither asthma (choice A) nor hyperthyroidism (choice D), nor diabetes (choice E) is a hypercoagulable state. Although drug abuse is a risk factor for PE, the drug must be taken intravenously (IV) rather than inhaled (choice C).

6–A. Leukotriene inhibitors (choice B) and cromolyn sodium (choice D) have no role in the treatment of acute asthma. Leukotriene inhibitors are used for maintenance therapy in moderate to severe asthmatics. Cromolyn sodium is used for maintenance therapy for exercise-induced asthma. Similarly, theophylline is also a maintenance drug. β-blockers would only exacerbate an acute asthma attack and are therefore contraindicated.

7–C. Hemoptysis associated with renal disease is seen in Wegener's granulomatosis and Goodpasture's disease. This association by itself is not life-threatening, unless the hemoptysis is associated with severe hypoxemia (choice B) or is massive in quantity (choice D), both of which are unusual in these diseases. Hemoptysis associated with pulmonary fungus balls known as mycetomas (choice A) is a well-known cause of life-threatening hemoptysis.

8–A. Although choice A represents the smallest induration among the choices, it is seen in a high-risk patient. The average risk of developing tuberculosis (TB) is approximately 10% per year in the human immunodeficiency virus (HIV) patient versus 10% per lifetime in the patient with no risk factors. Asthma (choice B), end-stage renal disease (choice C), and institutionalization (choice D) also are risk factors, but lesser than HIV, so a 10-mm induration would be required in those patients to make a diagnosis of TB.

9–A. Altered mental status, as seen in alcoholism and drug overdose, is a risk factor for aspiration. Stroke (choice C) also can be a risk factor, but only if it leads to the patient being force-fed or if the patient is unable to protect the airway. Asthma (choice B) and diabetes (choice D) and influenza A (choice E) on their own are not risk factors for aspiration.

10–C. Sputum with bacterial pneumonia usually is green and purulent, not white (choice A). Bacterial pneumonia is associated with increased cardiac and respiratory rates, not decreased rates (choice B).The radiographic pattern in bacterial pneumonia is that of a localized patchy infiltrate. A diffuse whiteout pattern (choice D) may be seen with hemothorax and ARDS. Hemoptysis and night sweats (choice E) are characteristic of tuberculosis (TB).

4

Gastrointestinal Emergencies

I. Overview

—Most gastrointestinal (GI) emergencies present with some **abdominal pain.**

—Abdominal pain can be approached by location. It may be localized to one or two quadrants or may be diffuse (Figure 4-1).

II. Peptic Ulcer Disease (PUD)

—Peptic ulcer disease is manifested by two types of peptic ulcers: gastric and duodenal (Table 4-1).

—Peptic ulcer disease may be complicated by perforation, obstruction, and hemorrhage.

A. PUD without perforation

1. **Symptoms** may include:

—burning midepigastric pain that begins either immediately after eating (gastric) or 1–3 hours after eating (duodenal)

—bloating

—abdominal distention

—eructation

—vomiting (gastric)

2. **Diagnostic tests**

—Diagnosis is made by endoscopy, usually on an outpatient basis.

3. **Treatment**

—Treatment is aimed at the multifactorial etiology of PUD.

a. **H_2 blockers** to decrease gastric acid production by blocking actions of histamine on parietal cell H_2 receptors (Table 4-2)

b. Proton pump inhibitors such as **omeprazole** or **lansoprazole** to block hydrogen ion production by parietal cell

c. **Sucralfate** to coat mucosal lining of stomach

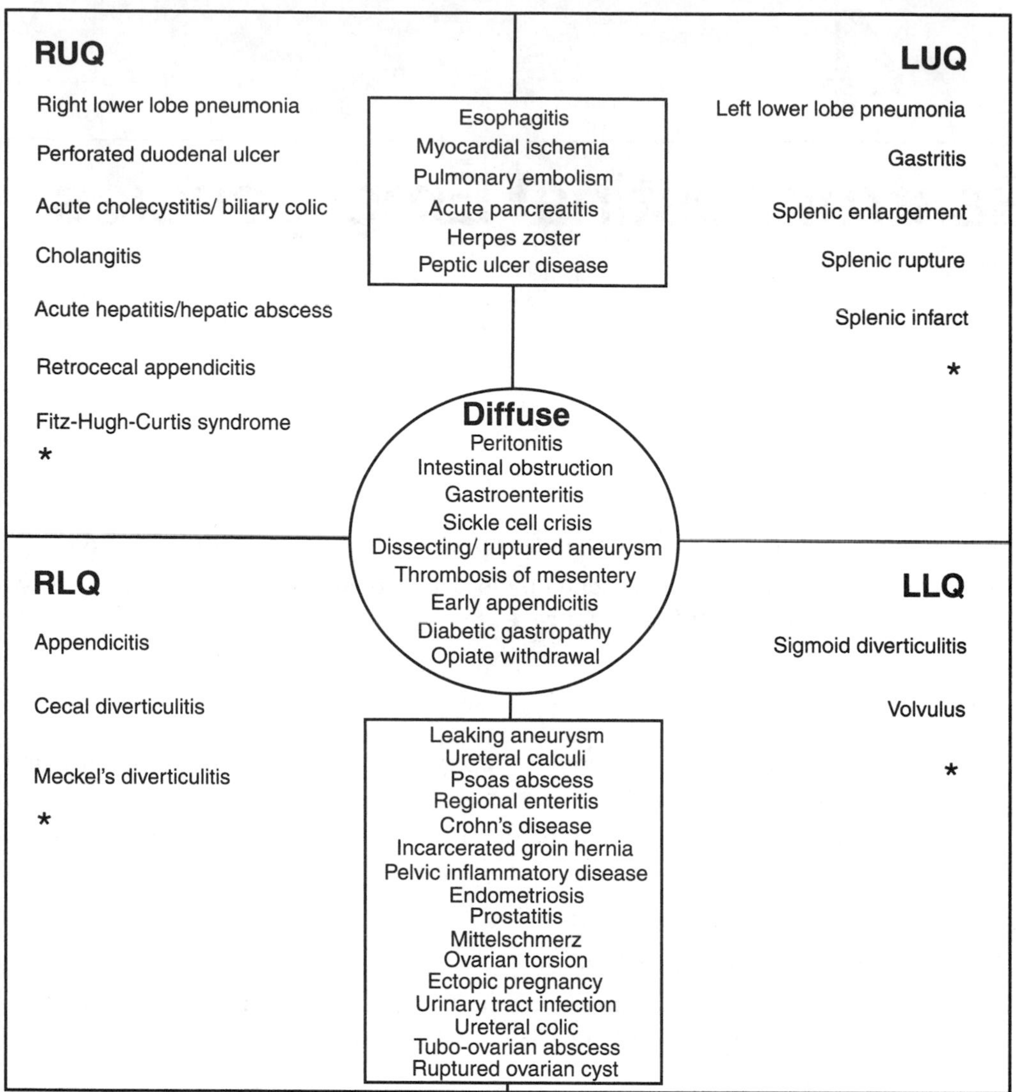

Figure 4-1. Localization of abdominal pain. *LLQ* = left lower quadrant; *LUQ* = left upper quadrant; *RLQ* = right lower quadrant; *RUQ* = right upper quadrant.

d. Eradication of *Helicobacter pylori* (Table 4-3)

e. **Misoprostol,** a prostaglandin analog thought to increase mucus and bicarbonate production, for patients who require concurrent NSAID therapy

f. Elimination of aggravating factors such as NSAIDs, nicotine, and certain foods

4. **Disposition**

—Patients with uncomplicated PUD can be discharged home with outpatient follow-up.

Table 4-1. Comparison of Gastric and Duodenal Ulcers

	Gastric	Duodenal
Occurrence	Less common	More common
Age at onset (y)	40–60	20–45
Response to food	Pain aggravated	Pain relieved
Location	Lesser curvature	Duodenal bulb
Associated with malignancy?	Yes	No

B. Perforated duodenal ulcer

1. Clinical presentation

a. Symptoms may include:

—**sudden onset of severe pain** in the midepigastrium and right upper quadrant (RUQ) pain with radiation to the right shoulder or back

—nausea

—vomiting, with or without hematemesis

—fever

b. Physical examination findings may include:

—a patient in acute distress lying immobile, perhaps in a fetal position to decrease pain

—tachypnea

—diffuse abdominal tenderness

—peritoneal/acute abdomen signs: **rigidity, guarding,** and **rebound**

—absent bowel sounds

—guaiac-positive stool

2. Diagnostic tests

a. Laboratory tests

(1) CBC to look for bleeding (dropping hematocrit)

(2) Chemistry panel to look for electrolyte disturbances secondary to vomiting

(3) Liver function tests (LFTs) and amylase—these are expected to be normal

b. Imaging studies

(1) Chest radiograph and **abdominal radiograph** (supine, upright, and right decubitus) to look for free air under the diaphragm, a sign that perforation has occurred

(2) Gastrograffin study if radiographs are negative, to look for ulcers and possible re-sealing

3. Treatment

a. Nothing by mouth

b. Intravenous fluids for hydration

c. Nasogastric suction if vomiting or abdominal distention is present

Table 4-2. H_2 Blockers

H_2 Blocker	Adult PO Dose	Adult IV Dose	Child Dose
Cimetidine	400 mg bid	300 mg q 6–8 h	5–7 mg/kg qid
Famotidine	20 mg qid or 40 mg qhs	20 mg q 12 h	1–2 mg/kg/day (maximum = 40 mg)
Nizatidine	150 mg bid	none	none
Ranitidine	150 mg qd or bid	50 mg q 6–8 h	1.5–2.0 mg/kg bid

bid = twice a day; *IV* = intravenous; *PO* = by mouth; *q* = every; *qd* = every day; *qhs* = at bedtime; *qid* = four times a day.

Table 4-3. Regimens for the Treatment of *Helicobacter pylori*

Regimen	Dosage	Estimated Rate of Eradication
Lansoprazole, and clarithromycin, and amoxicillin (PrevPac)	30 mg PO bid × 14 days 500 mg PO bid × 14 days 1 g PO bid × 14 days equals 1 PrevPac dose PO bid × 2 weeks	86%
Omeprazole, and clarithromycin, and amoxicillin	20 mg PO bid × 14 days 500 mg PO bid × 14 days 1 g PO bid × 14 days	80%–86%
Lansoprazole, *or* omeprazole, and clarithromycin, and metronidazole	30 mg PO bid × 14 days *or* 20 mg PO bid × 14 days 500 mg PO bid × 14 days 500 mg PO bid × 14 days	≥ 80%
Lansoprazole, *or* omeprazole, and BSS, and metronidazole and tetracycline	30 mg PO qd × 14 days *or* 20 mg PO qd × 14 days 525 mg PO qid × 14 days 500 mg PO tid × 14 days 500 mg PO qid × 14 days	83%–95%
Famotidine, *or* ranitidine, *or* nizatidine, and BSS, and metronidazole, and tetracycline**	40 mg/d PO qd or bid × 28 days *or* 300 mg/d PO qd or bid × 28 days *or* 300 mg/d PO qd or bid × 28 days 525 mg PO qid × initial 14 days 250 mg PO qid × initial 14 days 500 mg PO qid × initial 14 days	≥ 80%
RBS, and clarithromycin, and amoxicillin, *or* metronidazole, *or* tetracycline	400 mg PO bid × 14 days 500 mg PO bid × 14 days 1 g PO bid × 14 days *or* 500 mg PO bid × 14 days *or* 500 mg PO bid × 14 days	≥ 80%

(From American College of Gastroenterology: American College of Gastroenterology guidelines. *Am J Gastroenterol* 93:2330, 1998.)
BSS = bismuth subsalicylate (Pepto-Bismol); *bid* = twice a day; *PO* = by mouth; *qd* = every day ; *qid* = four times a day; *RBS* = ranitidine bismuth citrate (Tritec); *tid* = three times a day. (*BSS, metronidazole, tetracycline available as Helidac.)

d. Intravenous H_2 blockers to decrease gastric acid production (see Table 4-2)

4. Disposition

—Patients with suspected perforation are admitted to the surgical service. Emergent operative intervention may become necessary.

III. Acute Cholecystitis and Cholangitis

A. Overview

1. Definitions

—**Cholecystitis** is inflammation of the gallbladder, usually secondary to gallstones.

—**Cholangitis** is inflammation of the hepatic and common bile ducts secondary to bacterial infection.

2. Risk factors

a. For **cholecystitis:**

—Advanced age
—Female gender
—Multiparity
—Obesity
—Diabetes
—Rapid weight loss
—Prolonged fasting
—Cystic fibrosis
—Drugs: clofibrate, oral contraceptives
—Positive family history
—Native American heritage

b. For **cholangitis:**

—*Escherichia coli*
—*Klebsiella* species
—*Bacteroides fragilis*
—Hepatitis
—HIV
—Herpes simplex virus
—Advanced age

B. Clinical presentation

1. Symptoms may include:

—**persistent, colicky pain that is exacerbated with food** and may radiate to the right inferior scapula or right shoulder.

—anorexia

—nausea and vomiting that follow the abdominal pain

—fever

—**Charcot's triad** (cholangitis): fever, RUQ pain, jaundice

—**Reynolds' pentad** (cholangitis): Charcot's triad plus shock and altered mental status

2. **Physical examination findings** may include:
   —**RUQ tenderness**
   —palpable gallbladder (GB)
   —**Murphy's sign:** inspiratory arrest and pain on palpation of the GB during inspiration

C. Diagnostic tests

1. **Laboratory studies**
   a. **CBC** to look for leukocytosis and left shift. Leukocytosis is markedly more elevated in cholangitis than in cholecystitis.
   b. **LFTs** to look for elevated alkaline phosphatase (3–4 times normal), bilirubin, gamma-glutamyl transferase (GGT), and alanine transaminase (ALT).
   c. **Blood cultures** if patient is febrile
2. **Imaging studies**
   a. **Abdominal radiograph** to look for air in the biliary tree, perforation (presence of free air), or obstruction. Gallstones also may be seen (20% are radiopaque).
   b. **Abdominal ultrasound** is done when the abdominal radiograph is negative. Sonographic findings suggestive of cholecystitis can be divided into major and minor criteria. The presence of a major criterion makes the diagnosis of cholecystitis about 80% likely. The additional presence of minor criteria makes the diagnosis even more likely.
      (1) Major criteria for diagnosis of cholecystitis include:
         —presence of gallstones
         —nonvisualized gallbladder (GB)
      (2) Minor criteria include:
         —GB thickening (>4 mm)
         —GB tenderness to ultrasound probe
         —GB enlargement (>5 cm in any dimension)
         —Round-shaped GB
         —Common bile duct dilatation
   c. **Radioisotope scintigraphy (HIDA) scan** can be performed if ultrasound is equivocal or negative in the face of high clinical suspicion. The patient should fast for the 4 hours before the scan. Normally, the GB should be visualized 60 to 90 minutes after administration of contrast. A **nonvisualized GB** is considered a positive test.
   d. **CT scan** to look for abscess or neoplasm. May demonstrate dilatation of distal common bile duct (but is not the first-line test for this).

D. Treatment

1. **Nothing by mouth**
2. Intravenous fluids for hydration
3. Nasogastric suction if vomiting or abdominal distention is present

4. Analgesia as needed
5. **Antibiotics** to decrease the incidence of septic complications and to treat cholangitis
   a. For mild cases, use 1st- or 2nd-generation cephalosporin (e.g., cefazolin or cefoxitin).
   b. For severely ill patients, add gram-negative and anaerobic coverage (e.g., cephalosporin + aminoglycoside + metronidazole/clindamycin).
6. **Cholecystectomy** for acute cholecystitis. Procedure may be delayed until patient is afebrile.
7. **Endoscopic retrograde cholangiopancreatography (ERCP)** with sphincterotomy to remove common bile duct (CBD) stones, and drain fluid collection (cholangitis)

E. Disposition

1. Patients with acute cholecystitis or cholangitis are admitted to the surgical service.
2. If the diagnosis is in question, the patient is either admitted or observed in the ED for serial abdominal exams to elucidate the diagnosis.

IV. Acute Hepatitis

A. Overview

1. **Hepatitis** is inflammation of the liver.
2. **Causes** include:
   a. Viral agents
      —Hepatitis A, B, C, D, and E (Table 4-4)
      —Cytomegalovirus (CMV)
      —Epstein-Barr virus (EBV)
   b. Drugs
      —Acetaminophen

Table 4-4. Etiologic Agents of Hepatitis

Hepatitis	Transmission Route	Antibodies Produced	Permanent Liver Damage?
A	Enteral	Anti-HAV IgM	No
B	Enteral and parenteral	Anti–HBc-IgM HbsAg	Yes
C	Parenteral	Anti–HCV	Yes
D	Parenteral Occurs only with hepatitis B	Anti–HDV IgM HD Ag	Yes
E	Enteral	Anti–HEV IgM	No

HAV = hepatitis A virus; *HBc* = hepatitis B core; *HCV* = hepatitis C virus; *HDV* = hepatitis D virus; *HEV* = hepatitis E virus; *IgM* = immunoglobulin M.

—Isoniazid
—Many others

c. Toxins
—Alcohol
—Carbon tetrachloride
—Mushroom poisoning

3. Complications

—See Table 4-5 for complications of hepatic insufficiency.

B. Clinical presentation

1. **Symptoms** depend on the phase of the disease, which may be limited to any one phase without further progression.

a. **Symptoms** during the **prodromal phase** may include:
—fever
—malaise
—anorexia
—nausea
—vomiting

b. **Symptoms** during the **icteric phase** may include:
—jaundice (including icteric sclerae)
—dark urine
—light-colored stool
—pruritus

c. **Symptoms** during the **fulminant phase** may include:
—hepatic failure
—coagulopathy
—encephalopathy
—worsening jaundice

Table 4-5. Complications of Hepatic Insufficiency

	Diagnostic Clues	Treatment
Encephalopathy	Altered mental state Elevated serum ammonia	Decrease protein intake Lactulose
Hyponatremia	Low serum sodium	0.9% NSS to correct to a Na^+ of 120; then water restrict
Portal hypertension	Esophageal varices (endoscopy) Increased systemic BP	Propranolol Portacaval shunt, stent
Spontaneous bacterial peritonitis	> 500 PMNs in ascitic fluid (paracentesis)	Antibiotics to cover enterobacteriaceae, *S. pneumoniae,* enterococci, anaerobes
Coagulopathy	Prolonged PT and bleeding time	Vitamin K (IV or SQ)

BP = blood pressure; *IV* = intravenous; *NSS* = normal saline solution; *PMN* = polymorphonuclear leukocyte; *PT* = prothrombin; *SQ* = subcutaneous.

2. **Physical examination findings** may reveal (listed from most to least common):
   —**icterus**
   —**RUQ tenderness** (due to distention of liver capsule)
   —**hepatomegaly**
   —**dependent edema**
   —**ascites**
   —spider angiomata
   —asterixis
   —altered mental status (encephalopathy)

C. Diagnostic tests

1. **LFTs** to look for elevations.
   —A 10-fold increase in both AST and ALT with ALT > AST suggests viral hepatitis, whereas a 2- to 3-fold elevation of AST alone with AST > ALT suggests alcoholic hepatitis.
   —Elevated GGT is the most sensitive marker for heavy alcohol use and a good screening test for alcoholism.
   —Serum bilirubin is increased if cholestasis is present.
2. Serum **albumin** to look for decrease; decrease results in decreased oncotic pressure, which causes ascites.
3. **APTT/PT** prolongation to look for coagulopathy
4. Serum **ammonia** to look for elevation; would be present with encephalopathy
5. Serologic studies to look for hepatitis (see Table 4-4)
6. **Chemistry panel** to look for electrolyte abnormalities. Hyponatremia often is present in liver failure.

D. Treatment

1. Treatment is supportive and consists of:
   —intravenous fluids for hydration
   —**antiemetics** (e.g., metoclopramide 10 mg orally, intramuscularly (IM), or intravenously (IV) every 4–6 hours as needed) for control of vomiting
   —**vitamin K** 10 mg IM once daily for 3 days for prolonged PT
   —**lactulose** (30–60 mg orally or 300 ml retention enema) to reduce enteric uptake of amino acids and control encephalopathy.
   —**aldactone** 50–300 mg orally, once daily, to reduce ascites (may be used in combination with another diuretic class)
2. It is important to remember that in the presence of decreased liver function, the clearance of many drugs is impaired.

E. Disposition

1. Most patients can be discharged home with outpatient follow-up.

a. Patients with alcoholic or toxin hepatitis:

—should be advised to abstain from alcohol, products containing acetaminophen and other hepatotoxins.

b. Patients with viral hepatitis:

—should be counseled on personal hygiene and sanitation

—should be offered prophylaxis for household and sexual contacts

c. Patients with hepatitis C should be offered referral to a hepatologist for consideration of liver biopsy and interferon therapy.

2. Patients with coagulopathy, encephalopathy, intractable vomiting, or severe dehydration should be admitted.

V. Acute Appendicitis

A. Clinical presentation

1. Symptoms may include:

—**abdominal pain** beginning around the umbilicus, **migrating to the right lower quadrant (RLQ),** and localizing to McBurney's point

—anorexia

—**pain** that precedes vomiting

—fever

—diarrhea

—urinary urgency and RUQ pain (retrocecal appendicitis)

—Extremes of age, high fever, marked leukocytosis, and presence of symptoms for more than 36 hours suggest perforation.

2. Physical examination findings may include:

—an acutely ill-appearing patient

—abdominal tenderness

—**muscular rigidity**

—voluntary, then involuntary, guarding and right-sided rectal tenderness

—Several signs may be elicited on physical examination.

a. Iliopsoas sign: the patient is supine, with the right knee extended. The patient is asked to flex the right thigh against downward pressure of the examiner. Pelvic pain (due to irritation of the psoas secondary to an inflamed retrocecal appendix) is considered a positive test.

b. Obturator sign: the patient is supine with the right thigh flexed to 90°. The examiner rotates the right thigh internally then externally. Pelvic pain is considered a positive test.

c. Rovsing's sign: pain in the RLQ when the lower left quadrant (LLQ) is palpated.

B. Diagnostic tests

1. Laboratory studies

a. CBC to look for leukocytosis and left shift

b. β-hCG in women of childbearing age to look for pregnancy.

2. **Imaging studies**
   a. **CT scan with contrast.** CT has > 90% sensitivity for diagnosing appendicitis. Use of triple contrast (PO, IV, and rectal) increases the sensitivity to > 95%. CT scan with contrast is the choice test to look for:
   —periappendiceal inflammation
   —streaky pericecal opacities suggestive of a phlegmon
   —appendicoliths
   —fluid collections suggestive of an abscess
   b. **Abdominal radiograph:** three views—upright, supine, and lateral. Nonspecific findings that may suggest appendicitis include:
   —dilated loops of small bowel in RUQ
   —cecal dilatation
   —obstruction of appendiceal lumen (appendicolith)
   —loss of psoas muscle margin
   —soft mass with air bubbles in the RLQ
   —scoliosis of the lumbar spine to the right
   c. **Sonogram** to look for a **noncompressible appendix** with a diameter of at least 6 mm.
   d. **Barium enema** to look for incomplete filling of the appendix

C. **Treatment**

1. Nothing by mouth
2. Intravenous fluids for hydration
3. Nasogastric suction if vomiting or abdominal distention is present
4. Surgical consult
5. Analgesia
6. Antibiotics
   a. For nonperforated appendix: 1st- or 2nd-generation cephalosporin with anaerobic coverage (e.g., cefazolin or cefuroxime plus metronidazole)
   b. For perforated appendix: add gram-negative coverage (e.g., cephalosporin plus aminoglycoside plus metronidazole/clindamycin)
7. **Appendectomy.** Even if the appendix is found to be normal at operation, it is still removed.

D. **Disposition**

—If the diagnosis of appendicitis is made or strongly suspected, the patient is admitted to the surgical service.

—If the diagnosis is in question, the patient is either admitted or observed in the ED for serial abdominal examinations to elucidate the diagnosis.

VI. Acute Pancreatitis

A. Overview

1. **Causes** include:

—biliary disease

—**alcohol** abuse

—**drugs:** diuretics (thiazides, furosemide, ethacrynic acid), valproic acid, tetracycline, sulfonamides, pentamidine, azathioprine, dideoxyinosine, estrogens

—**infection:** mumps, coxsackievirus group B, HIV, mononucleosis, rubella, Epstein-Barr virus, cytomegalovirus, *Echovirus* species, *Ascaris lumbricoides, Clonorchis sinensis,* and many others

—malnutrition

—obstruction

—immediate postoperative state

—trauma

—end-stage renal disease

—cystic fibrosis

—scorpion evenomation

—collagen vascular disease

—burns

—pregnancy and postpartum period

—idiopathic

2. Prognosis

—The prognosis can be estimated by **Ranson's criteria.** Presence of a single criterion carries a mortality risk of 1%; the presence of 3 or 4 criteria increases the mortality risk to 15%; and the presence of 6 or 7 criteria increases the risk to nearly 100%. The criteria are as follows:

a. At admission

—Age > 55 years

—WBC count > 16,000/mm^3

—Serum glucose > 200 mg/dl

—Serum LDH > 350 IU/L

—AST > 250 U/L

b. At 48 hours

—Drop in Hct > 10%

—Rise of BUN > 5 mg/dl

—PO_2 < 60 mm Hg

—Base deficit > 4 mEq/L

—Sequestration of > 6 L fluid

3. Complications

a. Local

—Pseudocyst

—Abscess

—Phlegmon

b. Systemic

—Hypovolemic shock

—Adult respiratory distress syndrome (ARDS)
—Disseminated intravascular coagulation (DIC)

B. Clinical presentation

1. **Symptoms** may include:

—**excruciating knifelike epigastric pain** with **radiation to the back** and **LUQ.** Pain also may radiate diffusely.

—pain exacerbated by food

—**retching**

—**vomiting**

2. **Physical examination findings** may include:

—a patient writhing in pain, who may be sitting up and **leaning forward** or on his or her side with the knees flexed (this decreases irritation)

—**epigastric tenderness**

—muscle rigidity

—**distended abdomen**

—diminished or absent bowel sounds

—palpable tender transverse mass (occasionally)

—jaundice (24 hours after onset)

—ecchymoses of the flank **(Grey-Turner sign)** and umbilicus (**Cullen sign**) secondary to extravasation of blood (48 hours after onset)

—tachypnea, hyperthermia, and hypotension if shock is present

C. Diagnostic tests

1. **Laboratory studies**
   a. Serum **amylase**—will be markedly elevated (10 × normal) but is not specific for pancreatitis
   b. Serum **lipase**—is most specific for pancreatitis, and remains elevated a little longer than amylase, making it useful for detecting late presentations
   c. **Chemistry panel** to look for electrolyte disturbances. Generally, hyperglycemia, hypocalcemia, and hypoalbuminemia are noted.
   d. **CBC** to look for leukocytosis
   e. **Urinalysis** to look for glycosuria
2. **Imaging studies**
   a. **Abdominal radiograph** to look for a single, dilated atonic loop of small bowel (sentinel loop) that occurs secondary to ileus and pancreatic enlargement
   b. **Chest radiograph:** may reveal a pleural effusion (usually left-sided) or an elevated hemidiaphragm
   c. **Abdominal ultrasound** for detecting pancreatic enlargement, gallstones, presence of pancreatic pseudocyst or abscess, and extrahepatic ductal dilatation. Ultrasonography may be limited by the gaseous distention that is often present

d. **CT scan**—preferred over ultrasound. Positive findings include pancreatic or peripancreatic inflammation, collections of peripancreatic fluid, and presence of gallstones.

D. Treatment

1. Nothing by mouth
2. **Intravenous fluids** for volume replacement. Note that hypovolemia in pancreatitis can be severe, despite apparently mild serum electrolyte imbalances.
3. **Nasogastric suction** if nausea or vomiting is present
4. **H_2 blockers**—may be helpful to prevent bleeding from stress ulcers
5. **Antiemetics**—may provide relief from retching
6. **Analgesia** as needed
7. Antibiotic therapy—controversial. If given, a 2nd-generation cephalosporin with anaerobic coverage is adequate.
8. Surgical consult, especially for patients who do not improve with medical management, because an abscess or pseudocyst may be present

E. Disposition

1. Patients with mild symptoms who can tolerate oral intake can be discharged home on pain medication and a clear liquid diet, with outpatient follow-up
2. Patients with severe pain requiring IM or IV medication and those unable to tolerate oral intake should be admitted for further management.
3. Patients with severe dehydration, hypotension, or shock should be admitted to the ICU.

VII. Abdominal Aortic Aneurysm

A. Clinical presentation

1. **Symptoms** may include:

   —no symptoms (asymptomatic), unless aneurysm is growing rapidly or rupturing.

   —**syncope** followed by **severe back pain.**

2. **Physical examination findings** may include:

   —a tender **pulsatile mass.**

   —LLQ or flank tenderness.

   —pulse deficits in upper and lower extremities.

B. Diagnostic tests

1. **Laboratory studies**

   a. **CBC** to look for bleeding (dropping hematocrit)

   b. **Type** and **crossmatch,** in case transfusion becomes necessary

   c. Urinalysis to look for hematuria

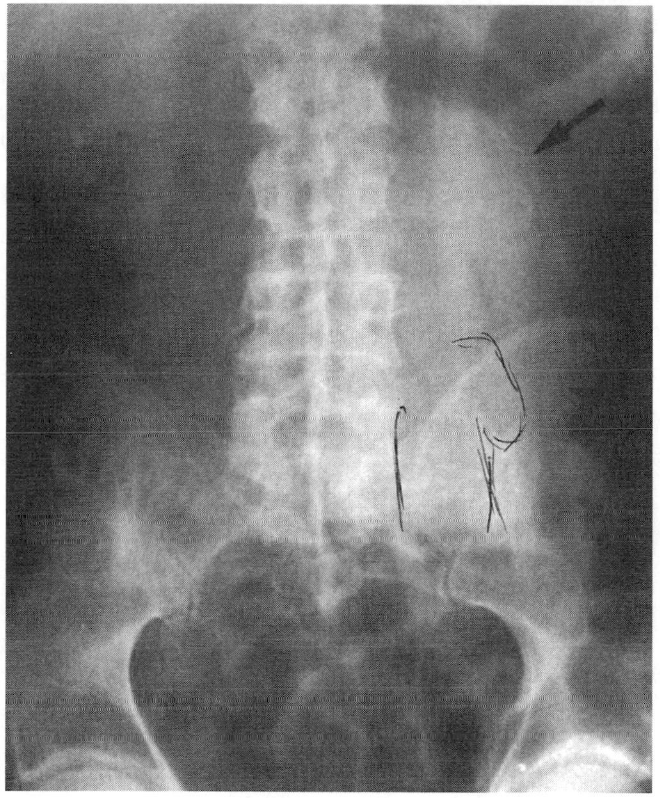

Figure 4-2. Abdominal radiograph demonstrating an abdominal aortic aneurysm. Note the ballooning of the aorta into the left abdomen. (Reprinted with permission from Harris JH Jr, Harris WH, Novelline RA: *The Radiology of Emergency Medicine,* 3rd ed. Baltimore: Williams & Wilkins, 1993, p 891.)

2. **Imaging studies**
   a. **Abdominal radiograph** or **CT scan** to look for calcified ballooning aorta (Figure 4-2)
   b. **Ultrasonography** to detect the presence of an aneurysm and measure its size

C. **Treatment**

1. Supplemental **oxygen**
2. Cardiac monitoring
3. Foley catheter to measure urine output (monitor of renal function)
4. Intravenous hydration
5. **Blood transfusion** as necessary to replace blood loss
6. **Nitroprusside** to lower blood pressure in the hypertensive patient
7. Indications for surgical repair include:
   a. Aneurysm > 5 cm in size
   b. Growth of > 0.5 cm in last 6 months
   c. Aortoiliac occlusive disease
8. Immediate surgical consult for ruptured or dissecting aneurysm

D. Disposition

1. Asymptomatic patients with an incidental finding of an AAA may be discharged home with outpatient referral to a vascular surgeon for elective repair.
2. Patients with a chronic contained rupture should be admitted for observation and work-up.

VIII. Bowel Obstruction

A. Causes

1. **Small bowel obstruction** may be caused by:
   —abdominal adhesions
   —incarcerated hernias
   —neoplasms
   —gallstones
   —inflammatory bowel disease (IBD)
   —abscess
   —radiation enteritis
   —bezoars
2. **Large bowel obstruction** may be caused by
   —sigmoid volvulus
   —colon carcinoma
   —diverticulitis
   —fecal impaction

B. Clinical presentation

1. **Symptoms** may include:
   —**waxing and waning abdominal pain** (due to peristalsis against obstruction)
   —bilious or feculent vomiting (elapsed time between eating and vomiting depends on location of obstruction)
   —**constipation**
   —obstipation
   —bloating
2. **Physical examination findings** may include:
   —presence of surgical scars
   —hernias
   —hyperactive, high-pitched bowel sounds (**borborygmi**), which may become hypoactive and eventually absent as the obstruction progresses
   —**abdominal distention**
   —initially normal vital signs

—tachycardia: secondary to dehydration due to sequestration of fluid

—hypotension: suggestive of strangulation and imminent peritonitis

—tender palpable mass (also suggestive of strangulation)

—pencil-thin stools

C. Diagnostic tests

1. **Laboratory studies**
   a. **CBC** to look for leukocytosis
   b. Serum **amylase**—may be elevated (nonspecific)
   c. **Chemistry panel** to look for electrolyte disturbances
   d. **Type** and **crossmatch,** in case blood transfusion becomes necessary
2. **Imaging studies**
   a. **Flat** and **upright abdominal radiograph** to look for free air under the diaphragm, in the gut, or in the peritoneum; to look for thickening of bowel wall and loss of mucosal pattern. Abdominal radiograph demonstrates a stepladder pattern in small bowel obstruction.
   b. **CT scan** to look for intramural gas, and thickening or edema of bowel wall (signs of ischemia)

D. Treatment

1. **Intravenous fluids** to replace fluid and electrolyte losses. In proximal or small bowel obstruction, the losses of K^+ and Cl^- are out of proportion to the fluid loss, resulting in a hypokalemic, hypochloremic metabolic acidosis. In contrast, in distal or colonic obstruction, the fluid and electrolyte losses are balanced.
2. **Nasogastric suction** to decompress the bowel
3. **Blood transfusion** if hematocrit is low or dropping
4. **Broad-spectrum antibiotics.** Examples of antibiotic regimens include:
   a. Cefotaxime 2 g IV every 8 hours
   b. Ticarcillin plus clavulanic acid 3.1 g IV every 6 hours
   c. Piperacillin plus tazobactam 3.375 g IV every 6 hours
   d. Ampicillin plus sulbactam 3.0 g IV every 6 hours
5. **Sigmoidoscopy,** both diagnostic (visualization of neoplasm, ability to biopsy) and therapeutic (decompresses bowel)

E. Disposition

—Patients are admitted to the surgical service. Emergent operative intervention is needed for complete obstruction.

IX. Acute Intestinal Ischemia

—must be detected, because it carries a high mortality.
—must be sought with a high degree of suspicion, especially in the patient at risk.

A. Risk factors

—Age > 50 years

—Recent myocardial infarction (MI)

—Cardiac arrhythmias (especially atrial fibrillation)

—Recent cardioversion

—Atherosclerosis

—Hypercoagulable states: congestive heart failure (CHF), malignancy

—Sepsis

B. Clinical presentation

1. **Symptoms** may include:

—pain out of proportion to the physical examination findings

—periumbilical pain radiating to RUQ or right iliac fossa

—pain worsened by eating

—insidious onset of pain if due to thromboses (nonocclusive); sudden onset of pain if due to emboli (occlusive)

—vomiting

—diarrhea

2. **Physical examination findings** may include:

—hyperactive or normal bowel sounds.

—abdominal distention.

—guaiac-positive stool.

—Acute intestinal ischemia is often difficult to diagnose because of the lack of significant findings on physical examination.

C. Diagnostic tests

1. **Laboratory studies**

a. **CBC** to look for leukocytosis and hemoconcentration. The hematocrit often is > 45%.

b. Serum **amylase**—will be elevated to 2–3 × normal

c. **Chemistry panel**—to look for electrolyte disturbances. Metabolic acidosis is commonly seen.

2. **Imaging studies**

a. **Abdominal radiograph** to look for a paralytic ileus and "thumbprinting" of colon

b. **CT scan** to look for:

—bowel wall thickening

—air in the bowel wall

—mesenteric portal vein gas (Figure 4-3)

c. **Angiography**—the diagnostic study of choice. Can identify clots within the mesenteric system.

D. Treatment

1. Treatment of underlying CHF or cardiac arrhythmias

2. **Intravenous fluids** to replace volume loss

3. Foley catheter to measure urine output

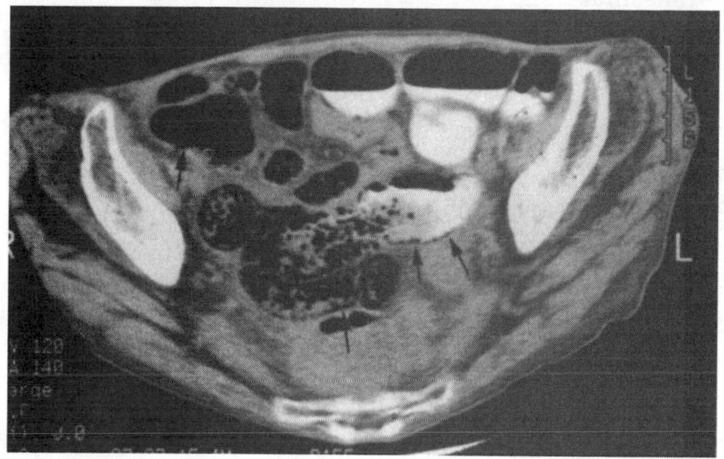

Figure 4-3. CT scan demonstrating bowel infarction. Note presence of portal venous gas *(arrows)*. (Reprinted with permission from Harris JH Jr, Harris WH, Novelline RA: *The Radiology of Emergency Medicine,* 3rd ed. Baltimore: Williams & Wilkins, 1993, p 852.)

4. **Vasopressors** for hypotension—contraindicated, because they may further exacerbate the ischemia via vasoconstriction
5. **Antibiotics** to cover bowel pathogens. An aminoglycoside with metronidazole or clindamycin is a good choice.
6. Surgical consult for probable exploratory laparotomy

E. Disposition

1. If the diagnosis of acute intestinal ischemia is made, the patient is admitted to the surgical service for imminent operative intervention.
2. If the diagnosis is in question, then serial abdominal examinations and observation in the ED may be appropriate. However, the mortality of acute intestinal ischemia is very high, and the diagnosis must be made as early as possible.

X. Diverticular Disease

—**Diverticulosis** is the presence of pouches or outpocketings of hollow organs (**diverticula**). **True diverticula** involve all layers of the bowel wall; **false diverticula** are limited to the mucosa and submucosa.

—**Diverticulitis** is the inflammation of diverticula secondary to bacterial proliferation.

—Both diverticulosis and diverticulitis are seen more commonly in people over 50 years of age, and are most often encountered in the sigmoid colon.

—Complications include perforation, abscess, fistula, and obstruction.

A. Clinical presentation

1. **Symptoms** may include:

—**constant LLQ pain** (sigmoid) or RLQ pain (cecal) exacerbated by food and relieved by a bowel movement or passage of flatus

—tenesmus

—malaise

—anorexia

—vomiting

—diarrhea

—urinary urgency and frequency (if a phlegmon is adjacent to the urinary bladder)

—Patients with cecal, ascending, and other right-sided diverticula tend to be younger, vomit less frequently, and have a more insidious onset of pain, which tends to be on the right versus the left.

2. **Physical examination findings** may include:

—fever

—tachycardia

—LLQ mass

—voluntary guarding

—rebound tenderness

—**guaiac-positive stool**

—decreased bowel sounds

—distended abdomen

B. **Diagnostic tests**

1. **Laboratory studies**

   a. **CBC** to look for leukocytosis

   b. **Chemistry panel** to look for electrolyte disturbances

2. **Imaging studies**

   a. The test of choice is **CT scan** of the abdomen to look for colonic wall thickening of > 5 cm, and streaking or inflammation in pericolonic fat.

   b. **Gastrograffin study** to look for diverticula, fistulas, ileus, or luminal narrowing. The presence of an extraluminal mass is indicative of an abscess.

   c. Sigmoidoscopy and colonoscopy usually are not appropriate in the setting of acute diverticular disease but may be performed with caution if the diagnosis is in question.

C. **Treatment**

1. **Intravenous fluids** to replace fluid loss

2. Nothing by mouth

3. **Nasogastric suction** if vomiting or abdominal distention is present

4. Analgesia: **meperidine** 50–150 mg IM or IV every 3–4 hours as needed. Meperidine is particularly useful because it also inhibits segmental contraction of the colon. Other opiates, such as codeine or morphine, should be avoided because they may increase intraluminal colonic pressure.

5. Antibiotics: many regimens are appropriate, including **cefoxitin** 2 g IV every 6 hours, plus **gentamicin** 1–1.5 mg/kg IV every 8 hours, or **tobramycin** 1.0–1.5 mg/kg every 8 hours plus either **metronidazole** 500 mg IV every 8 hours or **clindamycin** 600 mg IV every 6 hours.

D. Disposition

1. Patients who improve with the steps outlined under Treatment may be discharged with antibiotics if vital signs and hematocrit are stable.
2. Patients who do not improve within 24 hours require surgical management, because complications are likely.

XI. Inflammatory Bowel Disease (IBD)

—IBD consists of two entities: Crohn's disease and ulcerative colitis (UC). Differences between the two are outlined in Table 4-6.

A. Clinical presentation

1. **Symptoms** common to both Crohn's disease and ulcerative colitis include:

—crampy abdominal pain

—fever

—weight loss

—changes in bowel habits

—a **feeling of incomplete evacuation**

—relief of abdominal pain after a bowel movement

—**diarrhea** or **constipation.** Either one may predominate, or they may alternate.

—passage of mucus per rectum

—excessive **bloating**

Table 4-6. Features of Inflammatory Bowel Disease

	Crohn's disease	**Ulcerative Colitis**
Epidemiology	Males > females	Females > males
Location	Involves entire GI tract from mouth to anus	Limited to colon, particularly rectum and anus
Complications	Fistulas more common Strictures Abscess formation	Rectal prolapse Massive colonic hemorrhage Toxic megacolon
Pathologic lesions	Full-thickness (transmural) lesions Skip lesions Lymphoid hyperplasia Endoscopy: "cobblestone" pattern	Lesions in mucosa and submucosa only Continuous lesions Pseudopolyps Barium enema: "lead pipe" pattern

—pain that tends to be localized to the lower abdomen (Crohn's disease)

—**rectal tenesmus** (UC)

—anal incontinence (UC)

—shock (toxic megacolon in UC)

2. **Physical examination findings** may include:

—abdominal tenderness

—increased frequency of bowel sounds

—guaiac-positive stool with or without frank blood

—**perianal irritation**

—tympanic abdomen with decreased or absent bowel sounds (toxic megacolon in UC)

—skin manifestations: erythema nodosum or pyoderma gangrenosum

—ocular manifestations: uveitis or episcleritis

—musculoskeletal manifestations: arthritis

B. **Diagnostic tests**

1. **Laboratory studies**
   a. **CBC** to look for anemia
   b. **B_{12} level** if anemia is macrocytic. Anemia can be seen secondary to malabsorption in Crohn's disease.
   c. **Type** and **crossmatch** may be necessary if profound anemia is present.
   d. **Chemistry panel** to look for electrolyte disturbances secondary to diarrhea
   e. **Stool work-up** for occult blood, ova and parasites, culture and sensitivity and WBC to rule out an infectious cause for the diarrhea
   f. A **lactose tolerance test** may be useful to rule out this cause for the bloating, abdominal pain, and diarrhea

2. **Imaging studies**
   a. **Flat** and **upright abdominal radiographs** to look for dilated loops of bowel. A transverse colon > 8 cm suggests megacolon (Figure 4-4).
   b. **Barium enema**
      (1) In UC, a barium enema may be done to look for:
      —fuzzy margins
      —loss of haustral markings
      —pseudopolyps
      —decreased luminal opening
      (2) In Crohn's disease, a barium enema may be done to look for:
      —presence of strictures
      —fistulas and mucosal irregularities ("skip lesions")
   c. **Colonoscopy** to look for mucosal abnormalities and ulcerations. May be done on an outpatient basis

C. **Treatment**

1. **In the ED**

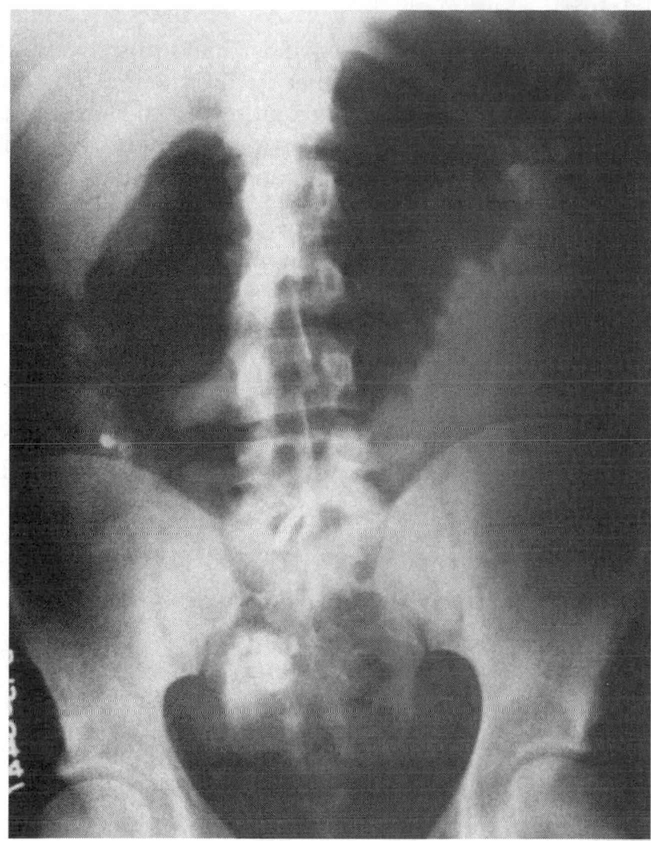

Figure 4-4. Abdominal radiograph demonstrating air-filled dilated transverse colon, suggestive of toxic megacolon in this patient with ulcerative colitis. (Reprinted with permission from Harris JH Jr, Harris WH, Novelline RA: *The Radiology of Emergency Medicine,* 3rd ed. Baltimore: Williams & Wilkins, 1993, p 855.)

   a. **Nothing by mouth**
   b. **Intravenous fluids** to replace fluid and electrolyte loss
   c. Broad-spectrum triple antibiotics for patients who appear toxic (see section X C 5)
   d. Corticosteroids: hydrocortisone 300 mg IV/day (adults) or **prednisolone** 0.5–2.0 mg/day (children). For patients who have never received steroids, ACTH 120 U/day is preferred.

2. Outpatient maintenance therapy may include:
   a. **Sulfasalazine** 2–4 g orally daily
   b. Antidiarrheals (Crohn's disease): **loperamide** 4 mg orally one time, then 2 mg after each loose stool, to a maximum of 16 mg/day; or **diphenoxylate** 5 mg orally every 6–8 hours until acute diarrhea is controlled, then 2.5–5 mg orally every 12 hours. Antidiarrheals are not recommended for UC, as they may precipitate toxic megacolon.
   c. Other helpful measures after acute attack is controlled include bulk-forming laxatives (psyllium 7.5 mg in one glass of water every 8–24 hours), a high-fiber diet, and reassurance. Anxiolytics and antispasmodics also may be helpful.
   d. For toxic megacolon, immediate GI and surgery consults

D. Disposition

1. Patients with severe exacerbations, including fever, significant weight loss, dehydration, or grossly bloody diarrhea, or those in whom complications are suspected should be admitted to the hospital for IV antibiotics, corticosteroids, and further management. Potential complications include perforation, obstruction, and hemorrhage.
2. Patients with toxic megacolon are admitted to the ICU.
3. All others can be discharged home with treatment as outlined and outpatient follow-up.

XII. Acute Gastroenteritis

—**Acute gastroenteritis** is the inflammation of the stomach and bowel secondary to an infectious agent, often ingested via contaminated food (Table 4-7).

A. Clinical presentation

1. **Types** include inflammatory and noninflammatory.
   a. Generally, viruses and many parasites produce a noninflammatory acute gastroenteritis (AGE).
   b. Bacteria may produce either kind.
2. **Symptoms**

   —The differences in the presentations of inflammatory and noninflammatory AGE are summarized in Table 4-8.

B. Diagnostic tests

1. **CBC** to look for leukocytosis and left shift
2. **Chemistry panel** to look for electrolyte disturbances. Hypernatremia and hypokalemia may be noted secondary to diarrhea and dehydration.
3. If an inflammatory process is suspected, **stool work-up** is appropriate. This includes stool culture and sensitivity, presence of WBC in stool, stool for ova and parasites and *C. difficile* toxin.

Table 4-7. Common Food-associated Pathogens that Cause Diarrhea

Food	Commonly Associated Pathogen
Honey	*Clostridium botulinum*
Shellfish	*Vibrio parahaemolyticus*
Reheated rice	*Bacillus cereus*
Mayonnaise	*Staphylococcus aureus*
Eggs, poultry	*Salmonella* spp
Home-canned foods	*Clostridium perfringens*
Ground beef	*Escherichia coli* 0157
Cheese	*Listeria* spp

Table 4-8. Inflammatory vs. Noninflammatory Acute Gastroenteritis

	Inflammatory/Invasive	Noninflammatory/Toxigenic
Causative pathogen	*Campylobacter jejuni* *Salmonella* spp *Yersinia pestis* *Clostridium difficile* *Entamoeba histolytica*	*Staphylococcus aureus* *Bacillus cereus* Enterotoxigenic *Escherichia coli* *Giardia lamblia* *Strongyloides* spp
Symptoms and clinical features	More gradual onset Symptoms last longer Small stool volumes Blood, pus, mucus in stools Fever may be present WBCs in stool	Sudden onset Symptoms last 24 h Large stool volumes No blood, pus, mucus in stools Fever is rare No WBCs in stool Nausea, vomiting more common
Treatment	Antibiotics Antidiarrheal agents contraindicated	Antibiotics contraindicated Antidiarrheal agents
Part of GI tract involved	Large bowel	Small bowel

C. Treatment

1. **Oral** or **intravenous fluids** to replace volume loss
2. **Antiemetics** if significant vomiting is present
3. Rehydration salts to replace electrolytes
4. **Antibiotics**
   a. Toxigenic bacterial diarrhea: contraindicated
   b. Invasive bacterial diarrhea: ciprofloxacin 500 mg orally twice a day for 10 days is a good broad-spectrum choice. Many other regimens also are suitable.
   c. Parasitic diarrhea: metronidazole 500 mg orally 3 times a day for 7–10 days is a good broad-spectrum choice
   d. *Clostridium difficile* colitis: metronidazole or vancomycin is effective
5. **Anticholinergics:** decrease intestinal motility and decrease abdominal cramps and may be useful in some cases
6. **Bismuth subsalicylate**—an antisecretory agent that decreases stool liquidity and frequency and is especially useful because of its few side effects
7. **Loperamide**—an opiate that increases transit time in the gut, thereby permitting increased resorption of water and salt. Antidiarrheals are contraindicated in inflammatory or invasive diarrhea, because they allow bacteria to remain in the GI tract for a longer time.

D. Disposition

1. Patients with stable vital signs who can tolerate oral rehydration may be discharged home with outpatient follow-up.

2. Patients who develop or have high risk of developing complications of AGE should be admitted. These complications include hypotension, shock, bowel perforation, renal failure, hemorrhage, and hemolytic-uremic syndrome.

XIII. Hernias

A. Overview

1. Definition

—A **hernia** is a protrusion of an organ or tissue out of the body cavity in which it normally lies.

—Hernias may occur anywhere in the body.

—The most common type is the inguinal hernia (indirect is more common than direct), followed by femoral and umbilical hernias

2. **Risk factors** include:

—congenital malformations

—family history

—undescended testes and other GU abnormalities

—pregnancy

—ascites

—chronic increased intraabdominal pressure

B. Clinical presentation

1. Most hernias are asymptomatic. **Symptoms,** when seen, may include:

—groin pain of acute onset and increasing intensity, suggestive of incarceration or strangulation

—nausea and vomiting if small bowel obstruction is present

—irritability, in infants

2. **Physical examination findings** may include:

—abnormal swelling and tenderness in the area of the hernia

—**an increase in size with increasing intraabdominal pressure**

—a mass that does not transilluminate, **differentiating** it from a hydrocele

—a protrusion of viscera through the external ring that is palpable via the scrotum in males during a Valsalva maneuver (inguinal hernia)

C. Diagnostic tests

1. Laboratory studies

a. **CBC** to look for leukocytosis and left shift

b. **Chemistry panel** to look for electrolyte abnormalities

2. Imaging studies

a. **Chest radiograph** to look for perforation (free air under the diaphragm)

b. **Flat** and **upright abdominal radiographs** to look for bowel obstruction

D. Treatment

1. Treatment consists of manual reduction of mass using minimal force, mild sedation, and local cool compresses.
2. A hernia that is not reducible may be strangulated or incarcerated. Treatment consists of:

—**nothing by mouth**

—**intravenous fluids** for hydration

—**nasogastric suction** if vomiting or abdominal distention present

—broad-spectrum **antibiotics**

—surgical consultation

—analgesia

E. Disposition

1. All patients with acutely incarcerated or strangulated hernias should be admitted to the surgical service for immediate repair.
2. Patients who are stable and in whom hernia was reduced can be discharged home with referral to a surgeon for elective repair.

XIV. Gastrointestinal Bleeding

—GI bleeding can be divided into upper and lower by the ligament of Treitz.

A. Causes

1. UGI bleeding

—Peptic ulcer disease

—Erosive gastritis

—Mallory-Weiss syndrome

—Arteriovenous malformations

—Esophageal varices

—Esophagitis

—Splenic vein thrombosis

2. LGI bleeding

—Diverticular disease

—Colon cancer

—Arteriovenous malformations

—Inflammatory bowel disease

—Hemorrhoids

Bowel ischemia (mesenteric thrombosis)

—Meckel's diverticulum (children)

—Anal fissure

B. Clinical presentation

1. **Symptoms of upper GI bleeding** (UGI) may include:
   —hematemesis
   —melena
2. **Symptoms of lower GI bleeding** (LGI) may include:
   —hematochezia
   —occult blood loss
3. **Physical examination findings** may include:
   —signs of alcohol abuse or cirrhosis such as facial rubor, ascites, spider angiomata, pallor, or jaundice
   —**guaiac-positive** stool, unless the onset of the bleed is extremely recent
   —palpable mass suggestive of tumor
   —**orthostatic hypotension**
   —**tachycardia, hypotension,** and **shock** in severe bleeds

C. Diagnostic tests

1. **CBC** to look for bleeding (dropping hematocrit) and platelet count
2. **Type** and **crossmatch** for 4–6 units of packed RBCs
3. **Chemistry panel** to look for electrolyte disturbances
4. **APTT/PT** to look for coagulopathies

D. Treatment

1. **Oxygen** by nasal cannula or face mask to optimize RBC saturation
2. **Intravenous fluids** for volume replacement
3. **Trendelenburg position** to maximize venous return of blood as tolerated
4. **Blood transfusion**
   a. Maintain Hb >10 g/dl in the elderly, who are prone to re-bleed.
   b. Maintain Hb >7 g/dl in young patients with no other comorbid disease.
   c. Maintain platelet count > 50,000/mm^3
5. **Nasogastric lavage**
   a. Blood-stained gastric contents or "coffee grounds" appearance are suggestive of UGI source of bleeding.
   b. Bile-stained gastric contents are suggestive of LGI source.
   c. No return of gastric contents is equivocal.
6. **Foley catheter** to measure urine output
7. Vitamin K for patients with coagulopathies
8. For UGI bleed:
   a. **Drugs to control bleeding**
      —Octreotide 100 μg bolus follwed by 50 μg/h drip

—Somatostatin 250 μg bolus followed by 250–500 μg/h drip
—Vasopressin 6–24 U/h drip

b. **Endoscopy** is the diagnostic treatment of choice. UGI bleed can be attenuated by endoscopic cauterization or sclerotherapy.

c. GI consult

9. For LGI bleed:

—Work-up depends on the rate of hemorrhage.

—Surgical consult is required for all LGI bleeds.

a. Slow/occult: **colonoscopy**

b. Moderate: anoscopy followed by colonoscopy and **tagged RBC scan** or angiogram, depending on severity

c. Fast: **angiogram** or operating room

E. Disposition

1. Patients with GI bleeding severe enough to produce hemodynamic instability should be admitted to the ICU.
2. Patients who are hemodynamically stable but are actively bleeding and symptomatic with hematocrits less than the recommended range should be admitted to the floor.
3. Asymptomatic patients with occult GI bleeds may be treated on an outpatient basis.

XV. Gastroesophageal Reflux Disease (GERD)

A. Clinical presentation

1. **Symptoms** may include:

—heartburn

—regurgitation

—angina-like chest pain

—dysphagia

—bronchospasm

—pain that worsens with recumbency, with bending over, and following meals

—relief obtained with antacids

2. **Physical examination findings** may include:

—a patient who is obese, with no other findings that are remarkable

B. Diagnostic tests

1. Work-up for MI as outlined in Chapter 2, section II A, to rule out pain of cardiac origin
2. Work-up for GERD (all may be done on an outpatient basis) includes:

—barium swallow

—endoscopy

—acid reflux test

Table 4-9. Factors that Aggravate Gastroesophageal Reflux Disease

Alcohol in excess
Cigarette smoking
Irritation of esophageal mucosa
Citrus fruits
Spicy foods
Lowering of LES pressure
Fatty foods
Chocolate
Yellow onions
Peppermint
Hiatal hernia
Drugs
Anticholinergics
Theophylline, caffeine
Progesterone
Calcium channel blockers
β-adrenergic agents
Diazepam
Meperidine

LES = lower esophageal sphincter.

C. Treatment

1. Avoidance of foods and medications that exacerbate reflux (Table 4-9)
2. Antacids
3. H_2 blockers (see Table 4-2)
4. Proton pump inhibitor such as **omeprazole** 20 mg orally per day

D. Disposition

1. If a cardiac etiology can be ruled out, the patient may be discharged home with outpatient follow-up.
2. If an underlying cardiac cause for the pain is possible, the patient should be admitted to the hospital until the possibility can be ruled out.

XVI. Foreign Bodies

A. Overview

1. **Incidence**

—Foreign bodies in the GI tract are seen primarily in children and, to a lesser extent, in special populations at risk, including edentulous adults and psychiatric patients.

2. **Complications** include:

—bleeding

—obstruction

—perforation

B. Clinical presentation

1. **Symptoms** vary depending on where in the GI tract the foreign body is located.
   a. Esophageal foreign bodies may cause **odynophagia** and **dysphagia.** **Sialorrhea** and **regurgitation** are seen with complete obstruction. In children, respiratory distress may be the presenting symptom.
   b. Gastric foreign bodies tend to be asymptomatic. If symptomatic, the most commonly reported symptom is **early satiety.**

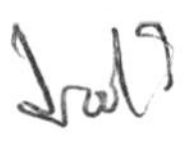

2. **Physical examination findings** may include:
   —**stridor, choking** and **coughing,** if the foreign body is lodged in the esophagus
   —It is important to remember that if one foreign body is found, it is necessary to search for others.

C. Diagnostic tests

—**Chest radiographs** (AP and lateral views), **neck radiographs** (lateral view), and **abdominal radiographs** to look for the foreign body itself (many are radiopaque), obstruction, or perforation. If perforation has occurred, the following features may be noted:

1. Subcutaneous air
2. Pneumomediastinum
3. Pleural effusion
4. Pneumothorax

D. Treatment

1. For blunt objects, observation to see if the object is passed is acceptable.
2. Sharp objects or objects larger than 5 × 2 cm must be removed endoscopically.
3. If a blunt object does not pass or if a sharp object cannot be removed endoscopically, surgical removal is necessary to prevent perforation.

E. Disposition

1. Once the foreign body is removed and there are no signs of complications (e.g., bleeding, perforation, obstruction), the patient can be discharged home with outpatient follow-up.
2. If complications have occurred or surgery is required to remove the foreign body, the patient should be admitted to the hospital.

Review Test

1. A 40-year-old, slightly obese woman presents with right upper quadrant (RUQ) pain of 2 days duration that is exacerbated by food, nausea, and vomiting. Which of the following findings is most suggestive for acute cholecystitis?

(A) Gallbladder thickening
(B) Elevated serum bilirubin
(C) A nonvisualized gallbladder
(D) Leukocytosis on CBC
(E) Right upper quadrant (RUQ) pain in the presence of fever and anorexia

2. Which of the following signs detected on physical examination is consistent with acute cholecystitis?

(A) Pelvic pain upon flexion of the extremity while the patient is supine
(B) Pelvic pain upon internal and external rotation of the flexed extremity
(C) Pain in the right lower quadrant when the left lower quadrant is palpated
(D) Pain and arrest of inspiration upon palpation of the right upper quadrant
(E) None of the above

3. Which one of the following types of hepatitis usually does NOT cause permanent damage to the liver?

(A) Alcoholic hepatitis
(B) Hepatitis A
(C) Hepatitis B
(D) Hepatitis C
(E) All of the above cause permanent liver damage

4. Which one of the following laboratory results is most specific for pancreatitis?

(A) Elevation of serum direct bilirubin
(B) Elevation of serum indirect bilirubin
(C) Elevation of eosinophils on peripheral smear
(D) Elevation of serum amylase
(E) Elevation of serum lipase

5. A 71-year-old woman is being admitted to the hospital from the emergency department for acute pancreatitis. Her complete blood cell count (CBC) shows a white blood cell (WBC) count of 13,000; her serum glucose is 171; and her serum lactate dehydrogenase (LDH) is 250. Which one of the following factors points to a poor prognosis for this patient?

(A) Her age
(B) Her gender
(C) Her white blood cell (WBC) count
(D) Her serum glucose
(E) Her serum LDH

6. Which one of the following is the most common cause of lower GI bleeding in adults?

(A) Arteriovenous malformations
(B) Peptic ulcer disease
(C) Diverticular disease
(D) Hemorrhoids
(E) Mesenteric thrombosis

7. Which of the following is the treatment of choice for a slow or occult lower gastrointestinal (GI) bleed?

(A) Angiogram
(B) Colonoscopy
(C) Endoscopy
(D) Surgical exploration
(E) Tagged red blood cell (RBC) scan

8. Which of the following treatments for inflammatory bowel disease represents first-line therapy, following reassurance and the fostering of a sound patient-physician relationship?

(A) Prednisone 40–60 mg orally every 24 hours
(B) Sulfasalazine 2–4 mg orally every 24 hours
(C) Psyllium 7.5 mg every 24 hours
(D) Metronidazole 750 mg orally every 24 hours
(E) Loperamide 4 mg orally every 24 hours

9. An 18-year-old woman presents with a sudden onset of diarrhea and vomiting of 8 hours duration. She reports six large-volume stools, which consisted mostly of "water," in the past 6 hours. On physical examination, she is febrile, tachycardic, and has dry oral mucosa. Which of the following treatments is contraindicated in this patient?

(A) Intravenous hydration
(B) Rehydration salts
(C) Antidiarrheal agents such as loperamide
(D) Antibiotic agents such as ciprofloxacin
(E) Antiemetic agents such as prochlorperazine

10. Which of the following is an indication for surgical repair of an abdominal aortic aneurysm (AAA)?

(A) Growth of the abdominal aortic aneurysm (AAA) of >0.5 cm in the past 6 months
(B) Size <5 cm
(C) History of valvular heart disease
(D) Patient age >55 years
(E) Presence of severe bleeding diathesis

Answers and Explanations

1–C. Although no one test can unequivocally demonstrate cholecystitis, of the choices listed, the presence of a nonvisualized gallbladder is the strongest factor in support of acute cholecystitis. Gallbladder thickening is nonspecific. An elevated serum bilirubin is seen secondary to obstruction of the biliary tract and is not necessarily due to cholecystitis. Leukocytosis on the CBC is seen in multiple conditions, including infection, inflammation, and neoplasia. Right upper quadrant (RUQ) pain in the presence of fever and anorexia is a common presentation of appendicitis in the pregnant patient.

2–D. Pain and arrest of inspiration upon palpation of the right upper quadrant represents Murphy's sign. Pelvic pain upon flexion of the extremity while the patient is supine (choice A), pelvic pain upon internal and external rotation of the flexed extremity (choice B), and pain in the right lower quadrant when the left lower quadrant is palpated (choice C) describe the iliopsoas, obturator and Rovsing's signs respectively, and are used to diagnose acute appendicitis, not cholecystitis.

3–B. Hepatitis A is a waterborne illness that is transmitted via the fecal-oral route and has an incubation period of 2 to 6 weeks. It generally is a self-limited illness and generally does not cause liver damage. Alcoholic hepatitis (choice A), hepatitis B (choice C), and hepatitis C (choice D) do cause permanent liver damage.

4–E. Of the tests listed, the most specific one for pancreatitis is the serum lipase. However, serum lipase also will be elevated in cancer of the pancreas, peptic ulcer disease (PUD), and bowel infarction. Serum amylase (choice B) also is elevated in pancreatitis but is much less specific than serum lipase. There are numerous causes for elevated serum amylase, including all of the causes for elevated lipase plus acute cholecystitis, acute appendicitis, peritonitis, salivary gland inflammation or neoplasm, carcinomatosis of the lung, burns, diabetic ketoacidosis (DKA), ruptured ectopic pregnancy, renal insufficiency, eating disorders, and acute ethanol intoxication. Eosinophilia (choice D) usually is noted with parasitic infection and allergic reactions. Elevated bilirubin (choices A and B) generally is not a feature of pancreatitis.

5–A. Age > 55 years is considered a poor prognostic factor in pancreatitis according to Ranson's criteria (see section VI A 2). Gender (choice B) is not a prognostic factor. WBC count (choice C), serum glucose (choice D), and serum LDH (choice E) are, in fact, criteria used to determine prognosis, but none are elevated enough to be considered poor.

6–C. The most common etiology for lower GI bleeding (defined as bleeding with origin below the ligament of Treitz) is diverticular disease, especially diverticulosis. Arteriovenous malformations (choice A) and mesenteric thrombosis (choice E) do cause lower GI bleeding, but are quite rare.

Peptic ulcer disease (choice B) is a cause for upper, not lower, GI bleeding. Hemorrhoids (choice D), although common, are not the most common etiology for lower GI bleed.

7–B. For a slow or occult bleed, the diagnostic test of choice is a colonoscopy. For moderate bleeds, colonoscopy followed by a tagged red blood cell (RBC) scan (choice E) is appropriate. Angiograms (choice A) and surgical procedures (choices C and D) are reserved for fast bleeds and bleeds in the setting of hemodynamic instability. See section XIV C for details.

8–C. The approach to treatment for inflammatory bowel disease (IBD), which is a chronic illness, is from least aggressive to more aggressive. The first-line agent to try is psyllium, which is a bulk-forming laxative. It is especially attractive because it has no major adverse effects. The next-line agent is sulfasalazine (choice B). Chronic suppression with corticosteroids (choice A) is considered a last resort due to its undesirable side effects. Loperamide (choice E) is used only in acute exacerbations that present with diarrhea, and not on a chronic basis. Metronidazole (choice D) and other antibiotics are of questionable benefit and should be reserved for cases in which infection is suspected.

9–D. Based on the description of this patient's symptoms and physical examination findings, she likely has a noninflammatory or toxigenic acute gastroenteritis, which is caused by elaboration of a toxin as opposed to the proliferation of bacteria in the gut. Therefore, antibiotics are contraindicated in this setting. All the other choices listed—intravenous hydration (choice A), rehydration salts (choice B), antidiarrheal agents such as loperamide (choice C), and antiemetic agents such as prochlorperazine (choice E)—are appropriate treatments.

10–A. Growth of the abdominal aortic aneurysm (AAA) by more than 0.5 cm in the past 6 months is an indication for surgery. Size <5 cm (choice B) is incorrect, because indication for surgery is AAA >5 cm, not <5 cm. Presence of valvular heart disease (choice C) and age of the patient (choice D) are not criteria for surgical repair of AAAs. The presence of a severe bleeding diathesis (choice E) usually is a contraindication to most major surgical procedures. See section VII C 7 for more information.

5

Genitourinary Emergencies

I. Acute Renal Failure

A. Overview

1. **Definition. Acute renal failure** is acute impairment of kidney function resulting in retention of substances that normally are excreted.
2. **Causes**
   a. **Prerenal causes** (due to inadequate perfusion) include:
      —Congestive heart failure (CHF)
      —Cirrhosis
      —Sepsis
      —Hypovolemia
      —Pulmonary edema
      —Severe burns
      —Pancreatitis
      —Nephrotic syndrome
      —Hypoalbuminemia
      —Pericardial tamponade
   b. **Renal causes** include:
      —acute tubular necrosis
      —allergic interstitial nephropathy (secondary to drugs/toxins/contrast dyes)
      —glomerulonephritis
      —renal vein or artery thrombosis
      —vasculitis
      —thrombotic thrombocytopenic purpura (TTP)
      —hemolytic-uremic syndrome
      —rhabdomyolysis
      —multiple myeloma
      —malignant hypertension
   c. **Postrenal causes** (due to outflow obstruction) include:
      —prostate enlargement

—bilateral renal vein occlusion
—ureteral stone obstruction
—neurogenic bladder
—phimosis

3. **Complications** include:
—hyperkalemia
—hypocalcemia
—pulmonary edema
—uremia
—pericarditis

B. **Clinical features**

1. **Symptoms**
   a. Secondary to electrolyte abnormalities—weakness
   b. Secondary to obstruction—urinary hesitancy, urinary frequency, and nocturia
   c. Secondary to volume overload—paroxysmal nocturnal dyspnea, dyspnea on exertion, orthopnea, and weight gain
   d. Secondary to uremia—confusion, agitation, seizures, lethargy, and coma
   e. Miscellaneous symptoms include nausea, vomiting, and fever.
2. **Physical examination findings**
   a. Signs of hypovolemia include:
   —orthostatic hypotension
   —tachycardia
   —decreased skin turgor
   b. Signs of volume overload include:
   —jugular venous distention (JVD)
   —rales
   —S3 gallop
   —peripheral or pulmonary edema
   c. Signs of renal urinary tract obstruction include:
   —distended bladder
   —suprapubic tenderness
   —**large post-void residual urine**
   —enlarged prostate

C. **Diagnostic tests** (Table 5-1)

1. **Laboratory studies**
   a. **Chemistry panel** to look for elevated blood urea nitrogen (BUN) and creatinine and electrolyte disturbances. Hyperkalemia, hypocalcemia, hyperphosphatemia, and metabolic acidosis are the abnormalities most commonly encountered.
   b. **Serum** and **urine osmolarity** and **electrolytes** to determine type of renal failure
   c. Blood and **urine cultures** if patient is febrile (acute renal failure predisposes to infection)

Table 5-1. Laboratory Findings in Acute Renal Failure

	BUN/Cr ratio	FE_{Na}	U_{osm}	U_{Na}
Prerenal causes	> 20:1	< 1.0	>500	<20
Renal causes	10:1 to 15:1	> 2.0	<300	>40
Postrenal causes	<10:1	> 2.0	<400	>40

BUN = blood urea nitrogen; FE_{Na} = fractional excretion of sodium; U_{osm} = urinary osmolality; U_{Na} = urinary sodium.

d. Urinalysis to look for:
—hematuria
—granular casts [indicative of acute tubular necrosis (ATN)]
—red blood cell (RBC) casts (indicative of acute glomerulonephritis)
—white blood cell (WBC) casts (indicative of acute interstitial nephritis)

2. Imaging studies

a. Chest radiograph to look for pulmonary edema, cardiomegaly, or pleural effusion

b. Sonogram to look for hydronephrosis

3. Electrocardiogram (ECG) to look for changes secondary to hyperkalemia (peaked T waves) hypocalcemia, or cardiac dysfunction

4. Formulas for assessing renal function

a. Creatinine clearance (CrCl). Normal is calculated as follows:

$$\text{CrCl} = \frac{(\text{urine Cr} \times \text{urine volume})}{(\text{serum Cr} \times \text{time})} \;/\; \frac{[(140 - \text{patient age}) \times (\text{patient weight})]}{(72 \times \text{serum Cr}) \times 0.85 \text{ (for women)}}$$

b. Fractional excretion of sodium (FE_{Na})

$$FE_{Na} = \frac{U_{Na}/\text{serum Cr}}{\text{serum Na}^{+} \times \text{urine Cr}} \times 100$$

D. Treatment

1. Intravenous fluids should be administered to hypovolemic patients; for euvolemic patients, intake should be matched to output.

2. Any offending medications should be discontinued.

3. Increase urinary output in anuric and oliguric patients with intrarenal failure. Treatment choices include:

a. Furosemide 2–5 mg/kg IV to a maximum of 400 mg

b. Dopamine 1–3 μg/kg/min IV

c. Mannitol 12.5–25 g IV

4. Relief of obstruction, if present. For lower tract obstruction, use 16-French Foley or coudé catheter. For upper tract obstruction, nephrostomy tubes may be required.

5. Treatment of hypocalcemia-induced tetany with 10 ml of 10% calcium gluconate. Dose can be repeated if necessary. Contraindicated in patients on digoxin therapy due to risk of cardiac arrest.

6. Treatment of hyperkalemia if >6.5 mEq/L or if ECG changes are present. Choices include:

a. 10 ml of 10% calcium gluconate or chloride. Hypercalcemia is a possibility, and should be watched for.
b. 10 U intravenous insulin with 50 g of glucose.
c. 25 g Kayexalate (resin) in 25 ml of 70% sorbitol. Hypernatremia is a possibility, and should be watched for.
d. 50 mg intravenous bicarbonate. Volume overload, alkalosis, and seizures are possibilities, and should be watched for.
e. Albuterol nebulizer treatment

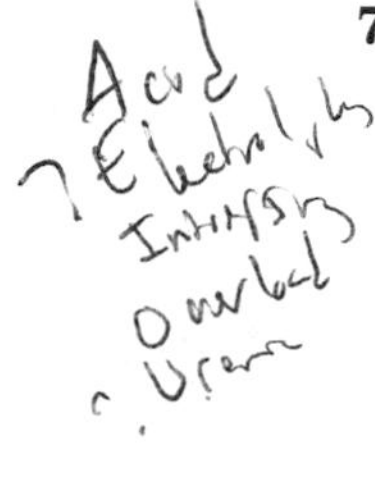

7. **Emergent hemodialysis** is indicated for:
   a. Severe refractory volume overload
   b. Symptomatic hyperkalemia refractory to medications specified in I C 6
   c. Acute, large, symptomatic elevation in blood urea nitrogen (BUN) and creatinine
   d. Certain toxic ingestions (see Chapter 18)
   e. Severe hypothermia

E. Disposition

1. Patients with new-onset acute renal failure should be admitted to the hospital for further work-up.
2. Patients with chronic renal failure who present with acute exacerbations may be discharged home if they have stable vital signs, have minimal fluid and electrolyte disturbances, have no signs of developing complications, and are able to follow up with their nephrologist or primary care provider (PCP).
3. All patients should be counseled regarding a high-calorie, low-protein, low-sodium, low-potassium diet.

II. Urolithiasis

A. Overview

1. **Urolithiasis** is the presence of calculi within the urinary tract. There are five major types of urinary stones: calcium oxalate (the most common, seen in >50% of cases); calcium phosphate; uric acid; struvite; and cysteine (the least common type).
2. **Causes** include:

   —increased absorption of calcium due to drugs or disease state

   —excessive dietary intake of calcium or uric acid

   —metabolic defects that produce an elevated uric acid level
3. **Risk factors**
   a. General risk factors include:
      —male gender
      —dehydration
      —hot climate
      —immobilization
      —family history
      —gout

—hyperparathyroidism
—inflammatory bowel disease
—sarcoidosis
—malignancy

b. Medications that may provoke urolithiasis include:
—hydrochlorothiazide
—acetazolamide
—allopurinol
—excessive consumption of vitamins
—antacid abuse

B. Clinical features

1. Symptoms may include:
—**sudden onset** of **severe colicky pain** in groin and flank
—**nausea**
—vomiting
—fever
—**hematuria**

2. Physical examination findings may include:
—an acutely ill-appearing patient writhing in pain
—tachycardia
—diaphoresis

C. Diagnostic tests

1. Laboratory studies

a. Urinalysis to look for hematuria and urinary pH. Presence of WBCs may indicate an infected stone. Uric acid stones are associated with a pH of 5.5 or less; a pH of >7.5 usually is seen with struvite stones.

b. Chemistry panel to look for hypercalcemia, hypophosphatemia, creatinine, and uric acid

2. Imaging studies

a. Plain radiograph of kidney, ureter, and bladder (**KUB**) to look for stones. Eighty-five percent of stones are radiopaque and are composed of calcium oxalate or calcium phosphate. A stone on radiograph appears approximately 125% of actual size.

b. Computed tomographic (CT) scan of abdomen without contrast to look for stones

c. Intravenous pyelogram if CT is not available to obtain both anatomic and functional information about the kidney. Positive findings include:
—dilatation and delayed filling of the affected collecting system
—hydronephrosis or hydroureter on the affected side
—contrast column cut-off

d. Ultrasonography (limited by operator's level of experience and patient's size) may be useful to detect:
—hydronephrosis
—a large ureteral stone

D. **Treatment**

1. **Intravenous (IV) fluids** for hydration, to maintain urine output at 100 ml/hr
2. **Analgesia:** IV for maximum efficacy, titratability, and speed of onset
   a. Meperidine 25–100 mg every 2–3 hours as needed
   b. Morphine 2–10 mg every 2–3 hours as needed
   c. Oxycodone 5–10 mg orally every 6 hours as needed
   d. Ketorolac 30–60 mg every 4–6 hours as needed intramuscularly (IM) or IV (non-opiate option)
3. **Antiemetics** if significant vomiting: prochlorperazine 10 mg IM or IV every 4–6 hours as needed
4. **Urologic consultation** for
   a. Intractable pain despite IV fluids and opiate analgesia
   b. Stone > 5 mm
   c. Patient with single kidney
   d. Persistent gross hematuria
5. **Surgical treatment** options
   a. Extracorporeal shock wave lithotripsy is indicated for
      —Renal stones < 2 cm
      —Stones in the renal pelvis or upper two thirds of the ureter
      —Non-infected stones
      —Patient with no coagulopathies
   b. Urethroscopy is indicated for
      —Stones in lower third of the ureter
      —Patient with no anatomical anomalies
   c. Open surgery is indicated for
      —Large obstructive stones
      —Infected stones

E. **Disposition**

1. Patients who have passed their stone while in the emergency department (ED) may be discharged home with outpatient follow-up.
2. Patients whose pain is adequately controlled and who are able to tolerate oral hydration may be discharged home with analgesia while waiting for the stone to pass. Patients should be instructed to strain their urine for stones and bring them for analysis.
3. Patients require admission to the urologic service if their pain is inadequately controlled or if they are unable to tolerate oral intake, are obstructed, have infected stones, have only one kidney, or are toxic.

III. Pyelonephritis

—Pyelonephritis is an infection of the upper urinary tract.

—Complications may include perinephric abscess, miscarriage in pregnant women, and urosepsis.

A. **Clinical features**

1. **Symptoms** may include:
   —**fever**
   —**chills**
   —**flank pain**
   —**dysuria**
   —frequency
   —urgency
   —hematuria
   —rigors
   —abdominal pain
2. **Physical examination findings** may include:
   —an acutely ill-appearing patient
   —flank and **costovertebral angle (CVA) tenderness**

B. **Diagnostic tests**

1. **Urinalysis.** Clean-catch midstream urine is centrifuged to look for **WBC casts.** (This test is more specific for pyelonephritis than for UTI.)
   a. **Bacteriuria** is indicated by the presence of >10 organisms per high-power field (HPF)
   b. **Pyuria** is indicated by the presence of >10 WBCs per HPF
   c. Hematuria may be seen with both UTI and pyelonephritis.
2. **Blood** and **urine cultures** to isolate specific organism
3. **Complete blood cell count (CBC)** to look for leukocytosis

C. **Treatment**

1. **Intravenous fluids** for hydration
2. **Antibiotics:** the drugs of choice are the fluoroquinolones. They can be given orally for outpatient therapy and IV for inpatients (Table 5-2).

Table 5-2. Antibiotic Regimens for Pyelonephritis

Outpatients
Ciprofloxacin 250 mg PO bid × 14 days
Enoxacin 400 mg PO bid × 14 days
Norfloxacin 400 mg PO bid × 14 days
Ofloxacin 200 mg PO bid × 14 days
Levofloxacin 250 mg PO once daily × 14 days
Lomefloxacin 400 mg PO once daily × 14 days
Hospitalized patients
Above fluoroquinolone regimens IV × 14 days
Ampicillin + gentamicin IV × 14 days
3rd-generation cephalosporin IV × 14 days

bid = twice a day; IV = intravenously; PO = by mouth.

D. Disposition

1. Most patients with pyelonephritis are sick enough to warrant admission. Patients who are not toxic and are able to tolerate oral fluids and antibiotics may be discharged home with outpatient follow-up.
2. All pediatric, geriatric, male, pregnant, or immunocompromised patients and those who appear toxic or are unable to tolerate fluids or antibiotics by mouth should be admitted.

IV. Urinary Tract Infection (UTI)

A. Overview

1. The term **UTI** is used to refer to infections anywhere in the urinary tract.
2. **Risk factors**
   a. Risk factors in women include:
      —sexual activity
      —pregnancy
      —postmenopausal state
      —use of spermicidal jellies
   b. Risk factors in men include:
      —anatomic abnormalities
      —prostatitis
      —genitourinary tumors
      —calculi
      —catheterization and other urologic procedures
   c. General risk factors include:
      —diabetes mellitus
      —infected urinary stones
      —urethral stricture

B. Clinical features

1. **Symptoms** may include:
   —**dysuria**
   —**frequency**
   —**urgency**
   —**nocturia**
   —**hematuria**
   —malodorous urine
2. **Physical examination findings** may include:
   —suprapubic tenderness
   —an enlarged prostate

C. Diagnostic tests

1. **Urinalysis.** Clean-catch midstream urine is centrifuged to look for:

a. **Bacteriuria** [>10 organisms per high-power field (HPF)]
b. **Pyuria** (>10 WBCs per HPF)
c. Hematuria (may be seen with both UTI and pyelonephritis)

2. **Urine culture** to isolate specific organism
3. **CBC** to look for leukocytosis
4. **β-hCG** in women of childbearing age to look for pregnancy (influences choice of antibiotics)

D. **Treatment**

1. **Intravenous fluids** are given to dilute urine.
2. **Antibiotics** are directed toward the specific offending organism, based on culture and sensitivity results. Empiric therapy may be begun while waiting for culture results (Table 5-3).
3. **Phenazopyridine** is a urinary tract analgesic that may be helpful with pain control. Patients should be warned that the drug will color their urine, sweat, and tears a bright orange. Generally, 1–2 days will provide adequate relief, because the infection will be under control by then.

E. **Disposition**

1. Patients with uncomplicated UTI who are not toxic can be discharged home with oral antibiotics and outpatient follow-up.
2. Patients who are toxic or who are suspected of having a concomitant up-

Table 5-3. Antibiotic Regimens for Urinary Tract Infections

Type of UTI	Recommended Antibiotic Regimen
First/uncomplicated/postcoital UTI	TMP/SX 160/800 mg PO bid × 3 days Ciprofloxacin 250 mg PO bid × 3 days Norfloxacin 400 mg PO bid × 3 days Ofloxacin 200 mg PO bid × 3 days Levofloxacin 250 mg PO bid × 3 days Fosfomycin 3 g in 4 oz of water × 1 dose
Complicated UTI (requiring hospitalization)	Ampicillin + gentamicin IV × 2–3 weeks, *or* Piperacillin + tazobactam IV × 2–3 weeks, *or* Imipenem IV × 2–3 weeks, 160/800 mg PO bid × 10 days followed by TMP-SX
Pregnancy-associated asymptomatic bacteriuria	Amoxicillin 500 mg PO tid × 3 days Nitrofurantoin 100 mg PO qid × 3 days Fluoroquinolones contraindicated
Pregnancy-associated UTI	Amoxicillin 500 mg PO tid × 10 days Amoxicillin + clavulinic acid 500 mg PO tid × 10 days Nitrofurantoin 100 mg PO qid × 10 days Fluoroquinolones contraindicated

bid = twice a day; IV = intravenously; PO = by mouth; qid = four times a day; tid = three times a day; TMP/SX = trimethoprim-sulfamethoxazole; UTI = urinary tract infection.

per UTI or complicated UTI obstruction or catheterization should be hospitalized to receive intravenous antibiotics.

3. All children presenting with a first-time UTI should be referred to a urologist to check for GU structural abnormalities.

V. Hematuria

A. Overview

1. Hematuria is defined as the presence of $\geq$5 RBC per mm^3 of unspun urine.
2. **Causes** may be summarized using the mnemonic TICS:

   T:

   —Trauma: instrumentation; direct blow; severe, prolonged exercise

   —Tumor: Wilms' tumor; hypernephroma; other tumors of bladder, prostate, and kidney

   —Toxins: phenols, turpentine, NSAIDs, sulfonamides; cyclophosphamide

   I:

   —Infections: *Schistosoma haematobium,* cystitis, prostatitis, UTI, glomerulonephritis, TB, yellow fever, black water fever

   —Inflammatory states: Goodpasture's syndrome

   C:

   —Calculi

   —Cysts

   —Congenital abnormalities: aneurysms, hemangiomas, arteriovenous malformations

   S:

   —Surgery

   —Sickle cell disease, and other hematological problems, e.g., hemophilia, thrombocytopenia, anticoagulants

   —(P)seudohematuria: bleeding from genitals, menses, factitious disorder, vegetable dyes, phenophthalein, phenozopyridine, porphyria

B. Clinical features

1. **Symptoms** may include dysuria, frequency, and urinary urgency.
2. Relation of hematuria to timing of the urinary stream may reveal the anatomical site affected.
   a. Initial hematuria: urethra distal to the urogenital diaphragm
   b. Middle hematuria: upper urinary tract or bladder itself
   c. Terminal hematuria: neck of the bladder or prostatic urethra
3. **Physical examination** findings may include

   —CVA tenderness

   —Enlarged prostate

C. Diagnostic tests

1. **Laboratory studies**
   a. Urinalysis, to look for
      (1) **RBCs.** Bloody-appearing urine that contains no RBCs may represent a pseudohematuria secondary to ingestion of certain foods (e.g., beets, rhubarb) or drugs, or may represent **myoglobinuria.**
      (2) **RBC casts:** suggestive of bleeding from upper urinary tract
   b. Urine culture, if an infectious cause is suspected
   c. CBC to look for leukocytosis
   d. PT/APTT to look for excessive anticoagulation
   e. CPK levels to look for rhabdomyolysis
   f. Chemistry panel to look for elevations in BUN and creatinine
2. **Imaging studies.** Abdominal CT scan, without contrast, to look for urolithiasis

D. Treatment

1. Intravenous fluids for hydration
2. Analgesics

E. Disposition

1. Patients whose pain is intractable should be admitted for intravenous analgesia and further work-up.
2. Patients who present with painless hematuria (or pain that can be adequately controlled with oral medications) and stable vital signs may be discharged home with outpatient follow-up to determine etiology.

VI. Urinary Retention

A. Overview

1. Urinary retention is the inability to void urine, or to void completely.
2. **Causes** include:
   a. Benign prostatic hypertrophy (the most common cause in men)
   b. Multiple sclerosis and diabetes mellitus (the most common causes in women)
   c. Obstruction of bladder outlet, which may be caused by:
      —benign prostatic hypertrophy
      —pregnancy
      —GU tract tumors
      —urolithiasis
      —urethral stricture
   d. Detrusor muscle instability or failure
   e. Neurogenic bladder, which may be caused by:
      —spinal shock
      —diabetes mellitus
      —multiple sclerosis

—Parkinson's disease
—cerebrovascular accident (CVA)
—brain tumor
—herniated disk

f. Medications
—Sympathomimetics
—**Anticholinergics**

3. **Complications** may include infection and post-obstructive diuresis.

B. **Clinical features**

1. **Symptoms** may include:
—urinary urgency
—frequency
—nocturia
—hesitancy
—a decrease in urinary stream
—dribbling
—feeling of incomplete emptying

2. **Physical examination findings** may include:
—suprapubic tenderness
—distended bladder
—enlarged prostate
—phimosis or paraphimosis of penis

C. **Diagnostic tests**

1. Urinary catheterization is both diagnostic and therapeutic. A post-void residual volume of >250 ml is diagnostic of urinary retention.

2. **Urinalysis** and **urine culture** to look for infection

3. A **chemistry panel** to look for renal insufficiency

D. **Treatment**

1. **Catheterization** with a 16-French Foley or coudé (curved tip) catheter provides immediate relief from the obstruction. Lubrication of the catheter with lidocaine jelly eases passage.

2. **Belladonna and opium suppositories** may provide relief from urinary urgency that occurs secondary to bladder spasm. The dose is 1 suppository every 4–6 hours as needed.

3. **Bethanechol** is a cholinergic agent used to treat nonobstructive urinary retention and retention due to neurogenic bladder. Dosage is 0.2 mg/kg orally twice daily (children) or 10–50 mg orally twice daily (adults).

4. **Neostigmine** is another cholinergic agent used to treat postoperative bladder distention and urinary retention in adults. The treatment dosage is 0.5–1.0 mg IM or subcutaneously every 3 hours for 5 doses, given after the bladder is emptied.

5. **Oxybutynin** is a urinary antispasmodic agent used to treat reflex neurogenic bladder. The dosage is 0.2 mg/kg orally 2 to 4 times per day (children) or 5 mg orally 2 or 3 times a day (adults).
6. Antibiotics are appropriate if infection is present, or if the catheter is to remain in place for more than a few days.
7. The underlying cause must be treated.

E. Disposition

1. Patients who are hemodynamically stable and able to care for themselves can be discharged home with an indwelling catheter with outpatient urology follow-up.
2. Patients who are toxic or in whom complications (e.g., infection, hemorrhage, postobstructive diuresis) are suspected should be admitted.
3. Patients in whom urinary retention is due to a neurogenic cause should be admitted for a thorough work-up and, possibly, intravenous antibiotics.

VII. Urethral Foreign Bodies

—Urethral foreign bodies are especially common in small children, but may be seen in adults of all ages as well, especially developmentally disabled or mentally ill adults.

A. Clinical features

1. **Symptoms** may include:

   —**bloody,** foul-smelling **discharge** from the urethra

   —dysuria

2. **Physical examination findings** may include a trapped foreign body.

B. Diagnostic tests

1. **Urinalysis** and **urine culture** to look for infection
2. **Radiograph** of bladder, urethra, and genitalia to look for foreign body

C. Treatment

1. Immediate referral to urology for removal of foreign object
2. Following removal, retrograde urethrography or endoscopy to confirm an intact nontraumatized urethra

D. Disposition

—Patients may be discharged home following removal of the foreign body, with outpatient follow-up.

VIII. Acute Scrotal Pain

A. Testicular torsion

—Testicular torsion occurs when a testicle or testicular appendage rotates on the pedicle axis.

—Torsion is 10 times more common in undescended testes and is more common in neonates and prepubertal boys. It has a bimodal age peak: once in neonates and again in boys aged 13–15 years.

—Torsion is more likely to occur in males in whom the pedicle is longer or in those who have a history of a previous episode.

—The prognosis for testis salvageability is nearly 100% if treated within 6 hours; 70% if treated within 6–12 hours; and 20% if treated within 12–24 hours. After 24 hours, the testis is not salvageable.

1. **Clinical features**
   a. **Symptoms** may include:
      —acute onset of severe unilateral pain
      —nausea
      —vomiting
      —abdominal pain
      —a history of similar episodes of abrupt pain with spontaneous resolution
      —anorexia
   b. **Physical examination findings** may include:
      —fever
      —edema or erythema of testis
      —absent cremasteric reflex
      —unilateral testicular elevation
      —long axis of testis in horizontal position
      —an affected testis that is swollen and larger than the unaffected testis
2. **Diagnostic tests**
   a. **Color Doppler ultrasound** (>90% sensitivity and specificity) to look for **decreased or absent** blood flow to testis. If the study is nondiagnostic, surgery is done right away. If clinical suspicion is high, the patient should be taken to the operating room immediately rather than waiting to perform an ultrasound study.
   b. **Urinalysis** to look for pyuria (rare)
3. **Treatment**
   a. **Immediate urology consult** before anything
   b. Analgesia: opiate (e.g., meperidine, morphine, oxycodone) or a nonsteroidal antiinflammatory drug (NSAID) (e.g., ketorolac)
   c. Attempted manual detorsion while waiting for consultant, Doppler study, or surgical repair. Rotate testes away from midline as if opening a book.
4. **Disposition**
   —Torsion must be reversed in patients with testicular torsion. Occasionally manual detorsion is successful, but this does not preclude surgical repair. Usually, surgery is necessary; when surgery is done, both testes are repaired to prevent future torsion.

B. Torsion of the appendix testis

1. Clinical features

a. Symptoms may include:

—more gradual onset of pain (usually for more than 24 hours)

—nausea and vomiting are rare

—no dysuria or discharge

b. Physical examination findings may include:

—palpable nodule

—positive cremasteric reflex

—isolated tenderness of the upper pole of the testis

—mild edema and erythema

2. Diagnostic tests

a. Color Doppler ultrasound to reveal normal or increased flow to testis

b. Transillumination of testis to look for **blue dot sign**

3. Treatment

a. Analgesia

b. Rest

c. Elevation of scrotum

4. Disposition

—Patients can be discharged with outpatient follow-up in 24 hours.

C. Epididymitis and orchitis

—**Epididymitis** is inflammation of the epididymis.

—**Orchitis** is inflammation of the testicle.

—The most common cause in men aged 20 to mid-40s is an STD; the most common cause in men aged 50 years and older is prostate disease.

—Risk factors include a history of STDs or risk factors for STDs; recent instrumentation; and a history of GU abnormalities.

1. Clinical features

a. Symptoms may include:

—gradual onset of pain

—dysuria

—penile discharge

—urinary retention

b. Physical examination findings may include:

—fever

—toxic appearance

—tender spermatic cord

—a normal cremasteric reflex

—normal testicular axis

2. **Diagnostic tests**
   a. **Laboratory studies**
      —Urethral swab (DNA probe) to look for gonorrhea or chlamydia infection
      —Urinalysis to look for WBC and bacteria
      —Urine culture to look for causative organism
      —CBC to look for leukocytosis
   b. Color Doppler ultrasound to exclude testicular torsion if clinical picture is confusing
3. **Treatment**
   a. Antibiotics to cover gonococcus, chlamydia, and *Escherichia coli*
   b. Analgesia: opiate (e.g., meperidine, morphine, oxycodone) or NSAID (e.g., ketorolac)
   c. Rest
   d. Scrotal elevation
   e. Urology consult for prepubertal boys to look for anatomic abnormalities of the urinary tract
4. **Disposition**
   a. Most patients can be discharged home with outpatient follow-up.
   b. Patients who are toxic or who have intractable pain should be admitted.

D. Hydrocele

—Hydrocele is accumulation of fluid in the scrotum (cavity of the tunica vaginalis) secondary to obstruction that impedes lymphatic drainage of the testicles

—Causes include congenital conditions, neoplasia, trauma, infection (e.g., elephantiasis), and congestive heart failure (CHF).

1. **Clinical features**
   a. **Symptoms** may include:
      —testicular swelling
      —absence of pain (usually)
      —association with an indirect inguinal hernia (sometimes)
   b. **Physical examination findings** may include:
      —a positive transillumination test
2. **Treatment**
   a. Underlying pathology such as a tumor should be sought.
   b. The patient should be observed for about 2 weeks.
   c. The hydrocele should be repaired surgically if it does not resolve spontaneously.

E. Varicocele

—Varicocele is dilatation of the veins of the pampiniform plexus, which act to keep the testes cool. Loss of the cooling mechanism impairs spermatogenesis.

—The **cause** is idiopathic.

1. **Clinical features** may include:

—Palpation of a "bag of worms" in the scrotum, a finding that becomes pronounced with Valsalva.

2. **Treatment**

—is surgical repair

3. **Disposition**

—Patients can be discharged home with outpatient follow-up in 24 hours for elective repair.

F. Fournier's gangrene

—Fournier's gangrene is polymicrobial infection of the scrotum, which can progress to arterial thrombosis in the skin and necrosis of the scrotum.

—Risk factors include diabetes mellitus, poor hygiene, immunocompromise, paraplegia, indwelling catheters, and hydrodermis suppurativa.

1. **Clinical features** may include:

—a toxic-appearing patient

—**pain in the genital area out of proportion to physical examination findings**

2. **Treatment**

a. ABCs, including intravenous fluids

b. Broad-spectrum antibiotics

—Triple therapy: ampicillin, gentamicin, *and* clindamycin

—Monotherapy: ticarcillin-clavulanate *or* ampicillin-sulbactam

c. Emergent wide surgical debridement

d. Hyperbaric oxygen (pre- and postoperatively)

e. Control of blood glucose, as needed

3. **Disposition**

—Patients are admitted to the surgical service for debridement.

IX. Problems of the Penis

A. Phimosis

—Phimosis is tightness of the foreskin, preventing it from being retracted over the glans.

—**Causes** may be physiologic (first 3 days of life), congenital, or acquired (e.g., infection, irritation).

1. **Clinical features** may include:

—inability to retract the foreskin

—pain on erection

2. **Treatment**

—Dorsal slit (incision of band of foreskin on the dorsal surface of the penis)

—Circumcision

3. **Disposition**

—Patients can be discharged home with outpatient follow-up in 24 hours.

B. **Paraphimosis**

—Edematous foreskin that constricts the glans penis

—may be caused by failure to retract the foreskin after cleansing or urologic procedures

1. **Clinical features** may include:

—swelling

—penile pain that worsens upon erection

—ulceration of foreskin

—penile drainage

2. **Treatment**

—1% lidocaine for anesthesia, followed by manual reduction attempt

—If manual reduction is unsuccessful, then dorsal slit

3. **Disposition**

—Patients can be discharged home with outpatient follow-up in 24 hours.

C. **Balanoposthitis**

—inflammation of the glans penis and foreskin

1. **Causes** may include:

—allergy to latex condoms

—infection, either fungal (*Candida* species) or bacterial (*B. vincentii,* streptococci)

—drugs: sulfonamides, tetracyclines, phenobarbital

—diabetes mellitus

2. **Clinical features** may include:

—tenderness to palpation

—swelling of prepuce

—penile pain

—erythema and ulceration of foreskin

—dysuria

—purulent, malodorous discharge

3. **Treatment**

—Area should be cleansed with soap and dried thoroughly.

—Antifungal cream may be applied. Antibiotics should be given if infection is present.

—Circumcision should be considered.

4. **Disposition**

—Patients can be discharged home with outpatient follow-up in 24 hours.

D. Priapism

—persistent, prolonged, painful erection

1. **Causes**
   a. Blood dyscrasias: e.g., sickle cell anemia, leukemia
   b. Drugs: e.g., trazodone, prazosin, chlorpromazine
   c. Pelvic vascular thrombosis, hematoma
   d. Spinal tumors
2. **Clinical features** may include:

   —loss of sexual function

   —pain

   —dysuria or inability to urinate
3. **Treatment**
   a. Reassurance
   b. Large-bore needle aspiration of blood from corpus cavernosum
   c. 0.25–0.50 mg terbutaline injected subcutaneously into corpus cavernosum
   d. For sickle cell disease: aggressive intravenous hydration. If symptoms still persist, then exchange transfusion to decrease percentage of sickled cells to less than 50%
4. **Disposition**

   —Most patients can be discharged home with outpatient follow-up in 24 hours.

   —Patients with sickle cell disease or other complicating conditions may need to be admitted for management.

E. Penile fracture

—Penile fracture is rupture of the tunica albuginea of the penis.

—It usually is caused by trauma during sexual intercourse.

1. **Clinical features** may include:

   —sudden onset of severe penile pain associated with a "click" sound

   —a swollen, discolored, tender penis
2. **Treatment and disposition**

   —Urologic consultation for surgical repair and evacuation of hematoma

X. Problems of the Prostate

A. Prostatitis

—Prostatitis is inflammation of the prostate.

—The **cause** usually is bacterial (e.g., infection with *E. coli*).

1. **Clinical features**
   a. **Symptoms** may include:

—fever, chills
—dysuria, urinary frequency, nocturia
—perineal and low back pain

b. **Physical examination findings** may include:
—a tender, boggy, tense prostate

2. **Treatment**
   a. Antibiotics: 2 weeks for acute infection, 12 weeks for chronic infection
   b. Analgesia
   c. Stool softeners

3. **Disposition**
—Most patients with prostatitis can be discharged home with antibiotics and outpatient follow-up in 24 hours.

B. Benign prostatic hypertrophy

—Benign prostatic hypertrophy (BPH) is an increase in the size of the prostate.

—The **etiology** is idiopathic.

1. **Clinical features**
   a. If caused by obstruction: decreased urinary stream, hesitancy, incontinence, urinary retention, distended bladder
   b. If due to irritation: dysuria, urinary frequency, urgency, nocturia

2. **Treatment**
   a. No emergency treatment is required for BPH.
   b. Outpatient options include:
   —surgical resection
   —alpha-adrenergic agonists (e.g., terazosin)
   —hormonal anti-androgens (e.g., finasteride)

3. **Disposition**
—Most patients with prostatitis can be discharged home with antibiotics and outpatient follow-up in 24 hours.

XI. Genitourinary Emergencies in Women.

See Chapter 16, "Obstetric and Gynecologic Emergencies."

Review Test

1. A 27-year-old woman presents with a complaint of feeling weak and light-headed. On physical examination you note a pale young woman with a pulse of 110 while supine and 90 when standing, and a blood pressure of 100/70 while supine and 70/50 while standing. Initial laboratory values report a blood urea nitrogen (BUN) of 32 and a creatinine of 1.5. Which of the following findings points to a prerenal etiology of her acute renal failure (ARF)?

(A) Fractional excretion of sodium = 0.8
(B) Urine osmolarity = 278
(C) Urine sodium = 47
(D) Blood urea nitrogen = 32
(E) All of the above are consistent with a prerenal ARF.

2. Which of the following is a plausible etiology for this patient's prerenal ARF?

(A) Kidney stone
(B) Systemic lupus erythematosus
(C) Ingestion of radiographic contrast dye
(D) Recent vomiting and diarrhea
(E) All of the above are plausible etiologies for prerenal ARF.

3. A 56-year-old man presents with the following laboratory data: blood urea nitrogen (BUN) = 45, serum sodium = 135, serum creatinine = 4.1, serum osmolarity = 280, urinary sodium (U_{Na}) = 50, urine creatinine = 56. Which of the following is the correct value for this patient's fractional excretion of sodium (FE_{Na})?

(A) FE_{Na} = .027
(B) FE_{Na} = 2.7
(C) FE_{Na} = 27
(D) FE_{Na} = 250
(E) The FE_{Na} cannot be calculated from the information given.

4. Which of the following types of renal failure does the patient described in question 3 likely have?

(A) Prerenal
(B) Renal
(C) Postrenal
(D) Acute
(E) Chronic

5. A 44-year-old man with acute renal failure has a serum potassium level of 6.0 mEq/L. He is currently asymptomatic, but his electrocardiogram (ECG) demonstrates peaked T waves as well as some nonspecific changes. Which of the following would be your preferred treatment choice?

(A) 5 g Kayexalate (resin) in 25 ml of 70% sorbitol.
(B) Intravenous saline via two large-bore peripheral lines at 150 ml/hr
(C) 10 ml of 10% calcium gluconate
(D) Ipratropium bromide via nebulizer
(E) There is no need to treat a potassium level of 6.0 mEq/L.

6. A 27-year-old male athlete presents with new-onset painless hematuria. Dipstick analysis of the urine shows blood, but microscopic analysis reveals no red blood cells. Which of the following possibilities would explain these findings?

(A) Factitious disorder
(B) Recent consumption of rhubarb pie
(C) Recent ingestion of phenazopyridine
(D) Myoglobinuria
(E) All of the above are plausible explanations

7. A 34-year-old man, currently under psychiatric treatment for depression, presents to the emergency department with a painful erection that has been present for the past 2 hours. He also reports dysuria and a feeling that he is unable to urinate. What is the most likely diagnosis?

(A) Phimosis
(B) Priapism
(C) Balanoposthitis
(D) Paraphimosis
(E) Penile fracture

8. A 37-year-old male diabetic patient presents to the emergency department with excruciating pain in his scrotum that extends into the rectal area. Findings on physical examination are unremarkable except for exquisite tenderness. The penis is without ulceration, and the foreskin has been removed by circumcision. Rectal examination reveals good sphincter tone, a slightly enlarged prostate, and guaiac-negative stool. Despite the paucity of findings, which of the following diagnoses must be considered?

(A) Priapism
(B) Phimosis
(C) Anal fissure
(D) Fournier's gangrene
(E) Chronic prostatitis

9. Which of the following findings confirms a diagnosis of urinary retention?

(A) Post-voiding residual volume > 250 ml
(B) A distended bladder
(C) Suprapubic tenderness
(D) Pyuria of catheterized urine
(E) Presence of red blood cell casts in urine

Answers and Explanations

1–A. Prerenal acute renal failure (ARF) is characterized by a fractional excretion of sodium (FE_{Na}) < 1.0, a blood urea nitrogen/creatinine (BUN/Cr) ratio of ≥ 20:1 (this patient's ratio is 21.3:1), a urine osmolarity > 500, and a urine sodium of <20. Of the choices listed, only choice A, fractional excretion of sodium = 0.8, is consistent with prerenal failure. For laboratory values of different types of acute renal failure, see Table 5-1.

2–D. Of the choices listed, only hypovolemia secondary to vomiting and diarrhea is a prerenal etiology of acute renal failure (ARF). Kidney stones are a postrenal (obstructive) cause of ARF. Systemic lupus erythematosus (SLE) and ingestion of radiographic contrast dye are renal etiologies of ARF. See Table 5-1 for further details.

3–B. The fractional excretion of sodium (FE_{Na}) is calculated as follows:

$$FE_{Na} = \frac{U_{Na} \times \text{serum creatinine} \times 100}{\text{Serum } Na^{+} \times \text{urine creatinine}} = \frac{50\ (4.1)\ (100)}{135\ (56)} = 2.7$$

4–B. This patient has a blood urea nitrogen/creatinine (BUN/Cr) ratio of 11, a fractional excretion of sodium (FE_{Na}) of 2.7 (>1), and a urinary sodium (U_{Na}) = 50 (>40). This places him in ARF of renal etiology (see Table 5-1). It is not possible given the information provided to determine whether this patient's renal failure is acute or chronic.

5–C. Although a potassium level of 6.0 mEq/L alone in an asymptomatic patient may not be sufficient reason to treat for hyperkalemia, the presence of electrocardiographic (ECG) changes does warrant treatment. The treatment of choice among those listed is calcium gluconate, because its onset of action is just a few minutes. Kayexalate resin also is an effective way to treat hyperkalemia, but it has a slower onset of action, at approximately 30 minutes. It is an incorrect answer to this question, however, because the dose specified, 5 g, is incorrect. The correct dose is 25 g in 25 ml of 70% sorbitol. Intravenous saline does nothing to displace potassium and therefore would not be a correct treatment for this patient. Albuterol, a common drug used in asthma, is also another treatment for hyperkalemia, but ipratropium bromide is not.

6–E. All of the choices are possible explanations. Painless hematuria can be the result of a factitious disorder, recent consumption of rhubarb pie, recent ingestion of phenazopyridine, or myoglobinuria, among other causes (see I A 2).

7–B. This patient most likely has priapism secondary to medication. Trazodone, a selective serotonin reuptake inhibitor (SSRI) commonly used to treat depression, is particularly notorious for having this adverse effect.

8–D. Pain out of proportion to physical examination findings is the hallmark of Fournier's gangrene. Priapism is painful prolonged erection. Phimosis is tightness of the foreskin of the penis, a diagnosis that is irrelevant in a circumcised patient. Anal fissure would produce pain on defecation and, often, a guaiac-positive stool secondary to fresh blood; in addition, it would not cause pain in the scrotum. Chronic prostatitis would not produce this degree of pain; in fact, chronic prostatitis often is asymptomatic.

9–A. Urinary retention is defined as a post-voiding residual volume of > 250 ml. A distended bladder and suprapubic tenderness are signs of urinary retention, but these findings alone do not make the diagnosis. Pyuria of catheterized urine simply suggests infection. The presence of red blood cell casts in the urine suggests hematuria of an upper urinary tract etiology.

6

Neurologic Emergencies

I. Altered Mental Status

A. Overview

1. Definitions

—**Altered mental status (AMS)** is an imprecise term that may denote delirium, dementia, or coma.

—**Delirium** is an altered or fluctuating level of consciousness, with or without global cognitive impairment, usually of acute onset.

—**Dementia** is altered cognitive function with preserved consciousness, usually of gradual onset.

—**Coma** is defined as a state of unarousable unresponsiveness.

2. Causes of delirium and coma can be loosely divided into metabolic/toxic causes requiring medical management, organic brain lesion causes potentially requiring surgical management, and psychogenic causes requiring psychiatric consultation (Figure 6-1).

—A useful mnemonic for the causes of altered mental status is AEIOU TIPS:

—**A:** Alcohol and other toxins

—**E:** Endocrine and environmental factors

—**I:** Insulin poisoning

—**O:** Oxygen deprivation

—**U:** Uremia

—**T:** Trauma

—**I:** Infection

—**P:** Psychiatric causes and porphyria

—**S:** Space-occupying lesions

B. Clinical features

1. Symptoms may include:

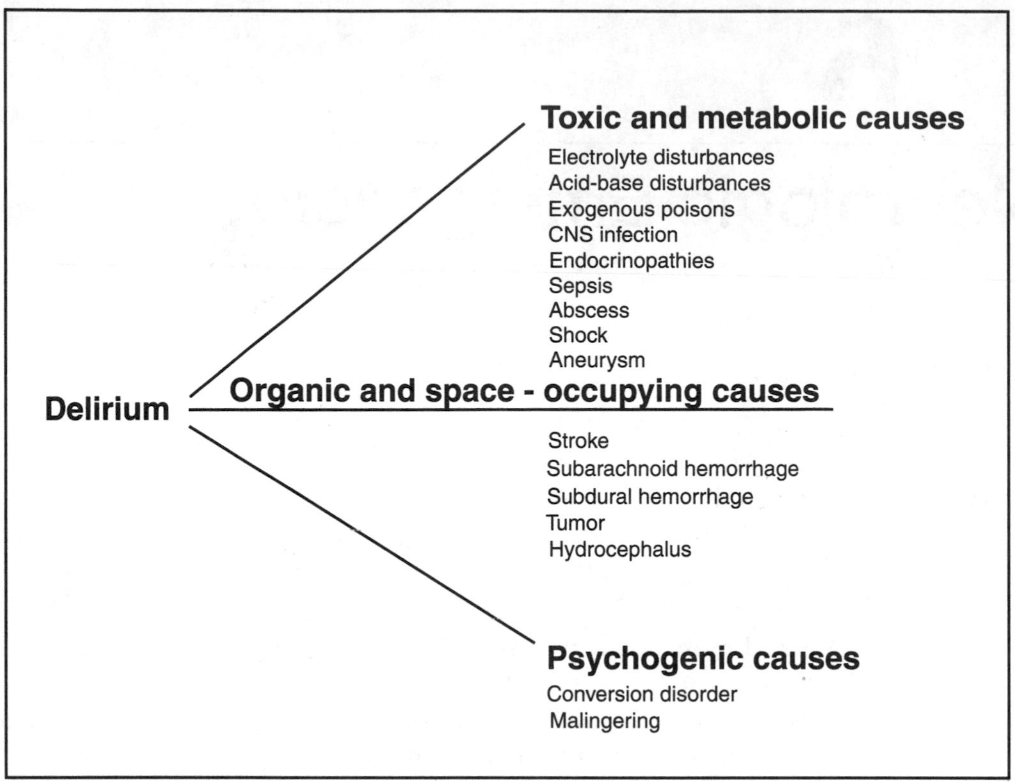

Figure 6-1. Causes of delirium. *CNS* = central nervous system.

—personality change

—vomiting

—headache

—dizziness

—confusion

—lethargy

2. **Physical examination findings may include:**

—**Skin:** pallor (anemia), jaundice (hepatic encephalopathy), cyanosis (hypoxemia), uremic frost (uremia), cherry red color (carbon monoxide poisoning), petechiae [(disseminated intravascular coagulation (DIC)], cold or hot temperature (hypo- or hyperthermia)

—**Breath:** acetone [diabetic ketoacidosis (DKA)], ethanol (see Table 18-2 in Chapter 18).

—**Pupils:** may be pinpoint (heroin), dilated (sympathomimetic), "blown" unilaterally with impaired extraocular movements (intracranial event, herniation). Metabolic coma usually preserves pupillary reaction and conjugate gaze. Oculocephalic (doll's eye) and oculovestibular (cold water) tests may be useful to document preservation of eye movements.

—**Funduscopic examination:** papilledema, diabetic or hypertensive retinopathy

—**Signs of head trauma:** raccoon eyes, Battle's sign (see Figure 17-2 in Chapter 17)

—**Disturbed respiratory pattern** (Table 6-1)

—**Tachycardia or bradycardia**

—**Fever** (sepsis/aspiration)

—**Asterixis** (hepatic encephalopathy; see Table 4-5 in Chapter 4)

C. Diagnostic tests

1. **Fingerstick glucose** determination to look for hypoglycemia
2. **Blood pressure** to look for hypertension, may be clue to elevated intracranial pressure (ICP)
3. **Pulse oximetry** to look for hypoxia
4. **CT scan** of the brain to look for space-occupying lesions, midline shift, intracranial bleed, elevated intracranial pressure
5. **Lumbar puncture (LP)** if meningitis is suspected or if subarachnoid hemorrhage is suspected and CT scan of the brain is negative

Table 6-1. Respiratory Patterns Associated With Altered Mental Status

Type of Respiration	Description	Associated With
Hypoventilation	< 8 breaths/min in an adult*	CNS depressants Renal coma (uremia) Diabetic coma ↑ intracranial pressure
Hyperventilation	> 18 breaths/min in an adult*	Hypoxia Metabolic acidosis Fever, sepsis Salicylate poisoning Hepatic coma
Kussmaul's	Deep, regular, sighing breathing Rate may be slow, normal, or fast	Diabetic ketoacidosis Uremia
Cheyne-Stokes (CSR)	Alternating periods of crescendo-decrescendo hyperventilation with apnea. Results in metabolic alkalosis. Patient not in imminent danger.	Bilateral cerebral disease Pre-transtentorial herniation Metabolic encephalopathy Upper brain stem lesions CHF, hypoxia
Cluster	Short-cycle CSR	Posterior fossa lesion ↑ intracranial pressure
Apneustic	Prolonged inspiratory pauses	Pontine infarctions
Ataxic or Biot's	Irregularly irregular rate and amplitude	Medullary lesions Pre–respiratory arrest

*Hypo- and hyperventilation rates for children are not specified because the normal respiratory rate in children varies by age.

6. **Arterial blood gas (ABG)** to look for acid–base disturbances
7. **Urinalysis** to look for bacteria (urosepsis) and calcium oxalate crystals (ethylene glycol poisoning)
8. **Liver function tests (LFTs)** if liver pathology is suspected
9. **Blood** and **urine cultures** if patient is febrile
10. **Coagulation studies** if disseminated intravascular coagulation (DIC) or thrombotic thrombocytopenic purpura (TTP) is suspected
11. **Complete blood count (CBC)** to look for infection, anemia, thrombocytopenia
12. **Toxicology** screen to look for toxins

D. **Treatment**

1. **Airway** secured
2. **Oxygen** by nonrebreather mask
3. **NTG** cocktail: naloxone 2 mg IV, thiamine 100 mg IV, glucose 25 mg IV
4. Charcoal and antidote if poisoning is known or suspected
5. Empiric **antibiotics** if meningitis is suspected (Table 6-2)

Table 6-2. Bacterial Etiologies of Meningitis by Age and Their Treatments

Age Group	Bugs	Drugs (IV)	Drugs (IV) for Penicillin-Allergic Patients	Consider Adding (all age groups):
<3 months of age (require follow up lumbar puncture in 24–36 hours)	Group B streptococci *Listeria* spp *Escherichia coli* *Klebsiella* spp *Enterobacter* spp *Staphylococcus aureus* *Haemophilus influenzae*	Ampicillin 50 mg/kg every 8 hours, AND Cefotaxime 50 mg/kg every 8 hours		For positive Gram stain or coma: Dexamethasone 0.4 g/kg every 12 hours for 2 days
3 months–50 years	*Streptococcus pneumoniae* *Neisseria meningitides* *H. influenzae*	Cefotaxime 2 g every 4–6 hours, OR Ceftriaxone 2 g every 12 hours	Vancomycin 15 mg/kg every 6 hours AND Gentamicin 2 mg/kg loading, then 1.7 mg/kg every 8 hours AND Rifampin 10–20 mg/kg every day	For drug-resistant *S. pneumoniae:* Vancomycin 15 mg/kg every 6 hours
> 50 years of age; debilitated or immunocompromised patients	*S. pneumoniae* *Listeria* spp Gram-negative bacteria	Ampicillin 2 g every 4 hours AND Cefotaxime 2 g every 4–6 hours OR Ceftriaxone 2 g every 12 hours		For drug-resistant *S. pneumoniae:* Vancomycin 15 mg/kg every 6 hours

IV = intravenous; *spp* = species.

6. Urgent neurosurgical consultation if warranted by CT scan findings

E. Disposition

—Disposition of the patient with delirium depends on the etiology. Refer to individual sections of the causes of delirium for specific dispositions.

II. Meningitis

A. Overview

1. Meningitis is an inflammation of the arachnoid and pia mater of the brain that may be caused by bacteria, viruses, or fungi.
2. The etiology of bacterial meningitis varies according to the age of the patient (see Table 6-2).
3. Viral meningitis generally has a less dramatic presentation and often has a more benign course than does bacterial meningitis.
4. Fungal meningitis usually is restricted to the immunocompromised host.

B. Clinical features

1. **Symptoms** may include:
   —**headache**
   —**stiff neck**
   —**fever**
   —chills
   —**photophobia**
   —**confusion**
   —phonophobia
   —nausea
   —vomiting
   —seizures (more common in children)
2. **Physical examination findings** may include:
   —irritable or floppy infant
   —**bulging fontanels** (due to increased ICP) in infants
   —tachycardia
   —tachypnea
   —fever > 38.3°C (101°F)
   —acutely ill-appearing patient
   —rash
   —petechiae
   —papilledema on funduscopic examination (not common)
   —hyperactive deep tendon reflexes
   —conjunctivitis, skin rash, and mouth sores (gonococcal meningitis)

—**Brudzinski sign:** flexion of hips and knees upon passive flexion of the neck

—**Kernig sign:** resistance to extension of knee when hip and knee are flexed to 90° angle in the supine patient

—Brudzinski and Kernig signs are highly suggestive for meningitis, but often are absent, especially in very young, very old, and immunocompromised patients

C. Diagnostic tests

1. **CBC** to look for leukocytosis
2. **Lumbar puncture**
   a. **Procedure:** an 18-gauge spinal needle is inserted into the L4 or L5 intervertebral space.
   b. **Opening pressure** is measured before collection of CSF. Normal opening pressures are < 20 mm H_20. Increased intracranial pressure can be seen in a variety of conditions, including pseudotumor cerebri, hydrocephalus, and brain stem herniation.
   c. Four tubes of fluid are collected:
      —Tube 1 is sent for cell count. In the event of a traumatic tap, a number of RBCs may be present. The presence of WBCs indicates infection.
      —Tube 2 is sent for glucose and protein content (Table 6-3).

Table 6-3. CSF Findings in Lumbar Puncture

	RBC	WBC; differential diagnosis (No./HPF)	Protein (mg/dl)	Glucose (mg/dl)	Appearance	Opening Pressure (mm H_2O)
Traumatic tap	Present, clear up by tube 4	Few or absent	Normal	Normal	Bloody, then clear	Normal
Subarachnoid hemorrhage	Many, *do not* clear up by tube 4 + xanthochromia	Few or absent	Normal	Normal	Bloody	High
Pseudotumor cerebri	Few or absent	Few or absent	Normal	Normal	Clear	Very high, 250–400
Bacterial meningitis	Few or absent, unless traumatic tap	Many, 2000–10,000; granulocytosis	High, >45	Low, <20	Turbid	High
Viral meningitis	Few or absent, unless traumatic tap	Many; lymphocytosis	Normal or slightly high	Normal	Clear	High
Tuberculous meningitis	Few or absent, unless traumatic tap	Many, 25–500; lymphocytosis	High, >45	Low, <20	Light yellow	High

CSF = cerebrospinal fluid; *HPF* = high-power field; *RBC* = red blood cells; *WBC* = white blood cells.

—Tube 3 is sent for Gram stain, culture and sensitivity, and serology.

—Tube 4 is sent for cell count. In the event of a traumatic tap, the number of RBCs will have decreased dramatically (to just a few cells) as compared to tube 1. If a significant number of RBCs still is present by tube 4, then subarachnoid hemorrhage must be suspected.

d. **Contraindications to LP** are infection/abscess of skin overlying the proposed puncture site and thrombocytopenia < 50,000. If the platelet count is < 20,000, platelets and/or fresh frozen plasma (FFP) should be administered before the tap. Platelets are contraindicated in TTP (see Chapter 15).

e. The most serious complication of the procedure is brain stem herniation.

3. **CT scan** of the brain should be performed before LP in the following situations:
   a. Suspected increase in intracranial pressure
   b. Change in level of consciousness or altered mental status
   c. Focal findings on neurologic examination
   d. New-onset seizure
   e. Recent head trauma (to rule out subarachnoid hemorrhage)

D. Treatment

1. **Viral** or **aseptic meningitis:** treatment is supportive and includes rest, increased fluids, a quiet darkened room, and analgesia as necessary. Certain drugs (e.g., carbamazepine, trimethoprim-sulfamethoxazole, metronidazole, and NSAIDs) may produce an aseptic meningitis picture. These should be discontinued if the patient has been taking them.
2. **Bacterial meningitis:** treatment depends on the causative organism, which varies depending on the age of the patient. Empiric therapies by age are summarized in Table 6-2.
3. **Prophylaxis** for bacterial meningitis is given to close contacts of the patient. Regimens include:
   a. Ciprofloxacin 500 mg orally, once
   b. Rifampin 10 mg/kg (children) or 600 mg (adults) every 12 hours for 4 doses
   c. Ceftriaxone 250 mg IM, once

E. Disposition

1. Patients who have bacterial meningitis or who appear toxic should be admitted to the hospital.
2. Patients with aseptic meningitis who appear well, are responsible, and are able to take care of themselves at home may be discharged home with analgesia and follow-up (with either primary care provider or return to ED) for repeat lumbar tap.

III. Pseudotumor Cerebri

A. Clinical features

1. **Symptoms** may include:

—**headache that is worst upon awakening;** improves as the day progresses; worsens with Valsalva, coughing, bending

—nausea

—relief after vomiting

2. **Physical examination findings** may include:

—**papilledema** on funduscopic examination

—sixth cranial nerve palsy

—**diplopia**

—**loss of acuity, visual field defects**

—tinnitus

B. Diagnostic tests

1. **CT scan** of the brain to look for signs of increased intracranial pressure in the absence of hydrocephalus or a mass lesion. Pseudotumor cerebri is a diagnosis of exclusion, so it is important to rule out other causes for clinical presentation.
2. **LP** to look for high opening pressure of 250–400 mm H_20. The CSF is otherwise normal. The procedure also is therapeutic.

C. Treatment

1. **Diuretic,** such as acetazolamide 250 mg orally 4 times a day
2. **Weight reduction** if patient is significantly over ideal body weight
3. **Optic nerve fenestration** if impending visual loss (in consultation with ophthalmology)
4. **Revision of patient's current medications** to look for any offending drugs
5. Dexamethasone 10 mg IV should be considered if cerebral edema is present acutely.

D. Disposition

—Once the diagnosis is made, the patient may be discharged home with outpatient referral to a neurologist.

IV. Normal Pressure Hydrocephalus

A. Overview

—Normal pressure hydrocephalus is a treatable cause of dementia.

—It often follows head trauma, SAH, or meningitis.

—It commonly is associated with a mass lesion.

B. Clinical features

1. **Symptoms** may include:

—the classic triad: **dementia, ataxic gait,** and **urinary incontinence**

—headache

—lethargy
—malaise
—ataxia
—**seizures** (more common in children)
—weakness

2. **Physical examination findings** may include:
—**no papilledema** on funduscopic examination
—altered mental status

C. Diagnostic tests

1. **CT scan** or **MRI** to look for enlarged ventricles without cerebral atrophy
2. **LP** to look for normal opening pressure

D. Treatment

1. Removal of 30 to 50 ml of CSF (CSF ventricular shunt)
2. Choroid plexectomy for papilloma (surgery)

E. Disposition

—Patients can be discharged home with outpatient referral to a neurologist.

V. Stroke

A. Overview

1. **Definitions**

—A **stroke** is a cerebrovascular accident that produces symptoms that last longer than 24 hours and usually results in permanent motor or sensory deficit. Figure 6-2 illustrates the different classifications of stroke.

—A **transient ischemic attack (TIA)** is a stroke the symptoms of which completely resolve within 24 hours and that does not result in any permanent deficit. TIAs are thought to herald an impending stroke and, therefore, deserve appropriate work-up.

2. **Causes**

a. **Thrombotic**
—Atherosclerosis
—Vasculitis
—Cerebral artery dissection
—Hypercoagulable states
—Syphilis
—Fibromuscular hyperplasia
—Cyanotic heart disease

b. **Embolic**
—Atrial fibrillation

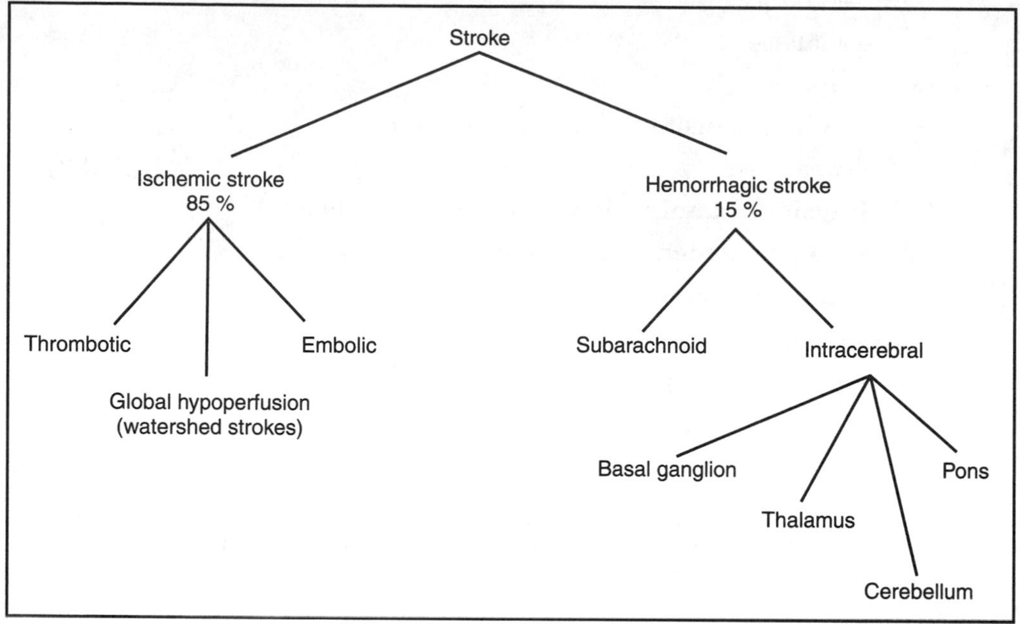

Figure 6-2. Classification of stroke.

—Myocardial infarction

—Cardiac arrhythmia

—Cardiac tumor (myxoma)

—Fat or septic emboli

c. **Hemorrhagic**

—Hypertension

—Arteriovenous malformation

—Amyloidosis

—Bleeding diathesis

—Iatrogenic anticoagulation

—Cocaine use

—Cigarette smoking

—Diabetes mellitus

B. Clinical features

1. **Thrombotic** ischemic stroke

—results from clot formation in a previously stenosed or otherwise damaged vessel.

—most commonly is caused by atherosclerosis.

—is marked by symptoms that wax and wane, develop over minutes to hours, and have a gradual onset.

—may occur in a patient who has had similar symptoms before (prior TIA) in the same distribution.

—may produce **carotid bruits,** noted on physical examination

2. **Embolic** ischemic stroke

—results from occlusion of a healthy distal vessel by intravascular material from a more proximal source.

—may occur in a patient with a history of prior TIAs in a different distribution.

—is marked by sudden onset of symptoms.

—**Atrial fibrillation** may be noted on ECG.

—Heart murmur and cutaneous signs of emboli such as Janeway lesions or Osler nodes (see Chapter 2 IX B) may be noted on physical examination.

3. **Hemorrhagic** stroke

—usually is associated with **hypertension.**

—is marked by sudden onset of symptoms.

—is accompanied by nausea, vomiting, headache, seizures, and coma more often than are other types.

—most commonly occur in the putamen.

—may have Cheyne-Stokes respiration noted with severe strokes.

—may lead to complications including seizures, increased intracranial pressure, hydrocephalus, and syndrome of inappropriate antidiuretic hormone (SIADH).

4. **Physical examination** findings in stroke depend on the vessel affected versus the type of stroke that occurred. Table 6-4 summarizes the signs and symptoms found in strokes of the major vessels.

Table 6-4. Patterns Seen in Stroke

Artery Affected	Deficit
Anterior cerebral	Sensorimotor loss on contralateral lower extremity, gait ataxia If B/L: abulia, primitive reflexes, bowel and bladder incontinence
Middle cerebral	Contralateral upper extremity hemiplegia Sometimes homonymous hemianopsia Left-sided lesion: language deficits, including aphasia, agraphia, dyslexia Right-sided lesion: spatial perception deficits, including hemineglect, prosopagnosia, asomatognosia, constructional apraxia
Posterior cerebral	Contralateral homonymous hemianopsia with macular sparing, CN III palsy If B/L: cortical blindness, visual agnosia
Internal carotid	Contralateral sensorimotor loss, ipsilateral blindness, aphasia, denial and hemineglect
Vertebrobasilar	Contralateral pain and temperature sense loss, ipsilateral paresthesias of face, diplopia, nystagmus, vertigo, dysarthria, dysphagia

B/L = bilateral; *CN* = cranial nerve.

C. Diagnostic tests

—Diagnostic testing is directed at confirming clinical suspicion of stroke as well as ruling out other etiologies for the neurologic deficits.

1. **Chemistry panel** to look for hypoglycemia and electrolyte abnormalities
2. **CT scan** of the brain to confirm presence of stroke and determine its etiology (ischemic vs. hemorrhagic). Hemorrhagic strokes larger than 1 cm and some ischemic events more than 6 hours old will be noted on CT. Many ischemic strokes can be visualized only on MRI in the first week.
3. Search for sources of thrombotic strokes:

   —**CBC** to look for polycythemia and/or thrombocytosis

   —Search (not necessarily in the ED) for indices of hypercoagulable states, including **antiphospholipid antibodies, antithrombin III, protein C,** and **protein S**

   —**Doppler ultrasound study of carotid artery** to look for carotid stenosis
4. Search for sources of embolic strokes:

   —**Electrocardiogram (ECG)** to look for atrial fibrillation, myocardial infarction (MI)

   —**Cardiac enzymes** to look for MI

   —**Echocardiogram** to look for valve vegetations and mural thrombi

   —Blood cultures if patient is febrile to look for endocarditis
5. Search for sources of hemorrhagic strokes:

   —**Coagulation studies** to look for a bleeding diathesis

   —**Toxicology screen** to look for cocaine or amphetamines

D. Treatment

—General supportive measures include **oxygen,** elevation of the head of the bed, and treatment of hypertension. Hypertension is treated with nitroprusside or labetalol, which can be easily titrated to a mean arterial pressure (MAP) of < 140 mm Hg.

1. **Thrombotic stroke**

   a. Anticoagulation with **heparin** if there is progressive worsening of neurologic symptoms

      —Loading dose: 80 U/kg bolus

      —Infusion: 18 U/kg per hour

   b. Prophylaxis

      —Aspirin 81 mg orally per day

      —Ticlopidine 250 mg orally per day

      —Clopidogrel 75 mg orally per day

   c. **Carotid endarterectomy** if stenosis is greater than 70% of carotid artery

   d. **Thrombolytic therapy**

      (i) Indications

      —Onset of symptoms within 3 hours of presentation

—No CT evidence of bleed

(ii) Dosing of recombinant TPA (rTPA): 0.9 mg/kg to a maximum dose of 90 mg

(iii) Contraindications

—Current or history of intracranial bleed

—Recent LP, arterial or central venous line

—Uncontrolled hypertension (HTN) (BP>185/110)

—Gastrointestinal (GI) or genitourinary (GU) bleed in last 21 days

—Presence of aneurysm or neoplasm

—Major neurologic deficit (risk outweighs possible benefit)

—Minor isolated neurologic deficit: sensory loss, dysarthria, mild weakness, mild ataxia

—Rapidly improving neurologic status

—Pregnant or lactating women

—Known bleeding diathesis (including iatrogenic anticoagulation)

2. Embolic stroke

a. Anticoagulation with **heparin** as for thrombotic stroke (see section V D 1 a)

b. Prophylaxis with ASA, ticlopidine, or clopidogrel as for thrombotic stroke (see section V D 1 b)

c. Treatment of any underlying endocarditis with antibiotics. Later valve replacement should be considered if necessary.

3. Hemorrhagic stroke

a. Control of hypertension (slowly) to prevent cerebral edema

—for dBP < 120: labetalol 10 mg IV over 2 minutes every 10–20 minutes, to a maximum dose of 150 mg

—for dBP > 120 or if labetalol not successful: nitroprusside 1.0–10.0 μg/kg/min

b. Mannitol and furosemide for increased intracranial pressure

c. Seizure prophylaxis: phenytoin loading dose 15–20 mg/kg IV or orally. Dosage for children and adults is the same.

E. Disposition

1. Patients with stroke are admitted to the hospital for monitoring of their neurologic status.

2. Patients with TIAs usually are admitted for work-up.

VI. Subarachnoid Hemorrhage

A. Overview

1. Definition

—A subarachnoid hemorrhage (SAH) is bleeding into the subarachnoid space and may occur as a result of trauma (more common) or spontaneously.

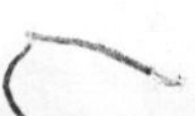

—The most common sites of hemorrhage are the internal carotid artery, the middle cerebral artery, and the anterior cerebral artery

2. **Causes** include:

—rupture of a saccular aneurysm (most common)

—arteriovenous malformation

—hypertension

—tumor

—blood dyscrasia

3. **Risk factors**

a. Substance abuse
—Ethanol
—Cocaine
—Cigarette smoking

b. Renal disease
—Polycystic kidney disease
—Fibromuscular dysplasia

c. Blood dyscrasias
—Sickle cell anemia
—Leukemia
—Hemophilia
—Thrombotic thrombocytopenic purpura

d. Vasculitis
—Systemic lupus erythematosus (SLE)
—Polyarteritis nodosa
—Henoch-Schönlein purpura

e. Collagen diseases
—Marfan syndrome
—Ehlers-Danlos syndrome
—Pseudoxanthoma elasticum

4. **Complications**

—Re-bleed

—Vasospasm

B. Clinical features

1. **Symptoms** may include:

—**sudden-onset headache: "thunderclap"** or **"worst headache of my life"**

—headache accompanied by stiff neck and photophobia (like meningitis)

—**loss of consciousness**

—**nausea, vomiting, and eye pain**

2. **Physical examination findings** may include:

—mental status ranging from alert and oriented x 3 to comatose

—positive Brudzinski and Kernig signs consistent with meningeal irritation

—**preretinal** or **subhyaloid hemorrhages** on funduscopic examination

3. Neurologic examination may reveal deficits that may help localize site of bleed (see section V)
4. Clinical status of patient may be classified as Grades I–V (Table 6-5).

C. Diagnostic tests

1. **CT scan** of the brain to look for blood in basal cisterns, sylvian fissure, intra- or extraparenchymal hematoma. Picks up 90% to 95% of positive bleeds. If clinical suspicion for SAH is high but CT is negative, then LP is mandatory to look for bleed.
2. **LP:** CSF on LP may be grossly bloody without significant drop in number of RBCs from tube 1 to tube 4. Supernatant will be xanthochromic 12 hours after bleed. High opening pressure, normal-high protein, and normal-low glucose also will be noted.
3. **Cerebral angiography** to look for aneurysms (gold standard)
4. **ECG** to look for broad inverted T waves and prolonged QT interval
5. CBC to look for leukocytosis
6. Urinalysis to look for proteinuria, glycosuria, and altered osmolarity as alternate reasons for patient's mental status

D. Treatment

1. **Immediate neurosurgical consult**
2. **Nimodipine** 60 mg orally every 4 hours for 21 days, start within 96 hours of SAH
3. **Dexamethasone** 10 mg IV, once, if significant edema is present
4. Norepinephrine, dopamine, or dobutamine to prevent hypotension
5. Nitroprusside, esmolol, or labetalol to prevent hypertension
6. Hyperventilation to a PCO_2 of 30–35 mm Hg to produce vasoconstriction and prevent cerebral edema
7. **Phenytoin** 15–18 mg/kg loading dose for seizure prophylaxis
8. Elevation of head of the bed to 30° if C-spine is not a concern.

E. Disposition

—Patients are admitted to the neurosurgical service.

Table 6-5. Classification of Subarachnoid Hemorrhage

Class	Symptoms and Signs
I	Mild headache +/− slight to no meningeal signs, no neurologic deficits
II	Severe headache, positive meningeal signs
III	Focal neurologic deficits, positive meningeal signs, confusion, lethargy
IV	Profoundly depressed level of consciousness, moderate to severe hemiparesis
V	Comatose with flaccidity or abnormal posturing

VII. Headache

—Causes are multiple; see discussions of migraine, cluster, and tension headaches that follow.

—Meningitis (section II), pseudotumor cerebri (section III), subarachnoid hemorrhage (section VI), and trigeminal neuralgia (section XI) are covered elsewhere in this chapter.

—Temporal arteritis is discussed in Chapter 11, I G.

—Acute angle closure glaucoma is discussed in Chapter 7, XXIV.

—Subdural and epidural hematomas are discussed in Chapter 17, II C.

—Other causes include post-lumbar headache, CNS masses and infections, and substance abuse or withdrawal.

A. Clinical features

—Figure 6-3 maps the distribution of pain for migraine, cluster, and tension headaches.

1. Migraine headaches

a. Types. There are two main variants of migraine headaches:

—Migraine may occur with a preceding aura **(classic migraine),** which is less common, or without an aura **(common migraine).**

—Auras are associated with **visual** or **olfactory disturbances** including scotomas, hemianopsia and, sometimes, hallucinations.

b. Incidence

—Migraines are more common in women by a ratio of 3 to 1.

—Approximately 75% of patients with migraine headaches have a **positive family history.**

c. Clinical features

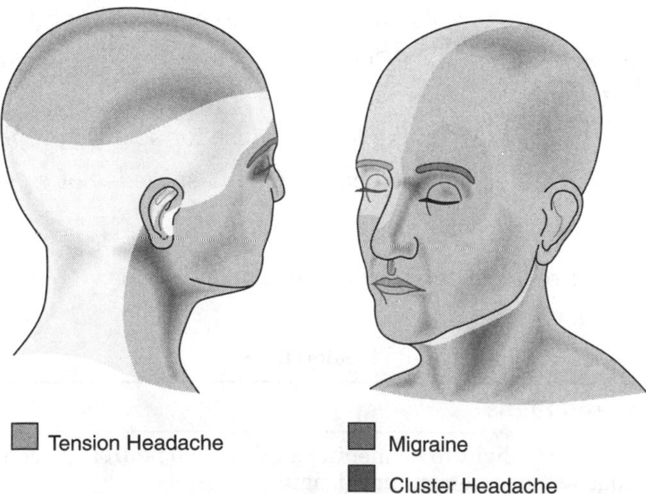

Figure 6-3. Map of the patterns of pain seen in migraine, cluster, and tension headache. (Adapted from LifeART Emergency Medicine Professional Collection. Copyright 1998, Lippincott Williams & Wilkins. All rights reserved.)

—Pain usually is **unilateral** and **pulsating,** and lasts from a few hours to a few days.

—Headache may be associated with **nausea, vomiting, photophobia,** phonophobia, lightheadedness, and vertigo.

—Headache is aggravated by physical activity.

—Headaches resolve on their own, often during sleep.

—Attacks may be precipitated or exacerbated by caffeine, excessive sleep, alcohol, specific foods, or emotional stress.

2. Cluster headache

—Cluster headaches are more common in men in their 30s, by a ratio of 6 to 1.

—Pain usually is **unilateral, piercing,** or **"exploding,"** localized to periorbital and oculofrontal areas (ocular cluster).

—Cluster headache lasts from 30 minutes to 3 hours.

—There are two main variants: episodic and chronic. In the episodic form, the attack-free interval is several months, whereas in the chronic form the attack-free interval is less than 1 week.

—Headache may be associated with ipsilateral lacrimation, ptosis, **nasal congestion, rhinorrhea,** nausea, bradycardia, and diaphoresis.

—Attacks may be precipitated or exacerbated by alcohol, bright lights, emotional stress, and (in women) menstrual cycle.

—Cluster headaches are not associated with a strong family history.

3. Tension headache

—There are two variants: episodic and chronic. The episodic variant is associated with an isolated stressor and generally is self limited. The chronic variant tends to occur daily and is associated with contraction of neck musculature.

—Pain is **bilateral,** of **dull, aching quality** in a bandlike distribution with varying intensity over the course of the day.

—Headache is associated with **insomnia, bruxism** (grinding of teeth), and tight neck muscles.

—Tension headache is not aggravated by physical activity.

—Tension headache is **associated with depression,** anxiety, poor posture, and excess caffeine intake.

—40% have **positive family history**

B. Diagnostic tests

—If the etiology of the headache is clear, laboratory testing is unnecessary.

—If underlying pathology is ambiguous, testing to rule out more serious causes may be warranted. Such tests include:

1. **CT scan** of the brain to look for increased intracranial pressure
2. LP puncture to look for meningitis
3. **Erythrocyte sedimentation rate (ESR)** to look for temporal arteritis if headache is temporal (see Chapter 11, I G)

4. CBC to look for infection
5. Radiographs of C-spine to look for injury (in cases of tension headache)
6. Radiographs of sinuses to look for sinusitis

C. Treatment

a. For all forms of headache, the following supportive measures often are helpful:

—Rest in a quiet, dark room

—Cold compresses over the eyes

—Hot shower

—Massage

—Biofeedback

b. Specific treatments vary for different types of headache.

1. Migraine headache

a. Treatment

—**Metoclopramide** 10 mg IV (first-line therapy)

—**Sumatriptan** 6 mg subcutaneously (also available as a nasal spray). Must be avoided in coronary artery disease (CAD), peripheral vascular disease (PVD), uncontrolled hypertension, and within 2 weeks of monoamine oxidase inhibitor (MAOI) usage.

—**Dihydroergotamine** (DHE) 1 mg IV (maximum 2 g/24 h) or IM (3 g/24 h). Pretreatment with prochlorperazine or metoclopramide to avoid nausea.

—**Ergotamine–caffeine** suppositories (2 mg) or tablets (1 mg) to a maximum of 6 mg/attack or 10 mg/week.

—**Acetaminophen** (500 mg)–**butalbital** (250 mg) combination: 1–2 capsules every 4 hours as needed, to a maximum of 6 capsules per 24 hours

b. Prophylaxis

—β-blockers: atenolol 50–100 mg orally per day or propranolol 80–320 mg orally per day

2. Cluster headaches

a. Treatment

—Use of opiates for analgesia must be avoided

—**100% oxygen** via nonrebreather mask for first 10–15 minutes of attack

—Sumatriptan 6 mg subcutaneously, to a maximum of 12 mg/24 h

—Dihydroergotamine 1 mg IM or IV

b. Prophylaxis

—Verapamil 80 mg orally 4 times a day during waking hours

—Lithium 600–1200 mg orally per day

—Methysergide 4–10 mg orally 3 or 4 times per day

3. Tension headache

a. Treatment

—NSAIDs (see Table 11-2 in Chapter 11)

b. **Prophylaxis**

—**Tricyclic antidepressants** for chronic variants

—β-blockers as for migraine headache (see section VII C 1 b)

D. **Disposition**

1. Most patients with headache in whom hemorrhage has been ruled out can be discharged home with outpatient neurology follow-up.
2. Patients who require IV medication for pain control or who have intractable vomiting are admitted to the hospital.

VIII. Seizures

A. **Overview**

1. **Definition**

—A seizure is a burst of electrical activity from the brain that results in involuntary movement, loss of consciousness, or both. Table 6-6 presents the classification of seizures.

2. **Risk factors**

a. **Serum electrolyte disturbances**

—Sodium < 120 mEq or >160 mEq

—Glucose < 60 mEq/L

—Magnesium < 1 mEq/L

—Calcium < 7 mEq/L

Table 6-6. Classification and Characteristics of Seizures

Generalized
(always LOC)
Convulsive (tonic clonic)
Postictal state
Urinary incontinence may occur
Tongue biting may occur
Nonconvulsive (absence, myoclonic)
Typical: no postictal state
Atypical: postictal state

Partial
Simple partial
No LOC
Focal clonic movements
Usually no postictal state
Visual/auditory/gustatory hallucinations
Déjà vu phenomenon
Ipsilateral signs, gaze away from side of seizure
Complex partial (psychomotor, temporal lobe seizure)
Higher cortical function preserved
Amnesia for ictal event
Postictal state common
Associated with an aura

LOC = loss of consciousness.

b. **Drugs**

—Amphetamines

—Cocaine

—PCP

—Ethanol

—TCAs

—Aspirin

—Theophylline

—Isoniazid

—Lithium

c. **Inborn errors of metabolism**

—Cerebral palsy

—Other congenital disorders

d. **CNS infections**

—Meningitis

—Encephalitis

—Human immunodeficiency virus (HIV)

—Syphilis

e. **Stress**

—Excessive sleep deprivation

—Posttraumatic stress (usually within first 24 hours)

f. **Miscellaneous**

—CVA

—CNS tumor

—Hypertensive encephalopathy

—Severe hypoxemia

B. Clinical features

—In general, seizures have **abrupt onset** and **last 1–5 minutes.** The postictal period, which is a period of altered mental status, can last up to 30 minutes.

—Unrecognized seizures may present as blank spells, unexplained injuries, and nocturnal tongue biting.

—**Status epilepticus** is defined as seizures lasting > 30 minutes or two or more seizures **without a lucid interval** in between.

C. Diagnostic tests

—Little testing is required if the patient has a well-documented history of seizure and the presentation is typical for this patient.

1. **Anticonvulsant drug blood level** should be checked. The level may be subtherapeutic if there has been:

—a recent change in dose

—a missed dose

—a change from brand-name to generic form

—addition of new medication that works via P_{450} system, accelerating clearance of the anticonvulsant

2. **Radiographs** to look for suspected fractures: posterior shoulder dislocations may occur during seizures and often are overlooked.
3. **Chemistry panel** to look for electrolyte disturbances
4. **Toxicology screen** if drug abuse is suspected
5. Theophylline level if patient is on this medication
6. **CT scan** or MRI of the brain if neurologic status is deteriorating or this is the first seizure presentation for the patient
7. Serum bicarbonate and prolactin levels to distinguish pseudo-seizures (levels are normal) from true seizures (HCO_3 is low, prolactin is high)

D. Treatment

1. Restraints as necessary to protect from self-injury
2. Patient side-turned to prevent aspiration in the event of vomiting
3. Airway secured once seizure stops
4. **Thiamin** (100 mg) and **glucose** (25–50 g) for hypoglycemic patients
5. Correction of any other electrolyte abnormalities
6. For status epilepticus and refractory seizures:
   a. **Diazepam**
      —Adults: 0.2–0.5 mg/kg IV every 15–30 minutes until seizures stop or maximum dose is reached. Maximum dose is 30 mg.
      —Children: 0.05–0.3 mg/kg every 15–30 minutes IM, IV or per rectum, until seizures stop or maximum dose is reached. Maximum dose: 5 mg for children under 5 years, 10 mg for children over 5 years.
   b. **Phenytoin**
      —Loading dose for both adults and children is 15–20 mg/kg IV slowly over 20–30 minutes
      —Phenytoin is not given IM due to erratic absorption
      —Must not be mixed with any glucose-containing IV fluid because it will precipitate
      —Hypotension and QRS widening possible
      —Fosphenytoin, a newer formulation of phenytoin, can be given IM or IV 3 times more rapidly.
   c. **Phenobarbital**
      —Loading dose for adults and children is 15–20 mg/kg IV. Maximum dose is 30 mg/kg.
      —Hypotension and respiratory depression are possible side effects.
   d. **Vitamin B_6 (pyridoxine)** for isoniazid-induced seizures. May be given empirically for refractory seizures. Dosages are 5 g IV, once, for adults and 10–50 mg IV, once, for children.
7. If patient continues to seize despite all of these measures, he or she should be intubated and general anesthesia should be administered.

E. Disposition

1. Patients with status epilepticus should be admitted for observation and airway management.
2. Patients with first-time seizure should be admitted for work-up.
3. A patient with previously diagnosed seizures who presents with an episode that is typical for that patient and responds to ED treatment can be discharged home with outpatient follow-up.

IX. Syncope

A. Clinical features may include:

—history of loss of consciousness

—no postictal state

B. Diagnostic tests

1. **CT scan of the brain** to look for cerebrovascular accident (CVA) or bleed
2. **ECG** to look for cardiac arrhythmia, particularly heart block
3. **Chemistry panel** to look for hypoglycemia and hyponatremia

C. Treatment

1. Electrolyte replacement as needed
2. Reassurance

D. Disposition

1. Patients who are stable may be discharged home with outpatient follow-up and Holter monitor.
2. Patients who are not at their baseline mental status should be admitted for further work-up.

X. Vertigo

—Vertigo is the subjective sensation that one is spinning in relation to one's surroundings.

—It has many causes (Figure 6-4).

A. Clinical features

1. **Peripheral vertigo**

—Acute onset, sometimes history of upper respiratory tract infection

—Intense dizziness, spinning or swaying sensation

—Nausea, vomiting, and diaphoresis common

—Hearing loss and tinnitus common

—Aggravated by position changes

—Nystagmus is **unidirectional,** horizontal, **fatigable,** and inhibited by ocular fixation

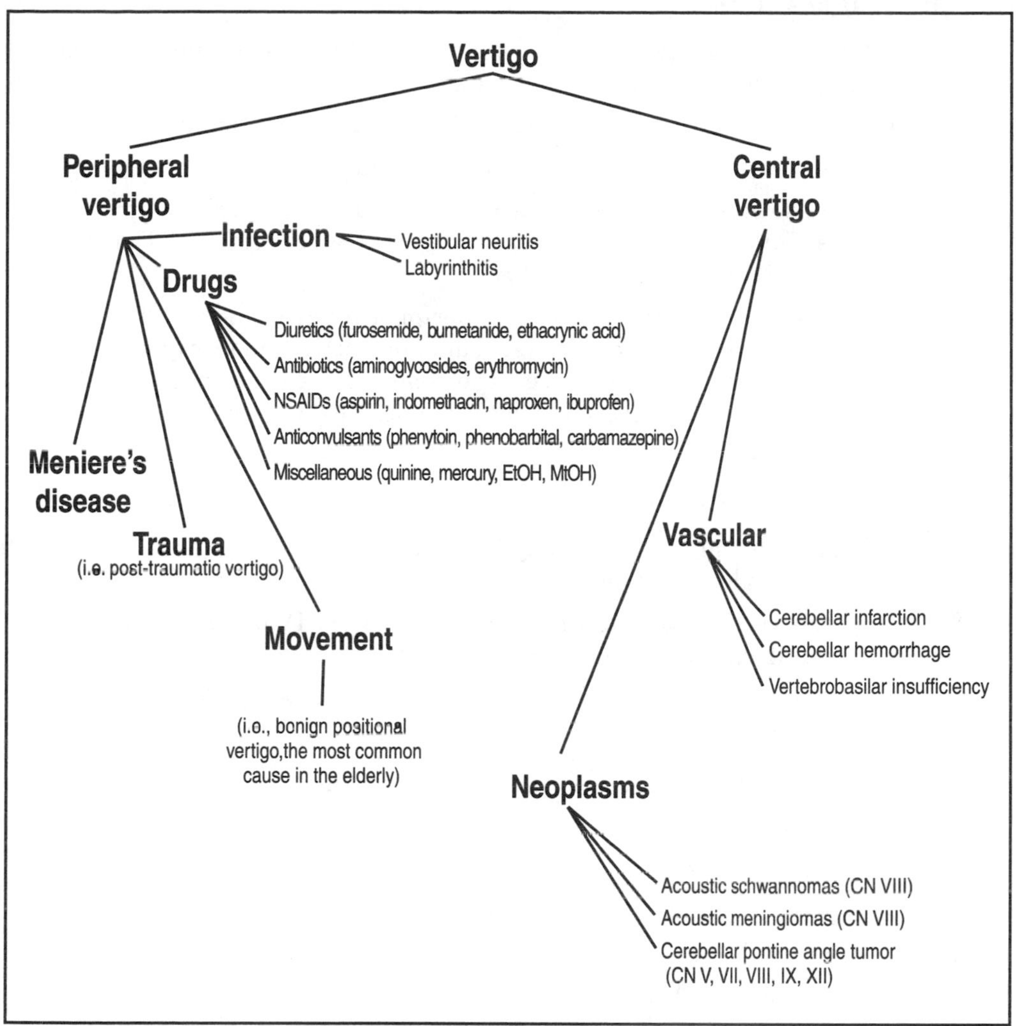

Figure 6-4. Causes of vertigo. *ASA* = aspirin; *CN* = cranial nerve; *EtOH* = ethanol; *MtOH* = methanol; *NSAIDs* = nonsteroidal antiinflammatory drugs

—Focal neurologic deficits uncommon

2. **Central vertigo**

—Gradual onset

—Generally less intense, vague symptoms

—Nausea, vomiting, diaphoresis uncommon

Hearing loss uncommon

—Not as affected by position changes and movement

—Neurologic deficits such as ataxia, hemiparesis, diplopia, dysphagia, or facial palsy may be noted

—Nystagmus is **multidirectional, nonfatigable,** and not inhibited by ocular fixation

B. Diagnostic tests

—Laboratory testing in cases of vertigo is not necessary unless the cause of the patient's "dizziness" is ambiguous.

1. CBC to look for leukocytosis, lymphocytosis and anemia
2. Chemistry panel to look for hypoglycemia
3. **MRI** to look for cerebellopontine angle tumors, cerebellar and posterior fossa infarcts, and hemorrhages. If MRI is not available, CT is acceptable to look for posterior fossa CVA.
4. **Barany maneuver** to look for peripheral vertigo. A positive test is defined as the presence of nystagmus or vertigo upon rapidly sitting up from the supine position with the head lifted and rotated 45° to the side. The test can be repeated to see if nystagmus is fatigable.

C. Treatment

1. Peripheral vertigo

   —Antihistamines: diphenhydramine 25–50 mg IM once, then orally, every 6 hours as needed

   —Antivertigo: **meclizine** 25 mg orally, IM, or IV per day as needed or **dimenhydrinate** 50 mg orally, IM, or IV

   —Antiemetics: promethazine 25–50 mg orally every 4–6 hours

2. Central vertigo

   —Neurology and neurosurgery consultations

D. Disposition

1. For peripheral vertigo:

   —Most patients can be discharged home with outpatient follow-up with an otorhinolaryngologist.

2. For central vertigo:

   —Patient is admitted to the hospital for work-up.

XI. Trigeminal Neuralgia

A. Overview

1. **Definition**

   —Trigeminal neuralgia, also known as **tic douloureux,** is a condition that results in paroxysms of pain along the distribution of the trigeminal nerve.

2. **Causes**

   —Idiopathic

   —Secondary to cerebellopontine angle tumors

   —Secondary to multiple sclerosis

B. Clinical features

1. **Symptoms** may include:

—**electric, shooting** kind of **pain in V2 distribution** of face (V1 and V3 also may be involved)

—pain that usually is **unilateral** (bilateral in 4% of cases)

—pain that lasts several seconds, followed by refractory period

—triggered by specific activities that employ facial muscles, such as applying cosmetics, eating, talking, smiling, crying, being tickled, and application of heat or cold

—decreased food intake and consequent weight loss from avoidance of above activities

—symptoms rarely occur at night

2. **No deficits are noted on physical examination.**

C. Diagnostic tests

—MRI to look for cerebellopontine angle tumors

D. Treatment

1. IV opiate analgesia for short-term pain relief
2. **Carbamazepine** 200 mg orally 3 times a day and **baclofen** 10 mg orally 3 times a day to prevent recurrence.
3. If medical treatment fails, surgical ablation of involved nerve branch can be considered.

E. Disposition

—Most patients can be discharged home following relief of the pain with outpatient follow-up.

XII. Multiple Sclerosis

—Multiple sclerosis is a disease in which demyelination of CNS axons occurs. It is most commonly seen in women in their twenties.

A. Clinical features

1. **Symptoms** may include:

—facial pain and **numbness**

—visual disturbances, including double vision and color blindness

—orbital pain with eye movement

—**urinary incontinence**

—general weakness

—tremor

—trigeminal neuralgia

2. **Physical examination findings** may include:

—**inability to explain the multiple neurologic deficits with a single lesion (key finding)**

—**optic neuritis**

—decreased motor strength

—facial nerve palsy

—**internuclear ophthalmoplegia**

—decreased vibration and position sense

—dysphagia

B. Diagnostic tests

—Multiple sclerosis is not an emergency department diagnosis, but its presence may be suspected clinically and should be considered in patients who present with neurologic deficits and complaints of such deficits in whom routine laboratory testing and even CT scan may be normal.

—The emergency physician's role in multiple sclerosis is to rule out a cerebrovascular or metabolic cause for the weakness, and to keep the differential diagnosis in mind and make the appropriate referral.

—LP may demonstrate **oligoclonal bands** in the CSF.

C. Treatment

—There is no cure for multiple sclerosis, so treatment (especially in the emergency department [ED]) is symptomatic.

1. Carbamazepine and baclofen for trigeminal neuralgia pain
2. Stool softeners for constipation
3. Neurology consult
4. Steroids—may be of benefit in some patients (given in conjunction with neurologist)

D. Disposition

—Patients can be discharged home with referral to a neurologist.

XIII. Myasthenia Gravis

—Myasthenia gravis is a disease in which antibodies to the acetylcholine (ACh) receptors are made, producing weakness of face and upper extremity muscles, especially upon repetitive stimulation.

—Although frustrating, it rarely is life-threatening (respiratory complications are unlikely), and mortality from the disease is low.

A. Clinical features

1. **Symptoms** may include:

   —weakness of face and upper extremity muscles

   —frequent eye blinking

   —difficulty chewing food

   —easy fatigability

2. **Physical examination findings** may include:

   —**fatigue produced by repetitive muscle stimulation**

   —facial muscle weakness

—ophthalmoplegia

—dysarthria

—dysphagia

B. **Diagnostic tests**

1. **Thyroid function tests (TFTs)** to look for thyroid dysfunction
2. **Anti-ACh receptor antibody** if diagnosis not previously made (outpatient)
3. **Edrophonium (Tensilon) test:** administration of this cholinesterase inhibitor produces marked improvement of symptoms. It is both therapeutic (short-term) and diagnostic.
4. Chest radiograph or CT scan of chest to look for thymoma

C. **Treatment**

1. Initial diagnosis and initiation of therapy is not done in the ED.
2. In previously diagnosed patients, the following may be administered for temporary relief (usually in consultation with neurology):

—**Pyridostigmine** 2 mg every 3 hours IM or IV or 60 mg orally every 6 hours

—**Dexamethasone** 10 mg IV, once

D. **Disposition**

—Reassurance and referral to a neurologist for outpatient management

XIV. Guillain-Barré Syndrome

A. **Overview**

1. **Definition**

—Guillain-Barré syndrome is an acute ascending demyelinating peripheral neuropathy, and the most common cause of acute neuromuscular paralysis.

2. **Incidence**

—An increased incidence of the disease is seen in elderly, postoperative, or pregnant patients and patients with Hodgkin's disease.

3. **Risk factors**

—Recent rabies or swine flu vaccination

—Certain drugs, such as gold, penicillamine, gangliosides, streptokinase, and captopril

B. **Clinical features**

—The typical presentation is acute-onset limb weakness preceded by a respiratory or gastrointestinal viral illness (especially with *C. jejuni*) 2 to 3 weeks earlier.

1. **Symptoms** may include:

—acute onset

—low back pain

—shoulder and thigh pain

—**ascending symmetric limb weakness**

2. **Physical examination findings** may include:

—**decreased deep tendon reflexes** in lower extremities (reflexes may be normal but, if increased, the diagnosis is extremely unlikely to be Guillain-Barré syndrome)

—decreased motor strength of lower extremities (ascending)

—decreased pain, vibration and position sense (ascending)

—usually no meningeal signs

—signs of autonomic dysfunction: labile BP, tachycardia, facial flushing

—**bulbar variant:** dysarthria, dysphagia, facial diplegia, descending paralysis

—**Miller-Fisher variant:** ophthalmoplegia, ataxia, areflexia, but no limb weakness

C. Diagnostic tests

1. **Lumbar puncture** to look for **increased CSF protein** with normal cell count and normal opening pressure
2. Peak flow or spirometry to assess respiratory effort
3. **Serologic testing** to look for prior infection with HIV, Epstein-Barr virus (EBV), or cytomegalovirus (CMV)
4. **Gadolinium MRI** of lumbar spine to look for enhancement of cauda equina roots (usually not done in ED)
5. **Nerve conduction studies** to look for decreased velocity, which may persist for months after clinical recovery (usually not done in ED)

D. Treatment

1. Neurology consult
2. Plasmapheresis
3. **Intravenous gamma globulins** decelerate the course of the disease and should be given especially to patients who cannot walk secondary to extreme lower extremity weakness.
4. Mechanical ventilation if respiratory muscle paralysis is present
5. Aspiration precautions
6. Analgesia as needed
7. Steroids have not been shown to be of any benefit.

E. Disposition

—Patients with Guillain-Barré syndrome should be admitted to the hospital for observation and management of the airway.

XV. Bell's Palsy

A. Overview

1. Definition

—Bell's palsy is palsy of the seventh cranial nerve. It may be peripheral or central.

2. Causes

—Idiopathic

—Lyme disease

—HIV

—Herpes

—Mumps

—Tumor

B. Clinical features

1. **Symptoms** may include:

—sudden-onset facial numbness

—unilateral symptoms

—hyperacusis

—impaired taste

—fullness or pain behind the mastoid

—decreased or increased tearing

2. **Physical examination findings** may include:

—inability to close eye on affected side

—less blinking on affected side

—sagging of eyelid on affected side

—intact corneal reflex

—edge of mouth appears drawn to contralateral side of insult

C. Diagnostic tests

1. CT scan of the brain to look for CVA or tumor
2. Viral serology if history is suggestive

D. Treatment

1. Reassurance that the condition will most likely resolve
2. Lubricating eye drops and eye patch to prevent corneal abrasion
3. **Prednisone** 30 mg orally 4 times a day for 5 days. May also give a tapered regimen.
4. Treatment for underlying etiology

E. Disposition

—Patients can be discharged home with outpatient follow-up with a neurologist or an otorhinolaryngologist.

Review Test

1. A 27-year-old woman presents with severe headache, stiff neck, and general malaise. Lumbar puncture reveals a pink CSF with few white blood cells, a normal protein, and glucose. You spin tubes 1 and 4 for cell count and obtain a yellowish supernatant in each. Which of the following is the most likely diagnosis?

(A) Traumatic tap
(B) Viral meningitis
(C) Subarachnoid hemorrhage
(D) Pseudotumor cerebri
(E) Tuberculous meningitis

2. Which of the following findings is diagnostic for pseudotumor cerebri?

(A) Papilledema
(B) Cranial nerve II, IV, or VI palsy
(C) Relief of headache after vomiting
(D) Increased intracranial pressure per CT scan
(E) None of the above

3. A 77-year-old man with past medical history significant for hypertension and coronary artery disease presents with sudden onset of right hemiparesis and dysarthria, which have become progressively worse over the past 5 hours. Which of the following is the most likely site of the lesion?

(A) Left middle cerebral artery
(B) Right middle cerebral artery
(C) Left anterior cerebral artery
(D) Right anterior cerebral artery
(E) Left vertebrobasilar artery

4. A 21-year-old woman presents with a severe left-sided headache of several hours' duration. She describes the pain as throbbing, and states that the previous evening she noted flashing lights. She has had these headaches before, and her mother and aunt have similar headaches. Which of the following is the most likely diagnosis?

(A) Cluster headache
(B) Subarachnoid hemorrhage
(C) Tension headache
(D) Migraine headache
(E) Pseudotumor cerebri

5. A 37-year-old woman presents with sudden-onset vertigo associated with right-sided hearing loss, nausea, vomiting, and a sense of loss of balance. She reports that she had an upper respiratory tract infection 2 weeks ago. Physical examination reveals a unidirectional fatigable nystagmus, and decreased hearing in her right ear. Which of the following diagnoses is most likely?

(A) Acute labyrinthitis
(B) Cerebellar pontine angle tumor
(C) Vestibular neuronitis
(D) Vertebrobasilar insufficiency
(E) Benign positional vertigo

6. A 48-year-old woman presents with acute vertigo, nausea, vomiting, hearing loss, and ringing in her left ear, which feels "full." She has a history of such attacks for the past 2 years. The attacks last about an hour and then resolve. Which of the following diagnoses is most likely?

(A) Benign positional vertigo
(B) Recurrent otitis media
(C) Posttraumatic vertigo
(D) Meniere's disease
(E) Vestibular neuronitis

7. A 33-year-old woman presents with complaints of weakness and tingling of her left side for 3 days. Three months ago she had right eye pain and blurred vision. One month ago she had an episode of urinary incontinence. Which of the following diagnoses is most likely?

(A) Guillain-Barré syndrome
(B) Viral syndrome
(C) Peripheral neuropathy
(D) Transient ischemic attack
(E) Multiple sclerosis

Directions: The response options for Items 8–11 are the same. You will be required to select one answer for each item in the set.

Questions 8–11

Match each description with the correct disease.

(A) Guillain-Barré syndrome
(B) Bell's palsy
(C) Myasthenia gravis
(D) Trigeminal neuralgia

8. Acute ascending peripheral neuropathy with symmetric limb weakness, frequently follows a viral illness

9. Acute unilateral severe facial pain, absence of neurologic deficits

10. Acute peripheral neuropathy with asymmetric involvement of face, often follows a viral illness

11. Facial muscle weakness, fatigability with repeated use

Answers and Explanations

1-C. The yellowish supernatant obtained is called xanthochromia, which is pathognomonic for subarachnoid hemorrhage. This yellowish color is not to be confused with the straw yellow color of cerebrospinal fluid (CSF) (unspun) seen in tuberculous meningitis. A traumatic tap also may present as a pink or red CSF, but this color and the number of red blood cells (RBCs) clear up by the last tube, and there is no xanthochromia. See Table 6-3 for more information on CSF findings in lumbar puncture.

2-E. Pseudotumor cerebri is a diagnosis of exclusion, so there are no findings that are diagnostic or pathognomonic for it. All choices listed are features of the disease, which is noted especially in young, overweight women. Differential diagnosis includes other causes for increased intracranial pressure such as papillitis, malignant hypertensive retinopathy, central retinal vein occlusion, ischemic optic neuropathy, vasculitis of the optic disc, sarcoid or tuberculous granuloma, or other tumor.

3-A. Contralateral hemiparesis and language deficits are seen with middle cerebral artery (MCA) lesions. Because the hemiparesis is on the right side of the body, the lesion is on the left side of the brain. Lesions of the anterior cerebral artery also can produce hemiparesis, but there usually are no associated language deficits. Homonymous hemianopsia also may be seen with MCA strokes. Vertebrobasilar artery strokes generally present with contralateral pain and temperature loss, not motor deficit.

4-D. This patient's presentation and history are typical of migraine headache (see section VII). Cluster headache is more common in men, and tension headache usually is bilateral. Subarachnoid hemorrhage is always a possibility and should be ruled out with CT scan and lumbar puncture if CT scan is negative. Pseudotumor cerebri is a diagnosis of exclusion, and usually is not accompanied by auras or a family history.

5-A. The sudden onset of the vertigo and unidirectional fatigable nystagmus suggest a peripheral cause of vertigo, which eliminates cerebellar pontine angle tumor and vertebrobasilar insufficiency. Benign positional vertigo is a diagnosis of exclusion, and is more common in the elderly. This leaves acute labyrinthitis and vestibular neuronitis. These can be distinguished by the fact that vestibular neuronitis does not present with hearing loss, which this patient does have; therefore, the diagnosis is acute labyrinthitis.

6-D. Meniere's disease is characterized by a triad of vertigo, tinnitus, and hearing loss. The vertigo of benign positional vertigo lasts only a few seconds, whereas in Meniere's disease it lasts for hours. Recurrent otitis media rarely produces acute vertigo and tinnitus, and also is uncommon in this patient's age group. Posttraumatic vertigo occurs post trauma, which is irrelevant in this chronic presentation. Vestibular neuronitis usually does not present with hearing loss.

7-E. Multiple sclerosis is best characterized by multiple neurologic deficits that cannot be accounted for by a single lesion. This patient's age and presentation are quite typical of MS. Although MS is a diagnosis of exclusion, MRI may demonstrate suggestive lesions and CSF studies may reveal oligoclonal bands. Guillain-Barré syndrome is an acute ascending neuropathy that usually follows a viral illness by a few weeks and does not match this patient's history or physical examination findings. A viral syndrome rarely produces this cluster of neurologic deficits. A peripheral neuropathy would not result in urinary incontinence. In a transient ischemic attack, symptoms resolve in 24 hours, by definition.

8-A. Guillain-Barré syndrome is an acute ascending peripheral neuropathy with symmetric limb weakness, which frequently follows a viral illness

9-D. Trigeminal neuralgia is characterized by acute unilateral severe facial pain and an absence of neurologic deficits.

10-B. Bell's palsy is an acute peripheral neuropathy with asymmetric involvement of the face, and often follows a viral illness.

11-C. Myasthenia gravis is characterized by facial muscle weakness and fatigability with repeated use.

7

Ocular Emergencies

I. Background

—Eye problems are a common reason for emergency department (ED) visits. Understanding the anatomy of the eye (Figure 7-1) allows for classification of these problems according to location of the injury. Evaluation of the eye begins with a thorough physical examination (Table 7-1) in addition to visual acuity testing (Figure 7-2).

II. Iritis

A. Overview

1. Definition

—Iritis is inflammation of the iris.

2. Risk factors

—Sarcoidosis

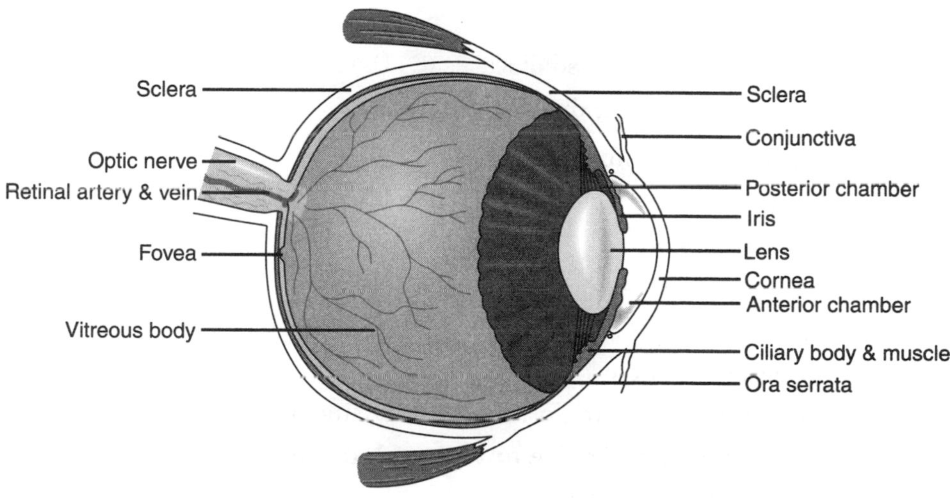

Figure 7-1. Anatomy of the eye. (From LifeART Super Anatomy 1 Collection. Copyright 1998, Lippincott Williams & Wilkins. All rights reserved.)

Table 7-1. Physical Examination of the Eye

Visual acuity testing
Vision is tested with patient's corrective lenses on, one eye at a time.
If patient does not have corrective lenses with him or her, pinhole may be used as substitute.
If pinhole testing does not improve visual acuity, retinal or optic nerve disease is possible.
If patient is unable to see Rosenbaum chart, ability to see number of fingers or hand movement or light perception at a distance of 3 feet should be documented.
Visual field testing
Defects are seen in glaucoma, retinal disease, and optic nerve damage.
Extraocular muscle testing
CN 3: Superior and inferior rectus, inferior oblique, and medial rectus muscles
CN 4: Superior oblique muscle
CN 6: Lateral rectus muscle
Defects are seen in diabetes, CNS masses, demyelinating diseases, trauma, and myasthenia gravis.
Funduscopic examination to look for
Optic disc swelling (papilledema) or cupping
Retinal hemorrhages and exudates
Presence of macular scarring
Dilation or attenuation of vessels, neovascularization, arteriovenous nicking
Slit-lamp examination under local anesthesia with fluorescein staining
Cobalt blue light to look for corneal abrasions, lacerations, and ulcerations
Green light to look for dendritic branching of herpes simplex ulcers
Lids everted to look for foreign bodies
Measurement of intraocular pressure
Normal IOP of 10–20 mm H_2O
IOP is increased in glaucoma, retrobulbar hemorrhage, benign intracranial hypertension, and hyphema.
IOP is decreased in ruptured globe, traumatic iritis, intraocular foreign body, and postoperative wound leak.

CN = cranial nerve; *CNS* = central nervous system; *IOP* = intraocular pressure.

—Sexually transmitted diseases (STDs)

—Collagen vascular disease

B. Clinical presentation

1. **Symptoms** may include:

   —blurred vision

   —**deep, aching eye pain** (Figure 7-3)

   —photophobia

   —a **red eye** (Table 7-2).

2. **Physical examination findings** may include:

   —**cells and flare in the anterior chamber**

   —conjunctival injection.

C. Diagnostic tests

—No special laboratory or imaging studies are necessary in the ED.

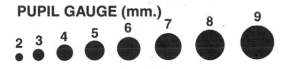

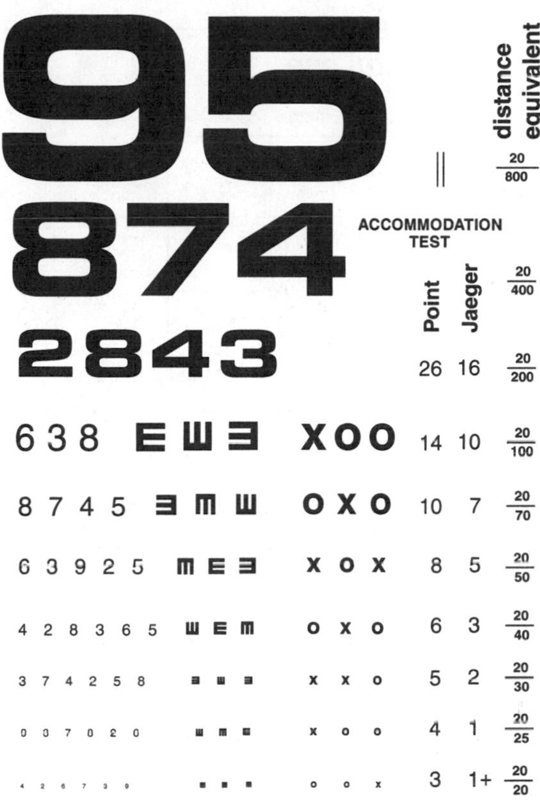

95
874
2843
distance equivalent
20/800
ACCOMMODATION TEST
Point Jaeger
20/400
26 16 20/200
638 XOO 14 10 20/100
8745 OXO 10 7 20/70
63925 XOX 8 5 20/50
428365 OXO 6 3 20/40
374258 XXO 5 2 20/30
4 1 20/25
3 1+ 20/20
Card is held in good light 14 inches from eye. Record vision for each eye separately with and without glasses. Presbyopic patients should read thru bifocal segment. Check myopes with glasses only.
PUPIL GAUGE (mm.)
2 3 4 5 6 7 8 9
Design Courtesy J.G. Rosenbaum, M.D., Cleveland, Ohio

Figure 7-2. Rosenbaum eye chart, read at 14 inches.

—Outpatient work-up should be done for collagen vascular disease, sexually transmitted diseases (STDs), and sarcoid, because iritis may be a manifestation of one of these illnesses.

1. Outpatient laboratory studies

—Rapid plasma reagin (RPR)

—Antinuclear antibody (ANA)

—Chemistry panel

—Complete blood count (CBC)

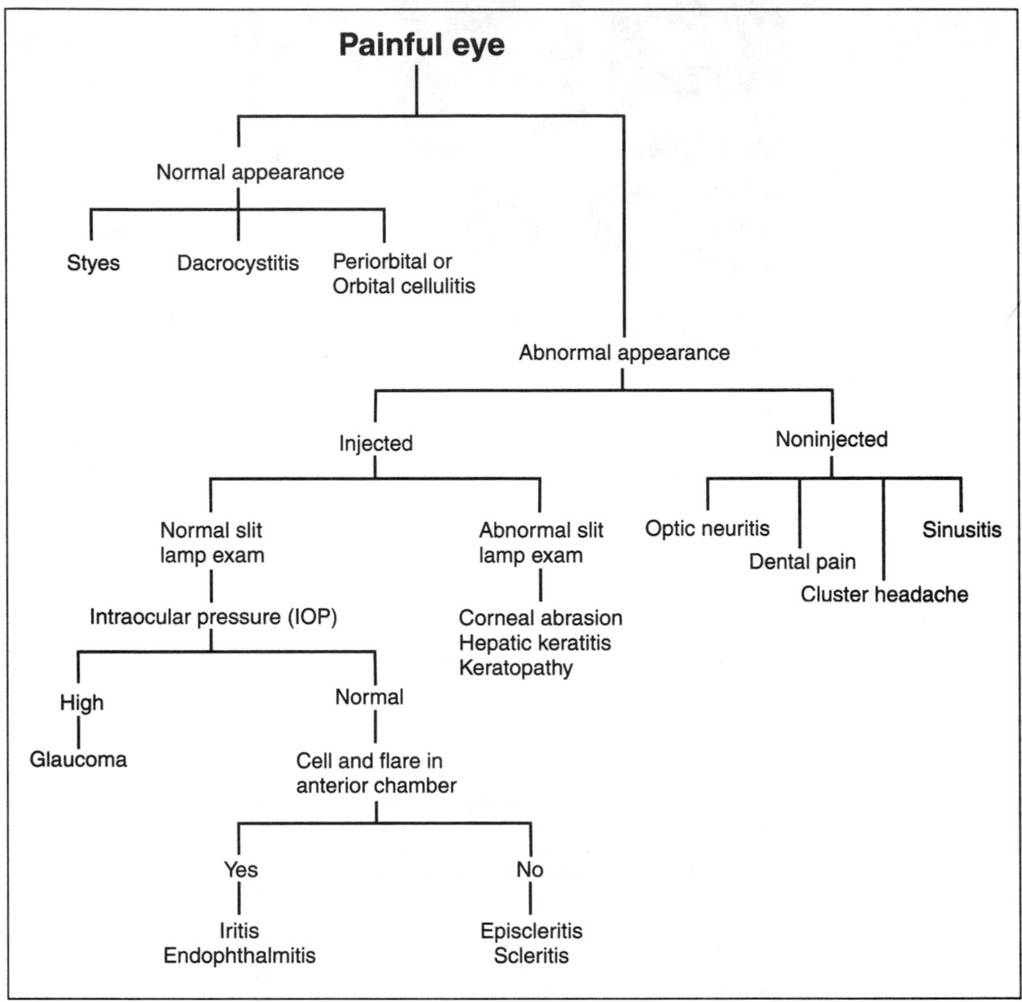

Figure 7-3. Differential diagnosis of the painful eye. *nl* = normal; *VA* = visual acuity.

2. **Imaging studies**

—Chest radiograph to look for changes associated with sarcoid, such as pulmonary fibrosis. Ninety percent of patients with sarcoid have an abnormal chest radiograph.

D. Treatment

1. Ophthalmology consult
2. Topical steroids in conjunction with ophthalmology
3. Cycloplegic eye drops (Table 7-3)

E. Disposition

—Patients can be discharged home with outpatient ophthalmology follow-up in 24–48 hours.

Table 7-2. Differential Diagnosis of the Red Eye

	Conjunctivitis	Acute Iritis	Corneal Trauma, Abrasion, Foreign Body	Keratitis	Acute Glaucoma
↓Acuity	If central lesion	+	+	No	++
Discharge	++		+	+	None
Pain	None	+	++		+++
IOP	Normal	Normal	Normal	Normal	High
Conjunctival injection	+	+	+	+	+
Cornea	Clear	Clear	Clear		Steamy
Pupil	Normal	Small	Normal	Normal	Dilated, fixed
Pupillary light response	Normal	Poor	Normal	Normal	None
Anterior chamber	Normal	Cells and flare	Normal	Normal	Shallow, narrow angle
Fluorescein	None	None	+	+	None

IOP = intraocular pressure.
+ = present; ++ = significant; +++ = severe.

III. Corneal Ulcer

A. Overview

1. Definition

—Corneal ulcer is an epithelial defect over the cornea, usually associated with infection.

—Corneal ulcers or infiltrates may be the result of bacterial, viral or fungal infections.

2. Causes

a. Bacterial

—Bacterial ulcers are the most common type.

—These most commonly occur following a traumatic break in the cornea, from either a tiny abrasion, a penetrating trauma, or an intraoperative wound.

—Bacterial ulcers also may develop as a consequence of decreased tear production and malnutrition.

—Contact lens wearers are particularly prone to pseudomonal ulcers.

b. Viral

—Viral ulcers usually develop on an intact cornea.

Table 7-3. Common Opthalmic Drugs

Class	Example	Brand Names	Strength	Dosage
Cycloplegic	Cyclopentolate	Cyclogyl, AK-pentolate	0.5%, 1%, 2%	1 drop × 1. May repeat × 1 in 5 min.
	Homatropine	Isopto- or AK-homatropine	2%, 5%	1 drop × 1. May repeat × 2 q 10 min.
	Scopolamine	Isopto hyoscine	0.25%	1–2 drops qid
	Atropine	Isoptoatropine	0.5%, 1%, 2%	1–2 drops tid
Mydriatic	Phenylephrine	Phenoptic, Neosynephrine, Mydfrin, AK-dilate	2.5%, 10%	1–2 drops × 1. May repeat × 1 in 15 min.
Antibacterial	Sulfacetamide	Bleph-10, Ocusulf-10, AK-sulf	10%	1–2 drops q 2–3 h
	Tobramycin	Tobrex, AK-Top	0.3%	1–2 drops q 4 h
	Bacitracin	AK-Tracin	–	1–2 drops q 4 h
	Ciprofloxacin	Ciloxan	–	1–2 drops q 2 h × 2 d then q 4 h × 5 d
	Erythromycin	Ilotycin Ophthalmic	0.5%	1–2 drops q 4 h
Artificial tears	Polyvinyl alcohol	Akwa tears, Murine Nu-tears, Refresh	–	1–2 drops q 6 h
Corticosteroid	Dexamethasone	Maxidex	0.1%	1–2 drops q 6 h
	Fluorometholone	Flarex, Fluor-Op, FML forte	0.1%, 0.25%	1–2 drops q 1–2 h × 2 d then q 4 h
	Prednisolone	AK-pred, Econopred, Inflamase, Pred Forte	0.125%, 1%	1–2 drops q 2 h × 2 d then q 4 h

q = every; *qid* = 4 times a day; *tid* = 3 times a day.

—The most common viral ulcer is caused by herpes simplex virus (HSV).

c. Fungal

—Fungal ulcers develop following corneal trauma with organic matter such as a tree branch or vegetable matter.

—Fungal ulcers may be seen in immunocompromised hosts, who are more prone to fungal infections in general, and in people who often use/abuse steroid eye drops.

B. Clinical features

1. Symptoms may include:

—pain
—red eye
—photophobia
—impaired vision
—headache

2. **Physical examination findings** may include:
   —**conjunctival injection**
   —**corneal thinning and ulceration**
   —stromal edema
   —cells and flare in the anterior chamber
   —**mucopurulent discharge**
   —folds in Descemet's membrane
   —constricted pupils (secondary to ciliary spasm)
   —decreased corneal sensation (especially with HSV and varicella zoster virus [VZV]).
3. **Slit-lamp examination findings**
   —**Pseudomonas ulcer fluoresces green under Wood's lamp** (no fluorescein dye needed).
   —**HSV** ulcer reveals a typical **branching dendritic pattern** with green light under slit lamp.

C. Diagnostic tests

—Culture of corneal scraping and discharge to look for causative organism

D. Treatment

1. Immediate consultation with an ophthalmologist is necessary.
2. Antibiotics should be given, as follows:
   - **a.** If epithelium is intact, and there is no staining of corneal epithelium and no conjunctival discharge, the patient can be given broad-spectrum antibacterial drops (see Table 7-3).
   - **b.** The presence of a large (>2 cm) corneal infiltrate, mucoid discharge, or pain warrants aggressive treatment. A suitable regimen includes fortified topical tobramycin or gentamicin drops (15 mg/ml) every hour plus fortified topical cefazolin or vancomycin drops (50 mg/ml) every hour, with dosage scheduled so that patient is using one antibiotic or the other every half hour.
3. Antiviral agents
   - **a.** 0.5% idoxuridine ointment 5 times a day or 1% drops every hour during the day and every 2 hours during the night
   - **b.** 1% trifluridine drops every 2 hours
   - **c.** 3% vidarabine ointment 5 times a day
4. Cycloplegic drops as needed (see Table 7-3)
5. Steroids are contraindicated in HSV ulcers, but may be used in other ulcers.
6. Antifungal therapy if the clinical scenario is suspicious for fungal infection
7. Tetanus prophylaxis if indicated
8. Patients are instructed not to wear contact lenses

E. Disposition

1. Hospital admission should be considered for patients with:

—large (>2 mm) corneal ulcers with significant stromal infiltration

—sight-threatening infections

—infections with *Pseudomonas aeruginosa, Neisseria gonorrhoeae,* or *Haemophilus influenzae*

—corneal perforation

2. Most other patients can be discharged home with outpatient ophthalmology follow-up within 24 hours.

IV. Scleritis

A. Overview

1. **Definition**

—Scleritis is inflammation of the sclera.

2. **Risk factors** include:

—collagen vascular disease

—sarcoid

—tuberculosis

—herpes zoster virus

—syphilis

—Lyme disease

—Crohn's disease

B. Clinical features

1. **Symptoms** may include:

—severe, boring pain that awakens the patient from sleep

—a gradual onset of pain and decrease in visual acuity

—photophobia

—a red eye

—tearing

—No discharge is present.

2. **Physical examination findings** may include:

—cells and flare in the anterior chamber

—a bluish hue to the sclera

—proptosis

—scleral thinning

—**No blanching of the vessels with phenylephrine** is seen.

C. Diagnostic tests

1. No special diagnostic or imaging tests are necessary.

2. However, because as many as 50% of patients have scleritis in association with a systemic illness, other tests may considered, including:

—CBC
—erythrocyte sedimentation rate (ESR)
—ANA
—RPR
—fluorescent treponemal antibody absorption (FTA-ABS)
—purified protein derivative (tuberculin) [PPD]

3. Chest radiograph may be considered.

D. Treatment

1. **Nonsteroidal anti-inflammatory agents (NSAIDs):** Indomethacin 25–50 mg orally three times a day or ibuprofen 800 mg orally three times a day for 7 days (see Table 11-2 in Chapter 11)
2. A **protective eye shield** should be worn to prevent perforation.
3. Oral steroid taper (60–120 mg orally per day tapered over 2 weeks)
4. Consultation with an internist or rheumatologist should be obtained if collagen vascular disease is also present or suspected.

E. Disposition

—The patient can be discharged home with outpatient ophthalmology follow-up in 24–48 hours.

V. Blepharitis

A. Overview

1. Definition

—Blepharitis usually is a chronic condition caused by oversecretion from the meibomian glands, resulting in excessive growth of normal lid flora (e.g., *Staphylococcus aureus, Staphylococcus epidermidis*)

2. **Risk factors** include:

—seborrhea

—**rosacea**

B. Clinical features

1. **Symptoms** may include:

—a gritty foreign body sensation when blinking
—burning lid margins
—itchy lid margins
—a dry eye sensation
—tearing
—intolerance of contact lenses

2. **Physical examination findings** may include:

—edema and erythema of the eyelid
—**scaling,** and a **greasy appearance of the lid margins**

—mucoid discharge

—loss of eyelashes

—inability to close the eyelids completely

C. Diagnostic tests

—No special diagnostic or imaging tests are necessary.

D. Treatment

1. Lid margins scrubbed daily with baby shampoo
2. Warm compresses applied to eyelid margins to help stimulate expression of secretions
3. Topical antibiotic ointment applied to lid margins 4 times a day for 2 weeks (see Table 7-3)
4. Systemic antibiotics for posterior eyelid margin blepharitis:
   a. Doxycycline 100 mg orally twice a day or tetracycline 500 mg orally 4 times a day for 1 month.
   b. For pregnant women and children under 10 years: erythromycin 250 mg orally 3 times a day, because doxycycline and tetracycline may interfere with bone and tooth development.

E. Disposition

—Patients can be discharged home with outpatient ophthalmology follow-up in 2 to 3 days.

VI. Chalazion

A. Overview

1. **Definition**

   —Chalazion is a chronic inflammatory granuloma of a meibomian gland.

2. **Risk factors** include:

   —acne

B. Clinical features

1. **Symptoms** may include:

   —a **painless nodule**

   —conjunctival injection

2. **Physical examination findings** may include:

   —a palpable, nontender, nonerythematous nodule on the eyelid.

   —no intraocular pathology (usually)

C. Diagnostic tests

—No special diagnostic or imaging tests are necessary.

—No cultures are necessary, because chalazion is a sterile inflammation.

D. Treatment

1. Warm compresses for 15 minutes 4 times a day
2. If the chalazion does not heal with conservative management or is cosmetically unacceptable, steroid injection of the chalazion or excision of the chalazion may be performed. These procedures usually are done by an ophthalmologist.

E. Disposition

—Patients can be discharged home with outpatient ophthalmology follow-up in 2 weeks.

VII. Hordeolum

A. Overview

1. **Definition**

—A hordeolum is a suppurative inflammation of a gland of the eyelid.

2. **Risk factors** may include:

—acne

B. Clinical features

1. **Symptoms** may include:

—a history of hordeola (common in diabetics and patients with chronic blepharitis)

—localized, red, painful swelling of one eyelid

2. **Physical examination findings** may include:

—a localized, erythematous, tender nodule on the inside or outside of the eyelid

—conjunctival injection

C. Diagnostic tests

—No special diagnostic or imaging tests are necessary.

—Discharge may be cultured, but yield often is low.

—If generalized eyelid cellulitis is present, CBC and blood cultures should be done.

D. Treatment

1. Warm compresses for 15 minutes 4 times a day
2. Incision and drainage of the hordeolum, with consultation with an ophthalmologist:

—A horizontal stab incision is used for external hordeola.

—A vertical stab incision is used for internal hordeola.

3. Antibiotics are given in severe cases: bacitracin or tobramycin 2 drops 4 times a day for 1 week

E. Disposition

—Patients can be discharged home with outpatient ophthalmology follow-up in 2 to 3 days.

VIII. Conjunctivitis

A. Overview

—Conjunctivitis is an infection of the conjunctiva.

—It may be bacterial, viral, or allergic.

—It is one of the most common eye complaints seen in the ED.

—STDs are a risk factor.

B. Clinical features

1. **Symptoms** may include:

—itchy eyes

—red eye

—discharge that is thick and **mucopurulent** (bacterial), thin and **seropurulent** (viral), or **clear** (allergic)

—sticky eyelids

—Onset usually is acute unless the conjunctivitis is related to an STD (e.g., chlamydial conjunctivitis).

2. **Physical examination findings** may include:

—preauricular adenopathy (viral, sometimes also bacterial)

—conjunctival injection

—chemosis

C. Diagnostic tests

1. Gram stain of discharge. Presence of **eosinophils** on Gram stain indicates an allergic conjunctivitis.
2. Culture of the discharge (unless clear). If gonococcus (GC) is suspected, the culture should be sent on Thayer-Martin medium.

D. Treatment

1. **For bacterial conjunctivitis:**

—Eye irrigation

—**Antibiotic eyedrops:** 2 drops in each eye every 2 hours for 2 days, then every 4 hours for 5 days, for a total of 1 week. Common choices include ciprofloxacin 3% or sulfacetamide drops.

—**Topical antibiotic ointment** every 4–6 hours: bacitracin, erythromycin, or tobramycin

2. **For gonococcal or chlamydial conjunctivitis,** treatment is the same as for bacterial conjunctivitis, with these additions:

—Treatment for STDs with **ceftriaxone 125 mg intramuscularly once,**

azithromycin 1 g orally once, or a 2- to 3-week regimen of doxycycline, erythromycin, or tetracycline if compliance is not a problem.

—Sexual partners of the patient should be treated simultaneously.

3. **For viral conjunctivitis:**

—**Artificial tears** for lubrication every 4 hours for 2 weeks

—**Cool compresses** to the eyes every 4 hours for 1 week

—Antihistamine eyedrops 4 times a day for 1 week if severe itching is present.

—Antiviral drops (e.g., trifluorothymidine 1%) or ointment (e.g., vidarabine 3%) 5 times a day for 7 days if co-infection with HSV is present

4. **For allergic conjunctivitis:**

—**Removal of the allergen**

—Artificial tears for lubrication every 4 hours for 2 weeks

—Cool compresses to the eyes every 4 hours for 1 week

—**Antihistamine drops** (e.g., naphazoline–pheniramine combination) 4 times a day for no more than 5 days (to prevent rebound vasodilatation)

—Oral antihistamine (e.g., cetirizine) 10 mg per day for 3–7 days

E. Disposition

1. Patients with simple conjunctivitis can be discharged home with outpatient follow-up in 24–48 hours.
2. Patients with gonococcal and *Chlamydia* conjunctivitis require immediate ophthalmology consult and may require hospitalization, because these types usually are manifestations of systemic disease.

IX. Periorbital and Orbital Cellulitis

A. Overview

1. **Definition**

   a. **Periorbital cellulitis**

   —refers to infection of the region anterior to the orbital septum.

   —does not extend into tissues within the orbit.

   b. **Orbital cellulitis**

   —refers to infection of the region posterior to the orbital septum.

   —involves structures within the orbit.

2. **Causes**

—Periorbital and orbital cellulitis often result from an extension of an existing sinusitis.

—*Staphylococcus aureus, Streptococcus pneumoniae,* and *H. influenzae* are the organisms most commonly involved.

3. **Risk factors** include:

—orbital trauma

—other facial infection (e.g., sinus, eye, dental, or ear infections)

—orbital surgery

4. **Complications** include:

—meningitis

—cavernous sinus thrombosis

—mucormycosis (a life-threatening infection that must be considered in any diabetic presenting with orbital cellulitis)

B. Clinical features

1. **Symptoms** may include:

—periorbital swelling

—periorbital erythema

—blurry vision

—purulent discharge

—fever

2. **Physical examination findings** may include:

—mild proptosis

—impaired extraocular movements in the affected eye (for orbital cellulitis) (Figure 7-4)

—chemosis

—conjunctival injection

—purulent discharge

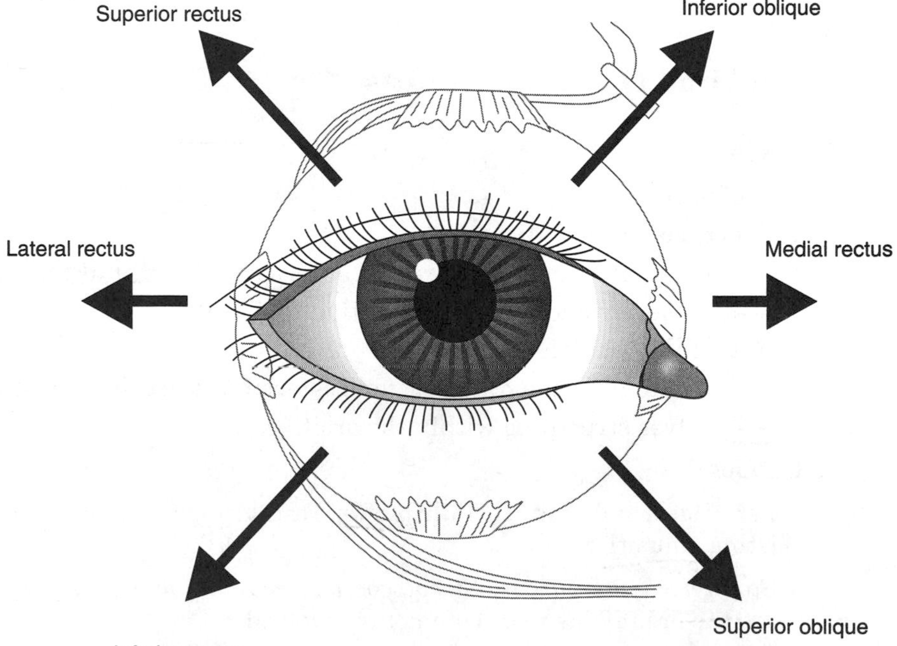

Figure 7-4. The healthy eye can perform all of the extraocular movements shown. (From LifeART Emergency Medicine Professional Collection. Copyright 1998, Lippincott Williams & Wilkins. All rights reserved.)

C. Diagnostic tests

1. Laboratory studies

a. CBC to look for leukocytosis

b. Blood cultures to identify causative organism

c. Chemistry panel to look for electrolyte disturbances

d. Gram stain of eye discharge

2. Computed tomographic (CT) scan to look for sinusitis, abscess, or foreign body

D. Treatment

1. Antibiotics

—Only the mildest cases of periorbital cellulitis should be treated with outpatient antibiotics. All orbital and most periorbital cellulitis should be treated with intravenous antibiotics. Many regimens are suitable.

a. Intravenous antibiotics (inpatient regimens)

—Ampicillin/sulbactam: 50 mg/kg (children) or 3 g (adults) every 6 hours

—Ticarcillin/clavulanic acid: 50 mg/kg (children) or 3.1 g (adults) every 6 hours

—Piperacillin/tazobactam: 100 mg/kg (children) or 3.375 g (adults) every 8 hours

b. Oral antibiotics (outpatient regimens)

—Amoxicillin/clavulanic acid: 20 mg/kg/day (children <5 years) or 875 mg (all patients >5 years) orally, twice a day for 10 days

2. Analgesia

3. Intravenous hydration

E. Disposition

1. Patients with very mild periorbital cellulitis may be discharged home with antibiotics and outpatient follow-up in 24–48 hours.

2. All other patients are admitted for intravenous antibiotics.

X. Ocular Chemical Burns

A. Overview

1. Definition

—An ocular chemical burn is caused by direct contact between the eye and chemicals such as alkali, acids, detergents, and solvents, or other irritant.

2. Risk factors include:

—working in a laboratory or industrial environment

—lack of protective eye goggles

3. Complications may include:

—corneal ulceration

—dry eye(s)

—visual impairment, including blindness

B. Clinical features

1. **Symptoms** may include:
   —burning of the eye and the skin around the eye
   —Burns due to ultraviolet light (corneal sunburn) may present with delayed pain.
2. Physical examination is deferred until copious irrigation is achieved.
3. **Physical examination findings** (with slit lamp) may include:
   —conjunctival chemosis
   —hyperemia
   —eyelid edema
   —acidic or alkaline pH (tested with Litmus paper)
   —punctate keratitis [especially with ultraviolet (UV) burns, common in welders]
   —corneal opacification

C. Diagnostic tests

—No special laboratory or imaging studies are necessary.

—Slit-lamp examination may be done to look for corneal abrasion.

D. Treatment

1. **Copious irrigation** with sterile water, saline, Ringer's lactate, or plain tap water for 30 minutes
   a. Anesthetic drops are administered prior to irrigation
   b. An eyelid speculum or Morgan lens attached to IV tubing is used to help keep the eye open and allow **maximum irrigation.**
   c. The pH of the eye is checked with litmus paper. Irrigation should be continued until a neutral pH is reached.
2. Cycloplegic drops may be given (see Table 7-3).
3. Topical antibiotic ointment (e.g., erythromycin)
4. A pressure **dressing over the eye**
5. Systemic analgesia as needed
6. Cold compresses and lubrication if eyelids or eyelashes are burned
7. Additional treatment for moderate to severe burns:
   a. Immediate ophthalmology consult
   b. Topical antibiotic drops (see Table 7-3)
   c. Treatment of intraocular pressure (IOP), if present (see Table 7-4)
   d. Debridement of necrotic tissue

E. Disposition

1. Patients with mild burns can be discharged home with a follow-up appointment with an ophthalmologist within 24 hours.
2. Patients with severe burns, especially alkali burns, should be admitted to the hospital for further management.

Table 7-4. Management of Increased IOP

Drug Class	Example	Dose	Mechanism of Action
β-Blocker	Timolol	0.5% bid	Decreases production of aqueous humor by inhibition of β adrenergic receptors in ciliary epithelium
Carbonic anhydrase inhibitor	Acetazolamide	500 mg IV, then 250 mg po qid	Decreases production of aqueous humor by inhibiting carbonic anhydrase in ciliary body
Topical vasoconstrictor	Epinephrine	1% bid	Decreases production of aqueous humor by vasoconstriction of ciliary body blood vessels; facilitates uveoscleral and trabecular outflow
Osmotic diuretic	Mannitol	20% 1–2 mg/kg IV over 45 min	Extracts water from aqueous humor back into plasma

bid = twice a day; *IOP* = intraocular pressure; *IV* = intravenously; *po* = orally; *qid* = four times a day.

XI. Globe Rupture

A. Overview

1. Definition

—A ruptured globe is a full-thickness tear of the sclera or cornea, usually secondary to trauma, and is a true emergency.

2. Risk factors

—Penetrating eye trauma

3. Complications may include:

—visual loss (blindness)

—retention of the intraocular foreign body

B. Clinical features

1. **Symptoms** may include **pain and sudden decrease in visual acuity.** This combination is a hallmark for globe rupture.
2. **Physical examination findings** may include:

—extrusion of ocular contents

—abnormally shaped pupil

—deflated appearance of the eyeball

—decreased IOP

—conjunctival edema or hemorrhage

—hyphema

—flattening of the anterior chamber

—periorbital ecchymosis

—dislocated or subluxed lens

C. Diagnostic tests

—CT scan of the orbits and brain to look for orbital wall fractures, foreign bodies, subdural hematomas, and other signs of orbital or head trauma

D. Treatment

1. Immediate ophthalmology consult
2. Use of a rigid protective eye shield
3. **Tetanus prophylaxis**
4. **Antibiotics** to prevent endophthalmitis. A cephalosporin with or without an aminoglycoside may be used, e.g., cefazolin 1 g intravenously every 8 hours.
5. Analgesia and sedation as necessary
6. Bed rest
7. Avoidance of Valsalva maneuvers
8. No oral intake

E. Disposition

—Patients with globe rupture should be admitted to the hospital for immediate surgical repair.

XII. Hyphema

A. Overview

1. **Definition**

   —Hyphema is the presence of blood in the anterior chamber (the area bordered anteriorly by the cornea and posteriorly by the iris and pupil) secondary to disruption of blood vessels in the iris and ciliary body.

2. **Risk factors** include:

   —ocular trauma

   —sickle cell disease

   —child abuse

   —postoperative period

3. **Complications** may include:

   —re-bleeding

   —glaucoma

   —corneal blood staining

B. Clinical features

1. **Symptoms** may include:

   —pain

   —blurred vision

   —photophobia

2. **Physical examination findings** may include:

—**blood in the anterior chamber** (layering or clotting)

—signs of orbital or facial trauma

C. Diagnostic tests

—CT scan of the orbits and brain to look for orbital wall fractures, foreign bodies, subdural hematomas, and other signs of orbital or head trauma

D. Treatment

1. Elevation of the head of the bed 30° to 45° (hyphema may not be seen when the patient is supine).
2. **Limitation of activities that involve extraocular muscle strain,** e.g., reading.
3. **Protection of the affected eye with a transparent shield.**
4. Cycloplegic drops (see Table 7-3).
5. Discontinuation of all products that contain aspirin.
6. Analgesia.
7. **Antiemetics:** prochlorperazine or metoclopramide 10 mg intramuscularly (IM)
8. Treatment of elevated IOP if present (see Table 7-4). This is especially important in patients with sickle cell disease.
9. Topical steroid drops if patient has photophobia or severe anterior chamber reaction; done in consultation with the ophthalmology department.
10. Prednisone, 5 mg orally, twice a day, for 5 days to decrease the chance of re-bleed.
11. **Surgical evacuation of hyphema.** Indications include increased IOP despite maximal medical therapy; significant decrease in visual acuity; blood filling the entire anterior chamber ("eight-ball" sign, or total hyphema); or a clot that persists beyond day 7.

E. Disposition

1. Reliable patients with small hyphemas (microhyphemas) may be discharged home with daily ophthalmology follow-up.
2. All other patients with hyphema must be admitted to the hospital for administration of aminocaproic acid (if not contraindicated) and management of intraocular pressure.

XIII. Traumatic Iridodialysis

A. Overview

1. Definition

—Traumatic iridodialysis is separation of the base of the iris from the ciliary body.

2. Risk factor

—Ocular trauma

B. Clinical features

1. **Symptoms** may include:
   —photophobia
   —tearing
   —deep eye pain
2. **Physical examination findings** may include:
   —conjunctival injection
   —cells and flare in the anterior chamber
   —pain in the affected eye when bright light is shone into it

C. Diagnostic tests

—No special laboratory or imaging studies are necessary.

D. Treatment

1. Paralysis of the iris and the ciliary body with a long-acting cycloplegic (e.g., homatropine).
2. Ophthalmology consultation
3. Administration of steroid drops (e.g., prednisolone acetate 1%) to alleviate inflammation.

E. Disposition

—Patients can be discharged home with outpatient ophthalmology follow-up in 1 week.

XIV. Intraocular Foreign Bodies

A. Overview

1. **Definition**
   —Foreign bodies may become lodged in the eye.
   —The most common site for entrapment of intraocular foreign bodies is the posterior segment, followed by the anterior segment, the lens and, finally, the orbit.
2. **Risk factors** include:
   —working with metal
   —lack of protective eyewear

B. Clinical features

1. **Symptoms** may include:
   —erythema
   —localized pain
2. **Physical examination findings** may include:
   —decreased visual acuity
   —conjunctival chemosis
   —hyphema
   —localized cataract

—vitreous hemorrhage

—**proptosis**

—**limitation of extraocular movement**

C. **Diagnostic tests**

1. **CT scan of the orbits** is the test of choice. It is especially recommended when:
   a. Plain films are negative but clinical suspicion for a foreign body is high
   b. The mechanism of injury puts the patient at risk for an intraocular foreign body, e.g., metal-on-metal grinding, or industrial or shop work where small particles are flying around at high speeds, especially if the patient was not wearing protective eyewear.
2. Plain films (Water's view and lateral skull views) of the orbits to look for radiopaque foreign bodies if CT is not available. Note that plain radiographs pick up only metallic objects.
3. MRI of the orbits may be useful in certain cases but is contraindicated in cases of known or suspected metallic foreign object

D. **Treatment**

1. **Removal of the foreign body** via irrigation or removal with a cotton swab or forceps. Surgical removal is indicated when the foreign body is an organic material (e.g., vegetable matter, wood) or a sharp object, or when signs of infection or optic nerve compression are present. Surgical removal is contraindicated in cases where it would cause more damage than would retention of the foreign body. This may be seen with inert objects such as stone, glass, plastic, and many metals.
2. **Tetanus prophylaxis**
3. **Antibiotics** to prevent endophthalmitis (see section XXV B 3 b)

E. **Disposition**

—Patients can be discharged home with outpatient ophthalmology follow-up in 24 hours.

—Use of safety goggles should be recommended.

XV. Orbital Fracture

A. **Overview**

1. **Definition**

—An orbital fracture is a fracture of any part of the orbital ring.

—Fracture of the orbital floor usually results from direct trauma to the globe and can result in increased IOP.

2. **Risk factors** include:

—direct facial trauma

B. **Clinical features**

1. **Symptoms** may include:

—**diplopia that disappears when one eye is covered**

—swelling of the eyelid after nose blowing

—pain on attempted vertical eye movement

—epistaxis

2. **Physical examination findings** may include:

—limitation of extraocular movements, especially upward and lateral gaze

—palpable step-off along the orbital rim

—decreased sensation in the ipsilateral cheek and upper lip (due to injury to infraorbital nerve)

—orbital edema

—subcutaneous or conjunctival emphysema

—ptosis

—enophthalmos

C. Diagnostic tests

1. CT scan of the orbits and brain to look for fractures, foreign bodies, subdural hematomas, and other signs of orbital or head trauma
2. Plain radiographs of the face to look for air–fluid levels if CT is not available

D. Treatment

1. **For all orbital fractures**
   a. Antibiotics
   b. Nasal decongestant
   c. Application of ice pack
2. **For orbital floor fractures**
   a. Ophthalmology consult
   b. Treatment of elevated IOP, if present
   c. Lateral canthotomy for decompression, if necessary
3. **For orbital roof fractures**

   —Neurosurgery and ophthalmology consults

E. Disposition

1. Patient can be discharged home with outpatient ophthalmology follow-up in 24 hours.
2. Patients should be instructed to refrain from nose blowing.
3. Surgical repair may be considered 1–2 weeks posttrauma if enophthalmos or cosmetic deformity is present.

XVI. Corneal Abrasion

A. Overview

1. **Definition**

   —A corneal abrasion is a scratching of the cornea.

2. **Risk factors** include:
   —blunt trauma to the eye
   —wearing contact lenses
3. **Complications**
   —corneal ulcer

B. Clinical features

1. **Symptoms** may include:
   —pain
   —photophobia
   — a sensation that a foreign body is in the eye
   —tearing
2. **Physical examination findings** may include:
   —injection of the conjunctiva
   —edematous eyelids
   —**epithelial staining defect** with fluorescein on slit-lamp examination

C. Diagnostic tests

—No special laboratory or imaging studies are necessary.

D. Treatment

1. Cycloplegic eye drops (see Table 7-3).
2. Antibiotic ointment (see Table 7-3), including pseudomonal coverage for contact lens wearers
3. Lid taped closed with protective gauze dressing
4. Analgesia as needed

E. Disposition

—Patients can be discharged home with outpatient ophthalmology follow-up in 24 hours.

XVII. Corneal Laceration

—**Risk factors** include penetrating eye trauma.

A. Clinical features

1. **Symptoms** may include:
   —visual loss
2. **Physical examination findings** suggestive of a full-thickness corneal tear may include:
   —a shallow anterior chamber
   —hyphema
   —teardrop-shaped pupil

3. Physical examination may be deferred if full-thickness laceration is suspected, to prevent further injury.

B. Diagnostic tests

—No special diagnostic or imaging tests are necessary.

C. Treatment

1. **Antibiotics to prevent endophthalmitis** (see section XXV B 3 b)
2. Repair under general anesthesia by an ophthalmologist

D. Disposition

—Patients with corneal lacerations are admitted to the surgical or ophthalmologic service for immediate surgical repair.

XVIII. Conjunctival Laceration

—**Risk factors** include penetrating trauma to the eye.

A. Clinical features

1. **Symptoms** may include:
   —a red eye
   —a sensation of having a foreign body in the eye
   —mild pain
2. **Physical examination findings** may include:
   —**fluorescein staining** of the conjunctiva on slit-lamp examination
   —conjunctival or subconjunctival hemorrhage
   —**exposed sclera**

B. Diagnostic tests

—Physical examination may be deferred if globe rupture is suspected, to prevent further injury.

—No special diagnostic or imaging tests are necessary.

C. Treatment

1. **Antibiotic ointment** 3 times a day for 4 to 7 days
2. **Pressure patch** for 24 hours
3. Repair of laceration: most lacerations heal on their own. If repair is needed, the ophthalmology department is consulted.

D. Disposition

—Patient can be discharged home with outpatient ophthalmology follow-up in 24 hours.

XIX. Eyelid Laceration

—**Risk factors** include penetrating trauma to the eye.

A. Clinical features

1. **Symptoms** may include pain and bleeding of the affected eye.
2. **Physical examination findings** may include:
   —globe injection
   —presence of a foreign object

B. Diagnostic tests

—CT scan or plain films of orbits if presence of foreign object is suspected

C. Treatment

1. If the laceration is simple and superficial, it is closed with 6–0 or 7–0 nylon.
2. The following lacerations require repair by an ophthalmologist:
   a. Lacerations involving lid margins, canalicular system, levator or canthal tendons, and orbital septum
   b. Lacerations with extensive tissue loss or severe distortion of anatomy
   c. Lacerations associated with ruptured globe or other trauma requiring surgery under general anesthesia

D. Disposition

1. Patients with superficial lacerations closed in the emergency department can be discharged home with outpatient ophthalmology follow-up in 48 hours.
2. Patients with complicated lacerations are managed by ophthalmology.

XX. Central Retinal Artery Occlusion (CRAO)

A. **Risk factors** include:

—temporal arteritis

—syphilis

—sickle cell disease

—connective tissue disease

B. Clinical features

1. **Symptoms** may include:
   —painless loss of monocular vision occurring over hours to days
   —visual field defects
2. **Physical examination findings** may include:
   —a **pale retina with a central cherry-red spot**
   —an afferent pupillary defect (paradoxic dilatation of pupil when light is shined from unaffected to affected eye)
   —carotid bruit
   —cardiac murmur

C. Diagnostic tests

—No special diagnostic or imaging tests are necessary to detect CRAO. However, testing may be directed at identifying the underlying cause, as follows:

1. CBC to look for polycythemia
2. Prothrombin time (PT), activated partial thromboplastin time (APTT), fibrinogen, antiphospholipid antibodies, protein C, protein S, antithrombin III to look for coagulopathies and hypercoagulable states
3. Lipid profile to look for atherosclerotic disease
4. Blood cultures to look for endocarditis if clinically suspicious
5. Electrocardiogram (ECG) to look for atrial fibrillation
6. ESR to look for elevation
7. Carotid Doppler ultrasound to look for carotid stenosis

D. Treatment

1. **Immediate ophthalmology consult**
2. Carbonic anhydrase inhibitor, e.g., **acetazolamide** 5–10 mg/kg every 6 hours IV (in children) or 250–500 mg every 2–4 hours IV (in adults)
3. Direct ocular massage: pressure is applied directly to the globe for 10 seconds, released for 10 seconds, then repeated, for 30 minutes. This prevents further dilation of the retinal vessels.
4. Topical β-blocker: timolol 0.5% or levobunolol 0.5%
5. Carbogen (95% oxygen and 5% carbon dioxide)

E. Disposition

1. Patient disposition is determined by ophthalmology consult. Usually, patients without comorbid disease may be discharged home with outpatient ophthalmology follow-up.
2. Patients with comorbid conditions may need to be admitted to the hospital for further management.

XXI. Central Retinal Vein Occlusion (CRVO)

A. Overview

1. Mechanisms thought to be responsible include:
   —external compression
   —thrombus formation
   —primary venous disease
2. **Risk factors**
   —diabetes mellitus
   —atherosclerosis
   —hypertension
   —hypercoagulable states

B. Clinical features

1. **Symptoms** may include:

 —painless loss of monocular vision occurring over hours to days

2. **Physical examination findings** include:

 —cotton wool spots

 —**papilledema**

 —dilated, tortuous retinal veins with streaks that represent hemorrhage

C. Diagnostic tests

—No special diagnostic or imaging tests are necessary to detect CRVO. However, testing may be directed at identifying the underlying cause.

D. Treatment

1. **Immediate ophthalmology consult**
2. Lowering of IOP to 15 mm H_20 (see Table 7-4). This allows for better perfusion of the retina and is thought to move the clot further down the vascular system.
3. Direct ocular massage
4. Anterior chamber paracentesis (done by ophthalmology)
5. Photocoagulation to prevent neovascularization (done by ophthalmology)
6. Hyperbaric oxygen

E. Disposition

1. Patients without comorbid disease may be discharged home with outpatient ophthalmology follow-up.
2. Patients with comorbid conditions may need to be admitted to the hospital for further management.

XXII. Retrobulbar Hemorrhage

A. Overview

1. **Definition**

 —Retrobulbar hemorrhage refers to bleeding behind the globe.

2. **Risk factors**

 —Blunt or penetrating trauma to the eye

B. Clinical features

1. **Symptoms** may include:

 —pain

 —visual loss

2. **Physical examination findings** may include:

 —an **acute increase in IOP**

 —central artery occlusion on funduscopic examination

—**diffuse subconjunctival hemorrhage**

—proptosis

—ecchymosis of the eyelids

—**limitation of extraocular movements**

—orbital emphysema

—chemosis

C. Diagnostic tests

—CT scan of the orbits to look for hematoma

D. Treatment

1. **Immediate ophthalmology consult**
2. Temporizing measures include **lateral canthotomy,** anterior chamber paracentesis, and decreasing the IOP (see Table 7-4).
3. Definitive therapy is surgical.

E. Disposition

—Patients are admitted to the hospital for further management.

XXIII. Retinal Detachment

A. Overview

1. Definition

—Retinal detachment is separation of the retinal layers secondary to one or more holes in the retina that allow for fluid accumulation in the potential space between the sensory and epithelial layers of the retina.

2. Mechanisms and risk factors

a. Rhegmatogenous detachment Surg

—the most common type

—associated with advancing age and degenerative myopia, especially with diopters > 6

b. Exudative retinal detachment photocoag

—occurs most commonly in association with systemic diseases such as hypertension, breast cancer, melanoma, glomerulonephritis, and the vasculitides, and local processes such as central retinal vein occlusion, papilledema, and choroid tumor

c. Tractional retinal detachment Surg

—associated with previous vitreous hemorrhage, diabetic retinopathy, sickle cell disease, and penetrating trauma

B. Clinical features

1. **Symptoms** may include:

—the **perception of intermittent flashing light, or flickering,** instead of normal image (indicates retinal tear until proven otherwise)

—absence of pain
—floaters
—distortion of images

2. **Physical examination findings** may include:

—decreased visual acuity if the macula is involved

—a **protruding, hazy, gray membrane of retina if anterior detachment has occurred**

C. Diagnostic tests

—No special diagnostic or imaging tests are necessary.

D. Treatment

—**Immediate ophthalmology consult**

E. Disposition

—Patients with retinal detachment are admitted to the ophthalmology service for emergent treatment, which may consist of surgical repair (rhegmatogenous and tractional types) or photocoagulation (exudative type).

XXIV. Acute Angle Closure Glaucoma

A. Overview

1. **Definition**

Angle closure glaucoma results from obstruction of the aqueous humor outflow and may present as acute, subacute, or chronic. The obstruction results in increased intraocular pressure and, if left untreated, can lead to blindness.

2. **Risk factors** (in patients with glaucoma) may include:

—stress

—adrenergics

—anticholinergics

B. Clinical features

1. **Symptoms** may include:

—**sudden onset of painful visual loss**

—headache

—nausea

—vomiting

—somnolence

2. **Physical examination findings** may include:

—**decreased visual acuity**

—conjunctival injection

—a **hazy cornea**

—a fixed, mid-position, or dilated pupil that is unreactive to light

—**increased IOP**

—rock-hard globe (secondary to increased IOP)

C. Diagnostic tests

—IOP should be measured, but no special diagnostic or imaging tests are necessary.

D. Treatment

1. **Immediate ophthalmology consult**
2. 1 drop pilocarpine 2% every 15 minutes until the pupil is constricted
3. Management of elevated IOP (see Table 7-4)

E. Disposition

—Patients with acute angle closure glaucoma are admitted to the ophthalmology service for surgical management.

XXV. Postoperative Ocular Emergencies

A. Overview

—Because many eye surgeries are now done as outpatient procedures, an increasing number of postoperative complications are being seen in the emergency department.

B. Postoperative endophthalmitis

—Endophthalmitis is a true ocular emergency that warrants immediate ophthalmology consultation.

—Delay in management of endophthalmitis is directly proportional to worsened prognosis.

1. **Clinical features** may include:

   —pain

   —photophobia

   —conjunctival injection

   —iritis

   —retinitis

   —vitreitis

2. **Diagnostic tests**

   —The diagnosis of endophthalmitis can be made only by an ophthalmologist.

   —No tests other than the laboratory studies required for admission are necessary in the ED.

3. **Treatment**

   a. Immediate ophthalmology consultation, preferably with the operating surgeon

b. Antibiotics should be started in the emergency department. The suggested regimen is ceftriaxone 1 g IV, plus fortified topical tobramycin drops 9.1–13.4 mg/ml every hour, plus fortified topical cefazolin drops 50 mg/ml every hour.

c. Definitive treatment includes instillation of antibiotics into the vitreous, which is done in the operating room by an ophthalmologist.

4. Disposition

—All patients should be admitted to the hospital for intravitreal antibiotics.

C. Post-laser in situ keratomileusis (LASIK)

1. Clinical features may include:

—a lost or displaced flap of cornea

—corneal infiltrate

—gross keratitis (discharge, pain)

—iritis

—retinal detachment (rare)

2. Diagnostic tests

—Culture of corneal scraping and discharge

3. Treatment

a. As with postoperative endophthalmitis, the operating surgeon should be called immediately when a patient presents with complications from this surgery.

b. Treatment as for corneal ulcer (see section III D)

4. Disposition

—As per recommendation of the ophthalmology department.

—If no ophthalmologist is available and the patient has no other comorbid conditions, the patient can be discharged with outpatient ophthalmology follow-up as soon as possible, but no later than 24 hours.

Review Test

Questions 1 and 2

A 27-year-old woman is struck in the left eye by a flying golf ball and presents to the emergency department (ED) complaining of left eye pain with diminishing vision. On examination of the eye, you note that there is severe proptosis and subconjunctival hemorrhage. The intraocular pressure (IOP) is 40 mm Hg. Extraocular movements are limited. The patient has light perception in the right eye.

1. Which of the following injuries does this patient most likely have?

(A) Globe rupture
(B) Retrobulbar hemorrhage
(C) Central retinal vein occlusion
(D) Central retinal artery occlusion
(E) Retinal detachment

2. Which of the following is the most appropriate immediate treatment for this patient?

(A) Direct orbital massage
(B) Ice pack to the orbit
(C) Prescription for miotic eyedrops
(D) Lateral canthotomy
(E) Prescription for sulfacetamide drops

3. A 33-year-old mechanic presents to the ED complaining of right eye pain. He had been pounding a piece of steel with a hammer the previous day while at work and reports a feeling that something is stuck in his eye. Visual acuity is 20/70 in the affected eye and 20/20 in the contralateral eye. On slit-lamp examination, no evidence of foreign body or corneal defect is noted. Which of the following is the most appropriate next step?

(A) CT scan of the orbits
(B) MRI of the orbits
(C) Ophthalmology follow-up in 24 hours
(D) Prescription for cycloplegic eye drops
(E) Prescription for tetracaine drops

Questions 4–7

A 65-year-old woman presents to the emergency department with sudden onset of painless loss of vision. On examination, the patient has hand motion vision in the right eye and 20/20 vision in the left eye. The cornea is clear, and slit-lamp examination of the anterior segment is unremarkable. The intraocular pressure (IOP) is 20 millimeters of water (mm H_2O).

4. Which of the following is the most likely diagnosis?

(A) Retrobulbar hemorrhage
(B) Retinal detachment
(C) Acute angle closure glaucoma
(D) Herpetic keratitis
(E) Endophthalmitis

5. Which of the following is the most appropriate management for this patient?

(A) Immediate consultation with the ophthalmology department
(B) Fluorescein angiogram of the retina
(C) Preparation for laser iridotomy
(D) Immediate measures to decrease intraocular pressure (IOP)
(E) Immediate administration of antibiotic drops

6. Examination of the posterior segment by the ophthalmologist shows a pale retina and pale optic nerve with a cherry-red spot in the macula. Which of the following is the most likely diagnosis?

(A) Central retinal artery occlusion
(B) Central retinal vein occlusion
(C) Acute ischemic optic neuropathy
(D) Retinal detachment
(E) Retrobulbar hemorrhage

7. If the patient had an erythrocyte sedimentation rate (ESR) of 135 and no cherry-red spot was found on direct ophthalmoscopy, which of the following would be the most appropriate management at this time?

(A) Admission for surgery to correct retinal detachment
(B) Discharge the patient home with ophthalmology follow-up in 24 hours
(C) Initiation of high dose steroid therapy
(D) Rheumatology consult
(E) Intravenous antibiotic therapy

Questions 8 and 9

A 70-year-old man who had glaucoma surgery with cataract extraction the previous day presents to the emergency department due to a painful red eye and some vision loss. Clinical examination reveals hand motion vision and red injected conjunctiva with a layered hypopyon (white cells) in the anterior chamber.

8. Which of the following is the most likely diagnosis?

(A) Temporal arteritis
(B) Retinal detachment
(C) Retrobulbar hemorrhage
(D) Endophthalmitis
(E) Central retinal artery occlusion

9. Which of the following is the most appropriate management for this patient?

(A) Preparation for laser iridotomy
(B) Immediate ophthalmology consult
(C) Initiation of topical antibiotics
(D) Initiation of topical steroids
(E) None of the above

10. A 25-year-old man presents to the emergency department with a history of trauma to the eye with a sharp object. On examination, his vision with pinhole is 20/80. There is a superior field defect on confrontation. Handlight examination reveals minimal chemosis in the lower part of the bulbar conjunctiva. The pupil reacts to light and accommodation, but is irregular and keyhole-shaped. Which of the following is the most appropriate management?

(A) Checking of intraocular pressure (IOP) with a Schiotz tonometer
(B) Instillation of antibiotic ointment every hour
(C) Instillation of steroid eye drops every hour
(D) Instillation of cycloplegic eye drops every hour
(E) Placement of a hard metal shield over the eye

Answers and Explanations

1-B, 2-D. Central retinal vein occlusion, central retinal artery occlusion, and retinal detachment are all causes of painless visual loss, and are not usually associated with trauma. Globe rupture is associated with trauma, but results in a decrease in intraocular pressure (IOP), due to extrusion of contents, resulting in a deflated appearance to the eyeball, not a proptotic one. Retrobulbar hemorrhage can occur following direct trauma to the eye and results in accumulation of blood behind the globe, resulting in elevated IOP. The increase in IOP causes proptosis, ischemia of the optic nerve, and, eventually, irreversible visual loss.

Decompression via lateral canthotomy is the treatment of choice to prevent these sequelae. Orbital massage would only worsen the pressure. Ice pack to the orbit is beneficial, but it is not the best treatment of those listed. Sulfacetamide drops (antibiotics) and miotic drops are not indicated.

3-A. Although the slit lamp examination for foreign body is negative in this patient, he has significant mechanism for an intraocular foreign body. Based on his sensation that a foreign body is present and the highly suspicious mechanism, the patient should be given a CT scan of his orbits to look for a foreign body that may have been missed on physical examination. The imaging study of choice is CT scan. MRI would be contraindicated for metallic objects. Plain radiographs may be helpful, but can only pick up certain types of foreign objects. A prescription for cycloplegic eyedrops is not necessary. A prescription for tetracaine drops is never appropriate for an intraocular foreign body. A prescription for antibiotic drops, however (not a choice listed here), is indicated in order to prevent endophthalmitis.

4-B. The most plausible, and only possible, choice of those listed is retinal detachment. All other diagnoses listed involve a painful eye. Endophthalmitis usually presents with pain and red eye. It is possible to have endophthalmitis without any of these signs, so this is a possible diagnosis, but not the most likely diagnosis. Additionally, retrobulbar hemorrhage and acute angle closure glaucoma present with elevated intraocular pressure (IOP). Herpetic keratitis shows dendritic staining on fluorescein examination. The differential diagnosis for painless loss of vision that manifests as a curtain-like defect (thus mimicking retinal detachment) is central retinal artery occlusion, central retinal vein occlusion, and acute ischemic optic neuropathy.

5-A. Retinal detachment is an ocular emergency that warrants immediate ophthalmologic consultation. A fluorescein angiogram of the retina for possible panretinal photocoagulation would be the treatment for central retinal vein occlusion, but is outside the realm of emergency medicine and should be done by an ophthalmologist. Laser iridotomy is the treatment for acute angle closure glaucoma. Because the intraocular pressure (IOP) in this case is normal, there is no need to institute measures to decrease it. Similarly, retinal detachment usually does not involve infection and, therefore, antibiotics would not be a priority.

6-A. The description of a pale retina with a central cherry-red spot is typical for central retinal artery occlusion. Direct ophthalmoscopy findings in central retinal vein occlusion include dilated tortuous retinal veins with hemorrhagic streaks (as opposed to a central spot), cotton wool spots, and papilledema. In retinal detachment, a detached retina is seen, and in acute ischemic optic neuropathy a pale optic disc without any signs of hemorrhage in the retina is seen. As in question 4, retrobulbar hemorrhage is unlikely in this patient given the clinical presentation. Retrobulbar hemorrhage does present within a pale retina. However, there is no central cherry-red spot.

7-C. A high erythrocyte sedimentation rate (ESR) with a painless loss of vision in a 65-year-old patient is suspect for temporal arteritis. The patient may have presented previously to medical attention due to the same symptom or, perhaps, with simply a headache over the temple(s). If temporal arteritis is suspected, treatment with prednisone is initiated to avert loss of vision in the other eye.

8-D. Any patient who presents postoperatively with a painful red eye has endophthalmitis until proven otherwise. Retinal detachment, temporal arteritis, and central retinal artery occlusion usually present with painless loss of vision and without red eye. Retrobulbar hemorrhage would not cause hypopyon.

9-B. Endophthalmitis is a true ocular emergency and requires immediate ophthalmology consultation, in this case preferably with the surgeon who performed the original surgery.

10-D. This patient has a penetrating eye injury. Instillation of any material by the emergency physician, whether saline, antibiotics, steroids, or cycloplegics, is contraindicated in an open eye injury. This patient probably has an inferior retinal detachment, given his superior field defect and chemosis in the inferior conjunctiva. Appropriate management consists of an immediate ophthalmology consult and placement of a hard, metal protective shield over the eye in the meantime. Checking the intraocular pressure (IOP) with a Schiotz tonometer is contraindicated, because this method actually requires pressure to be applied to the eyeball, which may further extrude the ocular contents.

8

Ear, Nose, and Throat Emergencies

I. Otitis Media (OM)

A. Overview

1. Definition

—OM is an infection of the middle ear.

2. Incidence and prognosis

—OM is most common in children, particularly those 6–8 months of age.

3. Risk factors include:

—daycare

—smoking in the household

—prior upper respiratory tract infection

—presence of siblings in the household

—winter

—pacifier use

—improper positioning of infant during bottle feeding (increases reflux of milk into the eustachian tube)

—teething

—craniofacial abnormalities

B. Clinical features

1. Symptoms may include:

—ear pain and a sense of fullness

—the perception of gurgling or rumbling sounds inside the ear

—decreased hearing

—vertigo

—fever

—purulent discharge

2. **Physical examination findings** may include:

—a bulging or erythematous tympanic membrane

—pain on retraction of the pinna

—poor feeding and irritability in infants

—an absent light reflex

—a **tympanic membrane that moves poorly to pressure changes on pneumatic otoscopy** (Table 8-1)

C. **Diagnostic tests**

—Laboratory testing usually is not performed, because the diagnosis is evident from the clinical examination.

—Culture of ear discharge may be considered if otitis is recurrent or only partially treated

—If the ear canal is occluded with wax, a few drops of hydrogen peroxide or 0.2 ml of docusate helps to soften wax for easy removal.

D. **Treatment**

1. **Antibiotics** x10d

—**Amoxicillin** is sufficient for most uncomplicated cases: 250–500 mg every 8 hours orally for 10 days (adults) or 40 mg/kg/day in divided doses every 8 hours orally for 10 days (children).

—If penicillin resistance is suspected, **amoxicillin-clavulanate** is used: 875 mg/125 mg every 12 hours orally for 7–10 days (adults) or 40 mg/kg/day in divided doses every 8 hours orally for 10 days (children).

—For penicillin-allergic patients, **trimethoprim-sulfamethoxazole** may be given: 1 double-strength (DS) tablet by mouth twice a day (adults) or 3–6 mg/kg by mouth twice a day (children) for 10 days

2. **Acetaminophen** for fever reduction and analgesia

3. For patients in extreme discomfort (especially children), a single dose of 2 drops of 2% lidocaine instilled in the ear may provide rapid relief.

4. **Tympanocentesis** [needle aspiration through the tympanic membrane (TM)] or **myringotomy** (3-mm surgical incision through the TM) is indicated for:

   a. OM refractory to antibiotic therapy.

Table 8-1. Pneumatic Otoscopy Findings

Normal ear	Tympanic membrane (TM) moves with positive pressure
Otitis media (OM)	TM moves poorly to positive pressure
Retraction of TM	TM moves to negative pressure
Rupture of TM	No movement of TM to positive or negative pressure

b. OM in newborns.

c. Suppurative complications.

d. Onset of OM in someone already on antibiotics.

E. Disposition

1. Patients with uncomplicated otitis media can be discharged home with antibiotics and outpatient follow-up in 48 hours.

2. Patients in the following categories should be admitted to the hospital:

—infants < 1 month old

—patients who appear toxic

—immunocompromised patients

—patients with suppurative complications such as mastoiditis, central nervous system (CNS) infection, or facial nerve palsy

II. Otitis Externa (OE)

A. Overview

1. Definition

—OE is an infection of the outer ear.

2. Causes

—Causes include trauma to the ear, foreign bodies in the ear, and psoriasis.

—A malignant form of OE called necrotizing OE is seen in insulin-dependent diabetics secondary to infection with *Pseudomonas* spp.

3. Risk factors include:

—prolonged exposure to water, as in swimming pools

—insulin-dependent diabetes

B. Clinical features

1. Symptoms may include:

—itching

—decreased hearing

—fever

2. Physical examination findings may include:

—pain on retraction of the pinna

—an edematous, tender, erythematous external ear canal

—furuncles noted in the external ear canal

—bullae noted on the tympanic membrane (bullous myringitis)

—lymphadenopathy

C. Diagnostic tests

1. Laboratory studies

—Laboratory testing usually is not performed, because the diagnosis is evident from the clinical examination.

—Culture of ear discharge may be considered if otitis is recurrent or only partially treated.

2. **Imaging studies**

—CT scan or MRI should be considered in patients with necrotizing OE to look for osteomyelitis.

D. **Treatment**

1. **Uncomplicated OE**

a. **Antibiotics:** Polymyxin B-Neomycin-Hydrocortisone suspension ear drops, 2 drops in affected ear 4 times a day for 10 days

b. **Acetaminophen** for fever reduction and analgesia as needed

2. **Necrotizing OE**

a. **Antibiotics.** Many regimens are suitable. Two suggested choices are imipenem, 500 mg every 6 hours intravenously (IV), and ciprofloxacin, 400 mg every 12 hours IV.

b. Surgical debridement

c. In diabetics, control of patient's diabetes

E. **Disposition**

1. Patients with uncomplicated OE can be discharged home with antibiotics and outpatient follow-up in 48 hours

2. Patients with necrotizing OE should be admitted to the hospital.

III. Mastoiditis

A. **Overview**

1. **Definition**

—Mastoiditis is an infection of the mastoid air cells.

2. **Causes**

—Mastoiditis occurs secondary to under-treated or partially treated otitis media (most common cause) and thus is seen more often in the pediatric and adolescent populations

—The organisms most frequently implicated include *Streptococcus pneumoniae, Streptococcus pyogenes, Staphylococcus aureus, Haemophilus influenzae,* and *Pseudomonas aeruginosa.*

3. **Risk factors** include a history of otitis media.

B. **Clinical features**

1. **Symptoms** may include:

—decreased hearing

—paresis of facial muscles

—vertigo

—ear pain

—discharge from the ear

—fever

2. **Physical examination findings** may include:

—bulging and erythema of the tympanic membrane secondary to antecedent OM

—retroauricular swelling and tenderness

—displacement of the earlobe

C. **Diagnostic tests**

1. **Laboratory studies**

—Gram stain and culture and sensitivity of ear fluid to isolate the causative organism

2. **Imaging studies**

—**CT** (test of choice) or plain radiographs of mastoid air cells to look for air–fluid levels, clouding of air cells, and destruction of temporal bone

D. **Treatment**

1. **Antibiotics**

—**Cefotaxime,** 1 g every 4 hours IV, or **ceftriaxone,** 1 g every 12 hours IV (adults)

—**Nafcillin,** 150 mg/kg/day in divided doses every 6 hours IV, or **cefuroxime,** 100 mg/kg/day in divided doses every 8 hours IV (children)

2. **Mastoidectomy** or **drainage of mastoid air cells.** Indications include:

—chronic drainage

—evidence of osteomyelitis per MRI or CT

—spread of infection to the CNS

3. Removal of cholesteatoma, if present

E. **Disposition**

—All patients with mastoiditis require admission to the hospital.

IV. Sinusitis

A. **Overview**

1. **Definition**

—Sinusitis is inflammation of any of the sinuses: ethmoid, frontal, sphenoid, or maxillary.

2. **Causes**

—The organisms most often implicated are *S. pneumoniae, M. catarrhalis,* and *H. influenzae.*

—The incidence of *H. influenzae* infection has decreased since the advent of the Hib vaccine.

B. **Clinical features**

1. **Symptoms** may include:

—fever

—general malaise

—anosmia

—headache and toothache (referred pain)

—mucopurulent discharge

—postnasal drip

—sore throat

—facial pain and pressure

2. **Physical examination findings** may include:

—opacity to transillumination of sinuses

—foreign body detected on rhinoscopy

—warmth and tenderness to percussion of sinuses

—halitosis

C. Diagnostic tests

—CT scan (test of choice) or plain radiographs of sinuses to look for **air–fluid levels** or **thickening of the mucosa** of 6 mm or more

D. Treatment

1. **Antibiotics** as for mastoiditis (see section III D)

—For uncomplicated cases, **amoxicillin** 875 mg orally twice a day for 14 days

—If penicillin resistance is suspected, **amoxicillin-clavulanate,** 875 mg orally twice a day for 21 days, or trimethoprim-sulfamethoxasole 1 DS tablet orally twice a day for 21 days

2. **Nasal decongestants,** but not for more than 4 days; otherwise, rebound nasal congestion may develop.

   a. Oxymetazoline 0.05% 1–2 drops every 6–12 hours

   b. Phenylephrine 0.05–1.0% 1–2 drops every 6–12 hours

3. **Acetaminophen** for fever reduction and analgesia, as needed

E. Disposition

1. Patients with simple maxillary sinusitis can be discharged home with antibiotics and outpatient follow-up in 48 hours.

2. Patients with frontal, ethmoid, or sphenoid sinusitis and patients who appear toxic should be admitted for intravenous antibiotics. These patients are at risk for developing complications such as brain abscess and CNS infection.

V. Pharyngitis

A. Overview

1. **Definition**

—Pharyngitis is an inflammation of the pharynx or throat.

2. **Causes**

a. Group A *Streptococcus* species—the most common cause in children
b. Adenovirus—the most common cause in adults
c. Bacterial causes
—*Streptococcus* spp
—*Mycoplasma* spp
—*Neisseria gonorrhoeae.*
d. Noninfectious causes
—Postnasal drip
—Smoking
—Chewing tobacco
e. *Corynebacterium diphtheriae*—a rare but potentially life-threatening cause of pharyngitis that affects nonimmunized and inadequately immunized individuals

B. Clinical features

—Clinical features cannot reliably differentiate among microbial etiologies.

1. **Viral pharyngitis** is characterized by:
—vesicles in the pharynx
—rhinorrhea
—cough
—low-grade or no fever
2. **Streptococcal pharyngitis** ("strep throat")
a. **Clinical features** include:
—exudates or pus in the pharynx
—petechiae in the pharynx
—scarlatiniform rash (in children)
—marked tonsillar edema
—abdominal pain (due to inflammation of Peyer's patches)
—fever as high as 41°C (106°F)
—lymphadenopathy
b. Peak ages are 5–6 years and the teenage years. It is extremely rare in patients younger than 2 years of age.
c. **Complications** include:
—abscess formation
—rheumatic fever
—poststreptococcal glomerulonephritis
3. **Diphtheria**
a. **Clinical features** include:
—pronounced cervical lymphadenopathy ("bull neck")
—a grayish-white pseudomembrane
—a characteristic breath odor
—drooling secondary to airway obstruction
—acutely ill-appearing patient
b. **Complications** of untreated infection include:

—bleeding diathesis of unknown etiology
—toxin-mediated myocarditis

C. Diagnostic tests

1. Laboratory studies

a. Complete blood cell count (CBC) to look for leukocytosis. Atypical lymphocytes are seen in mononucleosis.
b. Chemistry panel to look for blood urea nitrogen (BUN) or creatinine elevations. Poststreptococcal glomerulonephritis should be kept in mind.
c. Rapid streptococcal detection test to look for streptococcal infection
d. **Throat culture** to isolate causative organism (may omit if rapid Strep test is positive)
e. Monospot test to look for heterophile antibodies (mononucleosis)

2. **Radiograph** of lateral soft tissue of the neck if airway obstruction is present

D. Treatment

1. **For viral pharyngitis,** treatment is supportive, and includes:
—gargling with warm salt water
—sucking on hard lozenges
—increased fluid intake
—acetaminophen for analgesia and fever reduction
—bed rest

2. For streptococcal pharyngitis

a. Supportive measures as for viral pharyngitis (see section V D 1)
b. Streptococcal pharyngitis is treated to prevent the complication of acute rheumatic fever:
—**Penicillin V** 25–50 mg/kg/day in 4 divided doses for 10 days, or **benzathine penicillin** 25,000 U/kg intramuscularly once (to a maximum of 1.2 million units), then 250 mg 4 times a day by mouth for 10 days
—For penicillin-allergic patients, **erythromycin** 250 mg orally 4 times a day for 10 days (adults) or 13 mg/kg orally every 8 hours for 10 days (children)

3. For diphtheria pharyngitis:

a. Supportive measures as for viral and streptococcal pharyngitis (see section V D 1), plus:
(1) **Diphtheria antitoxin**
—20,000–40,000 U if presentation within preceding 48 hours
—40,000–60,000 U if nasopharyngeal lesions are present
—80,000–100,000 U if presentation more than 72 hours ago
(2) **Erythromycin** 20–25 mg/kg every 12 hours IV for 7–14 days, or penicillin G 25,000–50,000 U/kg every 24 hours IV for 2 weeks
b. **Reimmunization of close contacts** if their last vaccination was more than 5 years ago
c. **Strict isolation**

E. Disposition

1. Patients with viral pharyngitis can be discharged home with outpatient follow-up in 1 week.
2. Patients with streptococcal pharyngitis can be discharged home with antibiotics and outpatient follow-up if they are over the age of 1 month, do not appear toxic, and do not have any suppurative complications.
3. Patients with diphtheria pharyngitis should be admitted to the hospital to an isolation bed.

VI. Peritonsillar Abscess (Figure 8-1)

A. Clinical features

1. **Symptoms** may include:

—severe throat pain

—a muffled "hot potato" voice

—tilting of the head to the affected side

—decreased oral intake secondary to dysphagia

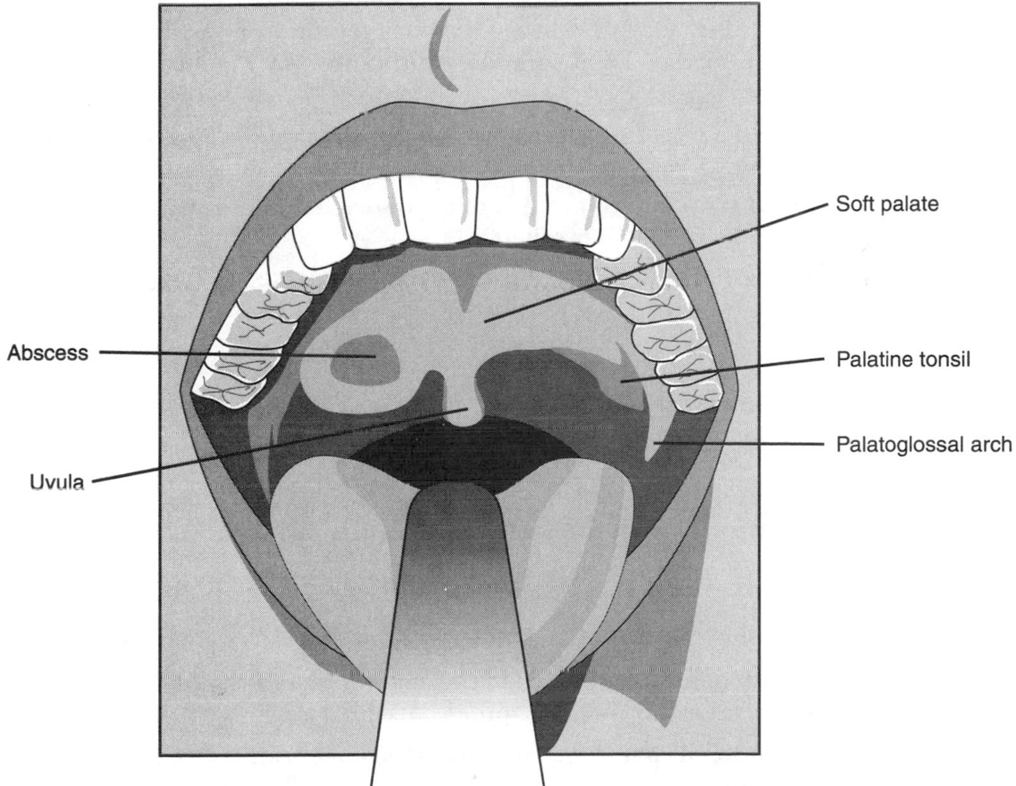

Figure 8-1. Peritonsillar abscess. (Adapted from LifeART Emergency Medicine Professional Collection. Copyright 1998, Lippincott Williams & Wilkins. All rights reserved.)

2. **Physical examination findings** may include:
   —a toxic appearance
   —**trismus** (especially with peritonsillar cellulitis)
   —**deviation of the uvula to the affected side**
   —a swollen, erythematous tonsil
   —a fluctuant soft palate mass
   —tender cervical lymph nodes

B. Diagnostic tests

1. **CBC** to look for leukocytosis.
2. **Culture** of abscess drainage to identify causative organism

C. Treatment

1. **The airway must be secured.** Up to one third of patients require intubation.
2. Consultation with an otolaryngologist for **incision** and **drainage** of the abscess. (Some centers do the incision and drainage in the emergency department and discharge the patient home with follow-up in 24 hours.)

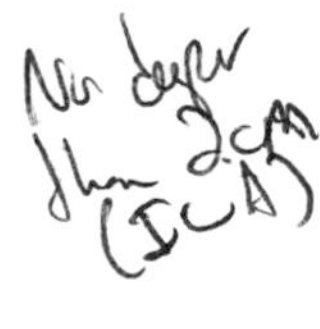

3. **Antibiotics** are directed against gram-positive organisms and anaerobes. The dosages are **penicillin** 2.4 million units IV by continuous infusion or in divided doses every 6 hours plus **metronidazole** 1 g IV loading dose, then 0.5 g IV every 6 hours (adults) or **penicillin** 50,000–100,000 U/kg/day IV plus **metronidazole** 7.5 mg/kg every 6 hours (children).
4. **Steroids** may be considered for severe edema or partial obstruction of the airway.
   a. If oral intake is tolerated, **prednisone** can be given, 40 mg orally (adults) or 1 mg/kg orally (children)
   b. IV alternatives include **methylprednisolone,** 1–2 mg/kg (children) or 125 mg (adults), and **hydrocortisone,** 100–500 mg (adults).

D. Disposition

—Most patients with a peritonsillar abscess are admitted to the hospital for incision and drainage, IV antibiotics, and hydration.

VII. Retropharyngeal and Parapharyngeal Abscess

A. Overview

1. **Definition**
   —The retropharyngeal space is the space between the posterior pharyngeal muscles and the paraspinal muscles.
   —The parapharyngeal space is the space between the pharynx and the masticator space (Figure 8-2).
2. **Risk factors** include recent dental procedures.

B. Clinical features

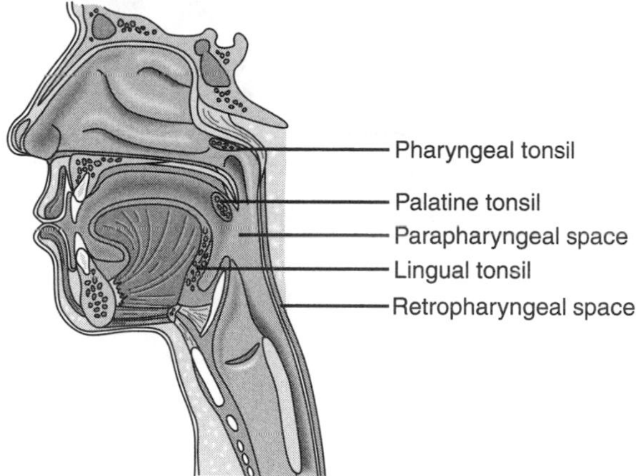

Figure 8-2. Anatomy of tonsils and pharyngeal spaces. (Adapted from LifeART Super Anatomy 1 Collection. Copyright 1998, Lippincott Williams & Wilkins. All rights reserved.)

1. **Symptoms** may include:
   —drooling
   —difficulty breathing
   —hyperextension of the neck
   —fever and chills
   —severe throat pain
2. **Physical examination findings** may include:
   —a toxic appearance
   —stridor
   —a swollen erythematous pharynx
   —tender cervical lymph nodes

C. **Diagnostic tests**

1. **Radiograph:** lateral view of neck to look for retropharyngeal soft tissue swelling. Prevertebral soft tissue should be < 7 mm at the level of C1-C3, < 5 mm at C3-C4, and < 22 mm between C4 and C7.
2. **Computed tomographic (CT) scan** or **magnetic resonance imaging (MRI) of neck and chest** to identify the location and extent of abscess

D. **Treatment**

1. **The airway must be secured.**
2. **Incision and drainage** of the abscess is performed in the operating room.
3. **Antibiotics** are given as for peritonsillar abscess (see section VI C 3).

E. **Disposition**

—Patients should be admitted to the surgical service for incision and drainage of the abscess.

VIII. Epiglottitis

A. Overview

1. Definition

—Epiglottitis is an infection of the epiglottis, vallecula, aryepiglottic folds, and arytenoids.

2. Causes

—*Haemophilus influenzae*

—Group A *Streptococcus*

—*Staphylococcus aureus*

—*Klebsiella pneumoniae*

3. Complications

—The most common complication of this infection is airway obstruction, making it a true emergency.

—Insertion of a tongue blade to obtain direct visualization is contraindicated, because doing so may precipitate airway obstruction.

B. Clinical features

1. **Symptoms** may include:

—fever

—**drooling**

—sore throat

—trismus

—dyspnea

—an acutely ill-appearing patient

2. **Physical examination findings** may include:

—an erythematous, edematous pharynx

—a **cherry-red epiglottis** (visualized on *indirect* laryngoscopy)

—**thick secretions**

—**stridor**

—cervical adenopathy

—positioning of head and neck in the "sniffing" position

C. Diagnostic tests

—Clinical suspicion is of prime diagnostic importance.

—Securing the airway is the first priority, as soon as the diagnosis is suspected.

1. Laboratory studies

a. CBC to look for leukocytosis

b. Blood culture to identify causative organism

2. **Radiograph of lateral soft tissue of the neck** to look for narrowing of posterior airway space and swelling of epiglottis—this is the most important test for epiglottitis

Thumb sign

D. Treatment

1. Securing of the airway. It may be necessary to do this in the operating room (an O_2-IV-monitor must be in place).
2. Dexamethasone may be given, in a single dose of 10 mg IV.
3. **Antibiotics** against the most common pathogens:
   —**cefuroxime** 1 g every 8 hours IV (adults) or 50 mg/kg every 8 hours IV (children), or
   —**cefotaxime** 2 g every 8 hours IV (adults) or 50 mg/kg every 8 hours IV (children), or
   —**ceftriaxone** 2 g IV every 24 h (adults) or 50 mg/kg IV every 24 hours (children)
4. Humidified air or oxygen
5. Acetaminophen for analgesia and fever reduction
6. Administration of *H. influenzae* B vaccine should be considered in unimmunized children < 5 years old.
7. Immediate otorhinolaryngology consult
8. Patient positioned upright

E. Disposition

—Patients with epiglottitis must be admitted to the hospital for observation, intravenous antibiotics, and airway management.

IX. Foreign Bodies in the Ear

A. Clinical features

1. **Symptoms** may include:
   —ear pain
   —a sense of fullness
   —hearing loss
   —a malodorous discharge
2. **Physical examination findings** may include:
   —a foreign body in the ear
   —perforation of the tympanic membrane
   —an acutely distressed patient if the foreign object is alive

B. Diagnostic tests

—Laboratory testing usually is not necessary, because the diagnosis is evident from clinical examination.

C. Treatment

1. **Removal of the foreign body** may be accomplished by irrigation with lidocaine (this is the safest method, and also kills bugs and provides analgesia), microforceps, or an ear hook. If removal is unsuccessful, consultation with an otorhinolaryngologist is necessary.

2. Analgesia with nonsteroidal antiinflammatory drugs (NSAIDs), as needed

D. Disposition

1. Patients in whom the foreign body is successfully removed and who have no complicating infection can be discharged home with outpatient follow-up in 1 week.
2. If the foreign body cannot be removed in the emergency department, the patient may need to be admitted for surgical removal.

X. Foreign Bodies in the Nose

A. Clinical features

1. **Symptoms** include:

   —unilateral epistaxis

   —a unilateral, foul-smelling discharge

2. **Physical examination** often reveals a foreign body to palpation or direct visualization.

B. Diagnostic tests

—Laboratory testing usually is not necessary, because the diagnosis is evident from clinical examination.

C. Treatment

1. **Removal of the foreign body** with a nasal speculum, a suction catheter, a nose hook, or a catheter with an inflatable balloon. Prior to manipulation, the nasal vestibule is prepared with an aerosol decongestant.
2. For smaller children, the parent can occlude the naris that does not contain the foreign body and blow a puff of air into the child's mouth, thereby causing the foreign body to be expelled.
3. If removal is unsuccessful, consultation with the otorhinolaryngology department is necessary.

D. Disposition

1. Patients in whom the foreign body is successfully removed and who have no complicating infection can be discharged home with outpatient follow-up in 1 week.
2. Patients in whom the foreign body cannot be removed in the emergency department may need to be admitted for surgical removal.

XI. Nasal Fracture

A. Overview

1. **Risk factors** include:

   —sports injuries

   —motor vehicle accidents

—falls

—domestic violence

2. **Complications** include:

—**septal hematoma**

—cribriform plate fracture with possible cerebrospinal fluid (CSF) leak

—blowout fracture

B. **Clinical features**

1. **Symptoms may** include:

—nasal pain

—nasal discharge (may be clear or bloody)

2. **Physical examination findings** may include:

—swelling

—tenderness or deformity of the nose

—ecchymosis and local crepitance

—evidence of facial trauma, including periorbital ecchymosis, epistaxis, rhinorrhea, or otorrhea

C. **Diagnostic tests**

—CT is the test of choice.

—If CT is not available, plain radiographs of the nose may be done to look for fractures.

D. **Treatment**

1. For **non-displaced fractures:**
   a. Analgesia
   b. Protective dressing
   c. Nasal decongestant
   d. Anterior nasal pack if **epistaxis** is present
2. For **displaced fractures:**
   a. Analgesia
   b. Nasal decongestant
   c. Ice
   d. Reduction of the fracture in the emergency department if swelling is not yet a problem. A protective dressing should not be placed, because significant swelling accompanies displaced fractures.
   e. The patient should see an oral or plastic surgeon or otorhinolaryngologist for follow-up once the swelling subsides (within 10–14 days).
3. For **septal hematoma:**

—The hematoma must be drained.

—If this is not done, permanent deformity of the nose secondary to damage to the cartilage, or infection leading to cavernous sinus thrombosis, which is life-threatening (50% mortality), may result.

E. Disposition

—Most patients can be discharged home with outpatient follow-up in 1 week.

XII. Epistaxis

A. Overview

1. Definition

—Nosebleeds in children are common, frequent, and usually benign.

—Nosebleeds in adults may herald underlying disease.

—Bleeding may be anterior (more common), from the inferior nasal septum (Kiesselbach's plexus), or posterior from the roof of the nasal cavity. (Posterior epistaxis is uncommon in children.)

2. Causes include:

—trauma

—infection

—nasal foreign body

—idiopathic causes

3. Risk factors include:

—abuse of NSAIDs

—alcohol abuse

—cocaine use

—blood dyscrasias

—hypertension

—anticoagulation

—dry, low-humidity air

B. Clinical features

1. Symptoms may include:

—bleeding

—lightheadedness

—pain if a nasal foreign object is present

2. Physical examination findings may include:

—dried blood clots

—a foreign object (blood may be mixed with pus)

—bruises on other parts of the body suggestive of a coagulopathy

—hepatosplenomegaly in patients with liver disease

—signs of head trauma

C. Diagnostic tests

—No special tests are necessary unless the history or physical examination suggests an underlying etiology.

1. **Laboratory studies**
   a. CBC to look for anemia and bleeding
   b. Liver function tests (LFTs) to look for liver disease
   c. Coagulation studies, including bleeding time, to look for coagulopathies
   d. Blood type and crossmatch if significant bleeding is present
2. **CT scan** of head and facial bones to look for head trauma, facial fracture, and foreign bodies.

D. **Treatment**

1. **Bleeding is stopped** via:
   a. Direct pressure, if technically feasible.
   b. Chemical cautery of the bleeding vessel with silver nitrate sticks.
   c. Topical vasoconstrictors such as epinephrine, thrombin, or topical cocaine.
   d. Anterior or posterior nasal packing.
2. **Antibiotics** to prevent sinusitis (see section IV D 1).

E. **Disposition**

1. Children with nosebleeds can be discharged home with outpatient follow-up in 1 week.
2. Adults with anterior epistaxis can be discharged home with antibiotics and outpatient follow-up in 48 hours to look for an underlying cause after bleeding is controlled in the ED.
3. Adults with posterior epistaxis should be admitted to the hospital because of the risk of asphyxiation.

Review Test

1. A 53-year-old man presents with new-onset epistaxis for which posterior nasal packing was required to attenuate bleeding. Which of the following is the most likely cause for this patient's nosebleed?

(A) Local trauma
(B) Hypertension
(C) Foreign body
(D) Upper respiratory tract infection
(E) Blood dyscrasia

2. A 3-year-old boy presents with fever and malaise and tugs at his right ear. Physical examination reveals a normal pinna and a bulging, erythematous tympanic membrane. Which of the following treatments should be instituted at this time?

(A) Steroid drops
(B) No treatment, because this probably is a viral syndrome
(C) Antibiotics against *Pseudomonas* spp
(D) Antibiotics against gram-positive organisms
(E) Antibiotics should be withheld until results of blood cultures are obtained.

3. Which one of the following statements regarding diphtheria pharyngitis is false?

(A) Complications include myocarditis and thrombocytopenia.
(B) Unimmunized children under the age of 12 should receive the diphtheria vaccine.
(C) Patients should be admitted to the hospital under strict isolation.
(D) Diphtheria antitoxin is administered to all patients.
(E) The first-line antibiotic is penicillin.

4. Which of the following is the first priority in the treatment of epiglottitis?

(A) Administration of dexamethasone 10 mg intravenously (IV)
(B) Securing the airway
(C) Administration of cefuroxime 1 g IV every 8 hours
(D) 100% oxygen
(E) Vaccination against *Haemophilus influenzae* type B

5. Which one of the following statements regarding mastoiditis is false?

(A) It results most often from under-treated otitis media.
(B) It may be caused by a cholesteatoma that blocks drainage.
(C) It occurs most commonly in elderly patients.
(D) Indications for mastoidectomy include osteomyelitis and spread to the central nervous system.
(E) The condition usually can be treated medically.

Answers and Explanations

1-B. The most common cause of nosebleeds in adults is hypertension. Posterior epistaxis accounts for only 10% of all nosebleeds, and usually is the result of laceration of the sphenopalatine artery. A blood dyscrasia most likely would have been discovered before the patient reached the age of 53 years. Local trauma is very difficult to inflict in the posterior septum. Foreign bodies in the nose are uncommon in adults. Upper respiratory tract infection can produce epistaxis, but it usually is anterior. Neoplasm, a choice not listed here, is another common cause of posterior epistaxis in adults.

2-D. Although otitis media may be viral, empiric antibiotic treatment against the most common organisms (gram-positive organisms) is the standard of care. Choices B, no treatment, and E, withholding of antibiotics until culture results are obtained, are inappropriate. Empiric therapy is instituted to avoid suppurative complications of otitis media such as mastoiditis and retropharyngeal and peritonsillar abscesses. Steroid drops are appropriate for otitis externa, not otitis media. Antipseudomonal coverage is required for malignant otitis externa, seen in diabetics, not for otitis media.

3-E. The antibiotic of choice is erythromycin. Penicillin can be used as an alternative in patients who cannot tolerate erythromycin. Nonimmunized or inadequately immunized children, adults, and close contacts of the patient who were vaccinated more than 5 years ago are (re)vaccinated.

4-B. As always, and especially in epiglottitis, the **a**irway, **b**reathing, and **c**irculation (ABCs) must be considered. Airway comes first. All of the other choices are correct treatments, but only after the airway is secured.

5-C. Mastoiditis is an infection that is seen predominantly in children and adolescents, not in elderly patients. All the other statements listed are correct.

9

Orofacial Emergencies

I. Dental Emergencies

A. Dental caries

1. Overview

—For purposes of describing pathology and identifying the specific tooth involved, each tooth is assigned a number (Figure 9-1).

a. Definition

—Dental caries is the most common cause of odontogenic pain.

b. Risk factors include:

—consumption of large amounts of sweets and hard candy

—poor oral hygiene

2. Clinical features

a. Symptoms may include:

—toothache

—jaw pain

—earache (referred pain)

—radiation of pain of MI to the jaw

b. Physical examination findings may include tenderness to percussion of the tooth.

3. Diagnostic tests

—Diagnosis is made on the basis of clinical examination, so laboratory testing is unnecessary.

—Extreme tenderness, especially at the periapical area, may represent a periapical abscess.

—If caries are not readily apparent, consider other diagnoses.

4. Treatment

a. Dental wax placed into the cavity to protect dentin and exposed pulp from irritation from heat, cold, and chemicals in food

b. Anesthetic nerve block for analgesia

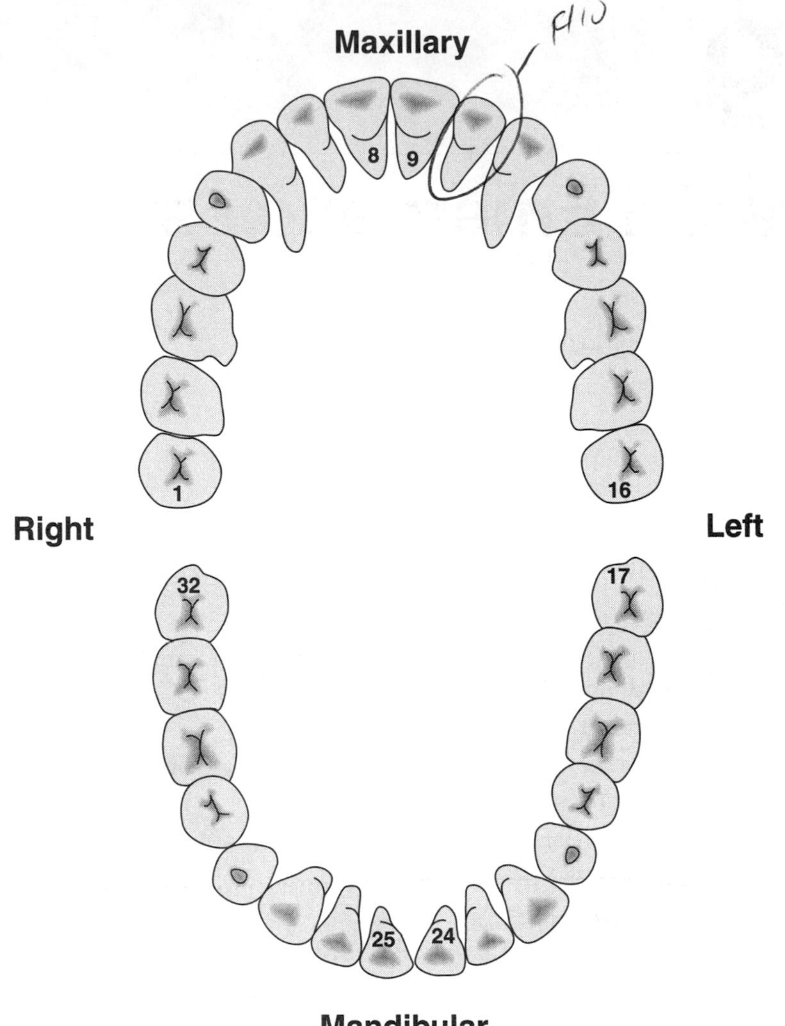

Figure 9-1. Numbering of the permanent teeth. (Adapted from LifeART Super Anatomy 3 Collection. Copyright 1998, Lippincott Williams & Wilkins. All rights reserved.)

c. Acetaminophen with codeine or oxycodone as necessary for further pain relief

d. Drainage of any periapical abscess

e. Definitive treatment is placement of a filling by a dentist.

5. Disposition

—Patients can be discharged home with outpatient follow-up in 24 hours.

B. Osteitis sicca (dry socket)

1. Overview

a. Definition

—Dry socket sometimes occurs after extraction of a tooth when the blood clot is lost or disintegrates, resulting in exposure of the bone in the socket.

b. **Risk factors include:**

—smoking (associated with poor wound healing)

—trauma to or infection of the alveolar bone

—excessive mouth rinsing (disrupts clot formation)

2. **Clinical features**

a. **Symptoms** may include:

—severe pain in the socket of the tooth that was extracted, due to loss of clot or poor clot formation

—pain that begins 24 to 96 hours after extraction and may last up to 3 weeks

—a foul odor emanating from the socket

b. **Physical examination findings** include an empty hole or space at the site where the clot should have been.

3. **Diagnostic tests**

—A **radiograph of the alveolar bone** and socket is obtained to look for retained debris or root tip

4. **Treatment**

a. **Local block** with long-acting anesthetic (e.g., bupivacaine) with a vasoconstrictor

b. Irrigation with warm saline

c. **Packing of socket** with petroleum gauze soaked in zinc oxide–eugenol mixture. This prevents food impaction, prevents infection, and prevents exposure to air, thereby decreasing pain.

d. Systemic analgesia. The pain often is refractory to nonopiate analgesics.

5. **Disposition**

—Patients can be discharged home with outpatient follow-up 24–48 hours after socket packing is placed.

—Packing must be replaced every 48–72 hours until granulation tissue begins to form and the patient starts to experience relief.

C. **Post-extraction bleeding**

1. **Clinical features**

a. **Symptoms** include:

—bleeding, either pulsatile (arterial) or oozing (venous)

—**primary bleeding,** which is bleeding from an injured vessel or soft tissue, or bleeding due to perforation of bone

—**secondary bleeding,** which is due to disruption of a clot or a coagulation defect

b. **Physical examination findings** may include:

—swelling of the soft tissues of the oral cavity.

—discolored or purplish soft tissue.

—signs of hypovolemia (a rare, late presentation)—e.g., tachycardia, a weak thready pulse, hypotension, and pallor.

2. **Diagnostic tests**
   a. **Local assessment** comes first, before any laboratory studies.
      —The field is debrided, suctioned, and cleared.
      —The area is visualized, and the bleed is localized.
      —If bleeding persists, laboratory and imaging studies are obtained.
   b. **Laboratory studies**
      —**Coagulation profile** to look for clotting factor defects (including bleeding time)
      —**Liver function tests (LFTs)** to look for liver disease as the cause of coagulation defects
      —**CBC** to look for drop in hematocrit and thrombocytopenia
   c. **Imaging studies** include an **arteriogram,** which may be necessary if arterial bleeding is not controllable (very rare).
3. **Treatment**
   a. Clearance and maintenance of patent airway
   b. **Isolation of the bleeding site:**
      —**Direct pressure is applied over the site for 45 minutes** using an absorbable gelatin sponge, with or without pressure packs containing hemostatic agents such as epinephrine, thrombin, or fibrinogen.
      —If bleeding persists, control may be obtained by electrocoagulation or, if technically feasible, by ligating the bleeding vessel.
   c. Placement of a deep suture across the soft tissue of the bleeding site
   d. Debridement of large obstructive hematomas
   e. Antibiotics if local infection is suspected
4. **Disposition**
   a. Patients whose bleeding has been successfully controlled may be discharged home with outpatient follow-up in 48 hours. Written postoperative care instructions should be given to the patient, as follows:
      —If re-bleeding occurs, bite on moist gauze for 45 minutes with constant pressure.
      —Avoid spitting, smoking, sucking through a straw, and eating hard candy.
      —Follow a soft mechanical diet (i.e., pureed foods) for 2–3 days.
   b. Patients in hypovolemic shock (very rare) must be admitted to the ICU.

D. Subluxed Tooth

—A subluxed tooth is a tooth that is loose, but still present in its socket.

1. **Clinical features**
   a. **Symptoms** include a loose or movable tooth or teeth.
   b. **Physical examination findings** include:
      —movement of the involved teeth
      —blood at the cementogingival junction
2. **Diagnostic tests**

—Diagnosis is made on the basis of clinical examination, so laboratory testing is unnecessary.

—Periapical radiographs may be considered if alveolar bone trauma is suspected.

3. **Treatment**
   a. Stabilization of teeth via wire ligatures or arch bars by a dentist, to be maintained for 2 weeks
   b. Temporizing measures, including stabilization of teeth with a resin-catalyst mixture (as if cementing) until dental consultation can be obtained
   c. Avoidance of hot liquids
   d. Soft mechanical diet

4. **Disposition**

—Patients can be discharged home with outpatient follow-up within 24 hours.

E. Avulsed tooth

—An avulsed tooth is one that has been expelled from its socket.

—This is a true dental emergency.

1. **Clinical features**
   a. **Symptoms** may include:
      —oral pain
      —bleeding
   b. **Physical examination findings** include:
      —blood in the empty socket
      —a missing tooth or teeth

2. **Diagnostic tests**

—Diagnosis is made on the basis of clinical examination, so laboratory testing is unnecessary.

—Periapical radiographs may be obtained if alveolar bone trauma is suspected.

3. **Treatment**
   a. Primary (deciduous) teeth in children younger than 6 years old are not replaced, to avoid ankylosing of tooth to alveolar bone
   b. The avulsed tooth is returned to its socket in adults and children older than 6 years old.
      —The best preservative until the tooth is replaced is saliva (the patient should be instructed to transport the tooth under the tongue or inside of the cheek) or Hank's solution, a commercially available pH-balanced solution.
      —The next best transportation medium is milk, followed by saline, and then by a wet handkerchief.
      —The worst transportation medium is none at all (dry).
   c. Once the tooth is replaced into the socket, stabilization is done as for a subluxed tooth (see I D 4).

d. Dental consult should be obtained if available

4. **Disposition**

—Patients can be discharged home with outpatient follow-up within 24 hours.

F. Tooth fracture

1. **Definition.** Tooth fractures (Figure 9-2) can be classified according to the extent of fracture penetration:

—**Ellis I:** into enamel only

—**Ellis II:** into dentin

—**Ellis III:** into pulp (true dental emergency)

2. **Clinical features**

a. **Symptoms** include tooth pain.

b. **Physical examination findings** may include:

—an obviously chipped tooth

—enamel that has a chalky white surface

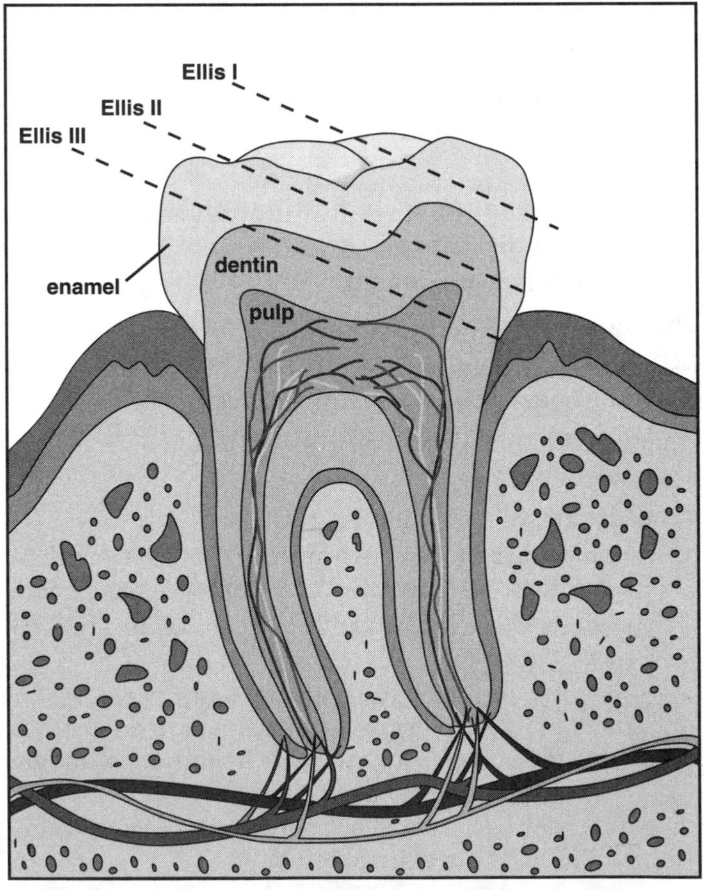

Figure 9-2. Types of tooth fractures. (Adapted from LifeART Super Anatomy 3 Collection. Copyright 1998, Lippincott Williams & Wilkins. All rights reserved.)

—dentin that has an ivory yellow color
—pulp that has a pinkish tinge to it
—frank bleeding vessels inside the pulp

3. Diagnostic tests

—Diagnosis is made on the basis of clinical examination, so laboratory testing is unnecessary.

—Periapical radiographs may be considered if alveolar bone trauma is suspected.

4. Treatment

a. For Ellis I fracture:

—Any sharp edges should be filed down with an emery board.

b. For Ellis II fracture:

—A calcium hydroxide dressing should be placed and covered with dental foil, a metal band, gauze, or enamel-bonded plastic.

c. For Ellis III fracture:

—Immediate consultation with a dentist or oral surgeon

—In adults, moist cotton should be placed over the pulp and then covered with dry dental foil. Pulpotomy should not be done. Nerve block may be considered for analgesia.

—In children, pulpotomy should be performed and the space packed with calcium hydroxide or commercially available root canal sealer. Nerve block or acetaminophen may be used for analgesia. Older children can have codeine.

5. Disposition

—Patients can be discharged home with outpatient follow-up with a general dentist or endodontist within 24 hours.

II. Infections

A. Ludwig's angina

1. Overview

a. Definition

—Ludwig's angina is a life-threatening cellulitis of the floor of the mouth involving the submental, sublingual, and submandibular spaces.

b. Causes

—The most common cause is infection of the 2nd or 3rd molars, which spreads into the spaces above the teeth

c. Risk factors include:

—recent dental work
—oral trauma
—salivary gland infection

2. Clinical features

a. Symptoms may include:

—moderate to severe pain

—dysphagia for both liquids and solids
—increased salivation
—glossitis

b. **Physical examination findings** may include:
—a swollen neck
—tachypnea
—**labored breathing**
—**edema of the oral cavity with elevation of the floor of the mouth**
—**drooling**

3. **Diagnostic tests**
   a. **Complete blood cell count (CBC)** to look for leukocytosis
   b. **Chemistry panel** to look for electrolyte abnormalities
   c. **Throat culture** and blood culture to look for the causative organism
4. **Treatment**
   a. **The airway must be secured.**
   b. IV fluids and **oxygen** are given, and the patient is placed on a cardiac monitor.
   c. **Antibiotics** against gram-positive organisms and anaerobes. Options include:
   —for adults: **penicillin** 2.4 million units intravenously (IV) by continuous infusion or in divided doses every 6 hours, plus **metronidazole** 1 g IV loading dose, then 0.5 g IV every 6 hours
   —for children: **penicillin** 50,000–100,000 U/kg/day IV, plus **metronidazole** 7.5 mg/kg every 6 hours
   —for penicillin-allergic patients, **clindamycin** 900 mg IV every 8 hours (adults) or 5 mg/kg IV every 6 hours (children)
   d. Immediate consultation with an oral surgeon or otorhinolaryngologist for **incision and drainage** of involved fascial planes followed by wide excision in the operating room. If odontogenic infection is present, the involved teeth are removed.
5. **Disposition**
—Patients should be admitted to the hospital for intravenous antibiotics and surgical exploration.

B. **Cavernous sinus thrombosis**

1. **Overview**
   a. **Definition**
   —Cavernous sinus thrombosis usually is a septic process that results from spread of infection from other sinuses or occurs as a suppurative process of infections of the upper half of the face.
   —It usually begins unilaterally and then spreads rapidly to become bilateral via the circular sinus.
   b. **Causes**
   —The organisms most commonly involved are *Streptococcus* spp, *Bacteroides* spp, and *Eikenella* spp.

c. **Risk factors** include:
—blowout fracture of the medial orbital wall
—ethmoid sinusitis
—infections of upper face (i.e., ear, dental, sinuses)

2. **Clinical features**
a. **Symptoms** may include:
—sudden onset of fever and chills
—headache
—purulent nasal discharge
—facial pain
—eye pain
—worsening of headache when head is down (e.g., when patient leans over)

b. **Physical examination findings** may include:
—**papilledema on funduscopic examination**
—proptosis due to orbital edema
—chemosis of conjunctiva and eyelids
—ophthalmoplegia
—**diplopia**
—ptosis
—exophthalmos
—decreased visual acuity
—periorbital tenderness
—swelling
—erythema

3. **Diagnostic tests**
a. **Laboratory studies**
—**CBC** to look for leukocytosis
—**Blood culture** to identify causative organism

b. **Computed tomographic (CT) scan** or **magnetic resonance imaging (MRI)** of cavernous sinus, orbit, and paranasal sinuses to look for fluid collections

4. **Treatment**
a. Antibiotics as for Ludwig's angina (see section II A 4 c)
b. Analgesia
c. Immediate consultation with an oral surgeon or otorhinolaryngologist
d. Incision and drainage in the operating room in cases of infected paranasal sinuses
e. Removal of involved teeth if odontogenic infection is present

5. **Disposition**
—Patients are admitted to the intensive care unit (ICU).
—The mortality rate is high (up to one third of cases), even with appropriate treatment

C. Acute Necrotizing Ulcerative Gingivitis

1. Overview

a. Definition

—Acute necrotizing ulcerative gingivitis is one of the few dental infections that actually penetrates non-necrotic tissue.

—The most common locations are the anterior incisor area and the posterior molar regions.

—Vincent's angina is an extension of this infection into the tonsils.

b. Causes

—The organisms most commonly involved are oral flora, *Spirochetes* spp, and *Fusobacterium* spp.

c. Incidence and prognosis

—It is commonly seen in adolescents and young adults.

2. Clinical features

a. Symptoms may include:

—oral pain

—fever

—malaise

—cervical adenopathy

—a metallic taste

b. Physical examination findings may include:

—edematous, ulcerated, bright red interdental papillae

—a **gray pseudomembrane** covering the gingiva, which bleeds when the membrane is removed

—halitosis

3. Diagnostic tests

—Diagnosis is made on the basis of clinical examination, so little laboratory testing is necessary.

—The following tests may be helpful:

a. **CBC** and **blood culture** in patients who may be immunocompromised and colonized with more than the typical organisms

b. Periapical dental radiographs to look for the extent of infection if further pathology is suspected

4. Treatment

a. Irrigation with warm saline solution

b. Antibiotics

(1) **Tetracycline** 250 mg orally 4 times a day (adults) or 20–50 mg/kg/day in divided doses 4 times a day (children > 8 years old)

(2) For children < 8 years old, **penicillin** 25–50 mg/kg in divided doses 4 times a day to avoid tooth discoloration

c. Topical viscous lidocaine for analgesia (maximum dose is 3 mg/kg)

d. Peroxide rinses

5. Disposition

—Patients can be discharged home with outpatient follow-up with a general dentist or periodontist in 48 hours

III. Fractures and Skeletal Disorders

A. Temporomandibular joint (TMJ) dislocation

1. Overview

a. Definition

—Temporomandibular joint dislocation occurs when the mandibular condyle is displaced forward from the articular eminence of the temporal bone.

b. Risk factors include:

—trauma

—yawning

—dystonic reaction

2. Clinical features

a. Symptoms may include:

—jaw pain

—dysarthria

—dysphagia

—inability to close down or bite on the anterior teeth (so the mouth stays open)

—malocclusion

b. Physical examination findings may include:

—tenderness to palpation

—inability to move or articulate the jaw

—in unilateral dislocation, deviation of the jaw toward the intact side

3. Diagnostic tests

—Mandibular radiographs to look for fracture

4. Treatment

a. Manual reduction

—The mandible is pulled downward, then posteriorly, then superiorly (Figure 9-3).

—Muscle relaxation with a benzodiazepine may be necessary before manual reduction can be done.

b. An elastic bandage wrapped circularly from the bottom of the chin to the top of the head may be used to keep the jaw closed for extra support, especially in recurrent dislocation.

5. Disposition

—Patients can be discharged home with outpatient follow-up in 1 week.

—Instructions include soft mechanical diet for 1 week, with muscle relaxants and NSAIDs as needed (see Tables 11-2 and 11-5 in Chapter 11).

B. Midface fracture

1. Overview

a. Definition

—Midface fractures include LeFort fractures (Figure 9-4) and the trimalar fracture.

Dislocated TMJ

Articular eminence

Mandibular fossa

Condyle

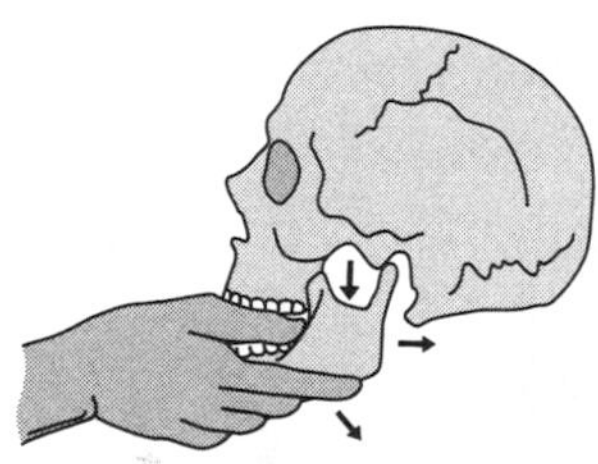

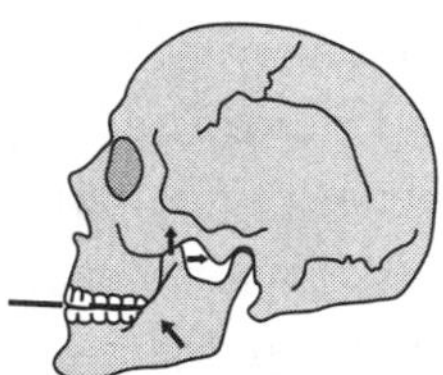

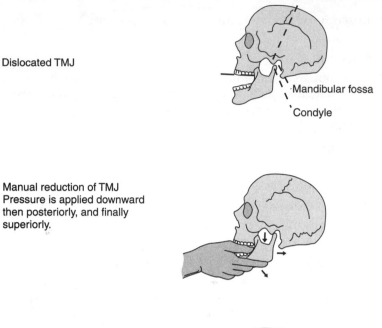

Figure 9-3. Manual reduction of a dislocated temporomandibular joint (TMJ). (A) Dislocated TMJ. (B) In manual reduction of TMJ, pressure is applied downward, then posteriorly and, finally, superiorly. (C) TMJ returned to normal position with the condyle sitting in the mandibular fossa behind the articular eminence. (Adapted from LifeART Super Anatomy 3 Collection. Copyright 1998, Lippincott Williams & Wilkins. All rights reserved.)

(1) LeFort I: separation of the lower maxilla, hard palate, and pterygoid processes from the rest of the maxilla (free-floating jaw)

(2) LeFort II: separation along the nasofrontal suture, the floor of the orbit, the zygomatico-maxillary sutures, and the pterygoid processes

(3) LeFort III: separation of the midface from the rest of the cranium.

(4) Trimalar: a complex fracture that involves the zygomatico-frontal suture, the zygomatic arches, the posterolateral wall of the maxillary sinuses, and the rim and floor of the orbit.

b. Risk factors include:

—motor vehicle accidents

—facial trauma

2. Clinical features

a. Symptoms may include:

(1) for LeFort fractures:

—jaw pain

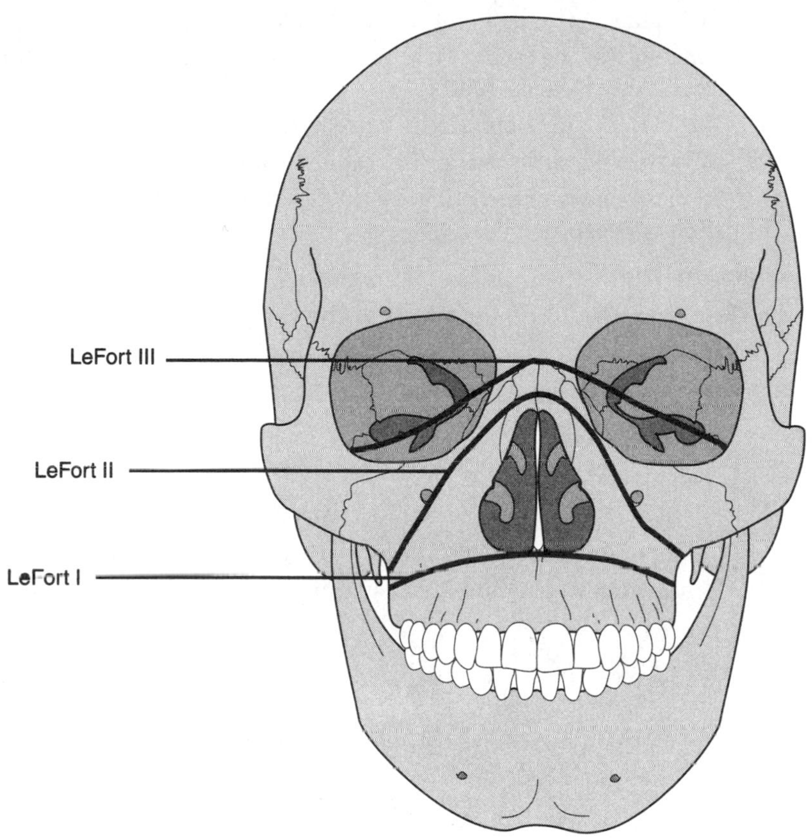

Figure 9-4. LeFort fractures. (Adapted from LifeART Super Anatomy 3 Collection. Copyright 1998, Lippincott Williams & Wilkins. All rights reserved.)

—diplopia
—bleeding

(2) for trimalar fractures:
—flattening of the cheek
—palpable step-off
—diplopia

b. Physical examination findings may include:
—CSF rhinorrhea (especially with LeFort I and II fractures)
—malocclusion of the teeth
—massive soft tissue swelling
—subconjunctival hemorrhage
—sensory deficits in the distribution of the trigeminal nerve

3. Diagnostic tests

—CT of the facial bones is done to look for air–fluid levels and fractures.

4. Treatment

a. The **airway** must be secured (this is especially important with LeFort II and III fractures).

b. The head of the bed should be elevated.
c. Antibiotics: **ceftriaxone** 2 g every 12 hours IV (adults) or 75 mg/kg/day IV (children).
d. Nasal packing if epistaxis is present.
e. **Tetanus prophylaxis** (see Table 19-5 in Chapter 19)
f. Neurosurgery consult if cerebrospinal fluid (CSF) rhinorrhea or otorrhea is present

5. **Disposition**

—Patients should be admitted to the oral or plastic surgery service for open reduction and internal fixation.

C. Mandibular Fracture

1. Overview

a. Definition

—The most common site of fracture is the angle of the mandible.

—The mandible often fractures in more than one location (Figure 9-5).

b. **Risk factors** include facial trauma.

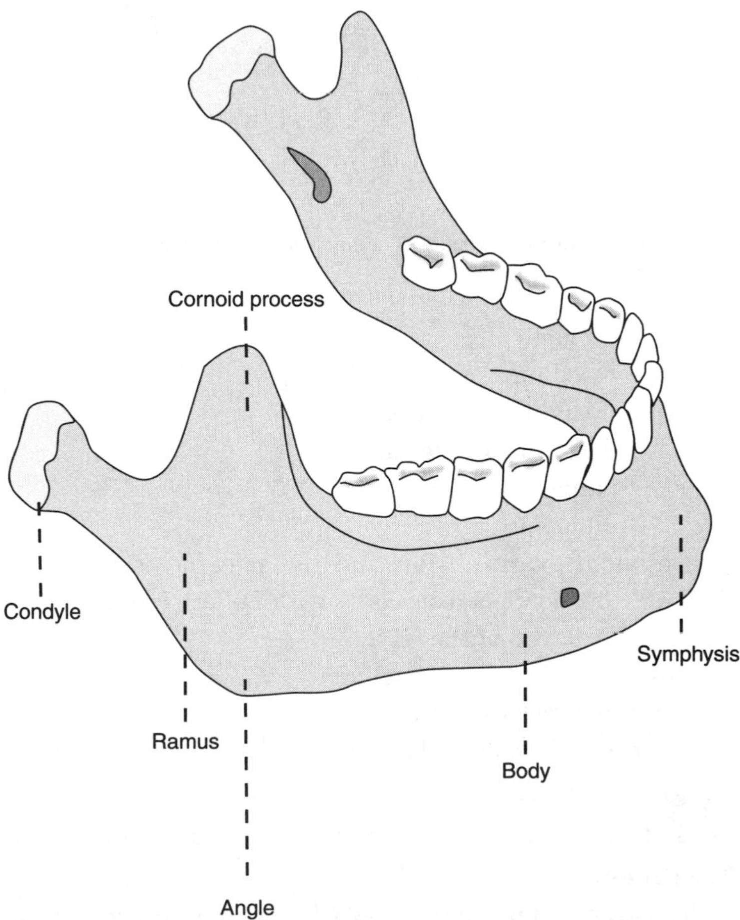

Figure 9-5. Sites of mandibular fractures. (Adapted from LifeART Super Anatomy 3 Collection. Copyright 1998, Lippincott Williams & Wilkins. All rights reserved.)

2. **Clinical features**
   a. **Symptoms** may include:
      —jaw pain
      —bleeding
      —inability to articulate the jaw
      —dysarthria
      —facial deformity
   b. **Physical examination findings** may include:
      —a step-off in dentition at the fracture site
      —malocclusion of the teeth
      —ecchymosis in the floor of the mouth
      —decreased sensation over the chin (mental nerve anesthesia)
3. **Diagnostic tests**
   a. A mandibular radiographic series to look for fracture
   b. A **CT scan** may be necessary to look for condylar fracture
4. **Treatment**
   a. The airway must be secured.
   b. Antibiotic prophylaxis using penicillin or a 1st-generation cephalosporin
   c. Tetanus prophylaxis (see Table 19-5)
5. **Disposition**
   —Patients should be admitted to the oral surgery service for open or closed reduction

IV. Soft Tissue Disorders

A. Sialolithiasis and sialoadenitis

1. **Overview**
   a. **Definition**
      —Sialolithiasis is the obstruction of one of the salivary glands by a stone composed of calcium deposits surrounding a foreign body, mucin, or bacterial nidus. Sialoadenitis results when the obstructing stone produces a local inflammation
   b. **Causes**
      —The organism most commonly involved is *S. aureus*.
2. **Clinical features**
   a. **Symptoms** may include:
      —pain and swelling over the infected salivary gland
      —exacerbation of pain on eating tart, sour, or bitter foods
   b. **Physical examination findings** may include:
      —an enlarged, tender, and indurated gland
      —a palpable firm mass (stone) along the duct of the salivary gland and floor of the mouth (submandibular gland)
      —purulence at the ductal orifice if infection is present secondary to obstruction

—expression of clear saliva on palpation of the duct if there is no infection

—pain and swelling that is reproducible with exposure to sour or bitter foods

3. **Diagnostic tests**

—Most cases are managed with antibiotics and warm compresses without any prior studies.

—The following tests are done in severe, chronic, or refractory cases:

a. **Occlusal radiograph** for the submandibular gland or CT for the parotid to look for radiopacity (stone) in the duct

b. In the absence of infection, **sialography** to check for a filling defect

4. **Treatment**

a. Analgesia with **nonsteroidal antiinflammatory drugs (NSAIDs)**

b. Antibiotics against *Staphylococcus* spp if infection is suspected

c. Warm compresses applied over the face

d. **The stone may be removed** via:

—dilatation of the duct with a lacrimal probe followed by manual removal of the stone (rarely successful)

—open incision over the site of obstruction (creates scar tissue)

—surgical removal of the stone by excising the involved portion of the gland

e. The gland may be removed (sialectomy) if the stone is impacted in the parenchyma of the gland.

5. **Disposition**

—Patients can be discharged home with outpatient follow-up in 48 hours.

B. Oral Ulcers (Table 9-1)

1. **Clinical features**

a. **Symptoms** may include:

—a blister in the oral cavity that may or may not be painful

—pain that is aggravated by salty, sour, or spicy foods

b. **Physical examination findings** may include a white fibrin clot surrounded by erythematous mucus.

2. **Diagnostic tests**

a. **CBC** if the lesion is suspicious for infection

b. Biopsy if the lesion is present for more than 2 weeks to look for malignancy

3. **Treatment** is supportive:

—gargling with warm salt water

—application of topical anesthetic gel as needed

—avoidance of aggravating foods

Table 9-1. Causes of Oral Ulcers

Trauma
Mechanical
Chemical (aspirin)
Temperature (hot foods)
Squamous cell carcinoma
Neoplasia
Autoimmune disease
Systemic lupus erythematosus
Pemphigous
Hereditary disease
Epidermolysis bullosa
Infection
Candidiasis
Herpes gingivostomatitis
Syphilis
Varicella zoster
Epstein-Barr virus
Acute necrotizing gingivitis
Miscellaneous
Aphthous stomatitis
Lichen planus
Drug reaction

4. Disposition

—Patients can be discharged home with outpatient follow-up in 1 week.

Review Questions

1. Which one of the following statements regarding the management of tooth fractures is true?

(A) Ellis III fracture in adults is treated with a pulpotomy.
(B) Ellis II fracture in children is treated by filing down exposed dentin.
(C) Ellis I and II fractures require immediate dental consult.
(D) Ellis III fractures in children are treated with a pulpotomy.
(E) Ellis II fractures are considered a true dental emergency.

2. Which of the following statements regarding avulsed teeth is false?

(A) It is especially important to replace avulsed teeth in toddlers and small children.
(B) The best medium for transporting an avulsed tooth is saliva or Hank s solution.
(C) The worst way to preserve an avulsed tooth is to let it dry out (no medium).
(D) Avulsed teeth are replaced directly into the socket as early as possible.
(E) All of the above statements are correct.

3. Which of the following is a risk factor for osteitis sicca (dry socket)?

(A) Cigarette smoking
(B) Alveolar bone trauma
(C) Multiple dental caries
(D) Excessive mouth washing
(E) All of the above

4. Which one of the following statements regarding cavernous sinus thrombosis is false?

(A) It is a life-threatening condition.
(B) Treatment consists of outpatient antibiotics, analgesia, and close follow-up.
(C) Incision and drainage of the sinuses may be necessary.
(D) The antibiotic of choice is nafcillin.
(E) Swelling of optic discs and double vision are common findings.

5. Which of the following statements regarding Ludwig s angina is true?

(A) Physical examination findings include papilledema, ptosis, and proptosis.
(B) The most common cause for this condition is oral trauma.
(C) It is a life-threatening condition.
(D) Treatment consists of outpatient antibiotics, analgesia, and close follow-up.
(E) None of the above statements are true.

Answers and Explanations

1-D. Ellis III fractures in children are treated with a pulpotomy. The key to this question is that the treatment for Ellis type fractures is different in children, who require pulpotomy, from that in adults, who do not. See section I F 1 for a description of Ellis fractures, types I through III, and their appropriate management.

2-A. Avulsed teeth are **not** replaced into the socket in children under the age of 6 years, to prevent ankylosing of the tooth to the alveolar bone.

3-E. Osteitis sicca occurs as a result of either poor clot formation or disruption of an existing clot. Poor clot formation is seen in smokers, diabetics, and patients by poor oral hygiene or trauma to the alveolar bone. An existing clot can be disrupted by sucking through a straw, excessive mouth washing, and eating hard candy. See section I B 1 for more information.

4-B. Cavernous sinus thrombosis usually is a septic process with a very high (30%) mortality despite appropriate treatment. Appropriate treatment consists of intravenous antibiotics and admission to the intensive care unit (ICU). See section II B 4 for further details.

5-C. Ludwig s angina is considered a life-threatening infection because of its potential for occluding the airway by raising the floor of the mouth. Papilledema, ptosis, and proptosis are findings on physical examination noted in cavernous sinus thrombosis, not Ludwig s angina. The most common cause for Ludwig s angina is odontogenic infection of the 2nd or 3rd molars, not oral trauma. Treatment consists of intravenous antibiotics and hospital admission, not outpatient management.

Answers and Explanations

10

Dermatologic Emergencies

I. Dermatitis

A. Acne

—Acne is an inflammatory condition of the skin that begins when the outlets of follicles are blocked.

1. Clinical presentation

—Acne presents primarily as red pustules on the face and trunk.

—**Comedones** (blackheads and whiteheads), papules, cysts, and scars also may be noted.

2. Diagnostic tests

—No special diagnostic tests are necessary.

3. Treatment

a. Tretinoin 0.025% cream for comedones, to be applied overnight and rinsed off in the morning

b. Protective sunscreen (SPF > 15) to be applied during the daytime

c. Antimicrobial rinse twice a day for mild acne

d. Antibiotics for moderate to severe acne (Table 10–1)

e. Isotretinoin for extremely severe cases, in consultation with a dermatologist. This drug is contraindicated in pregnancy. (A pregnancy test should be administered to women of childbearing age before this drug is given.)

4. Disposition

—Patients can be discharged home with outpatient follow-up with their primary care provider (PCP) or a dermatologist in 2 weeks.

B. Atopic dermatitis

Atopic dermatitis commonly occurs in conjunction with allergic rhinitis, asthma, or food or drug allergies. Patients with these conditions have an immune system that makes them slightly more susceptible to cutaneous infections.

Table 10-1. Antibiotics Used for Acne

Drug	Dose	Disadvantages/side effects
Tetracycline*	500 mg PO bid	Must be given on an empty stomach, 2 h before or 1 h after eating
Erythromycin	500 mg PO bid	GI upset
Doxycycline*	100 mg PO bid	Photosensitivity
Minocycline*	100 mg PO bid	Dizziness
Clindamycin	150 mg PO bid	Pseudomembranous colitis

*not recommended for pregnant or lactating women or children under age 8
bid = twice a day; *GI* = gastrointestinal; *PO* = orally

1. **Clinical presentation**
   a. The major **symptom** is **pruritus** (itching).
   b. **Physical examination findings** may include:
      (1) **rash**
         —usually present only in areas the patient can reach and scratch or areas that come in contact with an irritant
         —most commonly seen on the **cheeks** (in children) or on the **antecubital** and popliteal fossae (in adults)
      (2) poorly demarcated red plaques
      (3) a thickened epithelium at the site of the rash with **lichenification**
2. **Diagnostic tests**
   —No special diagnostic tests are necessary.
3. **Treatment**
   a. **Hydrocortisone 1.0–2.5% cream** applied twice a day for mild to moderate disease, on the face (adults) or for all disease (in children)
   b. **Triamcinolone 0.1% cream** applied twice a day for severe disease in adults (not on the face)
   c. **Greasy moisturizer** such as petroleum jelly or Eucerin cream applied to the skin as needed
   d. Avoidance of **known allergens**
   e. Avoidance of **irritants** such as soap, perfume, deodorant, and restrictive clothing
   f. Oatmeal baths for symptomatic relief
   g. **Nighttime sedation** if necessary to prevent scratching and the resulting excoriation and to ensure rest:
      (1) Diphenhydramine: 25–75 mg orally (adults) or 1–5 mg/kg orally (children)
      (2) Hydroxyzine: 25–75 mg orally (adults) or 0.75 mg/kg (children)
   h. Oral corticosteroids such as **prednisone** used for severe cases. Dosages are 40–60 mg orally daily for 7–10 days (adults) or 1–2 mg/kg orally daily for 7–10 days (children).

i. Any bacterial superinfection should be treated with antibiotics such as **cephalexin.** Dosages are 500 mg orally twice a day for 7–10 days (adults), or 25–50 mg/kg (to a maximum of 4 g/day) orally 4 times a day for 7–10 days (children).

4. Disposition

—Most patients can be discharged home with outpatient follow-up with their PCP or a dermatologist in 2 weeks.

—Follow-up should be in 1 week if oral corticosteroids were given in the emergency department (ED).

C. Contact dermatitis

1. Clinical presentation

—The clinical presentation of contact dermatitis is very similar to that of atopic dermatitis in both symptomatology (**pruritus**) and appearance of rash.

—The difference is that atopic dermatitis is caused by an immunologic reaction, whereas contact dermatitis is caused by a **specific irritant** coming in contact with the skin, producing a **local reaction.** Affected areas correspond to these contact areas rather than the typical areas of atopic dermatitis.

2. Diagnostic tests

—No special diagnostic tests are necessary unless the cause is not obvious and it becomes necessary to identify the allergen in order to avoid it (if possible). In this case, allergy testing may be warranted.

3. Treatment

—Treatment is the same as for atopic dermatitis (see I B 3).

4. Disposition

—Disposition is the same as for atopic dermatitis (see I B 4).

D. Stasis dermatitis

—Stasis dermatitis is eczema precipitated by lower extremity edema. The edema stretches the skin, producing inflammation and fissuring of the skin, which leads to pruritus.

1. Clinical presentation

a. **Symptoms** may include:

—**pruritus**

—**lower extremity edema**

b. **Physical examination findings** may include:

—erythema and edema of the legs

—ulcerations

—**hyperpigmentation of the skin**

—**red scaling plaques**

2. Diagnostic tests

a. **Laboratory studies**

(1) In patients with fever, a diagnosis of stasis dermatitis is inherently incomplete.

(2) A complete work-up should be done. This should include:
—a **complete blood cell count (CBC)** to look for leukocytosis
—a **blood culture** if the patient is febrile to look for the causative organism

b. **Imaging studies**

(1) **Doppler** ultrasound to look for underlying deep vein thrombosis (DVT)

(2) **Chest radiograph** or **echocardiography** if congestive heart failure (CHF) is suspected as the cause of edema

3. **Treatment**

a. The cause of the edema should be established and corrected.

b. Control of local edema:

(1) Diuretics: **furosemide** 40 mg orally or by intravenous (IV) push (adults) or 1–2 mg/kg orally or IV (children)

(2) Compression elastic stockings

(3) Elevation of the affected leg

(4) Avoidance of dependent positions

c. Topical corticosteroids administered to the area. One recommended agent is triamcinolone 0.1% to the area twice a day.

d. A moisturizer such as petroleum jelly or Eucerin cream applied to the area

e. Nighttime sedation as necessary

f. Treatment of any bacterial superinfection

4. **Disposition**

—Most patients can be discharged home with outpatient follow-up with their PCP or a dermatologist in 2 weeks.

E. **Psoriasis**

—Psoriasis is a chronic disease.

—It is worse in winter.

—There is a strong familial predisposition.

—Psoriasis can be triggered by severe sunburn, streptococcal infection, and stress.

1. **Clinical presentation**

a. There are several subforms of psoriasis:
—the **guttate** form, characterized by small papules over the trunk. It is more common in children.
—the **inverse** form, restricted to the skin folds
—the **erythrodermic** form, which covers most of the skin
—the **pustular** form, which can be life-threatening secondary to sepsis

b. **Symptoms** may include:
—**pruritic rash**
—psoriatic **arthritis**
—scattered **pitting of the nails**

c. **Physical examination findings** may include:
   (1) thick **sharply demarcated plaques** with **silvery scale**
      —Plaques may be large, >10 cm.
      —Lesions typically are located on the **scalp, knees, elbows, gluteal cleft, umbilical folds,** and **extensor surfaces.**
   (2) small papules

2. Diagnostic tests

—If presentation is indistinguishable from tinea (see section VI B 1), a potassium hydroxide (KOH) prep or fungal culture can be done.

3. Treatment

a. Hydration of the skin

b. **Topical corticosteroids** twice daily. Recommended agents are:
   —triamcinolone 0.1% cream (medium potency) or fluocinonide 0.05% cream (high potency) for the body
   —betamethasone 0.1% lotion for the scalp
   —hydrocortisone 1.0–2.5% cream for the face

c. **Topical tar 5% gel** for the body and **lotion** for the scalp applied twice daily

d. Other therapies available for severe and refractory cases of psoriasis include calcipotriene, anthralin, ultraviolet (UV) light, and psoralens. However, these are outside the realm of emergency medicine.

4. Disposition

—Patients with pustular or erythrodermic psoriasis should be admitted to the hospital for further management.

—Most other patients can be discharged home with outpatient follow-up with their PCP or a dermatologist in 2 weeks.

F. Seborrhea

1. Clinical presentation

—Seborrhea is marked by **nonpruritic,** poorly demarcated, erythematous **scaly plaques** with a greasy, **yellowish** appearance.

—The most common locations are the scalp at the hairline, the ears, and the retroauricular area.

2. Diagnostic tests

—If presentation is indistinguishable from tinea (see section VI B 1) , a KOH prep or a fungal culture can be done.

3. Treatment

a. For adults, an **antiseborrheic shampoo** may be used every other day. The shampoo is left on for 5 minutes, and the scales are then scrubbed off vigorously.

b. For infants, scalp scales should be softened with mineral oil or baby shampoo and then manually brushed or picked off. A fine-toothed comb is very helpful.

c. For severe cases (children and adults), topical hydrocortisone 1.0–2.5% may be used twice daily.

4. **Disposition**

—Patients can be discharged home with outpatient follow-up with their PCP or a dermatologist in 2 weeks.

II. Maculopapular Lesions

A. Pityriasis rosea

1. **Clinical presentation**
   a. Pityriasis rosea is **asymptomatic** except for occasional mild pruritus.
   b. **Physical examination findings** may include:
      —an **oval-shaped papulosquamous pink rash** over the **trunk** and **proximal extremities** in **linear eruptions** along skin lines ("Christmas tree" pattern)
      —a **herald patch,** which is a larger annular plaque, preceding eruption
      —no involvement of the palms of the hands and soles of the feet
   c. Pityriasis rosea usually is seen in adolescents and young adults.
2. **Diagnostic tests**
   —If the presentation is indistinguishable from that of secondary syphilis (see Table 14–3), a **reactive plasma reagent test (RPR)** for syphilis may be done.
3. **Treatment**
   a. **Hydrocortisone** 1.0–2.5% or **triamcinolone** 0.1% cream applied twice daily if the rash is itchy
   b. Exposure to natural sunlight may hasten recovery.
   c. Reassurance that the condition is benign
4. **Disposition**
   —Patients can be discharged home with outpatient follow-up with their PCP or a dermatologist in 2 weeks.

B. Lichen planus

1. **Clinical presentation** may include:
   —closely adherent shiny pink scale
   —hyperpigmentation at the sites of old lesions
   —white lesions on the mucous membranes
2. **Diagnostic tests**
   —No special diagnostic tests are necessary.
3. **Treatment**
   a. **Triamcinolone** 0.1% twice a day for the body
   b. **Fluocinonide** 0.5% liquid gel for mucous membranes
   c. **Prednisone** 40–60 mg orally daily for 7 days (adults) or 1–2 mg/kg/day (children) for severe oral lesions
   d. Topical analgesia with lidocaine jelly as needed
   e. Systemic analgesia with acetaminophen

4. **Disposition**

—Patients can be discharged home with outpatient follow-up with their PCP or a dermatologist in 2 weeks.

III. Vesiculobullous Lesions

A. Pemphigus vulgaris

—Pemphigus vulgaris is a rare autoimmune blistering disease.

—It results in death 80% of the time if left untreated.

1. **Clinical presentation**
   a. **Symptoms** may include:
      —oral erosions (almost always present) that are especially prominent on the gingiva and posterior palate
      —dysphagia secondary to oral lesions
      —lesions that progress to cover non–mucous membrane surfaces of the body.
   b. **Physical examination findings** may include:
      —large flaccid bullae on a background of non-inflamed skin
      —patients who do not appear acutely ill
2. **Diagnostic tests**
   —Diagnostic tests are not usually performed in the ED.
   a. Skin biopsy to look for intraepidermal bullae and eosinophils
   b. Immunofluorescent staining to look for IgG autoantibodies
3. **Treatment**
   a. **Prednisone** 60–200 mg (adults) or 1–2 mg/kg/day (children) orally or IV until new lesions stop appearing
   b. Nonsteroidal anti-inflammatory drugs (NSAIDs) for analgesia (see Table 11-2 in Chapter 11)
   c. Local wound care
4. **Disposition**
   —Most patients can be discharged home with outpatient follow-up with their PCP or a dermatologist the following day.
   —Patients who appear toxic or who are immunocompromised should be admitted to the hospital for intravenous fluids and corticosteroid therapy.

B. Staphylococcal scalded skin syndrome (SSSS)

1. **Overview**
   a. **Definition**
      —SSSS is a syndrome of exfoliation caused by a staphylococcal exotoxin.
      —It resembles toxic epidermal necrolysis (TEN; see III C) in physical appearance, but the treatment is different, and it is therefore important to distinguish between these entities (Table 10–2).

Table 10-2. Differences Between SSSS and TEN

	SSSS	TEN
Age group	Children under 5 years	Adults
Appear acutely ill	No	Yes
Focus of infection	Usually present	No
Mucous membranes	Spared	Involved
Skin biopsy shows	Epidermal blister	Subepidermal blister
Tzanck smear	Epithelial cells with small nuclei	Cuboidal cells with large nuclei
Antibiotics	Yes	No
Disposition	Most discharged	All patients admitted to ICU

ICU = intensive care unit; *SSSS* = staphylococcal scalded skin syndrome; *TEN* = toxic epidermal necrolysis.

b. **Incidence**
—SSSS is seen almost exclusively in children under the age of 5 years and immunocompromised adults.

2. **Clinical presentation**
a. **Symptoms** may include:
—a prodrome of fever, skin tenderness, and irritability
—superficial loss of skin but adequate barrier against fluid loss and bacterial superinfection
b. **Physical examination findings** may include:
—crusting of the skin around the mouth
—radial cracking of the skin
—dehydration
—skin that is warm and tender to palpation
—morbilliform rash with flaccid bullae (as with TEN, section III C)
—**Nikolsky's sign,** caused when gentle rubbing of the skin results in separation of the epidermis at the granular cell layer

3. **Diagnostic tests**
a. **Skin biopsy** to look for superficial blister in epidermis (not usually done in the ED)
b. Tzanck smear to look for epithelial cells with small nuclei
c. CBC to look for leukocytosis
d. Blood cultures to look for *Staphylococcus* organisms. (Results often are negative in children.)
e. **Chemistry panel** to look for electrolyte abnormalities

4. **Treatment**
a. Antibiotics against *Staphylococcus* spp: **cephalexin** or **nafcillin** 50 mg/kg 4 times a day for 7 days

b. Local skin care: wet to dry dressings, then Bacitracin (or other topical antibiotic) ointment

5. **Disposition**

—Most patients can be discharged home with outpatient follow-up with their PCP or a dermatologist in 2 weeks.

—Patients with major fluid and electrolyte imbalances may need to be admitted to the hospital for correction.

C. Toxic epidermal necrolysis (TEN)

1. **Overview**

a. **Definition**

—Toxic epidermal necrolysis (TEN) is a severe form of **erythema multiforme** caused by immune complex–mediated **hypersensitivity** to a drug.

b. **Causes**

—The most common offending agents are sulfonamides, penicillins, cephalosporins, anticonvulsants, and barbiturates.

—The most common infectious triggers are herpes simplex virus (HSV) and *Mycoplasma* spp.

c. **Incidence and prognosis**

—TEN usually is seen in adults.

d. **Complications** include:

—blindness

—phimosis

—renal failure

—sepsis

—gastrointestinal (GI) bleed

2. **Clinical presentation**

a. **Symptoms** may include:

—a prodrome of low-grade fever, headache, malaise, and anorexia

b. **Physical examination findings** may include:

—rapid onset of generalized painful erythematous **morbilliform rash** with **flaccid bullae**

—exfoliation of the skin at the dermo-epidermal junction, resulting in underlying **denuded skin**

—blistering of the mucous membranes

—**severe conjunctivitis**

3. **Diagnostic tests**

a. **Skin biopsy** to look for subepidermal blister with inflammation (not usually done in the ED)

b. Tzanck smear to look for cuboidal cells with large nuclei

c. **Chemistry panel** to look for electrolyte abnormalities and elevated blood urea nitrogen (BUN), creatinine, and CK

d. Urinalysis to look for hematuria and proteinuria if renal involvement is present

e. CBC to look for leukopenia

4. **Treatment**
   a. Discontinuation of the offending agent
   b. **Fluid and electrolyte replacement**
   c. Consultation with the burn service to debride necrosed skin and apply 0.5% silver nitrate wet dressings
   d. Treatment of conjunctivitis, if present (see Chapter 7, section VIII D)
   e. Steps taken to avert superinfection (prophylactic antibiotics are not indicated)
   f. Consultations with critical care, ophthalmology, and dermatology specialists should be considered.
   g. Use of systemic corticosteroids is controversial.

5. **Disposition**

   —Patients with toxic epidermal necrolysis should be admitted (or transferred) to the burn unit.

IV. Bacterial Infections

A. Cutaneous abscess

—An abscess is a collection of pus surrounded by an area of inflamed tissue in which hyperemia and infiltration of leukocytes are present.

—A **furuncle** is an abscess in a hair follicle or sweat gland.

—A **carbuncle** is a multilocular suppurative extension of a furuncle. Abscesses may occur on any area of the body.

1. **Clinical presentation**
   a. **Symptoms** may include:
      —pain
      —edema
      —erythema
      —warmth of the abscess area
      —fever
   b. **Physical examination findings** may include:
      —a tender fluctuant mass
      —localized erythema and lymphangitis

2. **Diagnostic tests**

   —No special diagnostic tests are necessary.

3. **Treatment**
   a. **Incision and drainage.** The wound should be packed with sterile or iodoform gauze.
   b. Antibiotics
      (1) In the ED: cephalexin 1 g IV once (adults) or 75 mg/kg once (children)
      (2) As outpatient therapy: 1st-generation cephalosporin, dicloxacillin or clindamycin for 10 days

(3) For diabetics: amoxicillin-clavulanic acid 500 mg orally 3 times a day; or other regimens that cover *Staphylococcus* spp, *Streptococcus* spp, gram-negative rods, and anaerobes.

c. NSAIDs for analgesia and fever reduction

4. Disposition

—Most patients can be discharged home with outpatient follow-up in 24 hours to remove packing and inspect the wound.

—Patients with systemic illness or who are severely immunocompromised may require hospitalization for administration of intravenous antibiotics.

B. Cellulitis

1. Overview

a. Definition

—Cellulitis is an infection of the **dermis and subcutaneous tissue.**

b. Causes

—The most common cause of cellulitis in general is *Staphylococcus aureus.*

—The most common cause of periorbital cellulitis is *Haemophilus influenzae.*

c. Risk factors include:

—**diabetes mellitus** or another immunocompromised state

—underlying local trauma or burn

—lymphedema secondary to tumor invasion or radiation therapy

—intravenous drug use

—having had saphenous veins removed for coronary artery bypass grafting

2. Clinical presentation

a. Symptoms may include:

—localized erythema and edema over a painful area

—fever, chills and malaise

—facial swelling if periorbital cellulitis

—local lymphadenopathy

—pruritus

b. Physical examination findings may include:

—borders of lesion that are not sharply demarcated

—rash that is most commonly located over the lower extremities and around the eyes

3. Diagnostic tests

a. CBC to look for leukocytosis

b. Blood cultures to identify causative organism

4. Treatment

a. Antibiotics

(1) In the ED: 1–2 g cefazolin IV

(2) For mild infections: dicloxacillin 500 mg orally every 6 hours for

10 days (adults) or penicillin V 25–50 mg/kg/day orally in 3 divided doses (children)

(3) For severe infections or infections in immunocompromised patients: nafcillin or oxacillin 2 g IV every 4 hours (adults) or 50 mg/kg IV every 6 hours (children). An alternative is cefazolin 1g IV (adults) every 8 hours or 25–100 mg/kg/day in divided doses (children).

b. Elevation of the extremity

c. NSAIDs for analgesia (see Table 11-2 in Chapter 11)

5. Disposition

a. Patients with mild or limited infection may be discharged home with outpatient follow-up in 48 hours.

b. Patients with severe infections, those who are immunocompromised, or those with facial cellulitis should be admitted to the hospital for intravenous antibiotics

C. Erysipelas

—Erysipelas is a **group A streptococcal** infection of the **superficial skin lymphatics.**

—It usually is acute, but it also may be chronic.

—It is most common in children and elderly patients.

1. Clinical presentation

a. Symptoms may include:

—a prodrome of fever, chills, and malaise

—pruritus

—facial erythema

—acute onset

b. Physical examination findings may include:

—lesions with **sharply demarcated,** deeply **raised** borders

—a rash that is most commonly located over the face and consists of an erythematous symmetric plaque

2. Diagnostic tests

a. CBC to look for leukocytosis

b. Blood cultures to identify causative organism

3. Treatment

—Treatment is the same as that for cellulitis. See section IV B 4.

4. Disposition

—Disposition is the same as that for cellulitis. See section IV B 5.

D. Impetigo Contagious

—Impetigo is a **staphylococcal** infection of the most superficial layer of the **epidermis.**

—It also can be caused by streptococcal infection.

1. Clinical presentation

—Impetigo begins as an erythematous tender papule and progresses to a **honey-colored, crusty, vesiculopustular rash.**

—It is most commonly located on the face.

—It may complicate insect bites.

—It may coexist with HSV.

2. Diagnostic tests

—No special diagnostic tests are necessary.

3. Treatment

a. For limited disease: **mupirocin** ointment to the area 4 times a day for 5 days

b. For more involved disease: **cephalexin** 25–50 mg/kg every 6 hours for 7 days (maximum dose is 4 g per day)

c. NSAIDs for analgesia (see Table 11-2 in Chapter 11)

4. Disposition

—Patients can be discharged home with outpatient follow-up in 2-3 days.

E. Scarlet fever

—Scarlet fever is a group A beta-hemolytic streptococcal infection caused by an **exotoxin.** It is transmitted via the airborne route. The peak incidence is in children aged 4 to 8 years.

1. Clinical presentation

a. **Symptoms** may include:

—abrupt onset of **fever**

—**sore throat**

—headache

—facial flushing

—vomiting

—abdominal pain

—**myalgias**

—a rash that appears 1 to 2 days after initial onset of symptoms

b. **Physical examination findings** may include:

—**"white strawberry tongue"** due to a white covering on the dorsum of the tongue with prominent red papillae; this progresses to a red strawberry tongue.

—red macules on the uvula and palate.

—purulent tonsillitis.

—bright red oral mucous membranes with a **circumoral pallor**

—a **sandpaper-like rash** due to punctate lesions on top of erythematous patches that is most prominent around the ears, axillae, and trunk

—Pastia's lines: linear petechiae in the skin creases

—desquamation of skin, occurring 1 week after resolution of the rash

2. Diagnostic tests

a. **Throat culture** or "rapid strep test" to look for streptococcal infection

b. Antistreptolysin O titer to look for group A streptococcal infection

c. **CBC** to look for leukocytosis and eosinophilia

3. **Treatment**
   a. **Benzathine penicillin** given intramuscularly is the drug of choice: 1.2 million units (adults) or 600,000 units (children under 25 kg). Oral penicillin V 4 times a day also may be given. Alternative drugs are macrolides and cephalosporins
   b. **Acetaminophen** to reduce fever: 325-1000 mg orally 3 or 4 times a day, to a maximum of 4 g/day (adults) and 10–15 mg/kg 4 times a day, to a maximum dose of 2.5 g/day (children)
   c. Treatment of potential complications is discussed in the sections referring specifically to those complications: otitis media (Ch. 8 I C); peritonsillar abscess (Ch. 8 VI C), sinusitis (Ch. 8 IV C); meningitis (Ch. 6 I C); pneumonia (Ch. 3 VI C), and rheumatic fever.

4. **Disposition**

   —Most patients can be discharged home with outpatient follow-up in 2–3 days.

   —Children should receive at least 1 day of antibiotics before they return to school.

V. Viral Infections

A. Varicella

—Varicella is a contagious, pruritic, viral infection that occurs most commonly in children.

1. **Clinical presentation** may include lesions that begin as pink, non-scaling papules, which develop pustules on top with eventual crusting. Lesions are present in **all stages of healing** and are scattered all over the body
2. **Diagnostic tests**

   —Chest radiograph to look for varicella pneumonia

3. **Treatment**
   a. **To control pruritus:** nighttime sedation with diphenhydramine or hydroxyzine. Oatmeal baths, cool compresses, talcum powder and calamine lotion also may be helpful
   b. Treatment of any bacterial superinfection
   c. **Acyclovir** for healthy hosts at risk for severe disease (e.g., patients with chronic dermatologic or respiratory conditions, or those who are older than 12)

      —800 mg orally 5 times a day for 5 days (adults) or 20 mg/kg orally daily (maximum dose 800 mg/day) for 5 days (children).

      —For high-risk groups (immunocompromised hosts, pregnant women in their 3rd trimester, and patients with evidence of pneumonia), 10–12 mg/kg (infused over 1 hour) every 8 hours for 7 days.

   d. Postexposure prophylaxis for high-risk groups with varicella immune globulin (VZIG)
   e. VZV vaccine is recommended as part of routine childhood immunizations and is given between the ages of 12 and 18 months. Susceptible unvaccinated adults should receive 2 doses of the vaccine 1 month apart.

4. Disposition

—Patients in high-risk groups should be admitted for intravenous antibiotics.

—Most other patients can be discharged home with outpatient follow-up in 2–3 days.

B. Herpes simplex

1. Clinical presentation may include painful scattered vesicles and pustules, most commonly on the mouth (usually HSV1) and genitalia (usually HSV2).

2. Diagnostic tests

—No specific tests are necessary.

—Tzanck smear does not differentiate between VZV and HSV.

3. Treatment

a. Antiviral agents: **acyclovir** 5 mg/kg up to 500 mg orally 5 times a day, or **famciclovir** 500 mg orally 3 times a day for 7 days, or **valacyclovir** 1000 mg orally 3 times a day for 7 days

b. NSAIDs or opiates for analgesia (see Table 11-2 in Chapter 11)

c. Topical **capsaicin** 0.25 % ointment to affected area 3 times a day for analgesia

d. Cool compresses, sitz baths, and Burow's solution for symptomatic relief

4. Disposition

—Most patients can be discharged home with outpatient follow-up in 2–3 days.

C. Herpes zoster

1. Clinical presentation

a. Symptoms may include:

—a prodrome of moderate to severe pain, which may precede the rash by 24–36 hours

—a blistering rash in **dermatomal distribution** (grouped vesicles on an erythematous base) with lesions that do not cross the midline

—lesions on trunk, face, and scalp (the most commonly affected areas)

b. Physical examination findings may include:

—lesions in the inner ear with involvement of the facial nerve (Ramsay-Hunt syndrome)

—lesions along the distribution of the ophthalmic division of the trigeminal nerve (ophthalmic zoster)

2. Diagnostic tests

—No specific tests are necessary.

—Tzanck smear does not differentiate between VZV and HSV.

3. Treatment

—Treatment is the same as that for HSV; see section V B 3.

4. Disposition

—Patients with ophthalmic zoster or involvement of multiple dermatomes should be admitted for intravenous antibiotics.

—Most other patients can be discharged home with outpatient follow-up in 2–3 days.

VI. Fungal Infections

A. Candida

—*Candida albicans* is a fungus that is part of the normal body flora that can overgrow secondary to diabetes, following therapy with antibiotics, and stress.

1. **Clinical presentation** may include:

   —oral lesions that manifest as white exudates that bleed when scraped

   —cutaneous lesions that manifest as red glistening plaques and are most prominent in skin folds and moist areas of the body

   —in **genital candidiasis,** a pruritic, beefy red vulva (in women) or balanitis (in men) and surrounding pustules

2. **Diagnostic tests**
   a. **KOH prep** to look for hyphae
   b. Fungal culture (optional)
   c. Chemistry panel to look for hyperglycemia if diabetes is suspected
   d. Urinalysis to look for glycosuria if diabetes is suspected

3. **Treatment**
   a. For cutaneous infections, a **topical antifungal** such as clotrimazole or miconazole applied once daily until the infection has cleared
   b. For oral thrush, nystatin oral suspension or fluconazole 150 mg orally, in a single dose (adults) or 6 mg/kg (children).
   c. For vulvar infections, either a topical antifungal for 3–7 days or a single dose of fluconazole 150 mg

4. **Disposition**

   —Most patients can be discharged home with outpatient follow-up in 2–3 days.

B. Tinea

—Tinea is a fungal infection that may occur in many places, notably on the head (tinea capitis), feet (tinea pedis), medial thighs (tinea cruris), and central trunk (tinea versicolor).

1. **Clinical findings**
   a. **Tinea capitis**

      —usually seen in children

      —associated with alopecia and a boggy scalp, and with annular lesions

   b. **Tinea pedis**

      —associated with fungal nail disease

      —well-demarcated lesions

c. **Tinea cruris**
—solid plaques
—penis, scrotum, and vulva usually spared

d. **Tinea versicolor**
—is not annular
—lesions occur mostly over the central trunk
—lesions are of many colors, including pink and skin-colored

2. **Diagnostic tests**
a. **KOH prep**
b. Fungal culture

3. **Treatment**
a. **Topical antifungal** such as clotrimazole or econazole once daily until clear
b. If pustules or blistering is present, or if hair follicles are involved:
—**griseofulvin** 500 mg orally twice a day (adults) or 20 mg/kg/day (children) with food, or
—**fluconazole** 200 mg/day (adults) or 3–5 mg/kg/day (children)
c. If severe inflammation is present: **prednisone** 40–60 mg per day orally in a single dose (adults) or 1 mg/kg/day for 7 days (children)

4. **Disposition**
—Most patients can be discharged home with outpatient follow-up with their PCP or a dermatologist in 2 weeks.
—If oral corticosteroids were given in the ED, follow-up should be in 1 week.

VII. Parasitic Infections

A. Scabies

1. **Clinical presentation**
a. **Symptoms** include eczema secondary to an immunologic reaction to mite infestation. The major symptom is **extreme pruritus.**
b. **Physical examination findings** include:
—linear erythematous burrows in characteristic locations: **web spaces of digits, axillae, groin, penis,** and **skin under breasts in women**
—no infestation above the neck
—lesions that are papulosquamous

2. **Diagnostic tests**
—Scraping of burrows may yield mites or mite feces.

3. **Treatment**
a. **5% permethrin cream** applied all over the patient's body and all household contacts and left on for 8–14 hours. Treatment to be repeated in 48 hours.

b. Ivermectin 200 mg given orally in a single dose (children and adults)

c. All linens and bedclothes that have come in contact with the patient in the previous 24 hours washed in hot water

d. Supportive measures for pruritus, including topical corticosteroids, skin lubrication, nighttime sedation, and treatment of bacterial superinfection (see section I B, atopic dermatitis).

4. Disposition. Patients can be discharged home with outpatient follow-up in 2–3 days.

B. Pediculosis

—Pediculosis is pruritus secondary to infestation by head lice.

1. Clinical presentation includes white nits (eggs) cemented to the hair shaft. A louse 3 cm long with an oval body and multiple appendages may be noted.

2. Diagnostic tests

—No special diagnostic tests are necessary

3. Treatment

a. Permethrin 5% cream applied for 10 minutes and then rinsed. Permethrin rinse should be repeated in 48 hours.

b. Lindane 1% shampoo is a cheaper alternative to permethrin; it is applied for 4 minutes, then rinsed. However, lindane is not recommended for children under the age of 2 years, or for pregnant or lactating women.

c. Ivermectin 200 mg is given orally in 1 dose (children and adults)

d. All household contacts and clothing must be washed in hot water.

4. Disposition

—Patients can be discharged home with outpatient follow-up in 1 week.

Review Questions

Directions: The response options for Items 1–6 are the same. You will be required to select one answer for each item in the set.

Questions 1–6

Match each description with the most appropriate disease.

1. Erysipelas
2. Varicella
3. Herpes zoster
4. Scarlet fever
5. Impetigo
6. Scabies

(A) A honey-colored, crusty, vesiculopustular rash
(B) Characterized by pruritic lesions in all different stages of healing
(C) Marked by linear petechiae in skin creases
(D) Characterized by a blistering rash in dermatomal distribution
(E) Marked by erythematous burrows in the web spaces of the hands
(F) Identified by the presence of a painful red rash with a sharply demarcated raised border

Directions: The response options for Items 7–11 are the same. You will be required to select one answer for each item in the set.

Questions 7–11

Match each definition with the most appropriate infection.

7. Erysipelas
8. Scabies
9. Candida
10. Cellulitis
11. Impetigo

(A) An infection of the dermis and subcutaneous tissue
(B) An infection of the superficial skin lymphatics
(C) An infection of the superficial layer of the epidermis
(D) Characterized by overgrowth of normal flora
(E) An infection associated with poor hygiene conditions

Directions: The response options for Items 12–16 are the same. Each item will state the number of options to choose. Choose exactly this number.

Questions 12–16

Match each item with the correct syndromes, diseases, or disorders.

(A) Stevens-Johnson syndrome
(B) Eczema
(C) Atopic dermatitis
(D) Psoriasis
(E) Seborrhea
(F) Pityriasis rosea
(G) Pediculosis
(H) Toxic epidermonecrolysis
(I) Herpes zoster
(J) Severe pemphigus vulgaris
(K) Scabies
(L) Pustular psoriasis

12. Parasitic infestation (select 2 disorders)
13. Intense pruritus (select 4 disorders)
14. Treated with corticosteroids (select 3 disorders)
15. Nonpruritic rash (select 2 disorders)
16. Requires hospitalization (select 4 disorders)

Answers and Explanations

1-F, 2-B, 3-D, 4-C, 5-A, 6-E. Erysipelas is characterized by the presence of a painful red rash with a sharply demarcated raised border. Varicella is characterized by the presence of pruritic lesions in all different stages of healing. Herpes zoster is characterized by a blistering rash in dermatomal distribution. One of the characteristic features of scarlet fever is linear petechiae in the skin creases. Impetigo presents as a honey-colored, crusty, vesiculopustular rash. Scabies is marked by erythematous burrows in the web spaces of the hands.

7-B, 8-E, 9-D, 10-A, 11-C. Erysipelas is an infection of the superficial skin lymphatics. Scabies is associated with poor hygiene conditions. Candida is characterized by overgrowth of normal flora. Cellulitis is an infection of the dermis and subcutaneous tissue. Impetigo is an infection of the superficial layer of the epidermis.

12-G, K; 13-B, C, D, G, K; 14-C, D, E, F; 15-E, I.; 16-A, H, J, L. Pediculosis and scabies are caused by parasitic infestation. Intense pruritus is a feature of eczema, atopic dermatitis, psoriasis, pediculosis, and scabies. Atopic dermatitis, psoriasis, seborrhea, and pityriasis rosea are treated with corticosteroids. Nonpruritic rash is a feature of seborrhea and herpes zoster. Stevens-Johnson syndrome, toxic epidermonecrolysis, severe pemphigus, and pustular psoriasis are all potentially life-threatening conditions that require hospitalization.

11

Rheumatology, Immunology, and Nontraumatic Musculoskeletal Emergencies

I. Collagen Vascular Diseases

A. Rheumatoid arthritis

1. Overview

a. Definition

—is a chronic syndrome characterized by inflammation of the peripheral joints, primarily the synovium, resulting in its destruction.

b. Incidence

—occurs most often in people between the ages of 25 and 50 years.

—is more common in women.

2. Clinical presentation

a. Symptoms may include:

—joint tenderness

—morning stiffness

b. Physical examination findings may include:

—deformities such as flexion contractures and ulnar deviation of the fingers

—soft tissue swelling in three or more joints

—synovial thickening

—symmetric involvement of proximal interphalangeal (PIP), metacarpophalangeal (MCP), or wrist joints

3. Diagnostic

a. Criteria (Table 11-1)

b. Tests

(1) Laboratory studies

Table 11-1. American College of Rheumatology Criteria for the Diagnosis of Rheumatoid Arthritis

1. Morning stiffness for at least 1 hour
2. Arthritis of at least 3 joint areas
3. Arthritis of hand joints (wrist, metacarpophalangeal or proximal interphalangeal joints)
4. Symmetric arthritis
5. Rheumatoid nodules
6. Serum rheumatoid factor, by a method positive in < 5% of normal control subjects
7. Radiographic changes (hand radiograph changes typical of rheumatoid arthritis that must include erosions or unequivocal bony decalcification)

Any 4 criteria must be present to diagnose rheumatoid arthritis; criteria 1 through 4 must have been present for at least 6 weeks.
(Reprinted with permission of the American College of Rheumatology, 1987.)

—Complete blood cell count (CBC) to look for normochromic (or slightly hypochromic) normocytic anemia

—Serum rheumatoid factor (RF): positive in >75% to 90% of cases

—Erythrocyte sedimentation rate (ESR): elevated in 90% of cases

—Aspiration of synovial fluid to look for a sterile but cloudy-appearing fluid with reduced viscosity; white blood cell (WBC) counts range from 3000–50,000

(2) Radiographs of involved joints may demonstrate:

—periarticular osteoporosis

—joint space (articular cartilage) narrowing

—marginal erosions

4. Treatment

a. Treatment in the emergency department (ED) may include:

(1) Nonsteroidal anti-inflammatory drugs (NSAIDs) for analgesia (Table 11-2)

(2) Splinting of painful joints

(3) Intraarticular steroids to relieve acutely painful joints. Approximate doses of methylprednisolone for various joints are 5 mg for PIP joints, 20 mg for wrists, 30 mg for elbows, and 40–80 mg for large joints such as the knee or shoulder. Steroids should be given only in instances where joint infection can be definitively excluded.

b. Outpatient treatment may include gold, methotrexate, and antimalarial agents.

5. Disposition

—Most patients can be discharged home with outpatient follow-up in 1–2 weeks.

B. Systemic lupus erythematosus (SLE)

—primarily affects young women between the ages of 15 and 45 years.

—may begin abruptly, or may develop insidiously over months or years with episodes of fever and malaise.

1. Clinical presentation

a. Symptoms may include:

—fatigue

Table 11-2. Nonsteroidal Anti-Inflammatory Drugs (NSAIDs)

Drug Class	Drug	Oral Dosage (Adults)	Oral Dosage (Children)
Salicylates	Aspirin*	MI, TIA: 325 mg qd AIF: 325 mg qid	Fever: 10 mg/kg qid AIF, Kawasaki disease: 20–30 mg/kg tid
	Diflunisal	250–500 mg bid	N/A
	Salsalate	1000 mg qd	N/A
Propionic acids	Fenoprofen	300–600 mg tid-qid	900–1800 mg/m²/day JRA
	Flurbiprofen	100 mg bid	N/A
	Ibuprofen	Dysmenorrhea: 200–400 mg tid-qid Arthritis and gout: 400–800 mg tid-qid (maximum dose = 2.4 g/day)	Fever: 10 mg/kg bid-tid JRA: 7.5–12.5 mg/kg qid max. dose = 2.4 g/day
	Ketoprofen	RA, OA: 50–75 mg tid maximum dose = 300 mg/day	fever: 0.5–1 mg/kg bid-qid
	Naproxen	250–500 bid (maximum dose = 1250 mg/day)	5 mg/kg bid max. dose = 1000 mg/day
	Oxaprozin	600–1200 qd	N/A
Acetic acids	Diclofenac	IR: 50 mg tid; DR: 75 mg bid; XR: 100 mg once daily	N/A
	Etodolac	400 mg bid-tid (maximum dose = 20 mg/kg)	N/A
	Indomethacin (also IV)	Arthritis and gout: 25–50 mg bid-tid (maximum dose = 200 mg/day)	PDA: 2 mg/kg × 2 IV Arthritis and gout: 0.5–1 mg bid-qid max. dose = 4 mg/kg/day
	Ketorolac (also IV, ophthalmic)	10 mg qid (maximum dose = 40 mg/day)	N/A
	Nabumetone	1000 mg qd-bid	N/A
	Sulindac	150–200 mg bid (maximum dose = 400 mg/day)	N/A
	Tolmetin	400 mg tid (maximum dose = 2 g/day)	5–10 mg/kg tid max. dose=30 mg/kg/day
Fenamates	Mefenaminic acid	250 mg qid	N/A
Oxicams	Piroxicam	10–20 mg/kg	0.2–0.3 mg/kg qd max. dose=15 mg/kg/day
Cox-2 inhibitor	Celecoxib	100 mg bid or 200 mg qd	N/A
	Rofecoxib	12.5–50 mg PO once daily	N/A
Other	Choline mg trisalicylate	500–1500 qd-tid	10–20 mg/kg tid
	Oxyphenbutazone	100 mg qid	N/A

Indications for one NSAID over another are not well defined. Drugs are grouped according to chemical class. If a patient does not respond to a particular NSAID, therapy with an NSAID from a different class is attempted.

*Note risk of Reye's syndrome with aspirin use in children. (See ch. 20(VII)F)

AIF = Anti-inflammatory; *bid* = twice a day; *DR* = delayed release; *IR* = immediate release; *IV* = intravenously; *JRA* = juvenile rheumatoid arthritis; *MI* = myocardial infarction; *OA* = osteoarthritis; *PDA* = patent ductus arteriosus; *qd* = once daily; *qid* = 4 times a day; *RA* = rheumatoid arthritis; *TIA* = transient ischemic attack; *tid* = 3 times a day; *XR* = extended release.

—facial rash
—arthralgias and arthritis
—headaches
—personality changes
—seizures
—psychoses if central nervous system (CNS) involvement is present

b. **Physical examination findings** may include:
—splenomegaly
—generalized adenopathy
—oral ulcers
—**malar (butterfly) rash:** typical of SLE, leaves no scar, may be photosensitive
—discoid rash: coin-shaped, can leave scars
—bullous lesions
—palpable purpura

2. **Diagnostic tests**

a. **Serum** antinuclear antibodies (**ANA**): positive ANA tests (usually in high titer) are found in > 98% of patients with SLE

b. **Chemistry panel** to look for blood urea nitrogen (BUN) or creatinine elevations

c. **Urinalysis** to look for hematuria (may be present in glomerulonephritis)

d. **CBC** to look for thrombocytopenia

3. **Treatment**

—New therapies for patients with SLE should be initiated only in consultation with a rheumatologist.

a. For mild disease:
—**NSAIDs** (see Table 11-2)
—**Antimalarial agents** (e.g., hydroxychloroquine)

b. For severe disease:
—**Corticosteroids** (e.g., prednisone, methylprednisolone)
—**Cytotoxic drugs** (e.g., azathioprine, cyclophosphamide, chlorambucil)

c. Anticoagulation therapy is needed for patients with antiphospholipid antibodies and recurrent thrombosis.

d. Indications for high-dose corticosteroids include:
—severe lupus nephritis
—central nervous system lupus
—thrombocytopenia with platelet counts <30,000/mm^3
—autoimmune hemolytic anemia
—sepsis

4. **Disposition**

—Disposition is individualized according to the systems involved and severity of symptoms.

C. Scleroderma

—Scleroderma can be localized with skin involvement only; can be limited to certain organs (as in CREST syndrome); or may manifest as a diffuse systemic illness with often fatal visceral involvement.

1. Clinical presentation

a. CREST syndrome

—**Calcinosis:** cutaneous deposits of calcium phosphate usually over the hands

—**Raynaud's phenomenon:** vasomotor disorder resulting in pallor, cyanosis, and, finally, erythema of fingers and toes. Ears and nose sometimes are involved.

—**Esophageal dysfunction:** neural dysfunction, smooth muscle involvement, and muscle fibrosis

—**Sclerodactyly:** induration of the fingers

—**Telangiectasia:** dilation of blood vessels appearing as small red areas

b. Symptoms of **systemic disease** may include:

—gastrointestinal (GI): esophageal dysmotility, dysphagia, acid reflux, biliary cirrhosis

—pulmonary: pulmonary hypertension, interstitial lung disease, pleurisy

—cardiac: cardiac arrhythmias, pericarditis with effusion, premature coronary artery disease, congestive heart failure (CHF)

—renal: acute or chronic renal failure

—musculoskeletal: resorption of bone, arthralgias, morning stiffness

2. Diagnostic tests

a. Laboratory studies

(1) **Serum anti-scl-70** : most specific test for scleroderma

(2) **CBC** to look for normocytic, normochromic anemia

(3) **ESR** to look for elevation

(4) **Pulmonary function tests (PFTs)** to look for decreased diffusion and vital capacity and increased residual volume

(5) **Urinalysis** to look for albuminuria and microscopic hematuria

(6) **Rheumatoid factor:** positive in one third of cases

(7) Serum ANA and serum nucleolar immunofluorescence tests will be positive

b. Imaging studies

(1) **Chest radiograph** to look for pulmonary fibrosis and diffuse reticular pattern

(2) Upper GI series to look for esophageal abnormalities

3. Treatment

—Treatment of scleroderma is difficult; no therapy has been consistently successful.

—Treatment is directed at alleviating symptoms.

a. For Raynaud's phenomenon:

—Hands must be kept warm.

—Smoking cessation

—Antiplatelet therapy: **aspirin** 81–325 mg orally (adults) or **dipyridamole** 25–125 mg 3 times a day orally (adults) or 1–2 mg/kg 3 times a day (children)

—Vasodilator: **isoxupride** 10–20 mg orally 3 times a day (adults)

b. For esophageal dysmotility:

—H_2 blockers (see Table 4-2 in Chapter 4, Gastrointestinal Emergencies)

—Motility agent: **cisapride** 10 mg 4 times a day 15 minutes before meals (adults)

—Antibiotics to treat bacterial overgrowth

—Supplemental vitamins

—Surgical dilatation of the esophagus

—Elevate head of bed to prevent reflux

c. Cardiac symptoms

—treat CHF (see Chapter 2 VII D)

d. Renal symptoms

—ACE inhibitors

4. Disposition

—Disposition is individualized according to the system involved and the severity of symptoms.

D. Sarcoidosis

—is a multisystem disorder.

—occurs most often between the ages of 20 and 40 years among people of northern European heritage and African-Americans.

—most often involves mediastinal and peripheral lymph nodes, lungs, liver, eyes, and skin.

1. Clinical presentation

a. Initial symptoms may include:

—fever

—weight loss

—arthralgias

—polyarthritis

—jaundice secondary to hepatic dysfunction

—diabetes insipidus

b. Later symptoms depend on the organ system involved.

c. Physical examination findings may include:

—uveitis

—granulomas of the nasal and conjunctival mucosa

—peripheral and mediastinal lymphadenopathy

—diffuse pulmonary infiltration

—cardiac abnormalities

—skin lesions

—CNS involvement

2. **Diagnostic tests**
   a. Laboratory studies
      (1) **Chemistry panel** to look for hypercalcemia and elevated uric acid
      (2) **Urinalysis** to look for hypercalciuria
      (3) CBC to look for leukopenia
      (4) **Liver function tests (LFTs)** to look for elevated serum alkaline phosphatase
      (5) **PFTs** to look for restrictive disease, decreased compliance, and impaired diffusing capacity
   b. **Radiographs** to look for bilateral hilar and right paratracheal adenopathy, which are virtually pathognomonic

3. **Treatment**
   a. Treatment of hypercalcemia
      (1) In the ED, **intravenous (IV) hydration** with normal saline to promote urinary excretion of calcium. May follow with a loop diuretic such as furosemide.
      (2) In outpatient setting:
         (a) **Calcitonin** (4 IU/kg intramuscularly (IM) or subcutaneously) to enhance urinary excretion of calcium
         (b) **Bisphosphonate derivatives** to inhibit resorption of calcium from bone:
            —Etidronate, 5 mg/kg orally
            —Pamidronate, 60 mg IV infusion over 2–24 hours
            —Alendronate, 40 mg orally
   b. To suppress **severe symptoms,** prednisone up to 1 mg/kg orally for 4 to 6 weeks

4. **Disposition**
   a. Most patients can be discharged home with outpatient follow-up.
   b. Patients with complications of CHF or hypercalcemia may need to be admitted to the hospital, depending on their hemodynamic status and response to treatment in the ED.

E. **Reiter's syndrome**

—Reactive arthritis associated with nonbacterial urethritis or cervicitis, conjunctivitis, and mucocutaneous lesions

—Commonly seen in men aged 20–40 years

—Initial illness typically resolves in 3–4 months

1. **Clinical presentation**
   a. **Symptoms** may include:
      —low-grade fever
      —conjunctivitis
      —arthritis
      —dysuria
      —back pain
   b. **Physical examination findings** may include:

—circinate balanitis and keratoderma blennorrhagicum

—ankylosis of the spine

2. Diagnostic tests

a. Laboratory studies

(1) Urethral or **cervical culture** to look for infection

(2) Synovial fluid analysis to look for normal glucose and presence of leukocytes

(3) Serum HLA B27 antigen: presence is strongly associated with Reiter's syndrome

b. Radiographs of sacroiliac joints to look for inflammation

3. Treatment

a. Antibiotics to treat initial infection: **ceftriaxone** 250 mg IM with **azithromycin** 1 g orally. This is the treatment regimen for sexually transmitted diseases (STDs), targeted at gonococcus and chlamydia.

b. Topical ophthalmic corticosteroids to treat severe iritis

c. NSAIDs for myalgias (see Table 11-2)

4. Disposition

—Most patients can be discharged home with outpatient follow-up.

F. Dermatomyositis and polymyositis

1. Overview

a. Definition

—Inflammatory changes in the muscles (polymyositis) and in the skin (dermatomyositis) with weakness and some degree of muscle atrophy, principally of the limb girdles.

b. Cause

—May be idiopathic, or may be associated with an underlying malignancy.

2. Clinical presentation

a. Symptoms may include:

—**symmetrical proximal muscle weakness**

—polyarthralgias

—difficulty climbing up and down stairs, kneeling, and raising arms

—Raynaud's phenomenon (See section I C)

b. Physical examination findings may include:

—**heliotrope rash** (V-sign over chest and neck)

—decreased deep tendon reflexes of proximal muscles

—cracking and fissuring of hands (mechanic's hands)

—nailfold abnormalities

—raised lesions over knuckles (Grotton's papules)

3. Diagnostic tests

a. ESR to look for elevation

b. ANA to look for elevation: >50% of cases

c. Chemistry panel to look for elevated creatinine kinase (CK) and lactate dehydrogenase (LDH)
d. LFTs to look for elevated aspartate aminotransferase (AST)
e. Outpatient tests may include:
—muscle biopsy to look for perifascicular muscle fiber atrophy and phagocytosis of muscle debris
—electromyogram (EMG) to look for polyphasic motor unit action potentials with short duration, low amplitude, and fibrillation.

4. **Treatment**
a. Physical activity should be limited until the inflammation subsides; then range-of-motion exercises should be initiated to prevent contractures.
b. Corticosteroids: prednisone 40–60 mg orally
c. Potassium supplements: 20–40 mEq orally daily
d. Immunosuppressive agents such as azathioprine or methotrexate should be considered for severe disease, in consultation with a rheumatologist.

5. **Disposition**
a. Most patients can be discharged home with outpatient follow-up.
b. Patients with acute complications such as respiratory impairment, pneumonia, or sepsis should be admitted to the hospital for further management.

G. **Temporal arteritis**

1. **Clinical presentation**
a. Symptoms may include:
—severe **headache,** especially over the temporalis muscle
—visual disturbances, including amaurosis fugax, scotoma, and blurred vision.
—**claudication** of the masseter, temporalis, and tongue muscles.
b. **Physical examination findings** may include:
—scalp tenderness
—**pulsating temporal artery** (in later stages, this may be absent)
—decreased visual acuity
—diplopia
—general weakness
—weight loss

2. **Diagnostic tests**
a. **ESR** to look for marked elevation
b. LFTs to look for elevated alkaline phosphatase
c. CBC to look for slight leukocytosis and thrombocytosis
d. Inpatient work-up may include a **temporal artery biopsy** to look for inflammatory infiltrates within the giant multinucleated cells.
—establishes a definitive diagnosis
—should be done within 96 hours of beginning steroid therapy
—3–5 cm needed for biopsy due to the possibility of skip lesions

—If biopsy is negative, the contralateral side should be biopsied; positive yield = 90%.

3. Treatment

—Due to the danger of blindness, any patient suspected of having temporal arteritis should be treated immediately with corticosteroids, even before a definitive diagnosis is established:

a. **Prednisone: 60 mg per day orally for 6 weeks**

b. Cytotoxic agents: azathioprine, methotrexate, dapsone (done in consultation with rheumatology)

4. Disposition

—Patients suspected of having temporal arteritis should be admitted to the hospital for further management.

II. Hypersensitivity Reactions

A. Anaphylaxis

1. Overview

a. Definition

—is an acute, often explosive, systemic reaction that occurs within seconds to minutes in a previously sensitized person who again receives the sensitizing antigen.

—can be aggravated or even induced de novo by exercise.

b. Causes

—Common causative antigens include serum, blood products, insect stings, certain foods such as shellfish and nuts, beta-lactam antimicrobials, and many other drugs.

c. Pathophysiology

—Histamine, leukotrienes, and other mediators are released when the antigen reacts with IgE on basophils and mast cells, causing smooth muscle contraction, vascular dilatation, urticaria, and angioedema. The resulting **effective decrease in plasma volume** leads to **shock.**

2. Clinical presentation

a. **Symptoms** may include:

—**pruritus**

—**agitation**

—**flushing**

—coughing

—sneezing

—palpitations

—hoarseness

—dyspnea

—nausea

b. **Physical examination findings** may include:

—tachypnea
—**wheezing**
—stridor
—**tachycardia**
—diffuse erythematous rash (hives)
—incontinence
—convulsions

3. **Diagnostic tests**

—The reaction is so quick and severe that there is no time for diagnostic tests. The presentation is dramatic enough that diagnosis is not difficult.

4. **Treatment**

a. **The airway must be secured.**

b. **Epinephrine** (1:1000) subcutaneously, 0.3–0.5 mL (adults) or 0.01 mL/kg (children)

c. **Diphenhydramine** 50–100 mg IV slowly over 3 minutes

d. H_2 blocker (see Table 4-2 in Chapter 4)

e. An oral antihistamine should be continued for 72 hours following resolution of symptoms.

f. Supportive measures such as oxygen, fluids, and vasopressors are given as needed.

5. **Disposition**

a. Patients with severe reactions should remain in the hospital under observation for 24 hours after recovery to ensure adequate treatment in case of relapse.

b. Following discharge, anyone who has had an anaphylactic reaction to a stinging insect should be provided with a kit containing a pre-filled syringe of epinephrine and an epinephrine nebulizer.

B. Angioedema and urticaria

1. **Overview**

a. **Definitions**

—**Urticaria:** local wheal and erythema with blanched centers, only in the dermis

—**Angioedema:** eruption similar to urticaria, but with well-demarcated, larger edematous areas that involve both dermis and subcutaneous structures

—Acute urticaria and angioedema are essentially anaphylaxis limited to the skin and subcutaneous tissues

—may occur separately or simultaneously

—are classified as IgE-dependent, complement-mediated, nonimmunologic, or idiopathic

b. **Causes**

—are similar to those for anaphylaxis (see section II A). ACE inhibitors, pollen, viral infections, heat or cold stimuli also are causes.

—If acute angioedema is recurrent, progressive, and never associated with urticaria, a hereditary enzyme deficiency should be suspected.

—Occasionally, urticaria may be the first or only visible sign of cutaneous vasculitis. It should be suspected when lesions persist for more than 24 hours.

2. **Clinical presentation**

   a. **Symptoms** and **physical examination findings** for **urticaria** may include:

      —pruritus

      —wheals

      —crops of hives that come and go.

   b. **Symptoms** and **physical examination findings** for **angioedema** include:

      —a more diffuse swelling present on the hands, feet, eyelids, lips, genitalia, and mucous membranes

      —edema of the upper airways

3. **Diagnostic tests**

   a. The rapid onset and self-limited nature of the rash is the mainstay of diagnosis.

   b. Serum C4 or C1 esterase inhibitor may be done to look for deficiency associated with hereditary angioedema (this usually is not done in the ED).

   c. Thyroid function tests (TFTs) to look for hypothyroidism (a few patients with intractable urticaria are hypothyroid)

4. **Treatment**

   a. For **urticaria:**

      —Removal of the causative agent

      —IV antihistamine: diphenhydramine, 50–100 mg every 4 hours (adults) or 5 mg/kg/day (children); hydroxyzine, 25–100 mg twice a day (adults) or 5 mg/kg/day (children); or cyproheptadine, 12–16 mg 3 times a day (adults) or 0.25 mg/kg/day (children).

      —**Prednisone** 30 to 40 mg orally daily for severe reactions

   b. **For angioedema:**

      —**airway must be secured (mainstay of therapy)**

      —**Epinephrine** 1:1000, 0.3 mL subcutaneously

      —IV antihistamine, as for urticaria [see section II B 4 a]

      —Fresh frozen plasma (contains C1 esterase inhibitor)

5. **Disposition**

   a. Patients without airway compromise whose symptoms resolve with ED treatment may be discharged home following observation for 4–6 hours with outpatient follow-up. See Table 11-3 for outpatient antihistamine prescriptions.

   b. Patients with hemodynamic compromise or who require ventilatory support should be admitted to the hospital.

Table 11-3. Outpatient (Oral) Antihistamine Regimens

Antihistamine for Acute Urticaria	Dosage for Adults	Dosage for Children
1st-generation		
Diphenhydramine	25–50 mg q 6 h	5 mg/kg/day
Hydroxyzine	25–50 mg q 6 h	5 mg/kg/day
2nd-generation		
Astemizole	10 mg once daily	<6 yrs: 0.2 mg/kg/day 6–12 yrs: 5 mg/kg/day
Acrivastine	8 mg once daily	None
Cetirizine	10 mg once daily	None
Fexophenadine	60 mg bid	None
Loratidine	10 mg once daily	None
Terfenadine	60 mg bid	3–6 yrs: 15 mg bid 6–12 yrs: 30 mg bid
For Perennial and Seasonal Allergic Rhinitis and Chronic Urticaria		
Azatadine	1–2 mg bid	None
Brompheniramine	4–12 mg qid bid (maximum dose = 24 mg/day)	<6 yrs: 0.5 mg/kg/day 6–12 yrs: 2–4 mg tid
Chlorpheniramine	4–12 mg qid-bid (maximum dose = 24 mg/day)	2–6 yrs: 0.1 mg qid 6–12 yrs: 2 mg qid
Clemastine	1.34 mg bid	0.67–1.3 mg q 8–12 h
Cyproheptadine	4–5 mg tid (maximum dose = 0.5 mg/kg/day)	2–6 yrs: 0.2 mg q 8–12 h 6–12 yrs: 4 mg q 8–12 h
Phenindamine	25 mg q 4–6 h	6–12 yrs: 12.5 mg q 4–6 h
Tripelennamine	25–50 mg q 4–6 h	5 mg/kg/day in divided doses q 4–6 h

bid = twice a day; *q* = every; *qid* = 4 times a day; *qid-bid* = 2–times a day; *tid* = 3 times a day.

III. Bony Abnormalities

A. Aseptic necrosis of the hip

1. Overview

a. Definition

—Necrosis is ischemic death of osteocytes and marrow.

—The bones that are most vulnerable have both limited vascular supply and restricted collateral circulation, such as the femoral head of the hip joint.

—Bilateral involvement occurs in 50% to 90% of cases.

b. Causes

(1) Traumatic

—Hip fracture

—Hip surgery

(2) Nontraumatic

(a) Children

—Slipped capital femoral epiphysis

—Legg-Calvé-Perthes disease (see Chapter 20 VII A, B)

(b) Adults

—immunosuppressive states (e.g., corticosteroid therapy, diabetes mellitus, alcoholism, malignancy, renal transplantation, Cushing's disease, radiotherapy, and SLE)

—pregnancy

—oral contraceptives

—blood dyscrasias

—decompression sickness

—carbon tetrachloride poisoning

2. Clinical presentation

a. Symptoms may include:

—unilateral pain that localizes to the groin, buttock, medial thigh, and medial aspect of the knee

—pain that worsens with ambulation and improves with rest

b. Physical examination findings may include:

—collapse of the articular surface

—secondary degenerative changes

—decreased range of motion

3. Diagnostic tests

a. Radiograph of joint to look for **bone islands, bone infarcts,** and **osteopenia.** Note that plain films initially may be normal. Early collapse of the cancellous bone is a pathognomonic radiolucent line referred to as the **crescent sign.**

b. Bone scan to look for a "hot-cold" region (demarcates vascularized versus nonvascularized bone)

c. MRI if radiographs are negative

4. Treatment

a. The goal is to restore joint function and relieve associated pain.

b. Weight-bearing should be discontinued until the condition is remedied.

c. NSAIDs for analgesia.

d. Core decompression of the femoral head

e. Total hip arthroplasty (replacement)

5. Disposition

—Patients may be discharged home with outpatient follow-up with an orthopaedist the next day if one is not available to see the patient in the ED.

B. Osteoporosis

1. Overview

a. Definitions

—is a generalized, progressive reduction in bone tissue mass.

—**Type I osteoporosis** (postmenopausal osteoporosis) occurs between ages 51 and 75 years and is 6 times more common in women than in men.

—**Type II osteoporosis** (involutional or senile osteoporosis) occurs mainly in those older than 70 years and may result from age-related reduction in vitamin D synthesis or resistance to vitamin D activity (Fig. 11-1).

—Types I and II may occur together in women.

b. Differential diagnosis

—includes osteomalacia, multiple myeloma, osteogenesis imperfecta, rheumatoid arthritis, hyperparathyroidism, renal failure, hyperthyroidism, idiopathic hypercalciuria, and Cushing's syndrome.

c. Risk factors

—include age, female gender, nulliparity, early menopause, low calcium intake, sedentary lifestyle, and high-dose corticosteroids.

2. Clinical presentation

—aching pain in the bones, particularly the back

—history of multiple fractures

—The most common fractures are **vertebral crush** and **distal radius** fractures.

3. Diagnostic tests

a. **Radiographs** to look for fractures

b. Chemistry panel and parathyroid hormone tests are done to look for other causes of bone loss.

c. Outpatient tests may include bone densitometry to look for decreased bone density from loss of trabecular structure

4. **Treatment** is preventive:

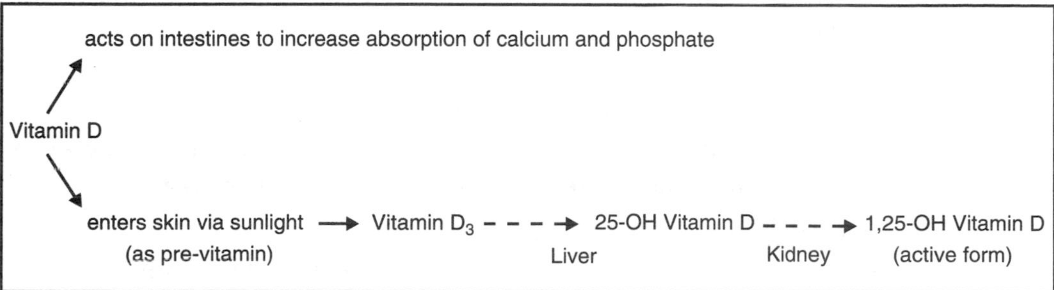

Figure 11-1. Metabolism of vitamin D.

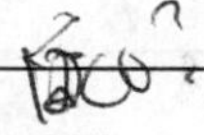

a. Dietary and **supplemental calcium:** calcium citrate 800 mg/day orally
b. **Estrogen replacement therapy**
c. Orthopaedic support
d. Analgesics for pain
e. Hyperextension exercises to strengthen paravertebral muscles
f. Avoidance of heavy lifting and falls
g. **Exercise**

5. **Disposition**
a. Patients with simple osteoporosis without acute fractures can be discharged home with the recommendations outlined above.
b. Vertebral crush fractures usually are managed conservatively; these patients also can be discharged home.
c. Other fractures require orthopaedic consultation or follow-up, depending on ED availability of orthopaedic consultation.

C. Osteomalacia

1. **Overview**
a. **Definition**
—results in soft bones due to impaired mineralization in mature bone.
b. **Causes**
—include vitamin D deficiency, intestinal malabsorption, liver disease, renal disease, and certain drugs (see Fig. 11-1).

2. **Clinical presentation**
—**Symptoms** and **physical examination findings** include pain and deformity, particularly in the long bones and pelvis.

3. **Diagnostic tests**
a. **Serum calcium** and **phosphate** to look for hypocalcemia and hypophosphatemia
b. **LFTs** to look for elevated serum alkaline phosphatase
c. Serum 25-hydroxyvitamin D levels: decreased in osteomalacia
d. **Urinalysis** to look for low urinary calcium and high phosphate excretion
e. Radiographs to look for pseudofractures (milkman's fractures, Looser's zones), which are seen at points where large arteries cross bones

4. **Treatment**
a. Underlying disease should be treated.
b. Vitamin D analog (e.g., ergocalciferol 25 μg orally daily) should be given.
c. Calcium and phosphate supplementation should be started.

5. **Disposition**
—Patients can be discharged home with outpatient follow-up.

D. Paget's disease of bone

1. **Overview**

a. Definition

—is a chronic disorder of bone remodeling resulting in disorganized mosaic patterns consisting of mixed trabecular (old) and woven (new) bone.

—The primary defect is increased bone turnover secondary to increased osteoclast activity.

—The new bone that follows is of woven rather than trabecular type, which is less strong.

b. Incidence

—increases with age.

c. Complications

—include CHF, hypercalcemia, cerebrovascular accident (CVA), and hypertension.

2. Clinical presentation

a. Symptoms and **physical examination findings** include:

—aching, deep pain and, occasionally, severe stiffness

—fatigue

—bowed lower extremities

—headaches

—decreasing auditory acuity

—increasing skull size with frontal bossing

b. Pathologic fractures may be the presenting finding. The pelvis, femur, skull, tibia, vertebrae, clavicle, and humerus are most commonly affected.

3. Diagnostic tests

a. Laboratory studies

(1) LFTs to look for elevated serum alkaline phosphatase

(2) Urinalysis to look for elevated urinary collagen cross-links (not usually done in the ED)

(3) Serum calcium to look for hypercalcemia

b. Radiographs to look for fractures, decreased bone density, and disorganized bone architecture

4. Treatment

a. NSAIDs for analgesia (see Table 11-2)

b. Treatment of hypercalcemia (see section I D 3 a)

c. For treatment of CHF: see Chapter 2, section VII D

d. For treatment of hypertension: see Chapter 2, section VIII E

e. For treatment of acute fractures, an orthopaedic surgeon should be consulted.

5. Disposition

a. Most patients can be discharged home with outpatient follow-up.

b. Patients with complications of CHF or hypercalcemia may need to be admitted to the hospital, depending on their hemodynamic status and response to treatment in the ED.

IV. Joint Abnormalities

A. Septic joint

—arthritis resulting from infection of the synovial tissues with pyogenic bacteria

—usually classified as gonococcal and nongonococcal

1. **Clinical presentation** (Table 11-4)
   a. **Gonococcal arthritis**
      (1) **Symptoms** may include:
      —fever
      —recent urethritis
      —salpingitis
      —hemorrhagic vesicular skin lesions
      (2) **Physical examination findings** may include:
      —migratory polyarthralgia
      —tenosynovitis
      —purulent arthritis
      —maculopapular or vesicular rash
      —urethral discharge
      —inguinal adenopathy
   b. **Nongonococcal arthritis**

Table 11-4. Features of Gonococcal and Nongonococcal Arthritis

	Gonococcal	Nongonococcal
Organism	*Neisseria gonorrhoeae*	*Staphylococcus aureus,* gram-negative bacilli, non-group A streptococci, anaerobes
Population	Young, healthy, sexually active adults	Small children, elderly, immunocompromised
Onset	1 day to several weeks after sexual encounter	Abrupt
Joints most commonly affected	Knee	Knee, hip
Arthritis	Migratory, polyarticular	Monoarticular
Symptoms	Fever, recent urethritis, salpingitis, hemorrhagic vesicular skin lesions	Fever, chills, acute joint pain, stiffness
Physical examination findings	Migratory polyarthralgia, tenosynovitis, purulent arthritis, maculopapular or vesicular rash, urethral discharge, inguinal adenopathy	Pain with passive motion of the involved joint Joint is warm, tender, and swollen, with evidence of effusion

(1) **Symptoms** may include:
—fever
—chills
—acute joint pain
—stiffness

(2) **Physical examination findings** may include:
—pain with passive motion of the involved joint
—joint that is warm, tender, and swollen, with evidence of effusion
—(The above findings are noted in any septic arthritis.)

2. Diagnostic tests

a. Laboratory studies

(1) **Synovial fluid aspiration (arthrocentesis)** to look for infection
—WBC count >100,000/μL with >90% polymorphonuclear cells (PMNs)
—Synovial fluid:blood glucose ratio <0.5
—Poor mucin clot
—Absence of uric acid or calcium pyrophosphate dihydrate crystals
—Culture almost always is positive in nongonococcal arthritis; in gonococcal arthritis it is positive only 20% of the time.

(2) **Urethral culture** to check for gonococcus.

(3) **ESR** to look for elevation (gonococcal arthritis)

(4) Tests for complement deficiency in patients with recurrent infections (not usually done in ED)

b. Imaging studies

(1) **Joint radiograph** to delineate effusion and rule out fracture

(2) Bone scans to demonstrate a "hot" joint, but usually unnecessary

3. Treatment

a. Empiric **intravenous antibiotics**

(1) For nongonococcal arthritis:
—1 g IV nafcillin plus gentamicin every 4 hours (adults)
—50–200 mg/kg/day nafcillin divided every 6 hours + 50–75 mg/kg/day ceftriaxone divided every 12–24 hours (children).

(2) For gonococcal arthritis:
—ceftriaxone, 1–2 g IM or IV daily until signs and symptoms resolve, then cefuroxime 500 mg orally twice a day or amoxicillin clavulanate 500 mg orally 3 times a day for 7 days (adults)

b. Surgical consult for joints that need surgical drainage (e.g., hips, joints affected by osteomyelitis, prosthetic joints; those that cannot be drained by other means)

c. NSAIDs for analgesia and to reduce fever

d. Patients with gonococcal arthritis and their sexual partners should also receive empiric treatment for possible coexistent *Chlamydia* infections (see Chapter 14, section IV B).

e. **Splinting** the joint may provide some analgesia during the acute stage.

f. **Physical therapy**

4. Disposition

—Patients with septic arthritis should go to the operating room for open washout.

B. Gout

1. Overview

a. Definition

—is a disease associated with overproduction or underexcretion of uric acid.

b. Causes

(1) **Factors associated with overproduction of uric acid** include obesity, alcohol consumption, drugs (e.g., thiazide diuretics), hemolytic events, and psoriasis.

(2) **Factors associated with underexcretion of uric acid** include:

—renal disease

—organ transplantation with cyclosporine use

—certain medications

—acidosis

—thyroid disease

—glucose-6-phosphatase deficiency

—fructose-1-phosphate aldolase deficiency.

2. Clinical presentation

a. Symptoms may include:

—pain, erythema, or edema of one or more joints

—pain or other symptoms that usually are monoarticular

—pain that occurs at night or early morning

—great toe most commonly initially affected (podagra)

b. Physical examination findings may include:

—**tophi** (nodular calcifications commonly seen on toes)

3. Diagnostic tests

a. Laboratory studies

(1) Joint aspiration to look for presence of **negatively birefringent crystals** in synovial fluid

(2) **Chemistry panel** to look for **elevated serum uric acid**

(3) CBC to look for leukocytosis, differentiate from septic joint

b. Radiograph of joint to look for soft tissue swelling and, in chronic cases, **tophi** or **erosions** of the bone (rat-bite erosions).

4. Treatment

a. NSAIDs: **Indomethacin** 75–150 mg/day

b. Colchicine 1 mg IV over 2 to 5 minutes followed by 1 mg IV in 12 hours if pain persists, then 0.5 to 1.5 mg/day

c. Intra-articular corticosteroids. See section I A 4.

d. Allopurinol is NOT indicated in acute gouty attacks

5. Disposition

—Most patients can be discharged home with outpatient follow-up.

C. Pseudogout

—is a microcrystalline arthritis

—is more common with advancing age

1. Clinical presentation

a. **Symptoms** may include:

—acute, episodic, gout-like attacks of synovial inflammation

—clinical history of recurrent, episodic acute attacks

b. **Physical examination findings** may include:

—pain in the large joints, especially the knee, although hip, wrist and elbow joints also have been involved.

2. Diagnostic tests

a. Synovial fluid analysis to look for

(1) intracellular and extracellular calcium pyrophosphate dihydrate crystals which are **positively birefringent** under polarized light.

(2) WBC count

b. **Chemistry panel** to look for hyperuricemia

c. Radiographs to look for chondrocalcinosis of the knees, the radial and ulnar joints, and the symphysis pubis

3. Treatment

—Same as for gout (see section IV B 4).

4. Disposition

—Patients can be discharged home with outpatient follow-up.

V. Low Back Pain Syndromes

A. Low back pain (LBP)

1. Definition

—pain in the lumbar, lumbosacral, or sacroiliac region

—pain may consist of ligamentous (sprain) or muscular (strain) symptoms.

2. Causes

—poor posture

—overuse

—obesity

—pregnancy

—direct mechanical nerve root pressure

—traumatic ligament rupture

—stress fracture

—infection

—tumor

—congenital defects

—spinal stenosis

—visceral disease

—psychosocial problems

3. **Incidence**

—Up to 80% of all individuals will develop back pain at some point during their life.

4. **Clinical presentation**

—**Symptoms** and **physical examination findings** depend on the etiology of the low back pain:

a. fibromyalgia: localized pain felt on firm palpation as point tenderness

b. spinal stenosis: pain that is worse with spinal extension and alleviated with spinal flexion, resulting in the classic "simian" posture. Positive straight leg raising test. Pain radiates to extremities.

c. infection or neoplasm: fever, chills, weight loss

d. spinal cord compression, central disk herniation, cauda equina syndrome: presence of neurologic abnormalities with the back pain

5. **Diagnostic tests**

a. Radiographs of lumbosacral spine to look for degenerative changes affecting disks at level L4–L5

b. Lumbar puncture if spinal tuberculosis is suspected

c. Bone scan to look for metastases, if indicated

6. **Treatment**

a. For uncomplicated LBP:

—local heat and massage

—abdominal and lumbosacral exercises and weight reduction

—smoking cessation

—bed rest with hips and knees flexed

—a lumbosacral support

—NSAIDs for analgesia

—avoidance of narcotics

—tricyclic antidepressants for chronic pain and depression

—muscle relaxants if musculoskeletal spasm is present (Table 11-5)

b. For LBP with neurologic findings:

—consultation with a neurosurgeon

—MRI to look for spinal lesions

7. **Disposition**

a. Patients with uncomplicated LBP may be discharged home with outpatient follow-up.

b. Patients whose LBP suggests an underlying complication should be referred to an appropriate specialist (infectious disease, trauma, neurosurgery, hematology-oncology)

B. Sacroiliitis

—often is a manifestation of ankylosing spondylitis, reactive arthritis, secondary syphilis, irritable bowel disease (IBD), Whipple's disease, or Reiter's syndrome.

Table 11-5. Muscle Relaxants

Drug	Oral Dosage (Adults)	Oral Dosage (Children)
Baclofen	5 mg tid	1–2 mg tid
Carisoprodol	350 mg tid-qid	N/A
Chlorzoxazone	250–500 mg tid-qid	20 mg/kg/day
Cyclobenzaprine	20–40 mg/day	N/A
Diazepam	2–10 mg bid-qid	0.12–0.8 mg/kg/day
Metaxalone	800 mg tid-qid	N/A
Methocarbamol	1500 mg qid	N/A unless for tetanus
Orphenadrine	100 mg bid	N/A
Quinine	200–300 mg qhs	N/A

bid = twice a day; *bid-qid* = 2–4 times a day; *qid* = 4 times a day; qhs = at bedtime; *tid* = 3 times a day.

—can begin anywhere along the lumbar spine.

1. **Clinical presentation**
   a. **Symptoms** may include:
      —sacroiliac joint pain
      —stiffness
   b. **Physical examination findings** may include:
      —pathologic sacroiliac joint pain produced by bilateral compression of the anterior iliac crests toward the midline, performed with the patient supine
      —pain arising from the contralateral pelvis as a result of Patrick's test. The patient **F**lexes, **AB**ducts, and **E**xternally **R**otates (FABER) the hip such that the ipsilateral heel rests on the contralateral knee. Then, pressure is exerted on the ipsilateral knee and the contralateral iliac crest.
      —sacroiliac discomfort provoked by **Gaenslen's maneuver:** The patient is positioned supine with both hips and knees in flexion. The patient is asked to move one buttock off the examining table edge while extending the leg over the side.
2. **Diagnostic tests**
   —Radiograph of the sacroiliac crests to look for blurring of the cortical margins of the subchondral bone and fibrosis of the articular surfaces, followed by erosions and sclerosis.
3. **Treatment**
   —Treatment is the same as for low back pain. See section V A 6.
4. **Disposition**
   —Patients can be discharged home with outpatient follow-up.

C. Sciatica

—is the compression of the lower lumbar and high sacral nerve roots that form the sciatic nerve resulting in pain in the buttocks, posterior lateral thigh, calf, and foot.

—Compression may result from a herniated disk, intraspinal tumor, intervertebral disk protrusion, epidural abscesses, or chronic meningitis, or from bony changes in rheumatoid arthritis (RA) or osteoarthritis (OA).

1. Clinical presentation

a. Symptoms may include:

—pain radiating down one or both buttocks or legs in the distribution of the sciatic nerve. The pain is sharp, lancinating, and burning.

—dermatomal numbness

—paresthesias of the lower limb

—low back pain

b. Physical examination findings may include:

—exacerbation of symptoms with Valsalva maneuvers on flexion or extension of the lumbosacral spine

—sensory or motor deficits, or both

—bladder or bowel dysfunction, or both

2. Diagnostic tests

a. CSF analysis to look for infection, neoplasia or bleed

b. Imaging studies

(1) MRI to look for spinal lesions is the best imaging test.

(2) Radiographs of spine to look for degenerative arthritis or metastatic disease

(3) CT scans to define the dimensions of the bony canal and lateral recess encroachment

(4) Myelography to outline soft tissue planes and delineate the level and extent of a disk protrusion or an intramedullary or extramedullary mass lesion

3. Treatment

a. Immediate neurosurgical consult should be obtained for disk protrusion, numbness, paresthesia, and bowel or bladder dysfunction.

b. NSAIDs, rest, and local supportive measures may be given as for low back pain. See section V A 6 and Table 11-2.

c. Incision and drainage should be done for abscesses.

4. Disposition

a. Patients with epidural abscesses should be admitted for intravenous antibiotics and surgical incision and drainage.

b. Patients with potential neurosurgical lesions are managed per recommendation with consulting neurosurgeon.

c. Most other patients can be discharged home with outpatient follow-up.

VI. Overuse Syndromes

A. Tendonitis and tenosynovitis

1. Overview

a. Definitions

—**Tendonitis** is the inflammation of a tendon.

—**Tenosynovitis** is the inflammation of the lining of the tendon sheath.

—The most common sites of inflammation are the shoulder capsule, wrist, and hip

b. Causes

—Repeated or extreme trauma, strain, or excessive exercise.

—Systemic diseases, most commonly RA, systemic sclerosis, gout, Reiter's syndrome, and disseminated gonococcal infection.

2. Clinical presentation

a. Symptoms may include:

—pain on movement of involved tendons

b. Physical examination findings may include:

—edema of the tendon sheaths

—friction rubs, either felt or heard with a stethoscope on movement of the tendon in its sheath

—pain on active range of motion

—no pain on passive range of motion

3. Diagnostic tests

—Radiographs to look for calcium deposition and to rule out fracture or foreign body

4. Treatment

a. Rest, ice, compression, elevation (RICE)

b. **Immobilization with a splint**

c. NSAIDs for 7–14 days (see Table 11-2)

d. Colchicine if patient's condition is caused by gout

e. **Injection of corticosteroid into the inflamed area:** can be given every 2–3 weeks for a few months

f. Surgical options include:

—removal of inflamed or calcific deposits

—release of fibro-osseous tunnels for de Quervain's disease

—tenosynovectomy of chronic inflammation, as in RA

g. Exercise and physical therapy after inflammation has subsided

5. Disposition

—Most patients can be discharged home with outpatient follow-up.

B. Bursitis

—is an acute or chronic inflammation of a bursa, a thin-walled sac lined with synovial tissue, located at sites where friction occurs.

—The most common sites are the shoulder (subacromial or subdeltoid bursitis), olecranon (miner's elbow), pre- or suprapatellar (housemaid's knee), heel (Achilles), ischial (tailor's or weaver's bottom), greater trochanteric, and first metatarsal head (bunion).

1. **Clinical presentation**
   a. **Symptoms** may include:
      —**pain** resulting from partial or complete tears and crystal release
      —**limitation of motion**
      —swelling and redness if the bursa is superficial (e.g., prepatellar, olecranon)
   b. **Physical examination findings** may include:
      —local pain aggravated by resisted flexion and supination of the forearm for bursitis of the elbow
      —tenderness proximally over the bicipital groove of the humerus and abduction of shoulder in an arc from 50° to 130° if shoulder bursitis
      —muscle atrophy if chronic bursitis
2. **Diagnostic tests**
   a. Aspiration of the joint if it is warm and erythematous to exclude infectious etiology and to look for crystals present with gout
   b. Radiograph of affected joint to look for subdeltoid calcific deposits
3. **Treatment**
   a. Antibiotics for infectious bursitis
   b. **Rest and splinting**
   c. Pendulum exercises: helpful for the shoulder joint
   d. **NSAIDs** for analgesia (see Table 11-2)
   e. Aspiration of bursa
   f. Intrabursal corticosteroids: 2.5–40 mg triamcinolone acetonide injected, depending on size of joint
   g. Systemic corticosteroids: prednisone 15 to 30 mg orally daily for 3 days for resistant cases
   h. **Physical therapy** to prevent muscle atrophy
4. **Disposition**
   a. Patients with infectious bursitis usually are admitted to the hospital for intravenous antibiotics
   b. All others can be discharged home with outpatient follow-up.

C. Fibrositis

—Describes pain and tenderness of muscle and adjacent connective tissue.

—The most common areas affected are the occiput, neck, shoulders, thorax (pleurodynia), lower back, and thighs.

—There is no specific histologic abnormality.

—It occurs mainly in women.

1. **Clinical presentation**
   a. **Symptoms** may include:

—gradual onset of pain
—stiffness
—pain exacerbated by overuse and systemic illness

b. **Physical examination findings** may include:
—tenderness
—local tightness or muscle spasm

2. **Diagnostic tests**
—No specific tests are necessary, but testing may be done to exclude other pathology.

3. **Treatment**
a. Supportive measures such as rest, massage, and heat
b. Stretching exercises
c. Low-dose tricyclic agents at bedtime (e.g., amitriptyline 10 or 25 mg) to promote deeper sleep
d. 1% lidocaine solution applied locally
e. NSAIDs for analgesia as needed

4. **Disposition**
—Most patients can be discharged home with outpatient follow-up.

D. Muscle sprains, strains, and injuries

1. **Definitions**

a. **Sprain**
—is an acute injury to a **ligament.**
—three grades: 1st-degree—mild, due to tearing a few ligamentous fibers; 2nd-degree—moderate pain, swelling, and disability; 3rd degree—severe pain from a complete rupture of the ligament causing joint instability.

b. **Strain**
—is an acute traumatic injury to the **muscle-tendon junction.**
—three grades: 1st-degree—mild; 2nd-degree—moderate, associated with a weakened muscle; 3rd-degree—complete tear of the muscle-tendon junction with severe pain and inability to contract the involved muscle.

c. **Overuse injuries**
—nonacute injuries, as compared to sprains and strains
—result from exercise, poor training methods, not allowing sufficient recovery time after strenuous activity, insufficient calcium or estrogen, and structural abnormalities.

2. **Clinical presentation**

a. **Symptoms** may include:
—pain
—swelling
—disability

b. **Physical examination findings** may include
—swelling

—ecchymosis
—inability to contract the involved muscle
—instability of the joint

3. **Diagnostic tests**

—Radiographs of the involved joint to rule out fracture

4. **Treatment**

a. **RICE**

b. **Immobilization with splinting**

c. **NSAIDs** and muscle relaxants as needed (see Tables 11-2 and 11-5)

d. Local corticosteroids: dose depends on size of joint, injected as described previously in this chapter

e. An appropriate exercise training program with warming up, stretching, cooling down, and alternating exercise intensity

f. Shoe inserts (orthotics)

g. Surgery

5. **Disposition**

—Patients can be discharged home with referral to an orthopaedist or sports medicine specialist.

E. **Carpal tunnel syndrome**

1. **Overview**

a. **Definition**

—is a syndrome of pain and motor and sensory symptoms that mainly affects the hand.
—may be unilateral or bilateral.
—should be differentiated from C-6 root compression caused by cervical radiculopathy.

b. **Cause**

—**compression of the median nerve** in the volar aspect of the wrist between the longitudinal tendons of forearm muscles that flex the hand and the transverse superficial carpal ligament.

c. **Risk factors**

—female gender
—elderly
—immunocompromised

2. **Clinical presentation**

a. **Symptoms** may include:

—paresthesias in the radial palmar aspect of the hand
—pain, which may be more severe at night
—pain in the wrist, the palm, or the area proximal to the compression site in the forearm and shoulder

b. **Physical examination findings** may include:

—a sensory deficit in the palmar aspect of the first three digits
—weakness and atrophy in the muscles responsible for thumb abduction and apposition

3. Diagnostic tests

—positive **Tinel's test** (hyperflexion of the wrists reproduces the symptoms)

—positive **Phalen's test:** numbness or tingling of thumb, index or middle finger upon flexing wrists upward 90°, indicative of median nerve compression

4. Treatment

a. Cock-up splint to affected wrist to help relieve pain

b. Intraarticular corticosteroid injection: 20 mg methylprednisolone IV for temporary (1–3 weeks) relief

c. Avoidance of tasks requiring forceful wrist flexion

d. Surgical decompression of the median nerve at the wrist

5. Disposition

—Patients can be discharged home with referral to an orthopaedist.

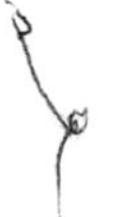

Review Test

1. Which of the following is an indication of rheumatoid arthritis?

(A) Evening stiffness
(B) Arthritis of < 3 joint areas
(C) Arthritis of distal interphalangeal (DIP) joints
(D) Asymmetric arthritis
(E) Rheumatoid nodules

2. What is the initial treatment for temporal arteritis?

(A) Prednisone
(B) Penicillin
(C) Ceftriaxone
(D) Morphine
(E) Nonsteroidal anti-inflammatory drugs (NSAIDs)

3. Which of the following is true of Paget's disease?

(A) It is an acute disorder of bone remodeling resulting in disorganized mosaic patterns in bone.
(B) Bacterial infection is suspected.
(C) Incidence of disease decreases with age
(D) Pain and aching are deep and occasionally severe.
(E) Increasing auditory acuity is a feature of the disease.

4. Which of the following is true regarding osteoporosis?

(A) Osteoporosis is characterized by an acute reduction in bone tissue mass.
(B) Type I osteoporosis (postmenopausal osteoporosis) occurs mainly in those older than 70 and may result from age-related reduction in vitamin D synthesis or resistance to vitamin D activity.
(C) Type II osteoporosis (involutional or senile osteoporosis) occurs between ages 51 and 75 years and is 6 times more common in women than in men.
(D) In men, types I and II may occur together.
(E) Aging is a risk factor.

5. A 25-year-old female office worker presents with pain in her right wrist and palm that is worse at night. On examination of the patient, you find a sensory deficit on the palmar aspect of the first three digits. Hyperflexion of the wrists for a minute reproduces the symptoms. Which of the following is your diagnosis?

(A) Tenosynovitis
(B) Carpal tunnel syndrome
(C) Fibrositis
(D) Tendonitis
(E) de Quervain's disease

Directions: The response options for Items 6–9 are the same. You will be required to select one answer for each item in the set.

Questions 6–9

Match the area of involvement with the name of the syndrome.

(A) Olecranon
(B) Suprapatella
(C) Retrocalcaneus
(D) Ischium

6. Miner's elbow

7. Achilles tendon

8. Tailor's bottom

9. Housemaid's knee

Answers and Explanations

1-E. The American College of Rheumatology proposed new, simplified criteria for the diagnosis of rheumatoid arthritis in 1987 (see Table 11-1). Rheumatoid nodules (E) are included on this list. Evening stiffness, arthritis of <3 joints, arthritis of the DIP joints, and asymmetrical arthritis are not criteria for the diagnosis.

2-A. Due to the danger of blindness, any patient suspected of having temporal arteritis should be immediately treated with corticosteroids, even before definitive diagnosis is established. There is no role for antibiotics in the treatment of temporal arteritis. Although morphine and NSAIDs may alleviate the headache associated with temporal arteritis, they only serve to mask the problem and are not considered appropriate therapy.

3-D. Paget's disease is a chronic disorder of bone remodeling resulting in disorganized mosaic patterns where normal bone marrow is replaced by fibrous connective tissue. This replacement results in a stiffening of the ear ossicles, which decreases, not increases, auditory acuity. The incidence of the disease increases, not decreases, with age. A viral, not bacterial, etiology is suspected. The disorder that results in disorganized mosaic patterns in bone is osteomalacia, not Paget's disease.

4-E. Aging is a known risk factor for osteoporosis. Osteoporosis is a progressive, not acute, reduction in bone mass. Type I, also called postmenopausal, osteoporosis, not type II osteoporosis, occurs between ages 51 and 75 years and is 6 times more common in women, not in men. Type II osteoporosis (involutional or senile osteoporosis), not type I osteoporosis, occurs mainly in those > 70 years and may result from age-related reduction in vitamin D synthesis or resistance to vitamin D activity. Both types may be seen together in women, not in men.

5-B. The reproducibility of symptoms upon hyperflexion of the wrist describes a positive Tinel's test, typical of carpal tunnel syndrome. The presence of pain at night and a sensory deficit along the distribution of the median nerve also are characteristic of this condition. Fibrositis (choice C) is not commonly seen in the hand. The usual areas affected by fibrositis are the occiput, neck, shoulders, thorax, lower back, and thighs. This patient's pain is present even at night, presumably when her hand and wrist are at rest. The pain of tendonitis and tenosynovitis usually occurs upon active ranging of the tendon involved and is frequently limited to one or two digits, which would be swollen. Such a presentation is not described here. De Quervain's disease is tenosynovitis of the extensor pollas brevis and abductor pollicis tendons.

6-A, 7-C, 8-D, 9-B. Miner's elbow affects the olecranon. Achilles tendon affects the retrocalcaneus. The ischium is affected in tailor's bottom. Housemaid's knee affects the suprapatellar region.

12

Endocrine, Metabolic, and Acid-Base Emergencies

I. Diabetic Ketoacidosis

A. Clinical features

1. **Symptoms** may include:
   —**polyuria**
   —**polydipsia**
   —nausea
   —vomiting
   —thirst
   —abdominal pain
   —weakness
   —blurry vision
   —weight loss
2. **Physical examination findings** may include:
   —dehydration
   —hypotension
   —reflex tachycardia
   —**fruity** or acetone odor on **breath**
   —hyperventilation or **Kussmaul's respiration**
   —abdominal tenderness
   —mental confusion or coma

B. Pathophysiology

1. **Insulin**
   —is produced by the pancreatic β-islet cells.

—is responsible for glucose uptake and conversion to glycogen in the liver.

—inhibits glycogenolysis and suppresses gluconeogenesis.

—increases lipogenesis, prevents lipolysis, converts free fatty acids to triglycerides, and stores fat in liver and adipose tissue.

—is involved in protein metabolism in the muscles, stimulates amino acid uptake, and mediates incorporation to muscle protein.

—prevents release of amino acids from muscle protein.

2. **Diabetic ketoacidosis (DKA)**

—results when there is not enough insulin to transport glucose into the cells.

—may be precipitated by infections, myocardial infarction, stroke, pregnancy, hyperthyroidism, pancreatitis, and dietary or medication noncompliance.

—The physiologic response to cellular starvation is the release of the counter-regulatory hormones glucagon, catecholamines, cortisol, and growth hormone.

—The counter-regulatory hormones are catabolic and essentially reverse the above-mentioned physiologic processes of insulin, resulting in hyperglycemia, ketonemia, and hyperkalemia.

C. Diagnostic tests

1. Arterial blood gases **(ABG)** or venous blood gases **(VBG)** to look for **metabolic acidosis with respiratory compensation**
2. **Chemistry panel** to look for an **elevated anion gap** (see Chapter 18, section I G 2 a for differential diagnosis), hyperkalemia, hypochloremia, and **hyperglycemia**
3. **Urinalysis (UA)** to look for glycosuria and **ketones**
4. **Chest radiograph** to look for infiltrates
5. **Serum acetone** level to look for > 2:1 dilution. (Note: a patient may be ketotic yet have a negative serum acetone level, because the serum acetone level measures only α-acetoacetic acid and does not reflect β-hydroxybutyrate.)
6. **Serum lactate** to distinguish from lactic acidosis

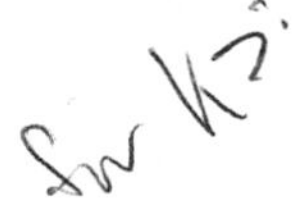

7. **Electrocardiogram (ECG)** to look for myocardial infarction or **hyperkalemia**
8. **Complete blood cell count (CBC)** to look for leukocytosis (may be elevated even in the absence of infection) and elevated hematocrit secondary to intravascular volume depletion
9. **Serum osmolality** to compare against calculated osmolality
10. **Glycosated hemoglobin (HbA1C)** to look for glucose control over last 3 months. Less than 8% indicates good diabetic control, whereas greater than 13% indicates poor control. This test is not necessarily done in the emergency department (ED).

D. Treatment

1. Calculation of water deficit: 0.6 × body weight [1–140/Na^+)]. Replace-

ment of fluids with 3 L normal saline (NS) over 3 hours, followed by continued infusion at 200 ml/h until serum electrolytes normalize and ketones are no longer present in the urine.

2. Corrected serum Na^+ = measured Na^+ + [1.5 × (Glu-150)/100]. Correction is not needed for glucose less than 150 mg/dl. Once the serum sodium level is 155 mEq/L, the IV fluid solution may be changed to 0.45 NS.
3. **Replacement of potassium deficits:** 100–200 mEq usually is required in the first 24 hours. An initial normal potassium level can be obtained even when intracellular potassium is severely depleted.
4. **Insulin drip** at 0.1U/kg/h (continuous infusion). When the glucose level falls below 250 mg/dl, the insulin drip is decreased to 1 U/h and glucose is added to the IV fluid.
5. **Replacement of serum phosphate** if <1.0 mg/dl. Add 5 ml of potassium phosphate to 1 L of IV fluid (about 20 mEq of potassium + 480 mg of phosphate).
6. Administration of sodium bicarbonate if pH <6.9, in modest amounts (44–100 mEq). Administration of bicarbonate decreases serum potassium.
7. Serum electrolytes and urinary ketones must be monitored every 1–2 hours, with aggressive fluid and electrolyte replacement. Urinary ketones may increase with treatment as acetoacetate is converted from β-hydroxybutyrate. Complete correction of hyperglycemia and ketonemia usually requires 8 to 16 hours of treatment.
8. Treatment of any underlying infections

E. Disposition

—Patients are admitted to the intensive care unit (ICU).

II. Nonketotic Hyperosmolar Coma (NKHC)

—is characterized by hyperosmolality and severe hyperglycemia without ketoacidosis.

—can occur in diabetics as well as non-diabetics.

—most commonly is seen in middle-aged, non-insulin-dependent diabetics.

—may be the initial presentation of diabetes.

—can be caused or exacerbated by certain medications, including diuretics (loop, thiazide, or osmotic), calcium channel blockers (CCBs), phenytoin, Thorazine, glucocorticoids, cimetidine, propranolol, and asparaginase.

A. Clinical features

1. **Symptoms** may include:

—polyuria

—polydipsia

—dry mouth

—altered mental status

—stupor

—coma

2. **Physical examination findings** may include:
   - —**significant dehydration** (patients have up to 4–6 L deficit)
   - —fever
   - —hypotension
   - —tachycardia
   - —shallow respirations, tachypnea
   - —**no acetone smell on breath** (in contrast to DKA)
   - —**obtundation:** directly proportional to serum osmolality
   - —hemisensory deficits and hemiparesis
   - —seizures (15%)
   - —aphasia, tremors, hyperreflexia, decreased deep tendon reflexes, flaccidity, positive Babinski's sign

B. Pathophysiology

—The mechanism behind the pathogenesis of NKHC is poorly understood.

—It is theorized that patients experience hyperglycemia due to elevated levels of glucagon, which promotes gluconeogenesis in the liver.

—These patients also have higher circulating levels of insulin, which are theorized to inhibit lipolysis, thus inhibiting the precursors required for ketone body formation.

—Hyperglycemia in these patients produces osmotic diuresis and fluid and electrolyte imbalances (potassium depletion may be as high as 400 to 1000 mEq).

—Calculation of corrected sodium: a decrease of 1.6 mEq/L of Na+ for each increase of 100 mg/dl of glucose or severe potassium depletion.

C. Diagnostic tests

1. **ABG** to look for **metabolic acidosis with respiratory compensation**
2. **Chemistry panel** to look for an **elevated anion gap** (see Chapter 18, section I G 2 a for differential diagnosis), **hyperglycemia,** elevated blood urea nitrogen (BUN):creatinine ratio (>30:1) and elevated CPK (which may reflect rhabdomyolysis)
3. **Serum osmolality** to compare against calculated osmolality
4. **URINALYSIS** to look for glycosuria and ketones
5. **Chest radiograph** to look for infiltrates
6. **Serum acetone** level to look for > 2:1 dilution (rarely present)
7. **Serum lactate** to look for lactic acidosis
8. **ECG** to look for myocardial infarction or hyperkalemia
9. **CBC** to look for leukocytosis
10. Lumbar puncture if meningeal signs are present. Expect normal opening pressure, CSF glucose = 50% of serum glucose, and normal or slightly elevated protein.

11. **HbA1C** to look for glucose control over last 3 months (not necessarily done in ED) if patient is diabetic
12. Serum drug levels if patient is on any medications, as needed
13. Other tests for work-up of altered mental status if cause is unclear (see Chapter 6, section I)

D. Treatment

1. Goals of treatment are glucose < 250 mg/dl, serum osmolality <320 mOsm, and urine output = 50 ml/h.
2. Water deficit must be calculated (see section I D 1)
3. Half of deficit is replaced in first 8 hours, with 2–3 L in first hour unless patient cannot tolerate high fluid load [e.g., patient with congestive heart failure (CHF)]
4. IVF of choice is 0.9% NaCl, unless serum Na^+ is > 145 or patient is severely hypertensive. Consider 0.45% NaCl in such cases.
5. Potassium is replaced with KCl 10–20 mEq/h for the first 24 to 36 hours early in the course of treatment.
6. IV drip is started, with 0.1U/kg/h of regular insulin until glucose level reaches 300. Note: larger doses of insulin may precipitate intravascular collapse, cerebral edema, and acute tubular necrosis secondary to large shifts of water into the cell.
7. IVFs are supplemented with glucose when the serum glucose <250 mg/dl. It is necessary to remember to evaluate for complications of cerebral edema (e.g., sudden hyperpyrexia, hypotension, and increased coma state).
8. Low-molecular-weight heparin should be considered for patients at increased risk of deep vein thrombosis.
9. Broad-spectrum antibiotic coverage is initiated if sepsis is suspected.

E. Disposition

—Patients must be admitted to the ICU for treatment and observation of complications.

III. Alcoholic Ketoacidosis

—presents similarly to DKA in that it is characterized by an increased anion gap acidosis as a result of high levels of ketoacids (β-hydroxybutyrate levels accumulate higher than acetoacetate).

—results when the rate of NAD reduction exceeds the rate of NADH oxidation, causing less NAD to be available for fatty acid oxidation, with resultant ketone body formation.

—**history** may include heavy alcohol consumption or binge drinking, with decrease in last 24–48 hours

A. Clinical features

1. **Symptoms** may include:

—nausea

—protracted vomiting
—abdominal pain
—anorexia for several days

2. **Physical examination findings** may include:
   —dehydration
   —tachypnea
   —orthostatic hypotension
   —decreased urine output
   —delirium tremens (withdrawal seizures)
   —hypothermia to mildly elevated temperature
   —may be accompanied by symptoms of sepsis, pyelonephritis, meningitis or pneumonia

B. Diagnostic tests

1. **ABG** to look for metabolic acidosis. pH may be low, normal, or high.
2. **Chemistry panel** to look for increased anion gap, hypoglycemia, hypokalemia, and hypochloremia.
3. **CBC** to look for leukocytosis
4. **Chest radiograph** to look for aspiration pneumonia
5. **Lactic acid level** to look for lactic acidosis (expect to be normal)
6. **Prothrombin time (PT)** and **activated partial thromboplastin time (APTT)** to look for coagulopathies
7. **Serum osmolality** to compare against calculated osmolality
8. **Serum ketone level** to look for elevation

C. Treatment

1. **Intravenous hydration** with D10-NS alternating with D10-½NS
2. **Thiamine** 50–100 mg IV to prevent Wernicke's encephalopathy
3. Use of exogenous insulin is not necessary
4. Sodium bicarbonate (start with 44 mEq or less), if pH <7.1. Supplemental potassium is given, and levels are monitored.
5. **Chlordiazepoxide** 50–150 mg intramuscularly (IM) or intravenously (IV) to prevent and control delirium tremens. Other sedatives may be used. Phenothiazines should be avoided, because they tend to lower the seizure threshold
6. Multivitamins including thiamine orally or IV
7. Folate 1 mg orally or IV
8. Magnesium sulfate 2 g IV in 50 ml NS

D. Disposition

1. Patients who have significant metabolic acidosis or who are unable to tolerate oral intake are admitted to the hospital for further management.
2. Patients who respond well to treatment in the ED may be discharged fol-

lowing observation for 6–8 hours and documented resolution of acidosis and ketonemia.

3. All patients should receive alcoholism counseling and referral for detoxification.

IV. Adrenal Insufficiency

—Adrenal insufficiency is a disease state due to decreased or absent levels of adrenal hormones.

—Primary insufficiency is due to failure of adrenal glands to secrete hormones. Clinical manifestations of failure do not become evident until 90% of the adrenal cortex has been destroyed.

—Secondary insufficiency is due to failure of the pituitary gland to produce adrenocorticotropic hormone (ACTH). Only cortisol production is affected; aldosterone production remains intact.

A. Pathophysiology

1. Aldosterone

—Aldosterone is the major mineralocorticoid hormone of the body.

—Aldosterone is produced in the zona glomerulosa of the adrenal cortex.

—Its main function is renal reabsorption of sodium in the distal tubule and collecting ducts, with subsequent excretion of potassium and hydrogen ions.

—The renin-angiotensin system is the most important regulator of aldosterone secretion.

—Deficiency results in **hyperkalemia** and **hyponatremia**.

2. Cortisol

—is the major glucocorticoid hormone of the body.

—is produced in the zona fasciculata of the adrenal cortex.

—has widespread effects on carbohydrate and protein metabolism.

—acts to counteract the effects of insulin and maintain blood glucose levels.

—governs body water distribution.

—enhances the pressor effects of catecholamine on heart muscle.

—inhibits inflammatory and allergic reactions.

—deficiency results in impairment of body's ability to handle stress.

B. Causes

1. Causes of **primary insufficiency** include:

—idiopathic causes (most common)

—autoimmune disorders

—tuberculosis

—sarcoidosis

—amyloidosis

—blastomycosis

—hemochromatosis

—AIDS

—neoplastic disease

—congenital adrenal hyperplasia

—fulminant septicemia in newborns (Waterhouse-Friderichsen syndrome)

—adrenalectomy

2. Causes of **secondary insufficiency** include:

—Suppression of the hypothalamic-pituitary-adrenal axis by exogenous steroids (most common)

—Sheehan's syndrome (postpartum pituitary necrosis)

—Pituitary infarct

—Autoimmune destruction of the pituitary

—Hypothalamic failure

C. Clinical presentation

1. **Symptoms** may include:

—anorexia

—nausea

—vomiting

—lethargy

—weakness

—fatigue on exertion

—weight loss

—abdominal pain

—diarrhea

2. **Physical examination findings**

a. **Systemic findings** may include:

—dehydration

—hypotension

—postural syncope

b. **Cardiac findings** may include:

—soft or almost inaudible heart sounds

—feeble tachycardic pulse

c. **Neurologic findings** may include:

—confusion

—rapidly ascending muscular weakness (secondary to hyperkalemia)

d. **Dermatologic findings** (with primary insufficiency) may include:

—increased pigmentation of skin and mucous membranes (secondary to increased melatonin production in primary insufficiency)

—longitudinal pigmented bands in nail beds
—mucocutaneous candidiasis
—alopecia
—decreased growth of axillary and pubic hair in women

D. Diagnostic tests

1. **CBC** to look for elevated hematocrit (secondary to dehydration), leukocytosis with lymphocytic predominance and eosinophilia
2. **Chemistry panel** to look for hyponatremia, hyperkalemia, hypoglycemia, and elevated BUN and creatinine with hypercalcemia and mild metabolic acidosis (secondary to dehydration)
3. **ECG** to look for flat or inverted T waves, prolonged QT interval, decreased voltage, and depressed ST segments. T waves may be peaked if significant hyperkalemia is present.
4. **Chest radiograph** to look for a narrow cardiac silhouette
5. **Abdominal radiograph** to look for adrenal calcifications
6. **Rapid corticotrophin stimulation test:**
   a. Baseline cortisol and ACTH levels are obtained.
   b. 250 μg (adults and children > 2 years) or 125 μg (children < 2 years) of synthetic ACTH (cosyntropin) is administered over 2 minutes.
   c. Cortisol and ACTH levels are measured at 30 and 60 minutes post-cosyntropin.
      —Cortisol level should rise by 10–20 μg/dl in a healthy person. If it does not, then adrenal insufficiency is present. ACTH level is used to distinguish between primary and secondary insufficiency.
      —ACTH level is > 250 μg/dl in primary insufficiency and less in secondary insufficiency.
7. **Head and abdominal CT scans or MRI** to look for pathology of pituitary and adrenal glands

E. Treatment

—Therapy consists of non-emergent replacement of deficient hormones.

1. Glucocorticoid: cortisol 20–37.5 mg orally daily
2. Mineralocorticoid: fludrocortisone 0.05–0.2 mg orally daily (for primary insufficiency)
3. Maintenance of adequate dietary salt intake
4. If decreased axillary and pubic hair is present, supplementation with fluoxymesterone 2–5 mg orally daily

F. Disposition

1. Patients may be discharged home with outpatient follow-up with an endocrinologist within 2–3 days.
2. Patients with severe hypotension and ECG changes or those in adrenal crisis (see section V) should be admitted to the hospital for further management.

V. Adrenal Crisis

—is a life-threatening condition seen in patients with adrenal insufficiency (primary or secondary) who are subjected to stress.

—may be precipitated by **infection** (most common), trauma, surgery, burns, pregnancy, alcohol withdrawal, hyperthyroidism, and drugs.

—most commonly is caused by prolonged use of steroids, especially in combination with a stressor such as trauma or infection.

A. Clinical presentation

1. **Symptoms** may include:
   - —acutely ill-appearing patient
   - —weakness
   - —confusion
   - —fever
   - —anorexia
   - —nausea
   - —vomiting
   - —abdominal pain
2. **Physical examination findings** may include:
   - —hypotension
   - —hyperthermia
   - —increased motor activity
   - —delirium
   - —seizures
   - —dehydration
   - —severe abdominal tenderness

B. Diagnostic tests

—No test is diagnostic in all cases. It often is necessary to treat presumptively.

1. **CBC** to look for elevated hematocrit (secondary to dehydration), leukocytosis with lymphocytic predominance, and eosinophilia
2. **Chemistry panel** to look for hyponatremia, hyperkalemia, hypoglycemia, and elevated BUN and creatinine with hypercalcemia and mild metabolic acidosis
3. **ECG** to look for flat or inverted T waves, prolonged **QT** interval, decreased voltage, and depressed ST segments. T waves may be peaked if significant hyperkalemia is present.
4. **Chest radiograph** to look for a narrow cardiac silhouette and **infiltrates**
5. Blood and urine cultures to look for source of infection
6. Serum cortisol level to look for deviation from baseline

7. Head CT scans to look for intracranial pathology (pituitary, bleed, mass, edema)

C. Treatment

—consists of **replacement of cortisol and aggressive volume resuscitation.**

1. Dexamethasone 4 mg or hydrocortisone 100 mg IV push. Dexamethasone is preferable because it does not interfere with results of corticotropin test or future cortisol measurements.
2. Rapid infusion of dextrose 5% in normal saline (D5NS) to correct dehydration, hypotension, hyponatremia, and hypoglycemia. Caution is necessary in patients prone to CHF.
3. Hydrocortisone 100 mg IV every 6 hours during the first 24 hours of therapy
4. When the total dosage of cortisol drops below 100 g/24 h, addition of desoxycorticosterone 5 mg IM daily is necessary to supplement mineralocorticoid deficiency.

D. Disposition

—Patients are admitted to the ICU.

VI. Thyroid Storm

A. Overview

1. Definition

—Thyroid storm is a rare complication of hyperthyroidism that is most commonly seen in patients with moderate to severe antecedent Graves' disease

—It is difficult to distinguish between thyrotoxicosis and thyroid storm, because they represent a continuum of symptoms on the same spectrum of disease.

2. Causes

—**sepsis (most common)**

—pulmonary emboli

—toxemia of pregnancy

—emotional stressors

—exacerbation of diabetes

3. Complications of untreated thyroid storm

—Congestive heart failure

—Refractory pulmonary edema

—Circulatory collapse

—Coma

—Death within 72 hours

B. Clinical features

1. **Symptoms** may include:
   —extreme irritability and anxiety
   —agitation, psychosis, mental confusion, obtundation, and coma
   —muscle weakness
   —myasthenia gravis (about 1% of patients)
   —diarrhea
   —heat intolerance
   —anorexia, weight loss
   —nausea, vomiting, and crampy abdominal pain
   —palpitations
   —in elderly patients, "apathetic storm," which presents with only lethargy and coma.
2. **Physical examination findings** may include:
   —fever
   —tachycardia
   —hypertension
   —delirium
   —diaphoresis
   —decreased muscle strength
   —systolic murmur
   —irregular heartbeat
   —widened pulse pressure
   —exophthalmos
   —pulmonary edema
   —jaundice (poor prognostic sign)
   —proximal muscle weakness

C. Diagnostic tests

—There are no laboratory tests that confirm thyroid storm, but the following tests may be useful in elucidating the diagnosis:

1. Thyroid function tests (TFTs) to look for elevations. T3 and T4 levels may be increased but do not distinguish hyperthyroidism from thyroid storm.
2. Admission laboratory studies, including CBC, chemistry panel, PT, APTT, and UA to look for sources of sepsis
3. ECG to look for atrial fibrillation, premature ventricular contractions (PVCs), and heart block (rare)
4. Chest radiograph to look for pulmonary edema and infiltrates

D. Treatment

1. Stabilization of airway, breathing, and circulation (ABCs), using **supplemental oxygen** if necessary

2. **Antipyretics** and cooling blanket (aspirin must be avoided due to increase in free T3 and T4 levels)
3. **Intravenous hydration** with saline and glucose
4. **Vitamin B complex**
5. **Dexamethasone** 2 mg every 6 hours (until T3 levels normalize and then taper) or any IV glucocorticoids equivalent to 300 mg of hydrocortisone per day
6. Digitalis and diuretics to control atrial fibrillation and CHF
7. **Propranolol** (1 mg/min IV to a total dose of 10 mg, or 40–80 mg orally every 6 hours) to blunt sympathomimetic activity
8. In consultation with the endocrinology department:

   —**Propylthiouracil** (loading dose is 900–1200 mg orally, and then 300–600 mg/24 h for 3–6 weeks) or **methimazole** (loading dose is 90–120 mg orally, then 5–30 mg/24 h for 3–6 weeks) to inhibit thyroid hormone synthesis

   —Potassium iodide 300 mg orally every 8 hours adults and children older than 1 year of age; half the dosage for children younger than 1 year of age to inhibit thyroid hormone release. This must not be given within 1 hour of administering propylthiouracil (PTU) or methimazole, or the exogenous iodine will be used up to make more thyroid hormone.

E. Disposition

—Patients with thyroid storm are admitted to the ICU. The definitive treatment of choice is radioactive iodine therapy

VII. Myxedema Coma

A. Overview

1. Definition

—Myxedema coma is associated with a **>50% mortality,** in spite of optimal therapeutic intervention.

—The usual presentation is in a patient with long-standing hypothyroidism who has been undertreated or undiagnosed and has had a recent stress.

2. Incidence

—It occurs more commonly in women and elderly patients.

3. Causes

a. of myxedema:

—cold exposure
—trauma
—infection
—central nervous system (CNS) depressants

b. of hypothyroidism:

—primary thyroid failure due to autoimmunity (most common)

—ablation of Graves' disease with radioactive iodine (second most common)

B. Clinical features

1. **Symptoms** may include:
   —fatigue and weakness
   —cold intolerance
   —constipation
   —weight gain without increased appetite
   —waxy swelling of skin and subcutaneous tissues
   —decreased hearing
   —decreased mentation
   —muscle cramps
   —deepened voice

2. **Physical examination findings**

   a. **Systemic findings** may include:
      —hypothermia without shivering (80%)
      —edema
      —hypotension
      —bradycardia

   b. **Neurologic findings** may include:
      —memory loss
      —hallucinations
      —grand mal seizures
      —delusions
      —cerebellar ataxia, intention tremor, and nystagmus
      —paresthesias
      —prolongation of deep tendon reflexes

   c. **Gastrointestinal (GI) findings** may include:
      —ascites
      —fecal impaction with abdominal distention
      —megacolon

   d. **Genitourinary (GU) findings** may include:
      —urinary retention

   e. **Dermatologic findings** may include:
      —dry, scaly, yellow skin
      —thinning of outer edges of eyebrows
      —scant body hair

C. Diagnostic tests

1. **Serum thyroid-stimulating hormone (TSH)** level to look for elevation in primary myxedema (thyroid) and decreased or normal levels in secondary myxedema (pituitary).

2. **Chemistry panel** to look for hyponatremia and hypochloremia and elevated serum creatinine
3. **ABG** to look for hypoxia and hypercapnia
4. **CBC** to look for leukocytosis and elevated mean corpuscular volume (MCV)
5. **ECG** to look for bradycardia, low voltage, flattening of T waves, and PR prolongation
6. **Echocardiography** to evaluate cardiac function and to look for presence of pericardial effusion
7. **Chest radiograph** to look for enlarged cardiac silhouette and infiltrates
8. Post-voiding urine residual to look for urinary retention
9. Blood and urine cultures if patient is febrile to look for source of infection
10. Lumbar puncture to look for meningitis or bleed. CSF protein levels may be >100 mg/dl, and opening pressure may be elevated.

D. Treatment

1. ABCs, including **supplemental oxygen**
2. Warm blankets to correct hypothermia
3. **Thyroxine**

   —is the drug of choice because it does not lead to abrupt T3 increases, which may be dangerous in the elderly patient.

   —is administered as a gradual infusion of 400–500 mg IV (loading dose) and then 50–100 mg IV daily

   —Serum T3 is a superior indicator of metabolism. Once the level is therapeutic, an oral dose of thyroxine, 100 to 200 μg/day, may be instituted.
4. **Hydrocortisone** 300 mg/day to protect against adrenal insufficiency
5. Broad-spectrum antibiotics if sepsis is suspected

E. Disposition

—Patients with myxedema coma should be admitted to the hospital for further management.

VIII. Hyponatremia

A. Overview

1. Definitions

—Hyponatremia is defined as a deficiency of sodium in the blood.

—There are three types of hyponatremia: hypovolemic, euvolemic, and hypervolemic.

—**Hypovolemic hyponatremia** is defined as loss of sodium > loss of water.

—**Euvolemic hyponatremia** is produced by a dilutional effect and occurs when there is an increase in extracellular fluid volume without shift (i.e., no edema).

—**Hypervolemic hyponatremia** exists when retention of water exceeds retention of sodium.

2. **Causes**
   a. Hypovolemic hyponatremia
      —vomiting
      —diarrhea
      —GI suction or drainage tubes or fistulas
      —burns
      —intraabdominal sepsis
      —bowel obstruction
      —pancreatitis
      —diuretics
      —renal tubular acidosis
      —mineralocorticoid deficiency
   b. Euvolemic hyponatremia
      —SIADH
      —hypoadrenalism
      —hypothyroidism
      —renal failure
      —psychogenic polydipsia
   c. Hypervolemic hyponatremia
      —CHF
      —cirrhosis
      —renal failure
      —nephrotic syndrome

B. Clinical features

Symptoms and **physical examination findings** may include:

—lethargy, apathy, confusion, disorientation, and agitation
—depression
—psychosis
—ataxia
—seizures
—muscle cramps
—anorexia, nausea
—weakness

C. Diagnostic tests

1. For hypovolemic hyponatremia:
   —Electrolytes
   —CBC
   —UA and urine electrolytes
   —Renal wasting: U_{Na} >20 mEq/dl

—Extrarenal wasting: U_{Na} <10 mEq/dl (usually GI losses and burns)

2. For euvolemic hyponatremia:

—Electrolytes

—CBC

—UA

—Patients with SIADH demonstrate concentrated urine with low serum osmolality

—Patients with psychogenic polydipsia have maximally dilute urine

3. For hypervolemic hyponatremia:

—Electrolytes

—CBC

—Serum osmolality

—Urine electrolytes to determine presence of renal vs. extrarenal wasting

D. Treatment

1. For hypovolemic hyponatremia:

—0.9% NS

—Replenishment of sodium, carefully and slowly, to prevent complication of central pontine myelinolysis

—3% hypertonic saline may be given for patients with severe neurologic findings.

2. For euvolemic hyponatremia:

—Free water intake is restricted.

—Determine cause.

—For SIADH, lithium or demeclocycline may be used.

—Sodium is replenished, carefully and slowly, to prevent complication of central pontine myelinolysis.

3. For hypervolemic hyponatremia:

—Fluid restriction

—Diuretics may be used, with caution

—Replenishment of sodium, carefully and slowly, to prevent complication of central pontine myelinolysis

E. Disposition

1. Patients with hyponatremia and neurologic findings or those with hemodynamic instability are admitted to the hospital for further work-up.
2. Patients whose hyponatremia has been corrected in the ED and those who remain asymptomatic may be discharged after 4–6 hours observation with outpatient follow-up in 2–3 days.

IX. Hypernatremia

A. Overview

1. Definition

—Hypernatremia is present when Na >145 mEq/L.

2. Causes

—decreased tolerance for oral fluids

—lack of access to water (e.g., nonambulatory patient)

—defective thirst mechanism

—depressed mentation

—protracted diarrhea, vomiting, or nasogastric tube (NGT) suctioning

—hyperglycemia, mannitol (osmotic diuresis)

—diabetes insipidus

—severe burns

—hyperventilation

—enteral or parenteral nutrition

—drugs (e.g., ticarcillin, carbenicillin)

—thyrotoxicosis

—large amounts of $NaHCO_3$ ingestion

—hyperaldosteronism

—hypertonic saline infusion (iatrogenic)

B. Clinical features

1. **Symptoms** may include:

—anorexia

—fatigue and irritability

—dehydration

—lethargy, confusion, stupor, coma

—hyperreflexia, spasticity

—tremor

—ataxia

—seizures

2. **Physical examination findings** may include:

—orthostatic hypotension

—tachycardia

—dehydration (i.e., flattened neck veins, dry mucous membranes)

C. Diagnostic tests

1. **UA** to look for urine specific gravity of <1.005 and low urine osmolality (diabetes insipidus)

2. **Chemistry panel** to look for other electrolyte imbalances and metabolic alkalosis
3. **Head CT** if source of altered mental status is not clear
4. Work-up for sepsis if patient is febrile

D. Treatment

1. If patient is **hypovolemic,** IV hydration with 0.9% NS infusion
2. If patient is **euvolemic,** IV hydration with 0.45% NS to increase free water intake and IV vasopressin or intranasal vasopressin for central diabetes insipidus
3. If patient is **hypervolemic,** establish increased renal sodium excretion with 20–40 mg **furosemide** IVP and maintain free water intake with 0.45% NS.

E. Disposition

—Patients are admitted to the hospital for further management.

X. Calcium Disturbances

A. Hypocalcemia

1. Definition

—a total serum calcium level < 8.0 mg/dl or an ionized calcium level < 2 mg/dl.

2. Causes

—parathyroid hormone (PTH) insufficiency

—severe magnesium disturbances

—drugs (e.g., cimetidine, ethanol)

—sepsis

—rhabdomyolysis

—pancreatitis

—renal or liver disease

—vitamin D deficiency (resulting from intestinal malabsorption, cholestyramine, primidone, or phenytoin)

—pseudohypoparathyroidism (e.g., Albright's hereditary osteodystrophy)

—citrate (transfusions, radiocontrast material)

—fluoride poisoning

3. Clinical features

a. **Symptoms** may include:

—CNS depression
—irritability
—confusion

—**seizures**
—**perioral paresthesia**
—muscle weakness
—anxiety
—psychosis

b. **Physical examination findings** may include:
—**fasciculations** and **tetany** (Chvostek's and Trousseau's signs)
—faint heart sounds
—bronchospasm (presence of rales and wheezing)

4. **Diagnostic tests**
   a. **Laboratory studies**
   —Ionized serum calcium to look for decrease
   —Serum PTH to look for hypoparathyroidism
   —CBC and peripheral smear to look for leukocytosis
   —Blood and urine cultures if patient is febrile
   —Serum toxicology to look for ethanol and any offending medications
   —Chemistry panel to look for hyperphosphatemia and magnesium abnormalities

   b. ECG to look for **QT prolongation**
   c. Chest radiograph to look for infiltrates

5. **Treatment**
   a. If patient is **symptomatic:**
   —IV bolus of $CaCl_2$ 1 ampule (10 ml of 10% solution = 360 mg Ca^{2+}) diluted in D5W or Ca is started
   —Gluconate, 3 ampules IV (10 ml of 10% solution = 93 mg Ca^{2+}) is given. Then a continuous infusion of 0.5–2 mg/kg/h is begun. In neonates and children, an initial bolus of 0.5–1 ml/kg of calcium gluconate is given IVP over 5 minutes.
   —Calcium infusion is discontinued if bradycardia develops.

   b. If patient is **asymptomatic:**
   —1–4 g calcium orally 3 times a day

   c. For **refractory** cases:
   —magnesium sulfate 10% 2–4 g IV

6. **Disposition**
   a. Patients who require IV therapy should be hospitalized for cardiac monitoring.
   b. Patients who are asymptomatic can be discharged home with outpatient follow-up.

B. Hypercalcemia

1. **Definitions**
   —Mild hypercalcemia = total serum calcium between 8 and 12 mg/dl
   —Severe hypercalcemia = total serum calcium >14 mg/dl

2. **Causes**

—include primary hyperparathyroidism (e.g., parathyroid adenoma, hyperplasia, or carcinoma)

—malignancies

—thiazides

—granulomatous diseases (e.g., sarcoidosis, tuberculosis, coccidiomycosis, histoplasmosis, leprosy)

—vitamin A intoxication

—milk-alkali syndrome

—long-term lithium treatment

3. Clinical features

a. **Symptoms** may include:

—CNS depression

—fatigue

—weakness

—confusion

—**lethargy**

—cardiac arrest

—anorexia

—nausea

—vomiting

b. **Physical examination findings** may include:

—bradycardia

—heart block

—dehydration

—ileus

—coma

4. Diagnostic tests

a. ECG to look for **shortened QT interval,** prolonged PR, widened QRS, sinus bradycardia, bundle branch block, high-degree AV block

b. Abdominal radiograph to look for **renal calculi**

c. Laboratory studies

—Ionized serum calcium to look for increase

—Serum PTH to look for hyperparathyroidism

—Chemistry panel to look for hypophosphatemia

—Blood cultures to look for infectious cause

—CBC and peripheral smear to look for neoplasia

—PPD panel to look for tuberculosis (TB)

5. Treatment

a. In the ED:

—**IV hydration** with normal saline to promote urinary excretion of calcium. May be followed with 10–40 mg of a loop diuretic such as furosemide.

b. Outpatient treatment:

—**Calcitonin** (4 IU/kg IM or subcutaneously) to enhance urinary excretion of calcium

—**Biphosphonate derivatives** to inhibit resorption of calcium from bone: etidronate 5 mg/kg orally; pamidronate 60 mg IV infusion over 2–24 hours; or alendronate 40 mg orally

6. Disposition

—Patients with calcium levels >12 mg/dl or who are symptomatic should be admitted to the hospital for further management.

XI. Potassium Disturbances

A. Hypokalemia

1. Definitions

—Hypokalemia is defined as potassium (K^+) level <3.0 mg/dl.

2. Causes

—exogenous insulin abuse or insulinoma

—renal tubular acidosis or interstitial nephritis

—drugs (e.g., cisplatin, amphotericin, penicillin, aminoglycosides, large doses of β-agonists, loop diuretics)

—leukemia

—hyperaldosteronism (Conn's syndrome)

—Bartter's syndrome

—villous adenoma

—renal artery stenosis

3. Clinical features

a. **Symptoms** may include:

—nausea and vomiting

—polyuria

—lethargy

—depression

—irritability

—confusion

—palpitations

b. **Physical examination findings** may include:

—irregular heartbeat

—abdominal distention

—paralytic ileus

—decreased or absent DTRs (areflexia)

—fasciculations, muscle weakness, or paralysis

—orthostatic hypotension

4. Diagnostic tests

a. ECG to look for **U waves,** extopy, 1st- and 2nd-degree heart block, atrial or ventricular fibrillation, PVCs, and asystole

b. Laboratory studies
—Chemistry panel to look for elevated CPK, hypomagnesemia, hypercalcemia, and metabolic alkalosis
—UA to look for myoglobin (rhabdomyolysis)
—Serum toxicology if patient is on any offending medications
—CBC and peripheral smear to look for leukocytosis and neoplasia

5. Treatment

a. Because 98% of K^+ is intracellular, a decreased K^+ actually reflects a much greater total body potassium deficit (decrease of 1.0 mEq/L serum K^+ = 370 mEq total body deficit of K^+)

b. For patients with ECG changes: KCl 10–20 mEq/h IV is given. Drip is stopped if patient develops PVCs, heart block, tachycardia, or widened QRS.

c. All other patients may be given 40 mEq K^+ orally every 4 hours.

6. Disposition

a. Symptomatic patients and those with serum $K^+ < 2.5$ mg/dl are admitted to the hospital.

b. Most other patients can be discharged with oral supplementation of potassium and outpatient follow-up within 48 hours.

B. Hyperkalemia

1. Definition

—a serum K^+ level >6.0 mg/dl

2. Causes

—large-volume blood transfusions
—renal insufficiency or failure
—hypoaldosteronism (Addison's disease)
—drugs (e.g., NSAIDs, ACE-inhibitors, heparin, cyclosporin, digitalis toxicity, carbenicillin, succinylcholine, β-blockers, trimethoprim-sulfamethoxazole [TMP-SMX], potassium-sparing diuretics)
—defects in tubular potassium secretion
—rhabdomyolysis
—tumor cell necrosis

3. Clinical features

a. **Symptoms** may include:
—muscle cramps
—muscle weakness
—paresthesias
—paralysis
—confusion

b. **Physical examination findings** may include:
—areflexia
—paralysis
—focal neurologic deficits

—respiratory insufficiency

—cardiac arrest

4. Diagnostic tests

a. ECG demonstrates progressively worsening changes of peaked T waves, loss of P waves, widened QRS, sine wave appearance, ventricular fibrillation or asystole, 2nd- and 3rd-degree heart block, and wide-complex tachycardia.

b. Chemistry panel to look for elevated CPK, hypermagnesemia, and metabolic acidosis.

c. Serum toxicology to look for medications

d. UA to look for myoglobin (rhabdomyolysis)

e. CBC to look for leukocytosis, thrombocytosis, hemolysis (pseudohyperkalemia)

5. Treatment

a. Patients are placed on a cardiac monitor.

b. Hyperkalemia is corrected as follows:

—For severe symptoms, 10 ml 10% calcium chloride or calcium gluconate IV by the most rapid method, which may be repeated once for a total of two times. This treatment is contraindicated in patients on digoxin.

—1 ampule sodium bicarbonate IVP over 5–15 minutes; must be used with caution in CHF or alkalosis

—10–20 U regular insulin IV bolus with D10-NS

—Albuterol nebulizer treatment (5–20 mg)

—Kayexalate 20 g orally or 50 g per rectum (1 g of Kayexalate removes 1.0 mEq of K+). Not very useful in the ED.

—Hemodialysis may be considered in patients with acute or chronic renal failure.

—Any underlying disorders must be treated.

—Any offending drugs must be discontinued.

6. Disposition

—Patients are admitted to a monitored hospital bed.

XII. Magnesium Disturbances

A. Hypomagnesemia

1. Definition

—serum Mg^{2+} level < 1.0 mEq/L

2. Causes

—may include diuretics, alcohol abuse, acute tubular necrosis, chronic glomerulonephritis, chronic pyelonephritis, interstitial nephropathy, post-renal transplant, decreased PTH production, chronic diarrhea, parenteral nutrition, acute pancreatitis, diabetes mellitus, hyperthyroidism, hyperaldosteronism, and drugs.

3. **Clinical features**

—mimic those of hypocalcemia

a. **Symptoms** may include:

—weakness

—tremor

—irritability

—dizziness

—seizures

b. **Physical examination findings** may include:

—tetany

—hyperreflexia

4. **Diagnostic tests**

—**ECG findings** may include prolonged PR, QRS, and QT intervals; flattened T waves; U waves; ST-T segment abnormalities; atrial fibrillation; **torsades de pointes;** and ventricular tachycardias.

5. **Treatment**

a. For asymptomatic hypomagnesemia: Magnesium hydroxide 200–600 mg orally

b. For symptomatic hypomagnesemia: 2–4 g magnesium sulfate IV over 30 minutes

6. **Disposition**

—Patients are admitted to the hospital.

a. Asymptomatic patients may be discharged with daily oral magnesium supplementation and outpatient follow-up in 48 hours.

b. Patients with cardiac or neurologic findings are admitted for further management.

B. **Hypermagnesemia**

1. **Definition**

—serum Mg^{2+}

2. **Causes**

—administration of antacids, laxatives, cathartics, or parenteral Mg^{2+} to patients with renal insufficiency

—colitis

—bowel obstruction

—gastric dilatation

—drugs (e.g., anticholinergics, opiates, lithium)

—rhabdomyolysis

—adrenal insufficiency

—tumor lysis syndrome

3. **Clinical features**

a. **Symptoms** may include:

—nausea

—vomiting
—weakness
—cutaneous flushing

b. **Physical examination findings** may include:
—**hyporeflexia**
—hypotension
—**respiratory depression**
—heart block
—asystole
—coma

4. **Diagnostic tests**
—ECG findings include **QRS widening,** QT and PR prolongation, and conduction abnormalities.

5. **Treatment**
a. All sources of exogenous magnesium are discontinued.
b. For severe symptoms: **0.9% NS** IV + 20–40 mg IV **furosemide** to increase elimination
c. For life-threatening symptoms: **calcium chloride** or **gluconate** 100–200 mg IV bolus, following which infusion is begun at 2–4 mg/kg/h
d. **Hemodialysis** for patients with respiratory failure or coma

6. **Disposition**
—Patients are admitted to a monitored setting for further management.

XIII. Phosphate Disturbances

A. Hypophosphatemia

1. **Definition**
—Hypophosphatemia is defined as follows:
—Mild: 2.5–2.8 mg/dl
—Moderate: 1–2.5 mg/dl
—Severe: <1 mg/dl

2. **Causes**
—DKA
—malnutrition
—diuretic or antacid therapy
—sepsis
—alcoholism
—acute renal failure
—renal transplant
—hyperparathyroidism
—hypoaldosteronism

—intestinal malabsorption

—respiratory alkalosis

—salicylate poisoning

—heat stroke

3. Clinical features

—Symptoms usually are present only in severe cases.

—**Symptoms** and **physical examination findings** include:

—ascending motor paralysis

—hypotension

—weakness

—confusion

—seizures

—coma

4. Diagnostic tests

a. Laboratory studies

—Chemistry panel to look for elevated CPK, **hypercalcemia,** hyperglycemia

—ABG to look for respiratory alkalosis

—CBC and smear to look for leukocytosis, anemia, and hemolysis

—Blood and urine cultures if patient is febrile

—PTH level to look for hyperparathyroidism

—Toxicology screen to look for salicylate poisoning

b. ECG to look for rhythm disturbances

c. Imaging studies

—Chest radiograph to look for infiltrates

—Echocardiogram to look for LV dysfunction

5. Treatment

a. For mild to moderate symptoms: potassium phosphate 250 mg (8 mmol phosphate), 2 tabs orally 4 times a day

b. For severe symptoms: potassium phosphate 10–40 mEq/h

6. Disposition

—Most patients can be discharged home with outpatient follow-up.

B. Hyperphosphatemia

1. Definition

—Hyperphosphatemia is defined as a phosphate level >5.0 mg/dl. The condition is rare.

2. Causes

—multiple myeloma

—hyperlipidemia

—renal failure

—rhabdomyolysis

—tumor lysis syndrome
—thyrotoxicosis
—hypoparathyroidism
—hemolysis and hyperbilirubinemia (pseudohyperphosphatemia)

3. **Clinical features**
   a. **Symptoms** may include:
      —paresthesias
      —seizures
   b. **Physical examination findings** may include:
      —**hyperreflexia**
      —**tetany**
      —hypotension
      —bradycardia
4. **Diagnostic tests**
   a. Laboratory studies
      —Chemistry panel to look for elevated CPK, BUN, creatinine, and **hypocalcemia**
      —LFTs to look for hyperbilirubinemia
      —TFTs to look for hyperthyroidism
      —UA to look for Bence Jones proteins (characteristic of multiple myeloma)
      —PTH level to look for hypoparathyroidism
   b. ECG to look for rhythm disturbances
   c. Imaging studies
      —Chest radiograph to look for CHF
      —Echocardiogram to look for LV dysfunction
5. **Treatment**
   a. Supportive care: 0.9% NS IV
   b. Hemodialysis may be considered for life-threatening symptoms
6. **Disposition**
   a. Most patients can be discharged home with outpatient follow-up.
   b. Patients with severe symptoms requiring hemodialysis may need to be hospitalized.

XIV. Acid-Base Disorders

A. General principles and approach

1. **Definitions**
   a. Normal pH = 7.37–7.44
   b. Acidemia = pH < 7.37
   c. Alkalemia = pH > 7.44
   d. A simple acid-base disorder (ABD) is a respiratory acidosis (RA), respiratory alkalosis (RK), metabolic acidosis (MA), or metabolic alkalosis (MK).

e. Respiratory disturbances have a primary abnormality of PCO_2 and are compensated by the renal (metabolic) system.

f. Metabolic disturbances have a primary abnormality of HCO_3 and are compensated by the respiratory system.

g. PCO_2 and HCO_3 (disturbance and compensation) go in the same direction (both increase or both decrease). If they do not go in the same direction, the ABD is a mixed one.

2. **Systematic approach to acid-base disturbances (Fig. 12-1)**
   a. Determine whether the disturbance is an acidemia or an alkalemia.
   b. Determine whether the disturbance is primarily respiratory or metabolic.
   c. Decide whether the degree of compensation is appropriate, keeping compensation limits in mind. If compensation is inadequate or limits are exceeded, a mixed disturbance is present.

3. **Diagnostic tests**
   a. ABG or VBG to look for pH, PCO_2, and HCO_3
      (1) Correlating VBG and ABG values:
      —pCO_2 5–7 mm Hg higher than arterial level
      —pH 0.03–0.05 units lower than arterial level
      —HCO_3 1–3 mEq lower than arterial level
      (2) The differences in VBG and ABG values may be greater in severe circulatory collapse.
   b. Chemistry panel to look for anion gap and electrolyte disturbances
      (1) Potassium
      —Alterations are more commonly seen in metabolic acid-base disturbances.
      —Levels generally are inversely related to pH and HCO_3
      (2) Chloride
      —is decreased in metabolic alkalosis
      —is elevated in non-anion gap acidosis
   c. CBC to look for leukocytosis (infection, sepsis)
   d. Toxicology screen to look for ingested poisons (see Chapter 18)
   e. Liver function tests (LFTs) to look for hepatic dysfunction
   f. Lactate level and serum ketones to look for cause of an elevated anion gap

4. **Treatment** for all disorders is correction of the underlying abnormality.

5. **Disposition**

   —is individualized based on the severity of the acid-base disturbance and underlying cause. General guidelines are:
   a. Patients with severe acidemia (pH <7.2) or hypoxemia ($PaO_2 < 60$ mm Hg) should be admitted to the ICU.
   b. Patients with toxic ingestions and suicidal intent should be transferred to the psychiatric unit once they are medically cleared.
   c. Patients whose ABD has been corrected in the ED and who are asymptomatic, alert, and oriented may be discharged with follow-up after observation for 4 to 6 hours.

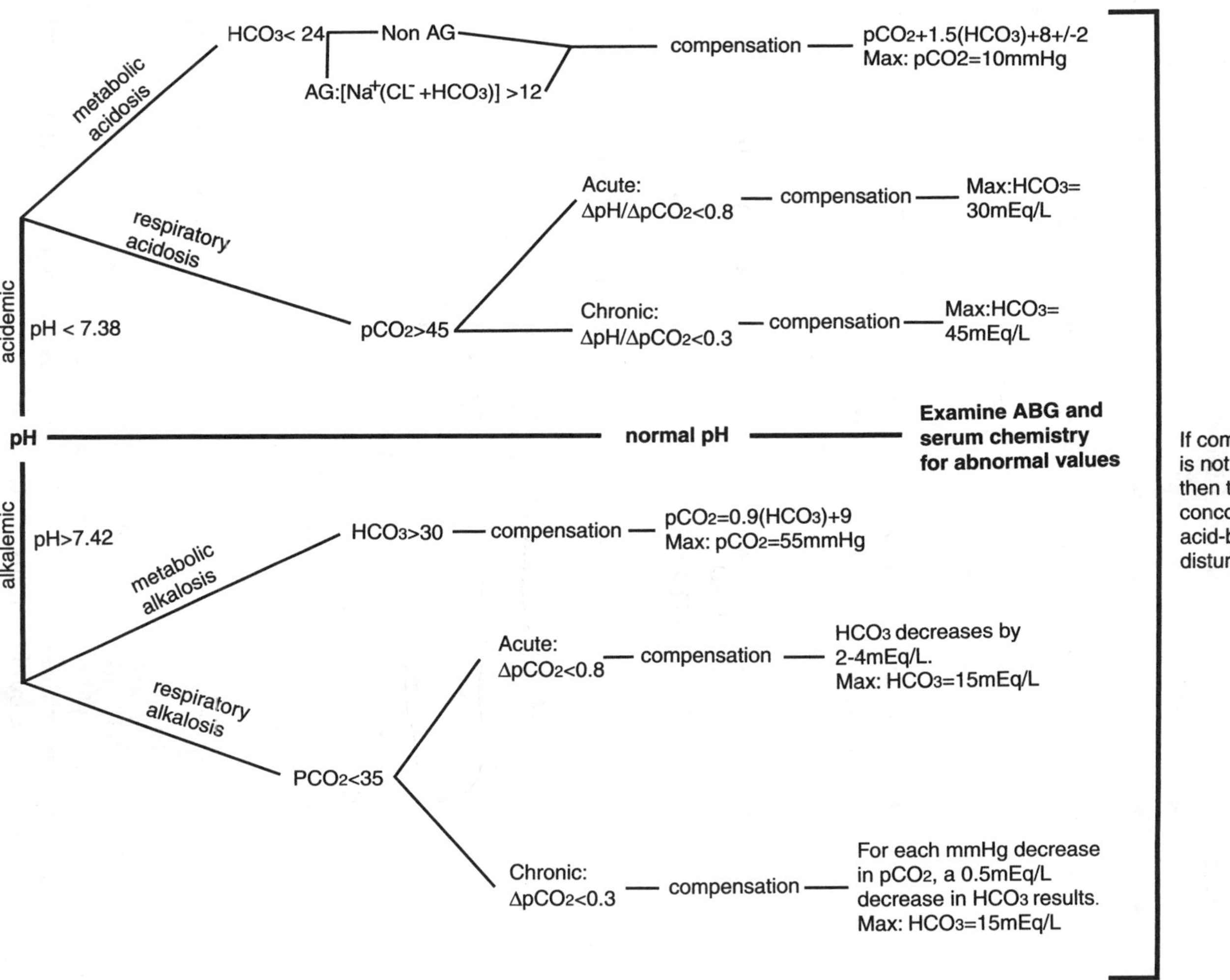

Figure 12-1. Systematic approach to acid-base disorders. *ABG* = arterial blood gases; *AG* = anion gap.

B. Respiratory acidosis

—Respiratory acidosis can be classified as acute or chronic. A helpful way to make the distinction is to calculate the difference in pH and pCO_2 from baseline:

—In acute RA, the expected decrease in pH = $[0.08 \text{ (measured } pCO_2 - 40)] \times 10$

—In chronic RA, the expected decrease in pH = $[0.03 \text{ (measured } pCO_2 - 40)] \times 10$

—Note that acute or chronic RA may also be present.

1. Causes

a. Pulmonary disease: COPD, severe pneumonia, and pulmonary edema

b. Airway obstruction: asthma, foreign body, laryngospasm

c. Mechanical: pneumothorax, flail chest, kyphoscoliosis, scleroderma, failure of mechanical ventilation

d. Neurologic: myasthenia gravis, muscular dystrophy, botulism, poliomyelitis, amyotrophic lateral sclerosis, Guillain-Barré syndrome, spinal cord injury, increased intracranial pressure, vertebral artery stroke

e. Drugs: opiates, salicylates, post-anesthesia

2. Treatment

a. Ventilation with supplemental oxygen

b. Correction of underlying disorder

c. Reversal of respiratory depression with naloxone if applicable

C. Respiratory alkalosis

—Chronic respiratory alkalosis is the only single defect in which compensatory correction to a normal pH can occur.

—If the pH is normal in the presence of an acid-base disorder, one is dealing with either a mixed acid-base defect (more common) or a chronic respiratory alkalosis

1. Causes

a. Drugs: salicylates (also cause simultaneous metabolic acidosis), thyroxine, epinephrine, xanthines, nicotine

b. Hyperventilation: anxiety, psychogenic, iatrogenic mechanical overventilation

c. Hypoxemia: pneumonia, pulmonary embolism, atelectasis, recent move to high altitude, late pregnancy

d. CNS: tumor, cerebrovascular accident (CVA), trauma

e. Hepatic encephalopathy

f. Gram-negative sepsis

2. Treatment

—Correction of underlying disorder

D. Metabolic acidosis

1. Classification

—Metabolic acidosis can be classified as elevated anion gap or nonanionic gap acidosis.

—Anion gap (AG) = $[Na^+ - (Cl^- + HCO_3)]$.

—An AG acidosis always represents a primary disturbance; it is never secondary to compensation

—For discussion of elevated anion gap acidosis, see Chapter 18 I G 2 a.

2. Calculating compensation

a. pCO_2 should equal $1.5[HCO_3] + 8$

—If pCO_2 is greater than expected, then a coexisting respiratory acidosis is present.

—If pCO_2 is less than expected, then a coexisting respiratory alkalosis is present

b. A simple way of determining appropriate compensation is to compare the last two digits to the right of the decimal point of the pH (must be > 7.0) with the pCO_2. They should be roughly equal.

3. Causes of nonanionic gap acidosis include:

—diarrhea

—fistula

—ileal loop

—renal tubular acidosis

—carbonic anhydrase inhibitor

—post-hypocapnia

4. Treatment

a. Correction of underlying cause

b. $NaHCO_3$ for pH < 7.2. Correct only one half of the deficit in the first 12 hours. HCO_3 replacement (in mEq) = [Base deficit × patient's weight in kg]/4

E. Metabolic alkalosis

1. Classification

—Metabolic alkalosis can be classified as chloride-responsive or chloride-resistant, based on the urinary chloride concentration:

—chloride-responsive: $U_{Cl} < 15$ mEq/dl

—chloride-resistant: $U_{Cl} > 15$ mEq/dl

2. Causes

a. Causes of **chloride-responsive** metabolic alkalosis include:

—stool losses secondary to laxative abuse or malabsorptive states

—vomiting

—diuretic abuse

—nasogastric suction

—massive blood transfusion

—exogenous alkali administration (e.g., antacids)

b. Causes of **chloride-resistant** metabolic alkalosis include:

—hyperaldosteronism
—hypokalemia
—hypomagnesemia
—Bartter's syndrome

3. **Treatment**

   a. Treatment for chloride-responsive metabolic acidosis includes:
   —IV hydration with 0.9% NaCl
   —correction of hypokalemia

   b. Treatment for chloride-resistant metabolic acidosis includes:
   —correction of the underlying abnormality
   —correction of hypokalemia
   —discontinuation of exogenous steroids, if applicable

Review Test

1. Which of the following is the most common cause of secondary adrenal insufficiency?

(A) Exogenous steroids
(B) Tuberculosis
(C) AIDS
(D) Pituitary infarct
(E) Idiopathic causes

2. Which of the following drugs is used to treat adrenal crisis?

(A) Propranolol
(B) Dexamethasone
(C) Methimazole
(D) Vasopressin
(E) Insulin

3. Which of the following features distinguishes diabetic ketoacidosis (DKA) from nonketotic hyperosmolar coma (NKHC)?

(A) Hyperglycemia
(B) Altered mental status
(C) Acidosis
(D) Acetone smell of breath
(E) Hyperkalemia

4. Which of the following drugs is the treatment of choice for delirium tremens?

(A) Phenytoin
(B) Ethanol
(C) Chlordiazepoxide
(D) Propranolol
(E) Normal saline

5. Which of the following causes of hypernatremia results from excess retention of water?

(A) Congestive heart failure (CHF)
(B) Syndrome of inappropriate secretion of antidiuretic hormone (SIADH)
(C) Psychogenic polydipsia
(D) Vomiting
(E) Burns

6. Which of the following features would be seen in the electrocardiogram (ECG) of a patient with hyperkalemia?

(A) Flattened T waves
(B) Loss of P waves
(C) Shortened QRS interval
(D) Prolonged QT interval
(E) U waves

7. A 33-year-old man is found unresponsive in the subway station. En route to the hospital, the paramedics administer naloxone, thiamine, and dextrose without response. The patient is agitated and unable to follow commands. His vital signs are: temperature (T) =102°F, blood pressure (BP) = 110/78, heart rate (HR) = 125, and respiratory rate (RR) = 40. His initial arterial blood gas (ABG) on 100% nonrebreather mask is: pH = 7.45, PCO_2 = 20, PO_2 = 197. His serum chemistry is: sodium (Na^+) = 131, potassium (K^+) = 3.4, chloride (Cl^-) = 91, bicarbonate (HCO_3)= 14, blood urea nitrogen (BUN) = 30, creatinine (Cr) = 1.5, and glucose (Glu) = 250. Which of the following best describes this patient's acid-base disturbance?

(A) Mixed metabolic acidosis and respiratory alkalosis
(B) Acute respiratory alkalosis with metabolic compensation
(C) Simple chronic respiratory alkalosis
(D) Mixed respiratory alkalosis with metabolic alkalosis
(E) Mixed respiratory alkalosis and respiratory acidosis

8. A 32-year-old woman who is 7 months pregnant presents to the emergency department (ED) complaining of nausea and vomiting and feeling very thirsty. Her vital signs are: temperature (T) = 98°F, blood pressure (BP) = 120/70, heart rate (HR) = 106, and respiratory rate (RR) = 30. Her initial arterial blood gas (ABG) on room air is: pH = 7.57, pCO_2 = 30, pO_2 = 95. Her serum chemistry is: Na^+ = 139, K^+ = 3.0, Cl^- = 100, HCO_3 = 32, BUN = 28, Cr = 0.8, Glu = 100. Which of the following best describes this patient's acid-base disturbance?

(A) Mixed metabolic acidosis and respiratory alkalosis
(B) Acute respiratory alkalosis with metabolic compensation
(C) Simple chronic respiratory alkalosis
(D) Mixed respiratory alkalosis with metabolic alkalosis
(E) Simple chronic metabolic alkalosis

9. A 41-year-old woman presents to the emergency department (ED) complaining of increased urination and thirst over the past 3 days with nausea and vomiting over the past day and a half. Patient also states she has fever and chills and is now feeling dizzy. Her vital signs are: temperature (T)= 101°F, blood pressure (BP) = 120/70, heart rate (HR) = 110, and respiratory rate (RR) = 24. Her initial arterial blood gas (ABG) on room air is: pH = 7.40, pCO_2 = 40, pO_2 = 80. Her serum chemistry is: sodium (Na^+) = 140, potassium (K^+) = 3.5, chloride (Cl^-) = 94, bicarbonate (HCO_3) = 25, blood urea nitrogen (BUN) = 24, creatinine (Cr) = 1.0, glucose (Glu) = 450. Which of the following best describes this patient's acid-base disturbance?

(A) Metabolic acidosis with respiratory compensation
(B) This patient does not have an acid-base disturbance
(C) Mixed metabolic acidosis and metabolic alkalosis
(D) Mixed respiratory acidosis with metabolic alkalosis
(E) Mixed metabolic acidosis and respiratory alkalosis

10. A 65-year-old woman with chronic obstructive pulmonary disease (COPD) and hypertension presents to the emergency department (ED) complaining of dizziness and shortness of breath. Her vital signs are: temperature (T) = 98°F, blood pressure (BP) = 140/90, heart rate (HR) = 80, and respiratory rate (RR) = 19. Her initial arterial blood gas (ABG) on 100% nonrebreather mask is: pH = 7.40, pCO_2 = 67, pO_2 = 247. Her serum chemistry is: sodium (Na^+) = 140, potassium (K^+) = 3.5, chloride (Cl^-) = 90, bicarbonate (HCO_3) = 40, blood urea nitrogen (BUN) = 24, creatinine (Cr) = 1.4, glucose (Glu) = 200. Which of the following best describes this patient's acid-base disturbance?

(A) Metabolic acidosis with respiratory compensation
(B) Mixed respiratory acidosis with metabolic alkalosis
(C) Mixed metabolic acidosis and metabolic alkalosis
(D) This patient does not have an acid-base disturbance
(E) Mixed respiratory alkalosis and metabolic acidosis

Directions: The response options for Items 11–16 are the same. Each item will state the number of options to choose. Choose exactly this number.

Questions 11–16

Choose the ECG findings associated with the specified electrolyte abnormalities.
(A) QRS widening
(B) Torsades de pointes
(C) U waves
(D) Flattened T waves
(E) QT prolongation
(F) Heart block

11. Hypermagnesemia (select 2 findings)

12. Hypomagnesemia (select 3 findings)

13. Hyperkalemia (select 2 findings)

14. Hypokalemia (select 3 findings)

15. Hypercalcemia (select 2 findings)

16. Hypocalcemia (select 1 finding)

Directions: The response options for Items 17–21 are the same. You will be required to select one answer for each item in the set.

Questions 17–21

Match the disorder with the correct pharmacologic treatment.
(A) Demeclocycline
(B) Etidronate
(C) Albuterol
(D) Vasopressin
(E) Calcium chloride

17. Syndrome of inappropriate secretion of antidiuretic hormone (SIADH)

18. Hyperkalemia

19. Diabetes insipidus

20. Hypercalcemia

21. Hypocalcemia

Answers and Explanations

1-A. The most common cause of primary adrenal insufficiency is idiopathic. The most common cause of secondary adrenal insufficiency is exogenous steroids. Overall, secondary adrenal insufficiency is more common than primary adrenal insufficiency, so, overall, exogenous steroids are the most common cause. Tuberculosis (choice B) formerly was the most common cause of primary adrenal insufficiency.

2-B. Adrenal crisis is treated by replacing corticosteroids and providing aggressive fluid resuscitation. Dexamethasone or hydrocortisone may be used. Propranolol and methimazole are used to treat thyroid storm. Vasopressin is used to treat diabetes insipidus. Insulin is used to treat diabetes mellitus.

3-D. The smell of acetone on the patient's breath is characteristic of diabetic ketoacidosis (DKA). Hyperglycemia, altered mental status, and acidosis are common to both DKA and non-ketotic hyperosmolar coma (NKHC). Serum potassium may be low, normal, or elevated in both DKA and NKHC.

4-C. Patients with tremors secondary to alcohol withdrawal are best managed with benzodiazepines. Phenytoin is not indicated because these are not true seizures, although they may progress to that point. Ethanol, although it would ablate the tremors, obviously is not the ED treatment of choice. Propranolol is a beta-blocker that may decrease heart rate and anxiety but would not control the tremors. Normal saline is an intravenous solution used to correct dehydration.

5-A. Hypervolemic hyponatremia results from excess retention of water in comparison to retention of sodium. Congestive heart failure, hepatic cirrhosis, and renal failure are examples of disease states in which this type of hyponatremia is observed. The syndrome of inappropriate secretion of antidiuretic hormone (SIADH) and psychogenic polydipsia result in euvolemic hyponatremia. In SIADH, there is a malfunction of the endocrine loop (often secondary to head trauma) such that excess antidiuretic hormone (ADH) is made, resulting in a very concentrated urine and excess retention of water. In psychogenic polydipsia, the patient drinks so much free water as to actually cause dilution of serum sodium. The urine, however, is maximally dilute, which can be used to differentiate this condition from SIADH. Vomiting and burns cause an excessive loss of sodium, resulting in hypovolemic hyponatremia.

6-B. A patient with hyperkalemia would demonstrate the following changes in progression: peaked T → loss of P waves → widening of QRS complex → sine wave appearance to QRS complexes → ventricular fibrillation → asystole. Note that a patient may have mild hyperkalemia without any electrocardiogram (ECG) changes. U waves (choice E) are seen in hypokalemia.

7-A. Approaching the problem systematically (see Figure 12-1), it is evident that the patient has an alkalemia (pH > 7.42). The PCO_2 is < 35 mm Hg, so this is a respiratory alkalosis. To determine whether it is chronic or acute, use the ΔpCO_2 value, which is $20/40 = 0.5$, suggestive of a chronic respiratory alkalosis, although the patient's (limited) history goes against this. Next, check whether the degree of compensation is appropriate. The maximum compensation for a chronic respiratory alkalosis is a HCO_3 of 15 mEq. Therefore, choices B (acute respiratory alkalosis with metabolic compensation) and C (simple chronic respiratory alkalosis) are incorrect. This patient's HCO_3 is below that level, which indicates that there is an additional acid-base disturbance. The additional disturbance can be either a metabolic acidosis or alkalosis. (It is not possible to have coexisting respiratory alkalosis and acidosis at the same time.) The bicarbonate level, which is quite low, indicates that this is a coexisting metabolic acidosis; therefore choice D, mixed respiratory alkalosis with metabolic alkalosis, is wrong. Calculation of the anion gap (AG) $[131-(91+14)] = 26$ indicates that this is an AG metabolic acidosis. Again, the compensation of this AG acidosis can be checked using the formula $[PCO_2 = 1.5(HCO_3) + 8 +/- 2] \rightarrow PCO_2 = 29 +/-2$. The PCO_2 does not equal $29 +/- 2$, so the AG acidosis is over-compensated.

One classic example of a mixed metabolic acidosis and respiratory alkalosis is salicylate poisoning. This is a likely scenario for this patient, who is comatose and has an elevated temperature. Other causes of a mixed metabolic acidosis and respiratory alkalosis are septic shock, central nervous system (CNS) disease, and fulminant liver or kidney failure.

8-D. Approaching the problem systematically (see Fig. 12-1), it is evident that the patient has an alkalemia (pH > 7.42). The pCO_2 is < 35 mm Hg, so this is a respiratory alkalosis. To determine whether it is a chronic or acute alkalosis, the pCO_2 value is used. It is 30/40, or 0.75, suggestive of a chronic respiratory alkalosis, although the acute form also is quite likely. The next step is to check whether the compensation is appropriate. In fact, it is not, because the HCO_3 is elevated rather than decreased. Therefore, the patient does not have acute respiratory alkalosis with metabolic compensation (choice B) or simple chronic respiratory alkalosis (choice C), and a coexisting metabolic alkalosis is present, so the patient does not have mixed metabolic acidosis and respiratory alkalosis (choice A). To double check, one can see if the metabolic alkalosis is appropriately compensated. Again, the pCO_2 is low instead of high, so the direction of the compensation itself is inappropriate.

This patient's respiratory alkalosis probably is due to her underlying increased ventilation, which is common in pregnancy. Her metabolic alkalosis probably is due to the vomiting. Other scenarios in which a mixed respiratory and metabolic alkalosis may be seen include patients on ventilators, nasogastric suction, diuretics, massive blood transfusions, and hepatic failure. The profound alkalemia that may result from these double alkaloses demands immediate attention. Severe alkalemia may impact perfusion hemodynamics and cardiac arrhythmias.

9-C. With a pH of 7.40, one cannot immediately tell if an acidemia or alkalemia is present. In this case, the next step is to inspect the serum chemistry. A few things are readily apparent. There is an elevated anion gap, the glucose is high, and the chloride is low. When the compensation for metabolic acidosis is checked, $pCO_2 = 1.5\ [HCO3] + 8 \pm 2 \rightarrow 44 \pm 2$. The pCO_2 does not equal 44 ± 2, so the acidosis is undercompensated by the respiratory effort. This means a second primary disturbance, which is making the patient more alkalotic, is present. The two choices are respiratory or metabolic alkalosis. The alkalosis obviously is not respiratory, because the pCO_2 is normal, so that leaves metabolic alkalosis as the coexisting disturbance. Generally, the presence of an AG acidosis with a normal bicarbonate usually means there is a coexisting metabolic alkalosis.

The differential diagnosis of an elevated anion gap can be recalled with the mnemonic "CART-MUDPILES" (see Chapter 18 I G).

Given this patient's elevated glucose, the likely cause of the AG acidosis is diabetic ketoacidosis (DKA). Treatment consists of aggressive fluid replacement. See section I for further discussion of DKA.

10-B. With a pH of 7.40, one cannot immediately tell if an acidemia or alkalemia is present. Looking at the arterial blood gases (ABG), one notes a very elevated pCO_2 despite 100% oxygen, which indicates that there is a primary respiratory acidosis. Because there is no change in pH from normal, one cannot use the formula to determine whether the acidosis is acute or chronic, although from the history of chronic obstructive pulmonary disease (COPD) this is most likely chronic or acute on chronic. The bicarbonate level, 40 mm Hg, confirms this, because the compensation is too high for pure acute respiratory acidosis. Therefore, the coexisting disturbance is a metabolic alkalosis.

This mixed picture commonly is seen in patients with chronic lung disease and CO_2 retention, with vomiting, or with treatment with diuretics and a low-salt diet. Although it is not necessary to correct the pH, it is important to treat the metabolic alkalosis with volume, chloride, and potassium, because the elevated HCO_3 may depress the respiratory rate even further.

Metabolic alkalosis often is accompanied by potassium depletion, which can, in turn, produce muscle weakness. When respiratory muscles are affected, hypoventilation superimposes a respiratory acidosis on the metabolic alkalosis. Potassium repletion can reverse this type of mechanical respiratory acidosis.

11-A, E. Hypermagnesemia is reflected by QRS widening and QT prolongation.

12-B, C, D. Hypomagnesemia produces torsades de pointes, U waves, and flattened T waves on electrocardiogram (ECG).

13-A, F. Hyperkalemia produces peaked T waves, QRS widening, and heart block on electrocardiogram (ECG).

14-C, D, F. Hypokalemia is reflected on electrocardiogram (ECG) by U waves, flattened T waves, and heart block.

15-A, F. Electrocardiographic (ECG) findings that point to hypercalcemia are QRS widening and heart block.

16-E. Hypocalcemia is indicated by a finding of QT prolongation on electrocardiography.

17-A. The syndrome of inappropriate secretion of antidiuretic hormone (SIADH) is treated with demeclocycline.

18-C. Hyperkalemia can be treated with albuterol, a β-agonist.

19-D. Vasopressin is used in the treatment of diabetes insipidus.

20-B. Hypercalcemia is treated with etidronate.

21-E. Calcium chloride is used in the treatment of hypocalcemia.

13

Psychiatric Emergencies

I. Overview

A. The American Psychiatric Association defines a psychiatric emergency as a situation that includes an acute disturbance of thought, behavior, mood, or social relationship which requires immediate intervention as defined by the client or family or social unit.

B. From 2%–10% of all patients presenting to the emergency department (ED) have an acute psychiatric disturbance in addition to their ostensible presenting complaint.

C. Most presentations occur at night. Up to 65% of patients presenting to the ED after midnight and before 8:00 A.M. have current or past psychiatric illness.

D. The following presentations of life-threatening psychiatric conditions must be prioritized for identification and management:

—Agitated, menacing, self-destructive, and out-of-control behavior

—Serious and chronic self-neglect

—Serious medical problems either coexisting with or causing psychiatric symptoms

—Organic causes of acute presentations must be ruled out. See Chapter 6 I for causes and management of altered mental status.

E. Criteria for involuntary commitment

1. Danger to self
2. Danger to others
3. Danger to health

F. Elements of emergency psychiatric care

1. Establishment of rapport
   —Response to client and family needs
   —Expression of empathy
2. Determination of physiologic status

—Medical history and vital signs are obtained.

—Necessary parts of physical examination are performed.

—Results of diagnostic tests are obtained and reviewed.

3. Physical and chemical restraints are used if necessary to provide safety to patient and others.
4. Psychiatric status is obtained:

—Precipitating events are identified.

—Past personal, family, and psychiatric histories are obtained.

—Mental status examination is performed.

—Data are collected from patient's family and current therapist.

—Provisional diagnosis is formulated.

5. Proper disposition must be determined.

—Inpatient or outpatient treatment, as appropriate, is arranged.

II. Approach to the Violent Patient

A. Factors predisposing to violence in the ED include:

—high-stress illnesses

—long waiting times

—uncomfortable waiting environment (uncomfortable seats, no distraction, poor staff-to-family communication)

—high-tension environment of ED

—perceived ready availability of drugs and hostages

—nonselective 24-hour open door policy with poor or absent security

—increased use of drugs and alcohol in population of ED frequenters

B. Causes of violence in patients include:

—acute organic brain syndrome (meningitis, encephalitis, brain abscess, or tumor)

—intoxication

—male gender

—drug or alcohol withdrawal

—acute psychosis or schizophrenia

—paranoid personality

—borderline personality

—antisocial personality

—depression with homicidal ideation

—temporal lobe epilepsy

C. Clinical features

1. **Historical clues to identifying the potentially violent patient (the 7 A's):**

—Absent roots: patient's childhood is marked by divorce, parental deaths, frequent moves, job changes, child abuse.

—Authority problems: patient has trouble taking orders from parents, teachers, and supervisors; gives nurses a hard time while they get vital signs.

—Arrest record

—Assaults: patient has multiple scars from chest tubes and exploratory laparotomies secondary to stab wounds. Patient states he is a fighter, is confrontational.

—Another's death: patient has been involved in another's death, either "accidental" or intentional.

—Alcohol or amphetamine abuse: patients are less inhibited.

—Access: patient has ability to obtain weapons.

2. **Symptoms** and **physical examination findings** may include:

—tense posture

—clenched fists

—loud, threatening, insistent speech

—psychomotor agitation

—jumpiness

D. Diagnostic tests

—Patient should be evaluated for the presenting complaint as well as for organic causes for the violent behavior. See Chapter 6 I for work-up of altered mental status.

1. Complete blood count (CBC) to look for infection
2. Chemistry panel to look for electrolyte abnormalities
3. Toxicology screen to look for substance abuse
4. Thyroid function tests (TFTs) to look for hyperthyroidism
5. Head computed tomographic (CT) scan to look for intracranial pathology
6. Lumbar puncture to look for brain infection and, when head CT is negative, for bleed

E. Treatment

1. Stance: Face the patient and **stand on patient's non-dominant side.** People will strike with the dominant hand and kick with the dominant leg. The following guidelines help to determine which is the non-dominant side:

—9 out of 10 people are right-handed

—People usually wear their watches on their non-dominant or "weak" side.

—The belt buckle usually points to the patient's "weak" side.

2. Distance: ED personnel should **stand 1½ leg-lengths from the patient,** out of kicking range.
3. Arms should hang at the side. Folded arms handicap a defensive attempt, and usually convey a hostile, domineering, authoritative stance.
4. **Limits must be established.** The team is brought to the patient (force in numbers) and he or she is told that it is necessary to regain control.
5. **Eye contact must be avoided.** Direct eye contact may put the patient on the defensive. The best place to gaze is at the upper chest, at the level of the first button of the collar or 9 inches below the chin.
6. **The exit must not be blocked,** and the patient must not be positioned between two walls (in a corner).
7. **Staff should try to distract the patient.** They may offer something to eat or drink.
8. The patient should be given a chance to save face. Options should be offered, if possible, e.g., "Would you prefer the medication orally or by injection?"
9. The patient should be offered **chemical restraint** (medical intervention): haloperidol 10 mg + lorazepam 4 mg intramuscularly (IM) or intravenously (IV).
10. If none of these strategies work, **mechanical restraint** is necessary. The team should establish a strategy, with one person assigned to each limb, one to the head, and a 6th person to put the restraints on.

F. Disposition

1. Patients are admitted to the psychiatric floor if psychotic features (e.g., hallucinations, delusions) are present.
2. If no psychotic features or suicidal or homicidal ideation are present and the patient calms down following treatment, he or she may be discharged home with outpatient psychiatric follow-up.
3. If the work-up yields any medical cause for delirium, the patient is admitted to the appropriate service for further management.
4. It is important to document that the patient has been properly handled.

III. Panic Attacks

A. Overview

—Panic attacks are a form of anxiety limited to **discrete episodes** that are associated with an impending sense of doom.

—Panic attacks may occur unexpectedly, or may be associated with specific situations.

B. Clinical presentation.

—**Symptoms** and **physical examination findings** may include:

1. **Motor tension**

—Trembling, twitching, or feeling shaky

—Muscle tension, aches, or soreness

—Restlessness

—Easy fatigability

2. **Autonomic hyperactivity**

—Shortness of breath

—Palpitations

—Sweating, or cold clammy hands

—Dry mouth

—Dizziness or lightheadedness

—Nausea, diarrhea, or other abdominal distress

—Flushes (hot flashes) or chills

—Frequent urination

—Trouble swallowing or "lump in throat"

3. **Vigilance and scanning**

—Feeling keyed up or on edge

—Exaggerated startle response

—Difficulty concentrating or "mind going blank" because of anxiety

—Trouble falling or staying asleep

—Irritability

C. Diagnostic tests

—No special diagnostic tests are necessary.

—Laboratory tests that may be appropriate to exclude an organic cause of anxiety include:

1. **TFTs** to look for hyperthyroidism
2. **Toxicology screen** to look for amphetamines and sympathomimetics
3. **Electrocardiogram (ECG)** to look for atrial fibrillation

D. Treatment

1. Reassurance
2. Encouragement to maintain control
3. **Breathing exercises** to control psychogenic hyperventilation
4. **Benzodiazepines:** the drug of choice in treating patients with anxiety. See Table 13-1 for specific drugs and dosages.

E. Disposition

1. Most patients with panic attacks can be successfully evaluated and treated in the ED.
2. Patients for whom an underlying medical disorder cannot be ruled out must be referred for further evaluation and therapy. If the suspected medical disorder is potentially life-threatening (e.g., unstable angina), the patient should be admitted to the hospital until it can be sorted out.
3. Patients with panic disorder and suicidal or homicidal ideation or with

Table 13-1. Benzodiazepines

Drug	Dosage	Half-life (hr)
Alprazolam	PO: 0.75–4 mg/24 h q 8 h	11–15
Chlordiazepoxide	PO: 15–100 mg/24 h in divided doses IM: not recommended	6–30
Clorazepate	PO: 7.5–60 mg/24 h in 1–4 divided doses	30–100
Diazepam	PO: 6–40 mg/24 h in 1–4 divided doses IV: 2.5–20 mg slowly IM: not recommended	20–50
Flurazepam	PO: 15–30 mg qhs	50–100
Halazepam	PO: 20–40 mg q 6–8 h	
Lorazepam	PO: 1–10 mg/24 h in 2–3 divided doses IV/IM: 0.05 mg/kg to 4 mg maximum	10–20
Midazolam	IV: 0.035–0.1 mg/kg prn IM 0.08 mg/kg	1–12
Oxazepam	PO: 30–120 mg/24 h in 3–4 divided doses	5–10
Prazepam	PO: 20–60 mg/24 h in divided doses or qhs	36–70
Temazepam	PO: 15–30 mg qhs	10

IM = intramuscularly; *IV* = intravenously; *PO* = orally; *prn* = as needed; *q* = every; *qhs* = at bedtime

major depression require urgent psychiatric consultation in the ED and admission to the psychiatry service.

4. If the phobic stimulus is known, patients are instructed to avoid it.

IV. Affective Disorders

A. Depression

—Depression may be connected with a history of a major life change such as the death of a spouse, retirement, or medical illness.

—In younger people, depression may be seen in the context of a history of substance abuse, relationship problems, or job loss.

1. Clinical presentation

a. Symptoms may include:

—loss of pleasure in daily activities (**anhedonia**)
—early morning awakening
—insomnia
—depressed mood (50% of patients with depression report this)
—sense of worthlessness
—many somatic complaints and chronic pain, especially in the elderly
—fatigue

b. Physical examination findings may include:

—stooped posture

—slow speech

—depressed facies

—dry mouth

—constipation

—impaired memory and concentration on mini-mental status exam

2. Diagnostic tests

—No specific diagnostic tests are necessary for depression. However, medical causes for symptoms must be excluded before this diagnosis is made, because they can exist concurrently.

a. **CBC** to look for infection

b. **Peripheral smear** to look for neoplasia

c. **Chemistry panel** to look for electrolyte abnormalities

d. **Serum toxicology screen** to look for substance abuse

e. **Serum medication levels** to look for toxicity (may not be intentional)

f. **Head CT** scan to look for recent CVA

g. **TFTs** to look for hypothyroidism

h. Serology for Epstein-Barr virus

3. Treatment

a. Antidepressants: Patient may be put on a selective serotonin reuptake inhibitor (SSRI) such as fluoxetine 20–60 mg/day. (SSRIs have the least potential for serious toxic effects from abuse.)

b. Therapy (outpatient)

4. Disposition

a. Most patients can be discharged home with outpatient psychiatric follow-up.

b. Patients who have active suicidal or homicidal ideation should be admitted to the psychiatry service.

B. Mania

—is a mood disorder that affects men and women equally.

—begins in the early 20s.

—has a familial predisposition: patients usually have a family history of affective disorders.

—confers an increased risk for substance abuse.

—often exists as part of bipolar disorder, an illness characterized by alternating periods of mania and depression.

1. Clinical presentation

a. **Symptoms** may include:

—euphoria

—elevated mood

—sense of increased or endless energy
—labile mood
—easy frustration
—demanding, egocentric behavior (grandiosity)
—insomnia
—poor judgment
—paranoia, delusions, and hallucinations

b. **Physical examination findings** may include:
—flight of ideas
—pressured speech
—psychomotor agitation

2. **Diagnostic tests**
   a. No specific diagnostic tests are necessary for mania.
   b. The differential diagnosis includes substance abuse and schizophrenia.
   c. The following laboratory studies may be helpful:
   —**Serum toxicology screen** to look for substance abuse
   —TFTs to look for hyperthyroidism
   —Serum ceruloplasmin if Wilson's disease is suspected
   —Serum lithium level if the patient is on that drug

3. **Treatment**
   a. Antipsychotics: haloperidol, 10–40 mg over the first 24 hours
   b. Benzodiazepines as needed (see Table 13-1)
   c. Consultation with psychiatry department
   d. Electroconvulsive therapy (ECT) in consultation with the psychiatry department, if none of the above control acute episode
   e. Lithium: begun at 300 mg orally every 6 to 8 hours (maximum dose is 2.4 g/day) to maintain remission (maintenance dose is 900–1800 mg/day; steady state is reached in 5 days); or carbamazepine, begun at 200 mg orally twice a day.

4. **Disposition**
   a. Patients who are acutely manic should be hospitalized, because they may be at risk of hurting themselves or getting into trouble with the law as a result of poor judgment.
   b. Patients who are hypomanic may be discharged home with outpatient psychiatric follow-up.

V. Psychosis

A. Overview

—The psychotic patient has a grossly impaired sense of reality.

—The most common psychosis is **schizophrenia.**

—Any underlying medical condition (organic cause) must always be ruled out.

B. Clinical presentation

—**Symptoms** and **physical examination findings** may include:

—no clouding of consciousness

—blunt, inappropriate, or labile affect

—thought disturbances in patient with clear sensorium

—short attention span

—speech that contains neologisms, echolalia, clanging

—presence of delusions

—presence of hallucinations

—unkempt appearance

C. Diagnostic tests

—No specific diagnostic tests are necessary for schizophrenia.

—As always, medical causes of symptoms must be excluded.

D. Treatment

1. Control of any violent behavior (see section II).

2. Sedation and chemical restraint:

—Haloperidol 2–10 mg orally or IM every 1–8 hours

—Droperidol 2.5–10 mg orally or IM every 3–4 hours

—Benzodiazepines as needed (see Table 13-1)

3. Minimal-stimulus environment

E. Disposition

—Acutely psychotic patients should be admitted to the psychiatry service.

VI. Conversion Disorder

A. Overview

—In conversion disorder, the patient has loss of function of a part of the nervous system, but no underlying organic cause can be identified.

—Primary gain may be involved: disability may be symbolic for other (nonphysical) pain that the patient has suffered and is trying to repress.

—Secondary gain may be involved (e.g., need to play sick role, wish to obtain worker's compensation).

—The relationship to the cause of the disorder may be obvious to the examiner, but the patient lacks insight, does not understand, and does not voluntarily produce symptoms.

—Conversion disorder often occurs abruptly, following a stressor.

B. Clinical presentation

1. Symptoms may include:

—paralysis

—seizures

—urinary retention

—blindness

—deafness

—unconsciousness

—paresthesias

2. **Physical examination** often is normal, although patients may develop contractures from presumed paralysis.

C. Diagnostic tests

—No special diagnostic tests are necessary, but diagnosis can only be made after organic causes for the patient's symptoms have been ruled out.

D. Treatment

—consists of reassurance.

E. Disposition

—Patients can be discharged home with outpatient follow-up.

VII. Eating Disorders

A. Anorexia nervosa

—Anorexia nervosa begins in adolescence and is seen 10 times more frequently in women.

—It involves a distorted body image (i.e., feeling fat when this clearly is not true).

—Patients often have poor family dynamics and a history of poor self-image, vigorous exercise, and laxative and diuretic abuse.

1. **Clinical presentation**

   a. **Symptoms** and **physical examination findings** may include:

   —weight loss (patients are underweight)

   —no appetite loss

   —amenorrhea

   —edema

   —bradycardia

   —hypothermia

   —chronic pain

   —fatigue

2. **Diagnostic tests**

   —No special diagnostic tests are necessary unless the diagnosis is unclear.

   —The differential diagnosis includes depression and schizophrenia.

   —Helpful laboratory tests may include:

a. CBC to look for anemia
b. Chemistry panel to look for metabolic acidosis
c. Urinalysis to look for ketones
d. ECG to look for rhythm and rate disturbances

3. Treatment

a. Individual therapy
b. Family therapy
c. For severe cases: IV fluids and hyperalimentation

4. Disposition

a. Patients who are not in immediate danger of starvation may be discharged home with outpatient follow-up.
b. Patients with severe anorexia nervosa should be hospitalized for IV hyperalimentation.

B. Bulimia nervosa

1. Overview

—Bulimia nervosa is a condition related to anorexia nervosa that involves binge eating followed by purging via vomiting, alternating with periods of self-starvation.

—It is 10 to 20 times more common in women overall, but more common in men than anorexia alone.

2. Clinical presentation

—**Symptoms** and **physical examination findings** may include:

—history of going to the bathroom immediately after meals (to vomit)

—**erosion of tooth enamel** (secondary to the acid produced with vomiting)

—**normal weight**

3. Diagnostic tests

—No special diagnostic tests are necessary unless the diagnosis is unclear.

—The differential diagnosis includes depression, schizophrenia, and borderline personality disorder.

4. Treatment

a. Antidepressants: may start an SSRI, such as fluoxetine 20–60 mg/day
b. Cognitive therapy

5. Disposition

—Most patients can be discharged home with outpatient follow-up.

VIII. Domestic Violence

—Domestic violence is defined by the American College of Emergency Physicians (ACEP) as "part of a pattern of coercive behaviors that an individual uses to establish and maintain power and control over another with whom he/she has had an intimate, romantic, or spousal relationship" (ACEP Policy Statement on Domestic Violence [No. 4163], Feb. 1999).

A. Clinical features

—**Symptoms** and **physical examination findings** of domestic violence are similar to those found in child maltreatment (see Chapter 20 IX) and, as in the case of suspected child maltreatment, are required to be reported by the physician. These may include:

—multiple injuries in different stages of healing

—injuries that are inconsistent with the reported mechanism of action

—maxillofacial trauma, especially periorbital ecchymosis

—bruises and fractures of the forearms

—chronic pain: pain in the pelvis, abdomen, and chest, and headaches

—symptoms of depression or mania

—term pregnancy without prenatal care, due to blocked access

—exacerbation of chronic illnesses due to blocked access to medications

B. Diagnostic tests

—No specific diagnostic tests are necessary. Underlying illnesses should be looked for, and injuries should be documented. Radiographs may be helpful in this regard.

C. Treatment

1. A safe environment is provided for the patient.
2. Psychiatry consult is arranged.
3. Social work consult is arranged.

D. Disposition

1. Patients whose acute injuries have been treated and who have a safe place to go (e.g., shelter, friend's home) may be discharged with outpatient follow-up.
2. Patients who do not have a safe place to go should be hospitalized until social services can be arranged.

IX. Elder Abuse

—As with child abuse and domestic violence, suspicion of elder abuse is required to be reported by the physician.

A. **Symptoms** and **physical examination findings** may include:

—physical neglect

—unkempt appearance

—malnourishment

—lack of adequate clothing (especially in winter)

—untreated medical conditions

—depressed facies

—sense of shame or guilt

B. Diagnostic tests

—No specific tests are necessary to diagnose elder abuse. However, all patients should receive baseline testing to exclude any underlying untreated medical conditions.

C. Treatment

1. Treatment of any infections, injuries, or electrolyte abnormalities
2. IV hydration
3. Psychiatry consult
4. Social work consult

D. Disposition

1. Patients whose acute injuries have been treated and who have a safe place to go (e.g., shelter, friend's home) may be discharged with outpatient follow-up.
2. Patients who do not have a safe place to go should be hospitalized until social services can be arranged.

X. Suicide

A. Clinical features

1. **Symptoms** may include:

   —frequent ED visits secondary to noncompliance with essential medications

   —self-inflicted wounds

   —overdose of medications or drugs of abuse

   —heavy alcohol drinking in a patient with alcoholic liver disease

   —motor vehicle accidents with single vehicle and single victim (patient)

   —symptoms of depression (see section IV)

2. **Physical examination findings** may include:

   —scars

   —wounds

   —occult weapons

B. Risk factors

—Caucasian race

—Male gender

—Age > 65 years

—Age group 15–24 years, especially in males

—History of psychiatric disorder

—Ongoing substance abuse

—History of prior suicide attempts

—Terminal or chronic illness

—History of personal abuse (inflicted by self or others)

—Family history of suicide

—Recent discharge from psychiatric hospital

—2- to 3-week "remission" period after starting antidepressant therapy

—Single, divorced, or separated status

—Living alone

—Recent loss of job or death of family member

—Access to firearms

—Feelings of worthlessness and excessive guilt

C. Diagnostic tests

—No specific diagnostic tests are necessary. Acute poisoning and trauma should be evaluated. Underlying medical diseases should be sought.

D. Treatment

1. Benzodiazepines to manage anxiety, as needed (see Table 13-1)
2. Reassurance

E. Disposition

—Patients who are actively suicidal or homicidal should be hospitalized for further management. See section I for criteria for involuntary confinement.

Review Test

1. A 23-year-old woman presents to the ED after slashing her wrists with a razor blade following an argument with her boyfriend. She has a past medical history for asthma, but takes no medications. She has presented to the ED previously for similar self-abuse and states she often has "relationship problems." What is the single most important question to ask this patient?

(A) Do you want to hurt or kill yourself or any other person?
(B) Do you use drugs or alcohol?
(C) Is there any possibility you might be pregnant?
(D) Is your boyfriend physically or sexually abusing you?
(E) Were you abused physically or sexually as a child?

Questions 2 and 3

A 41-year-old Wall Street executive is brought to the ED by his worried family. A few days ago, he came home proclaiming he had discovered the secret to happiness. The family states he has had boundless energy since then, finishing all the chores on his "life's to-do list" in a single evening. They became extremely worried when he quit his job yesterday and liquidated his hard-earned savings to buy a very expensive yacht.

2. Which of the following medications is likely to be most helpful to this patient?

(A) Phenytoin
(B) Droperidol
(C) Lorazepam
(D) Lithium
(E) Amitryptylline

3. Which of the following is the second medication to use if the first drug is not effective in controlling this patient's symptoms?

(A) Lithium
(B) Droperidol
(C) Carbamazepine
(D) Lorazepam
(E) Iimipramine

4. Which of the following is the drug of choice in the treatment of panic disorder?

(A) Nortryptaline
(B) Haloperidol
(C) Lithium
(D) Alprazolam
(E) Fluoxetine

5. Which of the following is a risk factor for successful suicide?

(A) Substance abuse
(B) Being married
(C) Having a demanding job
(D) Female gender
(E) Lack of underlying medical illness

Directions: The response options for Items 6–9 are the same. Each item will state the number of options to choose. Choose exactly this number.

Questions 6–9

Match the symptoms that often are present with the illness.

(A) Anorexia
(B) Distorted body image
(C) Anhedonia
(D) Insomnia
(E) Poor concentration
(F) Endocrine abnormalities
(G) Fatigue
(H) Vomiting
(I) Diarrhea

6. Depression (select 5 symptoms)

7. Anorexia nervosa (select 5 symptoms)

8. Bulimia (select 4 symptoms)

9. Anxiety (select 4 symptoms)

Answers and Explanations

1-A. Although all the questions suggested probably will be helpful in evaluating this patient, the most urgent question to ask is about suicidal or homicidal ideation, which is a psychiatric emergency. Patients who are suicidal or homicidal should be on a 1:1 hold (observed at all times), searched for weapons, restrained (for their own protection and the protection of others) if necessary, and admitted to the psychiatry service after medical clearance. Information regarding drug or alcohol use, possible pregnancy, and physical or sexual abuse, either current or in the past, can be obtained later.

2-D and **3-C.** Lithium is the first-line drug for the treatment of mania. If lithium does not work, carbamazepine may be effective. Other anticonvulsants such as phenytoin are not effective. Lorazepam and droperidol will not help the mania, although they may produce a slight sedating effect. Amitryptylline and imipramine are tricyclic antidepressants that are used to treat many disorders, but not mania.

4-D. The drug of choice for simple panic disorder (without concurrent depression) is a benzodiazepine. Alprazolam is the only benzodiazepine listed in the answer choices. (Other benzodiazepines are listed in Table 13-1.) Nortryptylline is a tricyclic antidepressant. Haloperidol is an antipsychotic. Lithium is used to treat mania. Fluoxetine is a selective serotonin reuptake inhibitor (SSRI) used to treat depression.

5-A. Substance abuse is a risk factor for suicide for more than one reason. First, substance abuse may have begun with a poor self-image and a need to fit in. Second, procurement of many drugs may put the abuser in dangerous places and situations. Finally, the addiction can create isolation, depression, and anxiety in the abuser. Single people and those who live alone are more prone to suicide than married people or those with a close circle of friends and family. Females are three times more likely to attempt suicide, but are only one third as likely to succeed at their attempts. The presence rather than the lack of a medical illness is more often associated with suicide. Finally, although having a demanding job may be stressful, unemployment is more often associated with suicide.

6-A, C, D, E, G. Depression may be marked by anorexia, anhedonia, insomnia, poor concentration, and fatigue.

7-A, B, E, F, G. Anorexia nervosa is marked by anorexia, distorted body image, poor concentration, endocrine abnormalities, and fatigue.

8-A, B, F, H. Bulimia nervosa is characterized by anorexia (patients go back and forth between binge eating and starving), distorted body image, endocrine abnormalities, and vomiting.

9-D, E, G, I. Anxiety is marked by insomnia, poor concentration, fatigue, and diarrhea.

14

Infectious Disease Emergencies

I. Septic Shock

A. Overview

—Septic shock is infection with a systemic response.

—It is mediated by a variety of cytokines.

—It is caused most commonly by gram-negative bacteremia.

—It is characterized by endothelial injury, marked decrease in vascular resistance, an initial "high-output state," and, ultimately, multi-organ system failure.

B. Clinical features may include:

—hyperventilation and apprehension (often the earliest clinical signs)

—fever and chills

—hypothermia

—altered mental status (ranging from agitation to coma)

—skin lesions: **ecthyma gangrenosum** ("bull's-eye" lesion of peripheral erythema and central necrosis, associated with *Pseudomonas* infection), vesicles and bullae, diffuse erythroderma

—hypotension

—warm extremities

—oliguria/anuria

—jaundice

—hemorrhagic manifestations: petechiae, epistaxis, disseminated intravascular coagulation (DIC)

—adult respiratory distress syndrome (ARDS)

—congestive heart failure (CHF)

C. **Diagnostic tests**

1. **Complete blood cell count (CBC)** to look for leukopenia or leukocytosis and thrombocytopenia or thrombocytosis
2. **Chemistry panel** to look for respiratory alkalosis (secondary to hyperventilation) and metabolic acidosis (secondary to anaerobic metabolism)
3. **Blood, urine, and wound cultures** to look for source of infection
4. **Chest radiograph** to look for infiltrate or ARDS
5. **Electrocardiogram (ECG)** to look for evidence of secondary ischemia
6. **Lactate level** to look for acidosis. A level > 4 mM indicates severe hypoperfusion.

D. **Treatment**

1. **Airway management:** supplemental oxygen and mechanical ventilation as needed
2. **Aggressive volume replacement**
3. Foley catheter to **monitor input** and **output**
4. **Intravenous (IV) antibiotics.** Empiric therapy should take into consideration the patient's age, comorbidities, and the suspected source. If there is no obvious source, many regimens are available. Some examples are listed below.
   a. For community-acquired, non-neutropenic infection: ceftriaxone 1 g IV every 12 hours plus gentamicin 1 mg/kg IV every 8 hours
   b. For nosocomial infection: mezlocillin, ticarcillin, or piperacillin 3 g IV every 4 hours plus gentamicin 1 mg/kg every 8 hours
5. Surgical débridement and removal of causative or potentiating devices such as indwelling Foley or vascular catheters
6. **Inotropic support:** dopamine or dobutamine starting at 5 μg/kg/min and titrated to mean arterial pressure (MAP) of 70 mm Hg and urine output > 1 ml/kg/hr
7. Routine monitoring of heart rate, blood pressure (BP), and pulse oximetry
8. Consider monitoring of central venous pressure for patients with concomitant CHF or end-stage renal disease (ESRD) or patients with no peripheral venous access.
9. Corticosteroids have **not** been shown to be useful.

E. **Disposition**

—Patients are admitted to the intensive care unit (ICU) for monitoring, aggressive fluid resuscitation, and IV antibiotics.

II. Central Nervous System (CNS) Infections

A. Tetanus

—Tetanus is caused by a toxin of ***Clostridium tetani,*** a gram-negative organism found in soil.

—Spores are introduced into the skin following trauma, "skin popping" (in heroin use), or surgery.

—The toxin blocks inhibitory neurons, resulting in unopposed muscle spasms (tetany).

1. **Clinical features** may include:

   —irritability

   —restlessness

   —**muscle spasms** ("lockjaw" is spasm of the jaw muscles)

   —tetany of the laryngeal and respiratory muscles

   —**opisthotonus**

   —**intact mental status**

   —difficulty sucking (infants)

2. **Diagnostic tests**
   - **a.** Anaerobic culture of wound: is positive in one third of cases.
   - **b.** CBC to look for leukocytosis: is normal in tetanus.
   - **c.** Lumbar puncture to look for meningitis: is normal in tetanus.
   - **d.** Computed tomography (CT) and magnetic resonance imaging (MRI) of the head to look for intracranial pathology: these are negative in tetanus.

3. **Treatment**
   - **a.** Airway, breathing, and circulation (ABCs), with particular attention to maintaining the airway
   - **b. Wound débridement** and irrigation with 3% hydrogen peroxide to create **aerobic** conditions
   - **c. Antibiotics**

     —Penicillin G 2.4 million units/day
   - **d. Muscle relaxants** (see Table 11-5)

     —Diazepam 10–30 mg IV every 1–3 hours as needed, or chlorpromazine 75–100 mg IV every 3–4 hours as needed

4. **Disposition**
   - **a.** Patients are admitted to the ICU.
   - **b.** An environment with minimal stimulation should be provided to prevent exacerbation of muscle spasms.

B. Rabies

—Rabies is caused by a rhabdovirus. Most cases reported in the United States since 1980 have resulted from exposure to bat saliva.

—Rabies has been acquired on all continents except Australia and Antarctica.

—More than 99% of all cases occur in developing countries, where canine rabies is still endemic.

—Rabies is a reportable illness.

—Patients who develop respiratory arrest or other complications, including cardiovascular, pulmonary, or neurological complications, ultimately will die.

1. Clinical features

—The incubation period usually is 3 weeks to 3 months (bites to the head are associated with shorter incubation periods). In the United States the average duration of illness is 13 days.

—Disease usually progresses according to the following three stages:

a. **Prodrome** (2–10 days)

—Malaise

—Fever

—Upper respiratory infection symptoms, e.g., sniffling, congestion

—Gastrointestinal (GI) symptoms

—Pain or paresthesias at the exposure site (50% of cases)

b. **Acute neurologic period** (2 forms; 2–7 days)

(1) **Furious rabies**

—Hyperactivity

—Disorientation

—Hallucinations

—Hyperthermia

—**Hypersalivation**

—Hypertension

—**Hydrophobia** (manifested as choking or gagging on drinking or even seeing water)

—**Aerophobia** (manifested as choking or gagging when air is blown on the face)

—Paralysis

(2) **Paralytic rabies**

—Paralysis is the main feature-at the exposure site, diffuse, or ascending, as in Guillain-Barré syndrome.

c. Progression to **coma** within 10 days of onset of clinical disease in all cases

2. Diagnostic tests

—Currently there are no tests that can diagnose rabies before the onset of symptoms.

a. CBC, cerebrospinal fluid (CSF), and chest radiograph: changes are nonspecific.

b. Immunofluorescent staining of hair follicle nerve ending from nape of neck to look for **antigen**

c. Serologic testing with rapid fluorescent focus inhibition test (RFFIT) of serum or CSF to look for positive **antibody** titer (useful only if patient has not been previously vaccinated). Serum usually is positive days 6–9; CSF is positive day 9.

d. Brain examination at autopsy to look for characteristic **Negri bodies**

3. Treatment (Table 14-1)

a. **Local wound care** with soap and water

b. Passive immunization with **human rabies immunoglobulin** (HRIG). A single dose of 20 IU/kg should be given on the first day: half

Table 14-1. Whom to Treat for Rabies

Animal exposure	Treatment
Bite or non-bite exposure to bats; dogs and cats in most developing countries and in the U.S. along the Mexican border; raccoons, skunks, foxes, groundhogs, and most wild carnivores	Treat. If suspicion is low and the animal's brain can be examined for rabies, treatment can be delayed for 48 hours.
Lagomorphs (squirrels and rodents except groundhogs) and dogs and cats in many Western states	Consult state or local health department. Treatment generally is not necessary.
Healthy domesticated cats, dogs, or ferrets	Confine animal for 10 days. Treat only if animal sickens or dies with signs of rabies in that time.

is infiltrated at the wound site and half is given intramuscularly (IM) in the gluteus or thigh. Effective until 7 days after postexposure prophylaxis (PEP) is begun.

c. PEP via **vaccine.** Human diploid cell rabies vaccine is given in the **deltoid** muscle in 5 doses on days 1, 3, 7, 14, and 28. It should be given immediately, but can be given anytime as soon as likelihood of exposure is discovered.

d. Steroids should **not** be given.

4. Disposition

a. Patients with confirmed rabies are hospitalized for supportive care.

b. Patients with suspected rabies may be treated as outpatients with close follow-up.

C. Botulism

1. Overview

a. Epidemiology

—Botulism is caused by the gram-positive rod ***Clostridium botulinum,*** an obligate anaerobe found in soil and water.

—Botulinum toxin is taken up in presynaptic nerve terminals and prevents acetylcholine release.

—Botulism has a 2-day incubation period.

b. Types

(1) Food-borne: the most common form, 90% of cases involve home-canned foods.

(2) Wound-borne: occurs after inoculation with spores during trauma or “skin-popping” (accompanies drug abuse).

(3) Infantile: occurs in infants 2–9 months old after ingestion of the spores, which germinate in the GI tract and release toxin (normal intestinal flora prevents this in older children and adults). Children younger than 1 year should not eat honey because of the danger of infantile botulism.

c. Differential diagnosis includes:

—Guillain-Barré syndrome

—myasthenia gravis
—Eaton-Lambert syndrome
—diphtheria
—sepsis (in infants)
—meningitis (in infants)
—Werdnig-Hoffman disease (in infants)
—infantile myasthenia (in infants)

2. **Clinical features** include the 8 D's:

—**D**escending paralysis

—**D**iplopia

—**D**yspnea

—**D**ysarthria

—**D**izziness

—**D**ry mouth

—**D**ysphagia

—**D**eath

3. **Diagnostic tests**

—Routine laboratory studies: results are normal.

—Laboratory detection of botulinum toxin from serum or stool

4. **Treatment**

a. **Airway must be secured.**

b. Equine **anti-A,B,E botulinum serum** 10 ml IV and 10 ml IM, repeated every 2–4 hours if disease continues to progress. Antitoxin can halt disease progression but does not reverse existing paralysis.

5. **Disposition**

—Patients are admitted to the hospital for further management.

D. Dengue

—also known as "break-bone fever"

—caused by a **flavivirus** and carried by the *Aedes aegypti* mosquito

—highest incidence in southeast Asia, India, and American tropics

—2–7 day incubation period

1. **Clinical features** may include:

—abrupt onset of fever and chills followed by 1–2 afebrile days, then fever again

—severe malaise

—retroorbital pain

—myalgia, arthralgia

—rash

—relative bradycardia

—generalized lymphadenopathy

—petechiae

—epistaxis

2. **Complications**

—Dengue hemorrhagic fever (DHF) is a potentially fatal complication in patients with previous exposure to dengue. It is characterized by dengue fever with thrombocytopenia and hemoconcentration that may progress to hypotension and shock.

3. **Diagnostic tests**
   a. **CBC** to look for neutropenia, thrombocytopenia, hemoconcentration
   b. **Chemistry panel** to look for electrolyte abnormalities
   c. **Prothrombin time (PT), activated partial thromboplastin time (APTT), bleeding time, d-dimer** to look for DIC
   d. **Liver function tests (LFTs)** to look for hepatic dysfunction
   e. **Blood** and **urine cultures** to identify causative organism
   f. Peripheral smear if malaria is suspected
   g. Immunoassay and polymerase chain reaction (PCR) to look for flavivirus or other suspected organism
4. **Treatment**
   a. **Acetaminophen** to decrease fever. Aspirin must be avoided: salicylates in the treatment of dengue have been associated with development of Reye's syndrome in children and bleeding diatheses in adults.
   b. Symptomatic treatment
   c. For hemorrhagic dengue:

      —vigorous IV hydration

      —blood and platelet transfusions as needed
   d. Heparin is contraindicated for DIC in dengue
5. **Disposition**

—Patients with dengue usually are admitted to the hospital for observation and monitoring for complications.

III. Human Immunodeficiency Virus (HIV) and Associated Infections

A. Overview

—HIV is a retrovirus that attacks the immune system, primarily CD4 T lymphocytes.

—Patients who present to the emergency department (ED) may have complaints related to the prodrome and the viral infection itself; opportunistic infections; or drug reactions and interactions of anti-HIV therapies.

B. Clinical features

1. Systemic symptoms: fever, malaise, headache, weight loss, lymphadenopathy

2. Skin: rash, vesicles, warts, pigmented lesions
3. Ophthalmologic: change in visual acuity, "floaters," photophobia, eye pain, redness
4. Head, eyes, ears, nose, throat (HEENT): pharyngitis, thrush, sinusitis, ulcers
5. Pulmonary: cough, hemoptysis, shortness of breath, chest pain
6. GI: nausea, vomiting, diarrhea, odynophagia, dysphagia, abdominal pain, perirectal pain and itching
7. Genitourinary (GU): vaginal discharge, itching and burning; dysuria; frequency
8. Neurologic: peripheral neuropathy, paresthesias, memory loss, focal neurologic deficits, seizures, altered mental status
9. Musculoskeletal: weakness, muscle wasting, myalgia, arthralgia

C. Diagnostic tests

—For reasons of confidentiality, counseling, and follow-up, definitive testing for HIV is performed infrequently in the ED setting. Rather, patients are referred for outpatient testing or, if admitted, can have testing done as inpatients.

—However, because of the need to treat needle-stick injuries (see Chapter 19) within hours of exposure, many EDs do perform definitive testing under these circumstances.

1. **CBC** to look for leukopenia, anemia, thrombocytopenia [important findings in antiretroviral toxicity and *Mycobacterium avium intracellulare* (MAI), among other entities]
2. **LFTs** to look for elevation, which is common secondary to antiretroviral therapy; coinfection with hepatitis B and C; and numerous opportunistic infections including cytomegalovirus (CMV), MAI, and *Mycobacterium tuberculosis* (MTB).
3. **Arterial blood gas (ABG)** to look for oxygenation parameters. Use of ABG in deciding *Pneumocystis carinii* pneumonia (PCP):
   a. A-a gradient > 35, $PO_2 < 70$
      —inpatient IV antibiotics and steroids
   b. A-a gradient < 35, $PO_2 > 70$
      —outpatient oral antibiotics
4. **Chest radiograph** to look for focal infiltrate (bacterial pneumonia), diffuse interstitial infiltrates [PCP, CMV, or Kaposi sarcoma (KS)], cavitary lesions (MTB, PCP, or fungal infections), or adenopathy (lymphoma, MTB or MAI, or KS). Chest radiographs are normal in up to 10% of patients with PCP.
5. **Lumbar puncture** with India ink examination or cryptococcal antigen testing to look for *Cryptococcus neoformans.* Gram stain and other fungal and viral cultures also are performed
6. **CT scan of the brain** with contrast to look for ring-enhancing lesions suggestive of toxoplasmosis, lymphoma, fungal infections, and tuberculosis

7. **Stool studies** for ova and parasites, leukocytes, and acid-fast bacteria to look for infection, if diarrhea is present
8. **Funduscopic examination** (CMV is described as white patches on a red background "like a pizza")
9. **Blood cultures** to look for source of infection. Fungal cultures for MTB and MAI are done in addition to the anaerobic and aerobic cultures.
10. **Sputum culture** for MTB if clinically indicated
11. **Tzanck smear** of any vesicles to look for herpes virus
12. **KOH prep** of oral lesions or vaginal discharge to look for *Candida* species

D. Treatment

1. Antiretroviral therapy is not initiated in the ED unless it is for postexposure prophylaxis of needle-stick injuries.
2. Supplemental oxygen as needed
3. IV hydration
4. Antibiotics (Table 14-2)
5. Consultation with an infectious disease specialist

E. Disposition

—Severity of findings dictates whether the patient requires admission and to what setting. Every effort should be made to ensure adequate follow-up of discharged patients, such as making sure they have a scheduled follow-up appointment when they leave the ED.

IV. Sexually Transmitted Diseases (STDs)

A. Gonorrhea

—History of unprotected sex or sex with a known infected partner is important.

1. **Clinical features**
   a. **Symptoms** may include:
      —urinary frequency
      —urinary urgency
      —dysuria
      —vaginal discharge
      —urethral discharge
   b. **Physical examination findings** may include:
      —**purulent yellow or green discharge** from urethral meatus or cervix
      —red or swollen distal portion of meatus
      —**friable cervix**
      —rectal discharge (gonococcal proctitis)
      —swollen knee joint (septic arthritis; see Chapter 11 IV A)

Table 14-2. Antibiotics for Commonly Seen Opportunistic Infections

Mild to moderate PCP	**TMP-SMX 2 DS tabs PO bid**
Moderate to severe PCP	TMP-SMX 12–15 mg TMP/kg day IV q 6 hrs + IV methylprednisolone 40 mg bid × 5 d, then taper
Toxoplasmosis	Pyrimethamine 100–200 mg PO × 1, then 50–100 mg PO qd + sulfadiazine 1–2 g PO qid × 6 weeks, then maintenance therapy
M. tuberculosis	INH 300 mg PO qd + rifampin 600 mg PO qd + pyrazinamide 20–35 mg/kg/day PO + ethambutol 15 mg/kg day PO × 9 months or 6 months past conversion of sputum culture (whichever is longer)
Cryptococcal meningitis	Amphotericin B 0.7 mg/kg/day IV (slow infusion), then maintenance therapy
Cytomegalovirus (CMV)	Induction therapy (should withhold other myelotoxic drugs during induction) ganciclovir 5 mg/kg IV over 1 hr q 12 hrs; daily CBC; G-CSF may be needed
Herpes simplex*	Acyclovir
Mucocutaneous, mild	200–400 mg PO 5×/day × 10 days
Mucocutaneous, severe	5 mg/kg IV over 1 hr tid × 10–14 days
Visceral organ involvement	10 mg/kg IV over 1 hr tid × 10–14 days
Herpes zoster	
Shingles	Acyclovir 800 mg PO 5×/day × 10 days
Disseminated infection	Acyclovir 10 mg/kg IV tid × 10 days
Candidiasis	
Oropharyngeal	Clotrimazole 10 mg troche 5×/day × 7–14 days
Esophagitis	Ketaconazole 200–400 mg PO × 14–21 days
Vulvovaginal	Fluconazole 150 mg PO × 1
Cryptosporidiosis	Supportive care

*may also use famcyclovir or valacyclovir. See section IV G.
bid = twice a day; *CBC* = complete blood cell count; *DS* = double strength; *G-CSF* = granulocyte colony stimulating factor; *INH* = Isoniazid; *IV* = intravenous; *PCP* = *Pneumocystis carinii* pneumonia; *PO* = orally; *q* = every; *qd* = per day; *qid* = 4 times a day; *tid* = 3 times a day; *TMP-SMX* = trimethoprim-sulfamethoxazole.

—cervical motion and adnexal tenderness [pelvic inflammatory disease (PID)]
—pharyngeal erythema and tonsillar exudate (gonococcal pharyngitis)
—petechial rash all over body or isolated erythematoid lesions and signs of shock (disseminated gonorrhea)

2. Diagnostic tests

a. The gold standard remains culturing of the discharge on modified Thayer-Martin medium

b. Gram stain of discharge to look for gram-negative intracellular diplococci. Yield is better in men than in women.

c. DNA probe culture of the discharge is more accurate than Gram stain, but results may not be immediately available.

3. Treatment

a. Antibiotics **should be administered to the patient and the patient's sexual contacts.** Options include:

—Ceftriaxone 125 mg intramuscularly (IM), once

—Cefixime 400 mg orally, once

—Ciprofloxacin 500 mg orally, once

—Ofloxacin 400 mg orally, once

—Azithromycin 1 g orally, once

—Spectinomycin 2 g IM, once

b. Due to a high rate (up to 60%) of concomitant *Chlamydia* infection, treatment for infection with *Chlamydia* spp always should be included (see IV B 3).

4. Disposition

a. Patients with mild symptoms may be discharged home with instructions to have their sexual partners examined and treated if necessary, and to refrain from sexual intercourse until they do.

b. Patients who are septic or have a septic joint are admitted for IV antibiotics.

c. Admission should be considered for patients with PID (see Chapter 16, section IV A).

d. HIV testing should be recommended.

B. Chlamydia

1. Clinical features

a. Symptoms may include:

—vaginal discharge

—dysuria

—frequency

—pelvic pain

—dyspareunia

b. Physical examination findings may include:

—yellow, mucopurulent discharge

—friable, erythematous cervix

—urethral erythema

—tender epididymis if infection is causing epididymitis

2. Diagnostic tests

a. Gram stain of discharge to look for multiple leukocytes without intracellular diplococci (the discharge may be difficult to differentiate from that of gonorrhea).

b. DNA probe, fluorescent antibody testing, and culture also can be used; results may not be available immediately.

3. Treatment. Antibiotics should be administered to both the patient and the patient's sexual contacts. Options include:

—azithromycin 1 g orally, once

—doxycycline 100 mg orally twice a day for 7 days

—ofloxacin 300 mg orally twice a day for 7 days

—erythromycin 500 mg orally 4 times a day for 7 days

4. Disposition

a. Patients with uncomplicated cervicitis/urethritis may be discharged with outpatient follow-up.

b. If the patient appears unreliable and may not take a full 7-day course of medication, single-dose therapy should be given before discharge.

c. Admission should be considered for patients with PID (see Chapter 16, section IV A).

d. HIV testing should be recommended.

C. Syphilis

1. Clinical features

—Syphilis presents with different clinical pictures, depending on the stage. The three stages are primary, secondary, and tertiary, with a latent phase between secondary and tertiary (Table 14-3).

2. Diagnostic tests

a. Serology, VDRL, fluorescent treponemal antibody absorption test (FTA-AB) to look for evidence of infection. May not be positive in primary syphilis. Any unknown (not easily recognizable as something else) genital lesion should raise the suspicion of syphilis.

b. Dark-field microscopy of suspicious lesion to look for the spirochete ***Treponema pallidum***

3. Treatment

a. For primary, secondary, latent for <1 year:

—Benzathine penicillin G 2.4 million units IM once (if penicillin-allergic, consider desensitization), or

—Doxycycline 100 mg orally twice a day for 14 days, or

—Tetracycline 500 mg orally 4 times a day for 14 days

b. For latent, unknown duration, tertiary (not including neurosyphilis):

—Benzathine penicillin G 2.4 million units IM weekly for 1 month or

—Doxycycline 100 mg orally twice a day for 1 month

c. For neurosyphilis, 3 different regimens are possible:

(1) Aqueous penicillin G, 2.4 million units every 4 hours for 10–14 days; or

(2) Procaine penicillin 2.4 million units IM daily for 10–14 days, plus Probenecid 500 mg orally 4 times a day for 10–14 days; or

(3) Ceftriaxone 1 g IV/IM daily for 14 days

4. Disposition

a. Patients with primary or secondary syphilis may be discharged after treatment with outpatient follow-up.

b. Repeat serologic testing should occur in 3–6 months.

c. Patients with tertiary syphilis typically present with other medical problems that require hospitalization.

d. HIV testing should be recommended.

Table 14-3. Syphilis Presentation by Stage

Stage	Symptoms and Physical Examination Findings	Time of Presentation	Serology
Primary	**Chancre:** painless papule at site of inoculation that becomes a painless ulcer Painless inguinal adenopathy	Onset about 3 weeks after exposure, lasts 2–6 weeks, then spontaneously resolves	−/+
Secondary	Generalized non-tender adenopathy Fever Sore throat Malaise Headache Weight loss Initially generalized macular, then maculopapular rash that includes palms and soles *Condyloma lata:* broad moist lesions found in warm moist regions such as genitalia or under breasts *Mucous patches* on tongue, oral mucosa, pharynx, perineum, and genitalia Healing chancre may be present in 15%–25% of patients Iritis Hepatitis Glomerulonephritis	6–8 weeks after healing of primary chancre	+
Early latent	Positive FTA with no signs/symptoms Normal CSF	< 1 yr after infection by history or serology	+
Late latent	Same as early latent phase	> 1 yr after infection	+
Tertiary	**Neurosyphilis** Meningovascular Headache Dizziness Blurred vision Confusion Cranial nerve palsies Stroke syndrome *Argyll Robertson pupil* (small pupil that reacts to accommodation but not to light) Parenchymatous Irritability/emotional instability Difficulty concentrating Seizures Aphasia Transient hemiparesis *Tabes dorsales* (Posterior column involvement with ataxia, wide-based gait, loss of position, deep pain and temperature sensation, decreased or absent deep tendon reflexes, urinary retention or incontinence, impotence, and sharp leg pain) **Cardiovascular** Aortic regurgitation Aortic aneurysm (typically thoracic and saccular) Aortitis Coronary artery ostial stenosis **Skin and other organs** *Gumma* (granulomatous, necrotic lesions on the skin, submucosa, or involving the palate, nasal septum, or any organs) Bone pain secondary to periostitis or osteitis with destructive or sclerosing lesions	6 mo–30 yrs	+

CSF = cerebrospinal fluid; *FTA* = fluorescent treponemal antibodies test

D. Trichomoniasis

1. Clinical features

a. Symptoms may include:
—copious, yellow-green, malodorous foamy vaginal discharge
—labial irritation or swelling
—dyspareunia
—dysuria
—may be asymptomatic (especially men)

b. Physical examination findings may include:
—copious, foamy discharge with pH > 5.5
—punctate red spots on cervix or vaginal wall ("strawberry cervix")

2. Diagnostic tests

a. Wet mount to look for motile trichomonads. These sometimes are picked up on urine microscopy when the patient complains of dysuria and denies any discharge.

b. "Whiff test": 2 drops of KOH are added to a slide of the discharge, which is then heated gently; when the clinician "takes a whiff," there is a fishy smell characteristic of trichomonas.

c. Urinalysis to look for concomitant urinary tract infection (UTI)

3. Treatment

a. Metronidazole 2 g orally once or 500 mg orally twice a day for 7 days

b. A pregnancy test should be given before treatment is prescribed. Treatment should not be given in first trimester of pregnancy, but if symptoms are severe, clotrimazole 100 mg intravaginally once daily for 14 days may be given.

4. Disposition

a. Patients may be discharged after treatment, with outpatient follow-up.

b. Patients should be instructed to refrain from sexual intercourse until treatment is finished and all partners have been examined and treated.

c. Patients should be instructed to avoid ingesting alcohol while taking metronidazole because it has a disulfiram-like effect, which results in violent vomiting, flushing, and headaches. (Note that only a small amount of alcohol, such as that found in a teaspoon of cough syrup, need be ingested to produce this effect.)

d. HIV testing should be recommended.

E. Lymphogranuloma venereum

—causative agent is ***Chlamydia trachomatis***

1. Clinical features

a. Symptoms may include:
—painful inguinal mass
—fever
—headache
—nausea

—vomiting
—joint pain
—back pain

b. **Physical examination findings may include:**
—initially unilateral tender inguinal node progressing to a large, tender, purplish indurated mass (bubo)
—sinuses with purulent or bloody discharge
—inguinal lymphadenopathy in males
—perirectal lymphadenopathy and rectal strictures in women

2. **Diagnostic tests**
   a. Serologic testing by complement fixation or microimmunofluorescence may be done.
   b. Culture is expensive and not often done.
   c. False-positives for syphilis can occur.

3. **Treatment**
—Treatment is not to be withheld pending serology results.
   a. Antibiotic options include:
   —Doxycycline 100 mg orally twice a day for 21 days
   —Erythromycin 500 mg orally 4 times a day for 21 days
   —Sulfamethoxazole 500 mg orally 4 times a day for 21 days
   b. Surgical consult should be considered for strictures and fistulas.

4. **Disposition**
   a. Patients who do not appear ill and are able to tolerate oral intake may be discharged with outpatient follow-up to reevaluate treatment and check serology results.
   b. HIV testing should be recommended.

F. Chancroid

—causative agent is ***Haemophilus ducreyi***

1. **Clinical features**
   a. **Symptoms** may include:
   —small painful papules or ulcers
   —painful inguinal adenopathy
   b. **Physical examination findings** may include:
   —tender, shallow ulcers with irregular reddish borders
   —tender inguinal nodes
   —inguinal mass/abscess from coalesced nodes (bubo)
   —sinuses from mass

2. **Diagnostic tests**
   a. **Gram stain** and culture of bubo aspirate or ulcer exudate
   b. **VDRL** to look for syphilis
   c. Immunofluorescence test for *H. ducreyi*

3. **Treatment**

a. **Aspiration of buboes** [(incision and drainage (I&D) should not be done]

b. **Antibiotics**

—Azithromycin 1 g orally once, or

—Ceftriaxone 250 mg IM once, or

—Erythromycin 500 mg orally 4 times a day for 7 days, or

—Ciprofloxacin 750 mg orally once

4. **Disposition**

a. Patients may be discharged with outpatient follow-up.

b. All the patient's sexual partners should be examined and treated if necessary. The patient should refrain from sexual intercourse until partners have been examined and treated and until the lesion is healed.

c. HIV testing should be recommended.

G. Herpes simplex virus (HSV)

—See Chapter 10 V B and C for discussion of dermal HSV and herpes zoster infection.

1. **Clinical presentation**

a. Prodromal **symptoms** may include:

—low-grade fever

—general malaise

b. **Physical examination findings** may include:

—painful, skin-colored vesicles on labia and vulvar vestibule (in women), or shaft of penis, penile foreskin, and perianal foreskin (in men)

—painless lesions inside vagina and on cervix

—inguinal adenopathy

—dysuria and urinary retention if bladder involvement present

2. **Diagnostic tests**

a. **HSV** culture of vesicular fluid or debris

b. Tzanck smear of vesicular fluid to look for multinucleated giant cells (does not differentiate between HSV and VZV)

c. Post-voiding residual urine collection if urinary retention is suspected

d. Screening for other STDs

3. **Treatment**

a. Antiviral agent: **acyclovir** 5 mg/kg up to 500 mg orally 5 times a day, or **famciclovir** 500 mg orally 3 times a day for 7 days, or **valacyclovir** 1000 mg orally 3 times a day for 7 days

b. NSAIDs or opiates for analgesia

c. **Capsaicin** or acyclovir topical ointments applied to skin for analgesia

d. Cool compresses, sitz baths, and Burow's solution for symptomatic relief

e. Abstinence from sexual activity as long as active lesions are present

4. **Disposition**

a. Patients can be discharged home with outpatient follow-up.

b. HIV testing should be recommended.

H. Condyloma acuminata (venereal warts)

—causative agent is human papilloma virus (HPV)

1. Clinical features

a. Symptoms may include:
—genital or perianal growths
—painful defecation
—abnormal urinary stream

b. Physical examination findings may include:
—soft, moist, pink, pedunculated growths on labia, vaginal wall, cervix, and perianal area (in women) or on penile shaft, urethra, and perianal area (in men). These growths may be solitary but often are multiple, located close together with a "cauliflower" appearance.

2. Diagnostic tests (outpatient)

—This condition is not an emergency. Definitive diagnosis and treatment usually are performed in the outpatient setting.

a. Colposcopy with 1% acetic acid to look for **white** lesions, which are suspicious for HPV. These lesions are biopsied for definitive diagnosis.

b. Darkfield microscopy of lesion scraping to look for syphilis.

3. Treatment (outpatient)

a. Recurrence is common, so treatment sometimes is problematic.

b. Outpatient options include:
—cryotherapy
—electrocautery
—1% topical Podophyllin solution (contraindicated in pregnancy)
—GU consult for large or obstructing lesions of the urethra
—Papanicolaou (Pap) smear for women, because HPV types 16 and 18 are associated with cervical cancer

4. Disposition

a. Patients may be discharged with outpatient follow-up.

b. Patients should refrain from sexual intercourse until lesions are gone. All sexual partners should be examined and treated.

c. HIV testing should be recommended.

V. Skin and Bone Infections

A. Toxic shock syndrome

—See Chapter 16 V C

B. Cellulitis

—See Chapter 10 IV B

C. Osteomyelitis

—Osteomyelitis is the infection of bone.

—It usually is bacterial in origin.

—It may be acute, subacute, or chronic.

—The most commonly affected area is the metaphyses of long bones.

—The most common causative organism is ***Staphylococcus aureus.***

—*Salmonella* is a common cause of osteomyelitis in asplenic patients.

1. **Clinical features**
   a. **Symptoms** may include:
      —pain
      —swelling
      —localized warmth
      —general malaise
   b. **Physical examination findings** may include:
      —fever
      —tenderness
      —decreased range of motion of adjacent joint
      —limping
      —normal neuromuscular exam
      —poor capillary refill in toes
      —poor distal pulses
2. **Risk factors** include:

   —diabetes mellitus

   —history of acute systemic illness within the preceding few weeks

   —trauma

   —soft tissue infection

   —surgery (e.g., internal fixation of a fracture)

   —ingrown toenail
3. **Diagnostic tests**
   a. AP and lateral radiographs to look for periosteal elevations, destruction of bone (radiolucent), and fading of cortical margins without surrounding reactive bone. These changes are evident 2 to 3 weeks after infection, but cannot be distinguished well from infarction or tumor.
   b. CT scan to look for intramedullary gas, early detection
   c. 99technetium bone scan
      —shows lesion 48 hours after infection
      —does not distinguish well between osteomyelitis and infarction or tumor
      —does distinguish well between bone and soft tissue infection
   d. **MRI** is the **most sensitive test.** It distinguishes bony infection from infarction, tumor, and soft tissue infection.
   e. **CBC** to look for leukocytosis
   f. **Blood cultures** to identify causative organism
4. **Treatment**

a. **Antibiotics**
—A 6-week course of IV antibiotics usually is necessary.
—If patient is not toxic-appearing at presentation, results of culture and sensitivity may be awaited to make it possible to begin specific therapy.
—If patient needs empiric coverage, therapy based on the most likely organisms should be started.

b. **Immobilization** of affected body part for 3 weeks

c. Antipyretics

d. **Orthopaedic consultation**

e. Surgical drainage if late presentation

5. **Disposition**
—Patients are admitted to the hospital for IV antibiotics.

VI. Parasitic Infections

A. Malaria

—is caused by four protozoa of the Plasmodium genus-***P. falciparum, P. vivax, P. ovale,*** and ***P. malariae***

—is transmitted by the *Anopheles* mosquito

—Risk factors include incomplete chemoprophylaxis, travel to endemic countries, and multiple *Anopheles* mosquito bites.

1. **Clinical features**

a. **Incubation period** typically is 10–14 days, but may be months to years in patients who have had partial prophylaxis.

b. **Symptoms** and **physical examination findings** may include:
—**classic triad: recurrent chills, fever, and sweats**
—malaise
—myalgia
—headache
—backache
—vomiting
—abdominal pain
—hepatosplenomegaly
—jaundice
—somnolence
—seizures
—coma

2. **Diagnostic tests**

a. **Giemsa-stained peripheral smear** to look for organism. **Slides must be read by hand.** Smears may be negative if the protozoa are sequestered in liver or if the patient has been partially treated with antimalarial drugs or broad-spectrum antibiotics, so if there is suspicion, smears must be repeated twice a day (during fever) for several days.

b. **CBC** to look for anemia
c. **LFTs** to look for hemolysis
d. **Chemistry panel** to look for elevated BUN and creatinine
e. **Urinalysis** to look for hematuria

3. **Treatment**
a. **Prophylaxis**
—for chloroquine-sensitive malaria: **chloroquine** 500 mg/week orally, starting 1 week prior to travel and ending 4 weeks afterward.
—for chloroquine-resistant malaria: **mefloquine** 250 mg/week orally, starting 1 week prior to travel and ending 4 weeks afterward. There are many contraindications to mefloquine, including pregnancy, epilepsy, and use of β-blockers.
b. **Acute illness**
—for chloroquine-sensitive malaria: chloroquine 600 mg orally for 2 days, followed by 300 mg orally for 1 day, then primaquine 15 mg/day for 14 days for *P. vivax* and *P. ovale.*
—for chloroquine-resistant malaria: quinine sulfate 650 mg orally 3 times a day for 3 days, or mefloquine 1250 mg orally once, or tetracycline 250 mg orally 4 times a day for 3 days, or clindamycin 900 mg orally 3 times a day for 3–5 days.
c. Exchange transfusion in severe disease

4. **Disposition**
a. Patients with *P. falciparum* and those who are severely ill, pregnant, or immunocompromised should be admitted to the hospital.
b. Malaria is more severe in children and pregnant women; severity is directly correlated with the degree of parasitemia.

B. Worm and fluke infections (Table 14-4)

C. Protozoan infections

1. **Giardiasis**
—transmitted by ingestion of *Giardia lamblia* cysts
a. **Clinical presentation** may include:
—diarrhea: chronic, foul-smelling stools; greasy, without blood or pus
—malabsorption syndrome
—stunted growth in children (reversible)
b. **Diagnostic tests**
—string test: gelatin-coated string is secured at mouth and swallowed. String is removed after 4–18 hours and examined for trophozoites.
—examination of stool for ova and parasites
—immunofluoresence or enzyme-linked immunosorbent assay (ELISA) tests for *Giardia* antigens
c. **Treatment**
(1) Non-pregnant adults: Metronidazole 250 mg orally 3 times a day for 5 days
(2) Pregnant adults:Paromomycin 10 mg/kg orally 3 times a day for 7 days (maximum = 500 mg/dose)

Table 14-4. Parasitic Worms and Flukes

Cestodes (tapeworms)	Intermediate host/Mode of transmission	Disease, symptoms, and signs	Treatment
Taenia solium	Pigs/eating undercooked pork	Adult tapeworms cause no symptoms *Cysticercosis:* symptoms depend on where the cysts are located (may be anywhere): Brain: seizures, strokes Eye: vision loss Muscle: myalgias, contractures	Praziquantel 10 mg/kg PO × 1
Taenia saginata	Cattle/eating undercooked beef	Usually asymptomatic Weight loss Nausea, vomiting, diarrhea	Praziquantel 10 mg/kg PO × 1
Diphyllobothrium latum	Fish/eating raw fish	Megaloblastic anemia	Praziquantel 10 mg/kg PO × 1
Echinococcus granulosus	Sheep (dogs are definitive host)/ ingestion of eggs	Hydatid cyst disease Lung and liver congestion Anaphylaxis secondary to cyst rupture	Surgical resection of cysts
Trematodes (flukes)			
Schistosoma mansoni, japonicum	Snails/via skin penetration	Cor pulmonale secondary to invasion of lung venules Hepatosplenomegaly Dermatitis	Praziquantel 20 mg/kg PO bid × 1 day
Schistosoma hematobium	Snails/via skin penetration	Hematuria Bladder carcinoma secondary to chronic GU irritation	Praziquantel 20 mg/kg PO bid × 1 day
Clonorchis simensis (liver fluke)	Snails, fish/eating undercooked fresh water fish	Usually asymptomatic Weight loss Abdominal pain Hepatomegaly	Praziquantel 25 mg/kg PO tid × 1 day
Paragonimus westermani (lung fluke)	Snails, crabs/fecal-oral	Paragonimiasis Hemoptysis	Praziquantel 25 mg/kg PO tid × 2 days
Intestinal nematodes			
Enterobius vermicularis (pinworm)	Hand-to-mouth	Perianal itching	Albendazole 400 PO × 1, or Mebendazole 100 mg PO × 3 days, or Pyrantel pamoate 11 mg/kg (maximum dose = 1 g PO × 1)
Trichuris trichuria (whipworm)	Fecal-oral	Usually asymptomatic Mild anemia Abdominal pain Diarrhea, tenesmus Perianal itching	Albendazole 400 mg PO × 1, or Mebendazole 100 mg PO × 3 days
Ascaris lumbricoides	Fecal-oral	Pneumonia Loeffler's pneumonitis	Albendazole 400 mg PO × 1, or

(cont.)

Table 14-4. (*Continued*).

Cestodes (tapeworms)	Intermediate host/Mode of transmission	Disease, symptoms, and signs	Treatment
		Intestinal infection/ obstruction Liver failure	Mebendazole 100 mg PO × 3 days
Necator Americanus (New World hookworm)	Skin penetration	Intense dermatitis Loeffler's pneumonitis Significant anemia GI symptoms Developmental delay in children (irreversible)	Albendazole 400 mg PO × 1, or Mebendazole 100 mg PO × 3 days
Ancylostoma duodenale (Old World hookworm)	Skin penetration	Same as for *Necator*	Albendazole 400 mg PO × 1, or Mebendazole 100 mg PO × 3 days
Strongyloides stercoralis	Skin penetration	Same as for *Necator,* plus: Diarrhea × 3–6 weeks Superimposed bacterial sepsis	Ivermectin 200 μg/kg/day × 2 days
Trichinella spiralis	Infected pork	Trichinosis Myalgias Facial and periorbital edema Conjunctivitis Pneumonia, myocarditis, encephalitis, nephritis, meningitis	Albendazole 400 mg PO bid × 14 days + prednisone 40–60 mg PO qd
Tissue nematodes			
Toxocara canis (dog hookworm)	Ingestion of eggs from infected soil	Visceral larva migrans Upper respiratory tract infections Pneumonia Diarrhea	Diethylcarbamazapine 2 ng/kg PO tid × 10 days
Wucheria bancrofti, Brugia malayi, Brugia timori	Mosquito bite	Elephantiasis (lymphatic obstruction of dependent parts including extremities, scrotum, testes)	Ivermectin 400 μg/kg × 1, or Diethylcarbamazapine 6 mg/kg/d in 3 divided doses × 21 d
Dracunculus medinensis (Guinea worm)	Drinking water containing infected copepods (crustaceans)	Dracunculiasis Allergic manifestations Local dermatologic lesions Syncope Nausea, vomiting	Diethylcarbamazapine or metronidazole for symptomatic relief; worm must be physically removed for cure (insert stick into ulcer and turn, allowing worm to wrap around it)
Onchocerca volvulus	Black fly bite	River blindness Varied ocular pathology secondary to intraocular microfilariae leading to blindness Onchocerciasis Dermatitis Lymphadenitis	Ivermectin 150 μg/kg PO × 1; repeat q 6 months; if eye involvement, start prednisone 1 mg/kg/day a few days prior to ivermectin
Loa loa	Deer fly bite	Loasis Fever, irritability Urticaria Conjunctivitis Recurrent subcutaneous inflammation	Ivermectin 400 μg/kg × 1, or Diethylcarbamazine 6 mg/kg/d in 3 divided doses × 21 d

bid = twice a day; *PO* = orally; *q* = every; *qd* = daily; *tid* = 3 times a day.

(3) Children: Furazolidone 1.5 mg/kg orally 4 times a day for 10 days (maximum = 100 mg/dose)

d. **Disposition**

—Patients can be discharged home with outpatient follow-up.

2. **Amoebiasis**

—acquired by ingestion of cysts of *Entamoeba histolytica* from contaminated food or water

a. **Clinical presentation** may include:

—fever

—bloody diarrhea

—lower abdominal and rectal pain

—enlarged liver

—weight loss

—Patients with noninvasive disease may be asymptomatic carriers.

b. **Diagnostic tests**

—examination of stool for ova and parasites

—immunofluorescence or ELISA tests for *E. histolytica*

—abdominal ultrasound to look for liver abscess

c. **Treatment**

(1) For asymptomatic cyst passers: paromomycin 25 mg/kg orally for 5–10 days (same dose for adults and children).

(2) For invasive amebic colitis and amebic liver abscess: metronidazole 500 mg orally 3 times a day (adults) or 35–50 mg/kg/day (children) plus paromomycin 25 mg/kg/day orally for 5–10 days.

VII. Tick-borne Infections

A. Lyme disease

—caused by the spirochete ***Borrelia burgdorferi***

—transmitted to humans from rodents and deer via the *Ixodes dammini* tick

—In the United States, most cases occur in the Northeast, Wisconsin, Minnesota, Oregon, and California.

1. **Clinical features**

—The disease is divided into 3 stages, but progression and manifestations vary widely.

a. **Stage 1**

—3 days to 1 month after the bite; classic sign is **erythema chronicum migrans** (ECM), a macule or papule at the tick bite site that expands into an erythematous, ring-like plaque with central clearing, found most commonly in the axillae, groin and thigh. The ECM rash is not universally present.

—resolves, untreated, after 3–4 weeks.

b. **Stage 2**

—develops weeks to months later

—involves the central and peripheral nervous systems in up to 20% of patients; symptoms range from peripheral neuropathy to meningoencephalitis.

—cardiovascular system involved in about 8% of patients; most common manifestation is A-V block

—involves musculoskeletal system in 60% of patients; a transient, asymmetric, oligoarthritis, especially of the knee, typically is seen.

c. **Stage 3**

—may occur years later; includes chronic arthritis, chronic skin lesions, or chronic neurologic syndromes. It is possible for the patient to present with Stage 2 or 3 without knowing that he or she had earlier stages of the disease.

2. **Diagnostic tests**

—Clinical diagnosis is the mainstay.

—Spirochetes can rarely be cultured from skin lesions.

—ELISA can be used as a screening test, but there are many false-positive results.

—Western blot is considered the "gold standard."

—The problem with all serologic tests is that they cannot distinguish patients with active disease from those with previous exposure.

3. **Treatment**

a. For erythema migrans, stage 1 or 2: amoxicillin 500 mg orally 3 times a day or doxycycline 100 mg orally 3 times a day for 3–4 weeks.

b. For patients with serious disease or those who have failed oral antibiotics: ceftriaxone 2 g/day IV or cefotaxime 2 g IV every 8 hours for 3–4 weeks.

c. Risks of empiric treatment outweigh benefits in those whose only evidence of disease is a positive serologic test.

4. **Disposition**

a. Patients with stage 1 disease can be discharged home with outpatient follow-up.

b. Patients with severe manifestations of stages 2 and 3 require hospitalization for IV antibiotics.

B. Rocky mountain spotted fever

—occurs most frequently in children and adolescents in the Mid-Atlantic states, but can occur throughout the eastern United States, and in some Western mountain states

—is caused by *Rickettsia rickettsi,* a gram-negative obligate intracellular organism transmitted by *Dermacentor* spp ticks that disseminates through the bloodstream and invades the endothelial lining of blood vessels, leading to a diffuse vasculitis and thrombotic occlusion of vessels

—Complications include shock, seizures, and death.

1. **Clinical features** may include:

—headache

—generalized malaise

—high fever [40°C (104°F)]

—rash appearing on day 3. Rash appears first on hands and feet and spreads axially. Eventually rash becomes purpuric.

—conjunctivitis

—periorbital or extremity edema

—splenomegaly (one third of cases)

—clouded sensorium, which progresses to coma

2. **Diagnostic tests**
   a. **CBC** to look for thrombocytopenia
   b. PT, APTT, d-dimer and fibrin split products to look for DIC
   c. **Chemistry panel** to look for hyponatremia
   d. **ECG** to look for ST segment elevation or PR prolongation
   e. Antibody titers for Rocky Mountain spotted fever. Results are not available immediately; treatment is begun before results are known.

3. **Treatment**

   —Antibiotics may be given orally (outpatient) or IV (inpatient):

   —Chloramphenicol 20 mg/kg every 6 hours for 7–10 days, or

   —Doxycycline 2–2.5 mg/kg every 12 hours for 14 days, or

   —Tetracycline 10 mg/kg every 6 hours for 7–10 days

   —*Note:* Tetracycline and doxycycline should be avoided in pregnant women and children younger than 9 years of age because they interfere with bone and tooth formation.

4. **Disposition**
   a. Most patients can be discharged home with outpatient follow-up.
   b. Patients with complications should be admitted for further management.

C. **Relapsing fever**

—causative organism is the *Borrelia* spirochete

—transmitted by the human body louse (**epidemic** disease) and by *Ornithodorus* ticks (**endemic** disease)

—if louse-borne, usually just one relapse

—if tick-borne, there may be several relapses

1. **Clinical features**
   a. **Symptoms** may include:

      —high fever

      —chills

      —myalgias and arthralgias

      —sudden resolution of symptoms 3–6 days after onset

—relapse of symptoms in 1 week

b. **Physical examination findings** may include:
—tachycardia
—tachypnea
—conjunctivitis
—petechiae
—hematuria
—hepatosplenomegaly

2. **Complications**
   a. Myocarditis
   b. Liver failure
   c. Intracranial hemorrhage
3. **Diagnostic tests**
   a. **Peripheral blood smear** prepared with Giemsa or Wright stain to isolate *Borrelia* spirochetes under dark-field microscopy
   b. **CBC** to look for thrombocytopenia
   c. **Urinalysis** to look for hematuria
   d. **PT, APTT,** and **bleeding time** to look for coagulopathies
   e. **LFTs** to look for hepatic dysfunction
4. **Treatment**
   a. **Antibiotics**
   —Doxycycline 100 mg orally twice a day or erythromycin 500 mg orally 4 times a day
   —given for 1 day if louse-borne disease, for 5 days if tick-borne disease
   b. The Jarisch-Herxheimer reaction occurs in many patients within 2 hours of starting antibiotics due to mass release of organisms into the bloodstream. This reaction consists of severe fever, rigors, drop in BP, and leukopenia. It is seen in many infectious diseases. Steroids are not helpful. Treatment is supportive with IV fluids for BP support and benzodiazepines for muscle relaxation.
5. **Disposition**
   a. Patients with mild disease can be discharged home with outpatient follow-up.
   b. Patients with severe disease or complications should be admitted to the hospital for further management.

D. Colorado tick fever

—causative organism is **coltivirus**

—transmitted by *Dermacentor andersoni* tick found in western United States and Canada

1. **Clinical features**
   a. **Symptoms** may include:
   —biphasic or "saddle-backed" fever
   —retroorbital headache
   —myalgias

—eye pain

b. **Physical examination findings** may include:
—conjunctival injection
—rash

2. **Complications**
—Meningoencephalitis
—Bleeding secondary to thrombocytopenia
—Pericarditis
—Myocarditis
—Epididymo-orchitis

3. **Diagnostic tests**
a. CBC to look for leukopenia and thrombocytopenia
b. Immunofluorescence test or ELISA for coltivirus
c. Standard laboratory studies if patient is admitted

4. **Treatment**
—is supportive
a. IV fluids
b. NSAIDs for analgesia (see Table 11-2)
—Aspirin must be avoided due to potential for Reye's syndrome (in children) and exacerbation of bleeding secondary to thrombocytopenia.

5. **Disposition**
a. Most patients can be discharged home with outpatient follow-up.
b. Patients with complications should be admitted to the hospital for further management.

E. Babesiosis

—caused by *Babesia* parasites, known as "piroplasms" because of their pear-shaped appearance during division

—transmitted from rodents to humans via the *Ixodes* tick

—because of the common tick vector, cotransmission of *B. burgdorferi,* the agent that causes Lyme disease, and *Ehrlichia,* the agent that causes human monocyte ehrlichiosis, is possible

—Disease usually is subclinical or mild in otherwise healthy people; it may be fatal in immunocompromised or asplenic patients, and in those with concurrent Lyme disease.

1. **Clinical features** may include:
—fever
—chills
—arthralgia and myalgia
—dark urine
—erythema chronicum migrans rash if concurrent Lyme disease

2. **Diagnostic tests**

a. **CBC** to look for anemia and thrombocytopenia
b. **Chemistry panel** to look for elevated blood urea nitrogen (BUN) and creatinine
c. **LFTs** to look for hemolysis
d. **Urinalysis** to look for hematuria
e. **Peripheral smear** to look for parasitized erythrocytes (resembling malaria)
f. **Indirect immunofluorescent antibody (IFA) test** or PCR to look for organism

3. **Treatment**
   a. Antibiotics
      —**Clindamycin** 600 mg orally or IV 3 times a day plus **quinine** 650 mg orally 3 times a day for 7–10 days
   b. Red blood cell (RBC) transfusion as needed

4. **Disposition**
   a. Most patients can be discharged home with outpatient follow-up.
   b. Patients with severe disease should be admitted to the hospital for IV antibiotics.

F. **Tularemia**

—also called "rabbit disease," "deerfly fever," and "marketmen's disease"

—caused by the gram-negative coccobacillus ***Francisella tularensis*** and transmitted to humans through ticks or contact with contaminated animal products

—Person-to-person transmission does not occur.

—More than half the cases reported in the United States are from Arkansas, Missouri, and Oklahoma.

1. **Clinical features** may include:
   —fever
   —chills
   —headache
   —malaise
   —rash
   —lymphadenopathy (ulceroglandular, most common type)
   —conjunctivitis (oculoglandular type)
   —pharyngitis (pharyngeal type)
   —pneumonitis (pneumonic type)

2. **Diagnostic tests**
   —If suspicious of tularemia, must alert laboratory workers to prevent occupational **exposure,** which may be **life-threatening.** A live attenuated vaccine is available for laboratory workers.
   a. **Chest radiograph** to look for patchy infiltrates or lobar consolidation with effusions

b. **CBC** to look for leukocytosis
c. **Blood** and **urine cultures** to look for causative organism
d. **ELISA** or **PCR** to look for causative organism

3. **Treatment**
a. **Streptomycin** 7.5–10 mg/kg (adults) or 15–20 mg/kg (children) IM every 12 hours for 10–14 days
b. Add 3rd-generation cephalosporin if meningitis also is present

4. **Disposition**
a. Patients with mild disease can be discharged home with outpatient follow-up.
b. Patients with severe disease should be admitted to the hospital for IV antibiotics.

VIII. Infections with Potential for Biological Disaster

A. Overview

—all are infectious with potential for airborne outbreak

—all are reportable illnesses

—examples include anthrax, plague, smallpox, Ebola, botulism, and others

B. Anthrax

—disease caused by *Bacillus anthracis,* a spore-forming, gram-positive bacillus

—3 types caused by:

inhalation of spores: pulmonary anthrax

ingestion of spores: GI anthrax

direct contact with infected skin lesions: cutaneous anthrax

1. **Clinical features**
a. Pulmonary anthrax
—prodrome of flu-like symptoms for 2–4 days
—abrupt onset of respiratory failure
—lymphadenopathy
—hemodynamic collapse
—high mortality despite early treatment
—person to person transmission usually does not occur
b. Cutaneous anthrax
—pruritus
—rash that progresses from papular → vesicular → deep black eschar
—most common sites for rash are head, forearms, and hands
—usually not fatal
c. GI anthrax
—abdominal pain

—nausea, vomiting

—fever

—may progress to sepsis

2. Diagnostic tests

a. Chest radiograph to look for widened mediastinum secondary to thoracic edema

b. Blood cultures to look for causative organism

c. Immunofluorescence or ELISA testing to isolate *B. anthracis*

3. Treatment

a. ABCs

b. Antibiotics:

—Ciprofloxacin 400 mg IV every 8–12 hours or doxycycline 200 mg IV once then 100 mg IV every 12 hours

—for children and pregnant women: penicillin 2 million units IV plus streptomycin 30 mg/kg IM every 12 hours

c. Prophylaxis:

—Ciprofloxacin 500 mg or doxycycline 100 mg orally twice a day for 4 weeks plus vaccine

—Vaccine is available commercially. An annual booster is required. It is administered routinely to military recruits.

4. Disposition

a. Patients with pulmonary or GI anthrax are admitted for IV antibiotics and monitoring of complications.

b. Patients with cutaneous anthrax can be discharged home with antibiotics and outpatient follow-up.

C. Pneumonic plague

1. Overview

—Plague is a disease caused by the gram-negative bacillus *Yersinia pestis.*

—It is transmitted by infected fleas, resulting in a possible airborne outbreak.

—Patient to patient transmission can occur with large aerosol droplets.

—Patients remain infectious until completing 72 hours of antimicrobial therapy.

—It carries 80%–100% mortality if untreated.

2. Clinical features

—fever

—cough with or without hemoptysis

—chest pain

—mucopurulent sputum

—shock

—bleeding diathesis

3. Diagnostic tests

a. Chest radiograph to look for patchy bronchial infiltrates
b. CBC to look for leukocytosis
c. LFTs to look for elevated AST and ALT
d. Serum antibody titers to *Y. pestis* in unvaccinated individuals
e. Immunofluorescence assay for *Y. pestis*

4. Treatment

a. ABCs
b. Antibiotics
—Streptomycin 30 mg/kg IM or doxycycline 100 mg IV twice a day
—for patients with meningitis: chloramphenicol
c. Prophylaxis (adults)
—Ciprofloxacin 500 mg or doxycycline 100 mg orally twice a day for 7 days

5. Disposition

—Patients are admitted to the hospital to receive 72 hours of antibiotics after which time they may be discharged if no complications develop.

D. Smallpox

—is an acute viral illness caused by the variola virus

—transmission route is airborne

—patients are infectious from the time of onset of the rash to the time the scabs disappear, approximately 3 weeks

1. Clinical features

—prodrome of fever and malaise (2–4 days) followed by

—rigors

—vomiting

—headache

—backache

—crops of vesicles more prominent on face and extremities and are all in the **same stage of eruption**

2. Diagnostic tests

—**PCR or ELISA testing to isolate the virus**

3. Treatment

a. is primarily supportive
b. quarantine of all infected patients
c. vaccine and vaccinia immune globulin (0.6 ml/kg IM) within 3 days of exposure. Supplies are limited.

4. Disposition

—Patients are admitted to isolation rooms with negative pressure ventilation. They are quarantined until they no longer are infectious.

Review Test

1. A 15-year-old boy who recently returned from a summer hiking trip to the Smoky Mountains presents to the emergency department. He complains of fever, severe headache, whole-body aches, and vomiting. No one else in the family is sick. Although the patient did not mention it, a rash is obvious on physical examination. Empiric therapy should include which of the following?

(A) Streptomycin
(B) Doxycycline
(C) Intravenous (IV) clindamycin
(D) Corticosteroids
(E) Erythromycin

2. A thin, HIV-positive man presents with progressive dyspnea on exertion and dry cough. His temperature is 101°F, pulse 112 beats per minute (bpm), blood pressure (BP) 120/80, respiratory rate (RR) 28–30, and oxygen saturation (0_2 sat) 96% on RA, drops to 92% on walking around the emergency department (ED). Physical examination reveals warm, dry skin; no lymphadenopathy; and lungs clear to auscultation. Complete blood cell count (CBC) shows a white blood cell (WBC) count of 3.6, chest radiograph is clear, $Pa0_2$ on RA is 85, and A-a gradient is 25. Which of the following should be included as first-line therapy in any empiric drug regimen?

(A) Trimethoprim-sulfamethoxazole (TMP-SMX)
(B) Dapsone
(C) Zidovudine, lamivudine, and indinavir
(D) Ceftriaxone
(E) TMP-SMX + IV methylprednisolone

3. An 8-year-old boy presents with a 2-day history of headache, sore throat, and "aching all over." The boy is scratching his leg, and physical examination reveals an annular lesion about 5 cm in diameter, red at the periphery with central clearing, and two adjacent similar smaller lesions. Which of the following antibiotics is recommended?

(A) Doxycycline
(B) Dicloxacillin
(C) Amoxicillin
(D) Trimethoprim-sulfamethoxazole (TMP-SMX)
(E) Ceftriaxone

4. Which of the following statements regarding rabies treatment is true?

(A) Passive immunization with human rabies immunoglobulin (HRIG) is still required in those previously immunized with human diploid cell rabies vaccine (HDCV) or rabies vaccine, adsorbed (RVA).
(B) Early administration of steroids may improve the outcome.
(C) Bites from domesticated dogs and cats should be routinely treated, because the risk of rabies outweighs the cost of empiric therapy.
(D) Vaccination dosage is not altered in pregnant women and children.
(E) Immunocompromised patients should receive only passive immunization.

Directions: The response options for Items 5–10 are the same. Each item will state the number of options to choose. Choose exactly this number.

Questions 5–10

Match the appropriate parasites to each antimicrobial agent:
(A) *Schistosoma hematobium*
(B) *Onchocerca volvulus*
(C) *Dracunculus medinensis*
(D) *Plasmodium vivax*
(E) *Wucheria bancrofti*
(F) *Toxocara canis*
(G) *Ascaris lumbricoides*
(H) *Necator americanus*
(I) *Clonorchis sinensis*
(J) *Trichuris trichiura*
(K) *Strongyloides stercoralis*
(L) *Diphyllobothrium latum*
(M) *Loa loa*
(N) *Giardia lamblia*

5. Albendazole (pick 3)

6. Praziquantel (pick 3)

7. Ivermectin (pick 4)

8. Diethylcarbamazine (pick 4)

9. Primaquine (pick 1)

10. Metronidazole (pick 2)

Directions: The response options for Items 11–19 are the same. You will be required to select one answer for each item in the set.

Questions 11–19

Match each disease with the most appropriate diagnostic test:
(A) Colposcopy
(B) ^{99}technetium bone scan
(C) Dark field microscopy
(D) Giemsa stain
(E) Whiff test
(F) Culture on Thayer-Martin medium
(G) Tzanck smear
(H) KOH test
(I) India ink examination of CSF

11. Herpes

12. Cryptococcal meningitis

13. Condyloma acuminata

14. Gonorrhea

15. Osteomyelitis

16. Malaria

17. Candida

18. Trichomoniasis

19. Syphilis

Answers and Explanations

1-B. Given the boy's history of travel to an endemic area and clinical findings of rash, headache, fever, myalgia/arthralgia, and vomiting, the physician should be suspicious of Rocky Mountain spotted fever (RMSF). Empiric therapy should include doxycycline, the preferred treatment for RMSF. If the physician suspects RMSF, treatment should be initiated immediately, because definitive test results are not readily available, and delays in proper antibiotic therapy can increase morbidity and mortality significantly. The differential diagnosis includes malaria, for which IV clindamycin is an acceptable treatment, and idiopathic thrombocytopenia, for which corticosteroids are an accepted therapy. Streptomycin and erythromycin are not indicated for the treatment of RMSF. Alternative antibiotics to doxycycline for RMSF include chloramphenicol or ciprofloxacin, not erythromycin or streptomycin.

2-A. The patient's history and physical and laboratory results are suggestive of mild to moderate *Pneumocystis carinii* pneumonia (PCP). Chest radiograph may be negative in up to 10% of cases of PCP; a clear chest radiograph does *not* rule out PCP, for which trimethoprim-sulfamethoxazole (TMP-SMX), 2 double-strength tablets orally per day for 21 days, is considered first-line therapy. Dapsone is considered second-line therapy in the treatment of PCP and should be initiated only if the patient has intolerable side effects with TMP-SMX and only after he or she has tested negative for G6PD deficiency. The choice of zidovudine, lamivudine, and indinavir is not an appropriate treatment, because the ED is not an appropriate setting to initiate antiretroviral therapy. Adequate follow-up of the patient once discharged from the ED or the hospital should, however, be ensured. Ceftriaxone would be appropriate for a bacterial, community-acquired pneumonia; however, the patient's clinical picture and chest radiograph are more consistent with PCP or a viral or atypical pneumonia than a bacterial pneumonia at this point. Intravenous (IV) methylprednisolone should be started within 72 hours of PCP therapy in cases of moderate-severe PCP ($PaO_2 < 70$ mm Hg and A-a gradient > 35 mm Hg) and stopped if definitive diagnosis of PCP is not made.

3-C. The clinical presentation points to Lyme disease. Amoxicillin 25–100 mg/kg/day given in 3 divided doses is the preferred treatment for Stage 1 Lyme disease in children younger than 12 years and pregnant women. Other options include cefuroxime 500 mg orally twice a day for 21 days; clarithromycin 500 mg orally twice a day for 14–21 days; or azithromycin 500 mg orally per day for 14–21 days. Doxycycline is incorrect, because it is the preferred treatment for Stage 1 Lyme disease in children older than 12 years old, adults, and nonpregnant women, and this patient is only 8 years old. Tetracycline antibiotics (including doxycycline) are contraindicated for children under 12 and pregnant women because they can cause tooth discoloration by interfering with the dental development process. Dicloxacillin and trimethoprim-sulfamethoxazole (TMP-SMX) are not indicated in the treatment of Lyme disease. Ceftriaxone may be indicated in treatment of Stage 2 Lyme disease with severe neurologic abnormalities, such as Lyme meningitis or encephalitis. The case presented here, however, is Stage 1 Lyme disease, identified by the typical erythema chronicum migrans rash.

4-D. Human diploid cell rabies vaccine (HDCV) or adsorbed rabies vaccine (RVA) should be given in 5 1-ml doses in the deltoid on days 0, 3, 7, 14, and 28 after exposure in adults, children, and infants. HDCV is an inactivated virus and is not contraindicated in pregnancy. People at high risk for exposure, such as veterinarians or spelunkers, may be given preexposure prophylaxis with HDCV or RVA. Passive immunization with human rabies immunoglobulin (HRIG) is *not* required in those who receive preexposure prophylaxis. Steroids actually are contraindicated in rabies, because animal studies have shown that steroids decrease the immune system's response to rabies vaccination. Routine treatment of bites from domestic dogs and cats is not required, because (except along the United States–Mexico border) the risk of rabies from domesticated dogs and cats is very low. Rabies immunoglobulin costs $565 to $725 per dose; rabies vaccine costs $141 per dose. The five rabies vaccine injections cause pain and induration at the site of inoculation in up to 80% of recipients and systemic reactions such as headache, malaise, nausea, and vomiting in up to 50%. Finally, immunosuppressed patients should receive both passive HRIG *and* vaccination with HDCV or RVA. However, because immunosuppression decreases the antibody response to the rabies vaccine, immunocompromised patients should have titers drawn after their last dose and receive additional doses if necessary.

5-G, H, J. Albendazole is recommended for treatment of infection by *Ascaris lumbricoides, Necator americanus,* and *Trichuris trichiura.*

6-A, I, L. Praziquantel is an appropriate treatment for infection by *Schistosoma hematobium, Clonorchis sinensis,* and *Diphyllobothrium latum.*

7-B, E, K, M. Ivermectin can be used to treat infection with *Onchocerca volvulus, Wucheria bancrofti, Strongyloides stercoralis,* and *Loa loa.*

8-C, E, F, M. Diethylcarbamazine is used to treat *Dracunculus medinensis, Wucheria bancrofti, Toxocara canis,* and *Loa loa.*

9-D. Primaquine is an accepted treatment for *Plasmodium vivax* infection.

10-C, N. Metronidazole is used to treat infection with *Dracunculus medinensis* and *Giardia lamblia.*

11-G. The Tzanck smear is used for diagnosis of herpes.

12-I. Cryptococcal meningitis may be detected via India ink examination of the cerebrospinal fluid (CSF).

13-A. Condyloma acuminata (venereal warts) can be detected with colposcopy.

14-F. Gonorrhea can be detected using culture on Thayer-Martin medium.

15-B. A ^{99}technetium bone scan can detect osteomyelitis.

16-D. Giemsa stain detects malaria.

17-H. The KOH test is used to detect infection with *Candida* spp.

18-E. The "whiff" test is used to detect trichomoniasis.

19-C. Syphilis may be detected via dark-field microscopy.

15

Hematology and Oncology Emergencies

I. Anemia

A. Overview

1. Definition

—**Anemia** is a decrease in red blood cell volume. Normal hematocrit is >37% in women and >42% in men.

2. Causes

a. Decreased red blood cell (RBC) synthesis

(1) Microcytic, hypochromic anemia may be caused by:

—iron deficiency

—sideroblastic anemia

(2) Normocytic, normochromic anemia may be caused by:

—anemia of chronic disease

—malignancy

—renal failure

—liver disease

(3) Macrocytic, normochromic anemia may be caused by:

—folate deficiency

—vitamin B_{12} deficiency

b. Increased RBC destruction may be seen in:

—autoimmune hemolytic anemia

—postoperative mechanical destruction of RBCs

—coagulopathies: thrombotic thrombocytopenic purpura (TTP), disseminated intravascular coagulation (DIC), hemolytic uremic syndrome (HUS)

—infections

—toxins (benzene, arsenic)

—inherited RBC abnormalities (hereditary spherocytosis, G6PD deficiency, sickle cell disease, thalassemia)
—Rh incompatibilities
—hypersplenism

c. **Acute blood loss (hemorrhage)** may result from:
—trauma
—GI bleed
—menorrhagia

B. Clinical features

—Clinical findings depend on the etiology of the anemia.

1. **Symptoms** may include:
—fatigue
—weakness
—dyspnea
—decreased exercise tolerance
—angina
—paresthesias, ataxia (B_{12} deficiency)
—sore tongue (folate deficiency)

2. **Physical examination findings** may include:
—pallor
—ecchymoses, petechiae
—guaiac-positive stool
—tachycardia
—tachypnea
—orthostatic hypotension
—jaundice
—splenomegaly
—lymphadenopathy

C. Diagnostic tests

1. For anemia secondary to acute blood loss

a. **Laboratory studies**
—**Complete blood count (CBC)** to look for low or dropping hematocrit
—Chemistry panel to look for elevated blood urea nitrogen (BUN) and creatinine to check for renal insufficiency; elevated direct bilirubin and lactate dehydrogenase (LDH) to check for hemolysis
—Urinalysis to look for hemoglobinuria

b. **Imaging studies**
—**Ultrasonography** of abdomen and pelvis to look for **splenomegaly** or **free fluid**
—Nasogastric lavage or endoscopy to look for upper gastrointestinal (GI) bleed

—Colonoscopy to look for lower GI bleed

2. If acute blood loss is not present, workup of other etiologies of anemia generally is not performed in the ED. Useful tests for other etiologies may include:

—**reticulocyte** count to calculate reticulocyte index (RI). An RI >2% suggests excess RBC destruction; an RI <2% suggests inadequate RBC production.

—**peripheral smear** to look for Heinz bodies (G6PD deficiency), spherocytes (hereditary spherocytosis), schistocytes (hemolysis) or Helmet cells (TTP)

—folate and B_{12} levels to look for deficiency

—direct Coombs test to look for autoimmune hemolytic anemia

—hemoglobin electrophoresis to look for sickle cell disease and thalassemia

—haptoglobin to look for decrease (hemolysis)

—iron level, ferritin, and transferrin iron-binding capacity to look for iron deficiency anemia

—bone marrow biopsy to look for malignancy

D. Treatment

1. Stabilization of airway, breathing, and circulation (ABCs), including supplemental oxygen
2. Intravenous (IV) hydration
3. Blood transfusion if symptomatic
4. Discontinuation of any toxins
5. Hematology consult
6. Outpatient therapies may include:

—corticosteroids

—B_{12}

—folate

—antithymocyte globulin

—erythropoietin

E. Disposition

1. Patients who are symptomatic (e.g., dyspneic, tachycardic, tachypneic, hypotensive) are admitted.
2. Most other patients can be discharged home with outpatient follow-up in one week.

II. Sickle Cell Crisis

A. Overview

1. **Definition**

—**Sickle cell disease** is an autosomal recessive disorder.

—People with **sickle cell disease** are homozygous for the sickle cell gene.

—People with **sickle cell trait** are heterozygous for the sickle cell gene.

2. **Risk factors** include:

—black race

—family history

3. **Complications (Table 15-1)** include:

—splenic sequestration

—acute chest syndrome

—transient aplastic crisis

B. Clinical features

1. **Symptoms** may include severe, poorly localized diffuse abdominal, extremity, or chest pain of acute onset, without other associated symptoms such as fever, vomiting or diarrhea.

2. **Physical examination findings** may include:

—an acutely ill-appearing patient who is writhing in pain

—no peritoneal signs

—normal bowel sounds

C. Diagnostic tests

1. **Laboratory studies**

—**CBC** to look for leukocytosis (>18,000/mL), left shift, and a decreased hematocrit (< 6 g/dL). Platelet count usually is normal or slightly elevated.

—**Chemistry panel** to look for electrolyte abnormalities.

—**LFTs** to differentiate sickle cell crisis from other diagnoses such as cholecystitis, pancreatitis, appendicitis, and bowel infarction

2. **Imaging studies**

—**Abdominal computed tomography (CT)** to differentiate sickle cell

Table 15-1. Complications of Sickle Cell Anemia

Complication	Symptoms and Treatment
Splenic sequestration	Usually occurs in growing children Symptoms: left upper quadrant pain, splenomegaly Can cause anemia and hypovolemic shock
Acute chest syndrome	Symptoms: chest pain, shortness of breath Chest radiograph: pulmonary infiltrates secondary to vaso-occlusion May require exchange transfusion
Transient aplastic crisis	Occurs secondary to viral infection, which greatly drops hematocrit Patients should be isolated to prevent spread to others with sickle cell disease

crisis from other conditions such as cholecystitis, pancreatitis, appendicitis and bowel infarction.

D. Treatment

1. **Intravenous fluids** for hydration
2. Supplemental **oxygen** if patient is hypoxic
3. **Analgesia**

—Acetaminophen with codeine or hydrocodone given orally may be adequate for moderate pain.

—IV opiate analgesia may be necessary for severe pain.

E. Disposition

1. Patients who improve after supportive treatment and analgesia and have stable vital signs may be discharged home.
2. Patients in whom pain persists after two doses of opiate analgesia should be admitted for further work-up.
3. The possibility of drug-seeking behavior should be considered in patients who present frequently.

III. Platelet Disorders

A. Idiopathic thrombotic thrombocytopenia (ITP)

1. Overview

a. Definition

—**ITP** is thrombocytopenia in the absence of any infection, toxin exposure, or underlying disease process that would account for it.

—It is a diagnosis of exclusion.

b. Cause

—ITP is caused by the presence of IgG autoantibodies on the surface of platelets.

c. Incidence

—ITP has two age peaks: in childhood, following infection (common), and in adulthood, as a chronic condition (less common)

—The adult form is more often noted in women.

2. Clinical findings

a. **Symptoms** may include:

—easy bruising

—gingival bleeding

—heavy menses

—spontaneous bleeding

b. **Physical examination findings** may include:

—petechial hemorrhages

—**absence of splenomegaly**

—guaiac-positive stool

—neurologic deficits (secondary to intracranial bleed)

3. Diagnostic tests

a. CBC to look for thrombocytopenia

b. **Imaging studies**

—CT scan of the head to look for intracranial bleed

—Abdominal ultrasonography to look for normal-sized spleen

4. Treatment

a. ABCs

b. Intravenous immune globulin (IVIG) 1–2 g/kg once

c. Prednisone 1–2 mg/kg IV

d. Platelet transfusion if actively bleeding (make sure patient does not actually have TTP [see section III B] rather than ITP)

e. Hematology consult

5. Disposition

a. Patients with active bleeding or those with platelet counts < 20,000 are admitted to the hospital for further management.

b. Asymptomatic patients may be discharged home with outpatient follow-up within 48 hours.

B. Thrombotic Thrombocytopenic Purpura (TTP)

1. Overview

a. **Definition**

—**TTP** is a disease process that results from deposition of von Willebrand factor multimers into microvasculature, which leads to platelet aggregation and shearing of RBCs as they pass through the vessel.

b. **Causes**

—The etiology is unknown.

c. **Risk factors** include:

—female gender

—age 10–45 years

—pregnancy

—drugs: ticlopidine, H_2 receptor antagonists, contraceptives, penicillin, chemotherapeutic agents

—autoimmune disorders

—infection (including *Escherichia coli* O157: H7)

—malignancy

d. **Prognosis**

—If diagnosed and treated, there is an 80% survival rate

—If the diagnosis is missed, there is an 80% mortality rate

2. Clinical features

a. The **diagnostic pentad** consists of:

—altered mental status (90%)

—thrombocytopenia: 5000–100,000 platelets/mm^3

—fever (seen in 50% to 90% of patients)

—renal dysfunction (seen in 50% to 85% of patients)

—anemia (microangiopathic hemolytic type)

b. Symptoms and **physical examination findings** may include:

—waxing and waning of mental status secondary to thrombosis in cerebral vessels

—petechiae, purpura, or ecchymoses secondary to thrombocytopenia

—oliguria secondary to renal dysfunction

—pallor and jaundice secondary to anemia

3. Diagnostic tests

a. Laboratory studies

—**CBC** to look for anemia and thrombocytopenia

—**Peripheral smear** to look for hemolysis, schistocytes, and helmet cells

—**Chemistry panel** to look for elevated BUN, creatinine, LDH, and bilirubin (unconjugated >conjugated).

—**Reticulocyte count** to look for elevation

—Haptoglobin to look for decrease

—**Urinalysis** to look for hematuria, red cell casts, and proteinuria

—Remainder of sepsis work-up if febrile: chest radiograph, urine culture, blood culture

b. Imaging studies

—CT scan of the head to look for infarcts

—Chest radiograph if patient is febrile

4. Treatment

a. Platelets *must not be transfused.*

—Platelets are thought to "fuel the fire," resulting in more thrombi in the microvasculature.

b. Daily plasmapheresis (PP) until platelet count normalizes

c. Fresh-frozen plasma (FFP) or cryoprecipitate transfusion until PP available

d. Packed red blood cell (PRBC) transfusion as needed

e. For refractory cases (but all of these are controversial):

—corticosteroids

—antiplatelet agents

—vincristine

—splenectomy

5. Disposition

—Patients are admitted to the intensive care unit.

C. Disseminated intravascular coagulation (DIC)

1. Overview

a. Definition

—DIC is an acquired coagulation disorder that may complicate diseases involving hemorrhage or tissue hypoperfusion.

—It occurs when normal hemostasis mechanisms "overshoot," producing persistently elevated levels of thrombin and consuming platelets and fibrinogen.

—Fibrinolysis results in the production of fibrin degradation products, causing hemostatic mechanisms to be re-triggered.

b. Risk factors include:

—obstetric complications: placental abruption, septic abortion, chorioamnionitis

—hemolysis: transfusion reactions, sickle cell disease

—congenital heart disease: aneurysms, vascular malformations

—hypoxia and hypoperfusion: cardiogenic shock, hemorrhage

—trauma: burns, tissue destruction

—envenomations

—sepsis

—malignancy

—hypo- or hyperthermia

2. Clinical findings

a. Patients at risk for DIC have worse bleeding or shock than would be expected from the underlying clinical condition.

b. Other features may include:

—acute renal failure

—generalized ecchymoses or petechiae

—central nervous system (CNS) or pulmonary bleeds

3. Diagnostic tests

a. CBC to look for thrombocytopenia

b. Coagulation profile to look for elevated prothrombin time (PT) and thrombin, variable activated partial thromboplastin time (APTT), and decreased fibrinogen.

c. Fibrin split products to look for elevation

d. Chemistry panel to look for elevated BUN and creatinine

e. CT scan of the head to look for intracranial bleeds

4. Treatment

—The fundamental tenet in treating DIC is to treat the underlying disorder.

—Other therapies have met with variable success and acceptance:

a. Heparin

—Activates the antithrombin III system, inhibits thrombin.

—Loading dose is 80 U/kg, followed by 18 U/kg/hr IV continuous drip

b. Cryoprecipitate: contains fibrinogen.

c. Platelets

—Transfusion for level $< 50,000$ for actively bleeding patients

—One unit of platelets raises the platelet count by 10,000.

5. Disposition

—Patients are admitted to the intensive care unit.

IV. Inherited Disorders of Coagulation

A. Hemophilia A and B

1. Overview

a. Definition

—The hemophilias are autosomal recessive X-linked disorders, and therefore occur almost exclusively in men.

—Patients often present with various forms of hemorrhage (see section IV A 2).

b. Risk factors include:

—family history

—male gender

2. Clinical findings may include:

—intramuscular bleed or compartment syndrome

—GI bleed

—retroperitoneal bleed

—neuropathy from local hemorrhagic nerve compression

—hemarthrosis

3. Diagnostic tests

—Most adult patients with hemophilia give a history of their disease.

a. Coagulation profile to look for abnormal PT, APTT, or bleeding time

b. CBC to look for thrombocytopenia

4. Treatment

a. Bleeding from minor trauma sometimes responds to simple compression

b. More severe complications, such as intracranial bleed, require replacement of the requisite clotting factor.

(1) Hemophilia A requires replacement of **factor VIII,** which is best given as **cryoprecipitate,** or factor VIII:C, which can be obtained separately.

—The dose to raise the level of factor VIII by 25% is about 15 units/kg. Each bag of cryoprecipitate contains 80–100 units.

—For acute bleeds, re-administration usually is needed at least every 24 hours until bleeding is controlled.

(2) Hemophilia B requires replacement of **factor IX,** which is found in **fresh frozen plasma (FFP).** A dose of 20 units/kg of factor IX raises the level 25%.

(3) **Desmopressin acetate** has been found to raise levels of factor VIII by 3- to 6-fold in some cases. The dose is 0.3–0.4 μg/kg IV over 30 minutes.

c. **Drainage of large hemarthroses** if the patient presents within the first few hours. Because infusion of clotting factor may promote intraarticular clot organization, any drainage should be done during or just after infusion. Joint aspiration is contraindicated in patients with antibodies to the depleted clotting factor. Clotting factor levels must be maintained above 25% for several days after drainage to prevent rebleeding. The joint should be immobilized.

d. Analgesia

—Pain control for these patients must exclude nonsteroidal anti-inflammatory drugs (NSAIDs) or intramuscular (IM) injections, due to the risk of bleeding complications.

5. Disposition

a. Patients with minor, controlled bleeding can be discharged into the care of their hematologist.

b. Patients with treated hemarthrosis can be discharged into the care of their hematologist and should be referred to physical therapy.

c. All other cases should be admitted with hematology involvement.

B. von Willebrand disease

1. Overview

a. Definition

—von Willebrand disease is an autosomal dominant disorder with incomplete penetrance that affects men and women equally.

—Possession of the gene does not always produce clinically significant bleeding.

—Because von Willebrand factor mediates platelet adhesion to subendothelium in cases of vessel wall compromise, its pattern of bleeding resembles that of platelet disorders.

b. Incidence

—von Willebrand disease is the most common inherited bleeding disorder, affecting up to 1% of the global population.

2. Clinical findings

a. Many patients are unaware that they have the disease until they experience excessive bleeding after trauma or surgery. Severe cases of von Willebrand disease can mimic hemophilia.

b. Symptoms and **physical examination findings** may include:

—pattern of easy and excessive bruising

—menorrhagia

—frequent epistaxis

—GI bleeding

3. Diagnostic tests

a. Coagulation profile to look for abnormal PT, APTT, or bleeding time

b. CBC to look for thrombocytopenia

4. Treatment

a. For severe bleeding, as in the case of trauma, administration of **factor VIII:vWF.**

—**Factor VIII:vWF** is different from the product used in hemophilia A (VIII:C); VIII:C has no utility in von Willebrand disease.

—Cryoprecipitate contains about 100 units of VIII:vWF per bag. The patient should receive about 10 units/kg to raise the level of vWF by 25%.

b. **Desmopressin acetate** will raise the level of von Willebrand factor in some cases. The dose is 0.3 μg/kg IV over 30 minutes.

5. **Disposition**
   a. Most patients with minor bleeding can be discharged with outpatient follow-up within 48 hours and restriction of NSAIDs.
   b. Patients with severe bleeding should be admitted with the involvement of a hematologist.

V. Transfusion Reactions

A. Overview

1. **Definition**

—Immunologic adverse reactions to transfusion of blood and blood products may take many forms. The emergency physician is most concerned with the immediate hemolytic reaction, most often seen with ABO blood group incompatibility.

2. **Complications** may include:

—renal failure

—shock

—DIC

B. Clinical findings

1. **Symptoms** may include:

—anxiety

—chest pain

—dyspnea

2. **Physical examination findings** may include:

—fever

—tachycardia

—hypotension

C. Diagnostic tests

1. Initial diagnosis is made by the clinical constellation of signs and symptoms.
2. Diagnosis can be confirmed by:

—repeat, careful comparison of hanging blood type to patient's blood type.

—comparison by the blood bank of patient's blood posttransfusion to hanging blood.

D. Treatment

1. Immediate discontinuation of the transfusion.
2. Hydration to prevent renal failure
3. Documentation of the number of milliliters of blood transfused followed

by return of the remainder of the incompatible blood (along with a new sample of the patient's blood) to the blood bank for analysis.

E. Disposition

1. Most patients receiving blood in the emergency department (ED) are admitted to the hospital for their underlying disorder.
2. Anyone receiving an "outpatient" transfusion in the emergency department must wait until blood bank analysis of the incompatible blood is complete before discharge can be considered.

VI. Neutropenic Fever

A. Overview

—Patients with a history consistent with immunocompromise who present with unexplained fever must be treated very aggressively. These patients can become extremely sick within hours.

1. **Definition**

   —Neutropenia is an absolute neutrophil count (ANC) of <500 cell/mm^3. It is often associated with more severe bacterial, viral, and fungal infections.

2. **Causes** of immunosuppression (Table 15-2) may include:

   —human immunodeficiency virus (HIV)

   —cancer

   —trauma

   —asplenia

   —anti–transplant rejection drugs

3. **Risk factors** include:

   —history of invasive procedures or indwelling devices

   —recent bacterial or fungal infection

   —recent use of oral antibiotics

   —chemotherapeutic agents associated with bone marrow suppression (e.g., busulfan, melphalan, nitrosoureas, cyclophosphamide, mercap-

Table 15-2. Causes of Immunosuppression in the Emergency Patient

Cause	Mechanism Causing Immunosuppression
HIV	Lack of CD4 cells
Cancer	Tumor load, chemotherapy
Trauma	Poor perfusion, burns
Asplenia	Infection with encapsulated organisms
Organ transplantation	Chronic steroid or immunosuppressive treatment

topurine, taxanes, anthracylines, anthraquinones, mithramycin, actinomycin D, methotrexate, cytarabine, cisplatin, and procarbazine)

B. Clinical findings may include:

—fever

—change in mental status

—dehydration

—hypotension

—tachycardia

C. Diagnostic tests (sepsis work-up)

1. Laboratory tests

a. Complete blood count to look for ANC and leukopenia

b. Blood and urine cultures to identify causative organism before giving antibiotics

c. Lumbar puncture to look for etiology of altered mental status

2. Imaging studies

a. Chest radiograph to look for infiltrates

b. CT scan of the head to look for etiology of altered mental status

c. Sinus films if other sources are negative

D. Treatment

1. Empiric treatment with broad-spectrum antibiotics, usually an aminoglycoside and antipseudomonal penicillin

2. Intravenous hydration

3. Antifungal therapy: may be considered for relapsed fever

4. Antiviral therapy: may be considered for suspected herpes encephalitis

E. Disposition

—Patients with neutropenia or immunocompromise and fever should be admitted to a reverse isolation bed.

VII. Tumor Lysis Syndrome

A. Overview

1. Definition

—**Tumor lysis syndrome** occurs when a large amount of neoplastic tissue is destroyed by chemotherapeutic agents, releasing intracellular contents into the bloodstream.

2. Risk factors

—It occurs most commonly in patients with a high tumor burden, such as in high-grade lymphomas and leukemias, and less commonly in solid tumors.

B. Symptoms and **physical examination findings** may include:

—muscle cramps

—tetany

C. Diagnostic tests

1. Chemistry profile to look for hyperkalemia, hyperphosphatemia, hypocalcemia, hyperuricemia and elevated BUN, creatinine, and LDH
2. Electrocardiogram (ECG) to look for arrhythmias secondary to electrolyte disturbances

D. Treatment

1. ABCs
2. Aggressive intravenous hydration
3. Correction of electrolyte abnormalities
4. **Early dialysis** should be considered for potassium >6mEq/L, phosphate >10mg/dL, creatinine >10mg/dL, uric acid >10mg/dL

E. Disposition

—Patients with tumor lysis syndrome are admitted to the hospital for further management.

VIII. Superior Vena Cava Syndrome

A. Overview

1. **Definition**

   —**Superior vena cava syndrome** is obstruction or infiltration of the superior vena cava by neoplasm or thrombosis.

2. **Risk factors** include:

   —cancers of lung, breast, and testes

   —lymphoma

   —thoracic aortic aneurysm

   —goiter

   —pericardial constriction

   —presence of central venous catheter

B. Clinical findings

1. **Symptoms** may include:

   —shortness of breath

   —cough

   —swelling of face, trunk, and upper extremities

   —dysphagia

   —chest pain

2. **Physical examination findings** may include:

   —periorbital edema

—jugular venous distention

—palpable supraclavicular mass

—papilledema on funduscopic examination

C. Diagnostic tests

1. CBC to look for leukocytosis, thrombocytosis
2. Radiograph or CT scan of chest to look for a mass, hilar adenopathy, or pleural effusion

D. Treatment

1. Temporary treatment in the ED for patients with SVCS includes:

—elevation of the head of the bed

—reduction of venous pressure with diuretics and glucocorticoids (e.g., furosemide, 40 mg IV, plus methylprednisolone, 125 mg IV)

—avoidance of IV access in upper extremities

2. Definitive treatment must be carried out by the patient's oncologist or hematologist and may include:

—chemotherapy

—localized radiotherapy

E. Disposition

1. Patients with early signs of superior vena cava syndrome may be treated as outpatients by an oncologist.
2. Patients with advanced signs of superior vena cava syndrome often require admission.

IX. Hyperviscosity Syndrome

A. Overview

1. **Definition**

—**Hyperviscosity syndrome** is characterized by increased viscosity of the blood due to an increase in formed elements (erythrocytes or leukocytes) or proteins.

2. **Risk factors** include:

—Waldenström's macroglobulinemia

—multiple myeloma

—cryoglobulinemia

—leukemia

—polycythemia vera

B. Clinical findings

1. **Symptoms** may include:

—**the classic triad: increased bleeding, visual changes,** and **neurologic changes**

—fatigue

—anorexia

—weight loss

—headache

—dizziness

—somnolence/lethargy/coma

—seizure

—auditory changes

2. **Physical examination findings** may include:

—venous engorgement in retina or bulbar conjunctiva

—retinal microaneurysms, hemorrhages, or exudates

—rales

—bleeding of mucosal surfaces

—respiratory distress

C. Diagnostic tests

1. Coagulation profile to look for abnormal PT or APTT
2. CBC to look for anemia (secondary to expanded plasma volume, which results in hemodilution) and leukocytosis
3. Peripheral smear or erythrocyte sedimentation rate (ESR) to look for rouleaux formation
4. Chemistry panel to look for electrolyte abnormalities

D. Treatment

1. Temporizing measures in the ED may include:

—IV hydration

—diuresis

—phlebotomy if recommended by hematologist/oncologist

2. Definitive treatment includes leukapheresis or plasmapheresis.

E. Disposition

—Patients are admitted to the hospital for further management.

X. Malignant Effusions

A. Overview

1. Definition

—**Malignant effusions** are exudates that occur when tumor disrupts capillary endothelium or impairs lymphatic drainage.

—Patients with malignant pericardial effusion usually cannot be distinguished at first from patients with pericardial effusion of other origin.

2. **Risk factors** include:

—congestive heart failure

—pneumonia

—malignancy

3. **Prognosis**

—The prognosis for malignant effusions is poor.

B. Malignant pleural effusion

1. **Clinical findings** may include:

—dyspnea

—tachypnea

—cough

—pleuritic chest wall pain

2. **Diagnostic tests**

a. Chest radiograph

—Blunting of the costophrenic angle corresponds to 175–500 ml of contained fluid.

—Opacification of a hemithorax corresponds to >1500 ml of contained fluid.

b. Pleural tap to look for malignant cells on cytologic examination. Malignant effusions are exudative in nature and often are bloody and lymphocytic. (See Table 3-2 in Chapter 3 for laboratory findings of exudates).

3. **Treatment**

a. ABCs, including supplemental oxygen

b. Drainage of pleural effusion.

—Patients experiencing respiratory distress should have effusion drained by tube thoracostomy or large-volume therapeutic tap.

—Removal of more than 1500 ml of pleural fluid may cause reexpansion pulmonary edema in some cases.

c. Definitive therapy may include:

—sclerotherapy

—pleural stripping

—chemotherapy or radiotherapy

—pleuroperitoneal shunt

4. **Disposition**

—Patients with newly diagnosed malignant pleural effusion should be admitted.

C. Malignant pericardial effusion

1. **Clinical findings**

a. **Symptoms** may include:

—anxiety

—chest pain

—dyspnea
—preference for sitting upright or leaning forward

b. **Physical examination findings** may include:
—jugular venous distension
—distant heart sounds
—pericardial friction rub
—pericardial tamponade (see Chapter 2 VI)
—pulsus paradoxus

2. **Diagnostic tests**
   a. ECG to look for tachycardia, low voltage, and nonspecific ST-T wave changes
   b. Chest radiograph to look for enlarged cardiac silhouette
   c. CT scan of chest to look for pericardial effusion, pericardial thickening, and adjacent mass
   d. Echocardiogram to localize effusion and assess cardiac wall motion
3. **Treatment**
   a. ABCs, including supplemental oxygen
   b. Analgesia as needed
   c. Pericardiocentesis for acutely symptomatic patients, preferably with echocardiography localization. Posterior effusions are particularly difficult to drain and may require surgical intervention.
   d. Cardiothoracic or oncology consultations as needed
4. **Disposition**

—Symptomatic patients with pericardial effusion should be admitted.

XI. Spinal Cord Compression

A. Overview

1. **Definition**

—Spinal cord compression occurs in patients with cancer when there is vertebral body collapse at the site of bony infiltration, or with direct epidural tumor extension.

2. **Risk factors** include:

—malignancy, especially with cancers of breast, lung and prostate, and lymphoma

B. Clinical findings

1. **Symptoms** may include:

—back pain: localized or radicular, not relieved by rest

—weakness: inability to get out of a chair, inability to ambulate

—urinary incontinence

—constipation

2. **Physical examination findings** may include:

—lower extremity weakness: inability to heel-walk or toe-walk, inability to do deep knee bends

—hyperactive deep tendon reflexes

C. Diagnostic tests

1. Radiographs of spine to look for bony degeneration at the level of neurological compromise: 70% of lesions occur in the thoracic spine, 20% are lumbosacral, and 10% are cervical.
2. Magnetic resonance imaging (MRI) is the diagnostic test of choice to look for specific location of lesion.

D. Treatment

1. Emergency treatment of spinal cord compression must be instituted early, often before the completion of definitive study, to preserve as much function as possible.
2. **Neurosurgery** and oncology consults are needed.
3. **Dexamethasone**

   —Initial loading dose recommendations range from 10 mg to 100 mg IV followed by 4 to 24 mg IV every 6 hours.

   —Dosing should be chosen in conjunction with neurosurgical or oncology consultant.
4. Definitive treatment for spinal cord compression may include:

   —laminectomy

   —radiotherapy

   —chemotherapy

E. Disposition

—All patients with initial diagnosis of spinal cord compression should be admitted.

XII. Paraneoplastic Syndromes

A. Overview

—The paraneoplastic syndromes are a diverse group of diseases associated with cancer, but not directly due to tumor invasion or spread.

—Most involve **ectopic production of endocrine hormones.**

—These syndromes are not treatable in the emergency department, but correct identification may aid in diagnosis of an underlying tumor.

B. Clinical findings

1. **Fever**

   —Fever occurs in many patients with cancer and often cannot be attributed to an infectious cause.

   —It is most commonly associated with Hodgkin's disease, renal cell carcinoma and osteogenic sarcoma.

—Until infectious causes are ruled out, cancer patients presenting with fever should be treated as immunocompromised and cared for accordingly.

2. **Weight loss** and anorexia

   —These findings are common in patients with cancer, leading to a wasting phenomenon not wholly explained by decreased intake.

   —Tumor necrosis factor is thought to be responsible for the reduction in fat stores that is commonly seen.

3. **Ectopic endocrine** hormone production is common (Table 15-3).

4. **Neurologic abnormalities** noted include:

   —amyotrophic lateral sclerosis

   —subacute motor neuropathy

   —peripheral and autonomic neuropathies, not directly due to local tumor invasion.

   —Occult cancer should be suspected in any patient with the diseases just listed above.

5. **Muscular abnormalities** associated with cancer include:

   —dermatomyositis

   —polymyositis

   —Eaton-Lambert syndrome. **Eaton-Lambert syndrome** can be differentiated from myasthenia gravis by an improvement of muscle strength with exercise, and a poor response to edrophonium

6. **Blood components** may be altered (Table 15-4).

Table 15-3. Common Endocrine Abnormalities Associated with Cancer

Ectopic peptide	Syndrome	Most commonly associated tumors
ACTH	**Cushing syndrome:** hypokalemia, hyperglycemia, hypertension, muscle weakness	Small cell carcinoma of lung
Antidiuretic hormone (vasopressin)	**Syndrome of inappropriate ADH production (SIADH):** water intoxication, change in mental status, coma, death	Small cell carcinoma of lung
Parathyroid hormone-like peptide	**Hypercalcemia** tetany obtundation	Multiple myeloma Lung and breast cancer Lymphoma Renal cell carcinoma
Gonadotropins (e.g.: hCG)	**Altered sex characteristics:** precocious puberty, gynecomastia, oligomenorrhea	Germ cell tumors Choriocarcinoma Pituitary tumors
Insulin and insulin-like growth factor	**Hypoglycemia** Altered mental status	Islet cell tumors Hepatocellular carcinoma

ACTH = adrenocorticotropic hormone; *ADH* = antidiuretic hormone; *hCG* = human chorionic gonadotropin

Table 15-4. Common Paraneoplastic Hematologic Abnormalities

Abnormality	Associated malignancy
Erythrocytosis	Renal cell carcinoma, hepatocellular carcinoma, others
Pure red cell aplasia	Thymoma
Autoimmune hemolytic anemia	B cell neoplasms, solid tumors
Paraneoplastic granulocytosis	Tumors secreting colony-stimulating-factor (CSF)
Eosinophilia	Hodgkin's disease
Thrombocytosis	All cancers

XIII. Complications of Radiotherapy (Table 15-5)

Table 15-5. Injury Associated With Radiotherapy

System Affected	Type of Injury
Eyes	Cataracts
Fetus	Microcephaly, growth retardation, hydrocephaly, microphthalmia, blindness, spina bifida
GI tract	Esophagitis, esophageal stricture, gastritis, proctitis
Heart	Myocardial fibrosis, constrictive pericarditis
Kidney	Nephritis
Lung	Pulmonary fibrosis
Reproductive system	Sterility
Skin	Radiodermatitis, poor wound healing, ulcers
Spinal cord	Transverse myelitis

XIV. Complications of Chemotherapy (Table 15-6)

Table 15-6. Common Toxic Effects of Chemotherapeutic Agents

Effect	Agent
Cystitis	Cyclophosphamide
Nausea, vomiting	Procarbazine, cisplatin, cyclophosphamide, anthracyclines, nitrosureas, busulfan, melphalan
Pulmonary fibrosis	Cyclophosphamide, bleomycin, busulfan, melphalan
Nephropathy	Streptozocin, nitrosureas, cisplatin
Mucositis	Methotrexate, actinomycin D, anthracyclines
Diarrhea	Actinomycin D, anthracyclines, fluorouracil
Encephalopathy	Cytarabine
Neuropathy	Vinca alkaloids, taxanes
Cardiomyopathy	Anthroquinones, anthracyclines
VIII nerve damage	Cisplatin

Review Test

1. A 21-year-old man presents to the emergency department with a large, swollen knee. He does not remember any recent injury. He gives a history of hemophilia A. Which of the following therapies will best promote clotting in this patient?

(A) Cryoprecipitate
(B) Dexamethasone
(C) Fresh frozen plasma (FFP)
(D) Heparin
(E) Platelets

2. A 32-year-old woman presents to the emergency department with a history of heavy vaginal bleeding for 14 days. She says she has always had heavy periods but she "just can't take it anymore." She has no past medical history except for frequent nosebleeds. She notes that her father also gets frequent nosebleeds, and bled a lot during a recent surgery. The patient has no fever. Serum pregnancy test is negative. Which of the following disorders is most likely to account for the patient's symptoms?

(A) Hemophilia A
(B) Hemophilia B
(C) Liver disease
(D) Vitamin K deficiency
(E) von Willebrand disease

3. A 38-year-old woman presents to the emergency department with fever and shortness of breath. The patient recalls being hospitalized as a child after a bicycle accident, but has no other medical history. Physical examination reveals temperature of 101.2°F, occasional crackles at the left lung base, and a small scar in the left upper quadrant of her abdomen. This patient is most likely to be at risk for infection from which of the following organisms?

(A) *Legionella pneumophila*
(B) *Mycoplasma pneumoniae*
(C) *Pseudomonas aeruginosa*
(D) *Staphylococcus aureus*
(E) *Streptococcus pneumoniae*

4. A 43-year-old woman with a history of intravenous (IV) drug abuse and hepatitis C presents to the emergency department with weakness. She is found to have a massive upper gastrointestinal (GI) bleed, with a hemoglobin of 6. Two units of blood are obtained from the blood bank. While the first one is being transfused, the patient develops fever, anxiety, and severe shortness of breath. The blood transfusion is halted. Which of the following is the most appropriate next step?

(A) Infusion of cryoprecipitate
(B) Infusion of the second pack of red blood cells
(C) Infusion of normal saline
(D) Infusion of platelets
(E) Infusion of heparin

5. Patients with tumor lysis syndrome are most likely to have which of the following laboratory abnormalities?

(A) Hypercalcemia
(B) Hyperuricemia
(C) Hyperglycemia
(D) Hypophosphatemia
(E) Hypokalemia

Questions 6 and 7

A 62-year-old woman with a history of breast cancer, status post-right-sided lumpectomy and radiotherapy, presents to the emergency department with a persistent cough, shortness of breath, and difficulty swallowing. She also notes that her "arms are getting fat" and her rings no longer fit.

6. Which of the following treatments is most appropriate at this time?

(A) Aggressive hydration
(B) Dexamethasone
(C) Elevation of the head of the bed
(D) Phlebotomy of 2 units
(E) Preparation for dialysis

7. The patient's chest film returns, showing complete opacification of the right hemithorax. Malignant cells are later identified from the diagnostic tap. Which one of the following statements is correct?

(A) Most malignant pleural effusions are transudates.
(B) Transudates generally have a protein content > 3 g/dL.
(C) Exudates generally have an LDH level >200.
(D) This patient should not have the pleural effusion drained due to the risk of reexpansion pulmonary edema.
(E) This patient probably will live at least 6 months.

8. A 54-year-old man with multiple myeloma presents to the emergency department with headaches and dizziness. On questioning, he reports that he bleeds from his gums when brushing his teeth. He also states that he needs a prescription for new glasses. Physical examination reveals a cachectic man, retinal hemorrhages on funduscopy, and brown heme-positive stool on rectal examination. Which of the following treatments is most likely to improve this patient's symptoms?

(A) Chemotherapy
(B) Dexamethasone
(C) Dialysis
(D) Plasmapheresis
(E) Radiotherapy

9. A 71-year-old man with a history of prostate cancer presents to the emergency department by EMS with severe back pain unrelieved by rest or prescribed pain medication. The patient missed his last outpatient appointment because he was "too weak to walk." Spine films show several collapsed thoracic and lumbar vertebrae. Which of the following is the most appropriate next step?

(A) Await neurosurgical consultation
(B) Give dexamethasone intravenously (IV)
(C) Diuresis
(D) Computed tomographic (CT) scan of the head
(E) Total spine magnetic resonance imaging (MRI)

Answers and Explanations

1-A. Patients with hemophilia A lack factor VIII, which is found in cryoprecipitate or a separate blood product, factor VIII:C. Factor VIII also can be increased in patients with hemophilia A by administration of desmopressin acetate (DDAVP). Fresh frozen plasma is the appropriate choice for patients with hemophilia B. Heparin would be considered in a bleeding patient only if he or she was thought to be in disseminated intravascular coagulation (DIC). Administration of platelets would not improve clotting in this patient.

2-E. This patient most likely has von Willebrand disease. Hemophilia A and B are exceedingly rare and occur almost exclusively in men. Although liver disease and vitamin K deficiency can cause prolonged bleeding, they do not account for the patient's family history of bleeding.

3-E. This patient appears to have had a splenectomy, and is therefore most at risk from encapsulated organisms. *Streptococcus pneumoniae* is the only encapsulated organism listed.

4-C. This patient is having a transfusion reaction. Hydration is critical in this patient for two reasons: (1) to maintain intravascular volume and (2) to prevent renal failure due to the transfusion reaction. Although hanging the second bag of blood may seem appropriate, it is relatively contraindicated until the patient has a repeat blood type sent for analysis by the blood bank, along with the suspected incompatible blood.

5-B. Tumor lysis syndrome is associated with release of intracellular contents of killed tumor cells into the bloodstream, and is, therefore, associated with hyperuricemia, hyperkalemia, hyperphosphatemia, and hypocalcemia.

6-C. At this time, the patient most likely has superior vena cava syndrome. Appropriate emergency department management includes elevation of the head of the bed, and cautious use of diuretics. Phlebotomy may be considered in patients with hyperviscosity syndrome.

7-C. Malignant pleural effusions are exudates, and therefore are characterized by high protein content and high LDH content. Although reexpansion pulmonary edema is a risk, it is much riskier to withhold treatment from this symptomatic patient. Eighty percent of patients with malignant pleural effusion die within 6 months.

8-D. This patient has hyperviscosity syndrome, which is characterized by neurologic changes, visual changes, and bleeding. Plasmapheresis will remove the abnormal paraproteins secreted by plasma cells in multiple myeloma and reduce the viscosity of the blood.

9-B. This patient has spinal cord compression. Although the dose of dexamethasone is controversial, there is no controversy about the timing of its usage; it must be started as early as possible to improve the neurological outcome of this patient. It is reasonable to obtain an MRI and a neurosurgical consultation, but the treatment of this patient should not be delayed to obtain such studies.

16

Obstetric and Gynecologic Emergencies

I. Vaginal Bleeding

—Vaginal bleeding is a common emergency department (ED) complaint.

—The differential diagnosis includes many diagnoses, the most important of which is ectopic pregnancy.

—It is important to ascertain that bleeding is actually vaginal in origin, and not from the genitourinary or gastrointestinal tracts.

A. Bleeding in early pregnancy (before 20 weeks)

—The most common cause of 1st-trimester bleeding is spontaneous abortion (Table 16-1).

—Spontaneous abortion most commonly occurs secondary to chromosomal abnormalities in the fetus.

B. Bleeding in late pregnancy (20 weeks or later)

1. Definitions

a. **Abruptio placentae:** premature separation of a normally implanted placenta. It is diagnosed clinically, and often occurs in the setting of trauma. Bleeding may be internal or external, bright red or dark.

b. **Placenta previa:** premature separation of an abnormally implanted placenta covering the cervical os. Bleeding is always external and bright red, and usually is painless.

c. **Vasa previa:** rare cause of bleeding secondary to velamentous insertion of umbilical cord into placental vessels. Imminent risk of fetal exsanguination.

d. **Uterine rupture:** full-thickness tear of myometrium. Bleeding usually is accompanied by pain.

2. Clinical features

a. **Symptoms** may include:

—vaginal bleeding, either painful (abruptio) or painless (previa)

Table 16-1. Types of Spontaneous Abortions

	Missed	Threatened	Inevitable	Incomplete	Completed	Septic
Symptoms and physical examination findings	May be asymptomatic	Painless vaginal bleeding	Progressive cervical dilatation	Same as with inevitable abortion, but with passage of tissue (products of conception)	History of vaginal bleeding and cramping	Fever, bleeding, cramping, pain Purulent discharge from cervix Boggy, tender, enlarged uterus
Vaginal bleeding	Scant brown discharge	Minimal	Profuse, heavy		Minimal if present	Variable
Cramping	No	Minimal	Severe		No	Variable
Internal os	Closed	Closed	Open		Open or closed	Open with passing of tissue (POC)
Diagnostic tests	Type & screen Quantitative β-hCG	β-hCG	Preoperative laboratory β-hCG	Preoperative laboratory studies β-hCG Fetal tissue pathology	Pre-op labs β-hCG	Pre-op labs, β-hCG Cervix C&S Blood C&S Fetal tissue pathology
Ultrasonography findings	Irregularly shaped or collapsed gestational sac Absent yolk sac No fetal heart activity	Normal ultrasound (IUP)	Irregularly shaped gestational sac low in the uterus	Some products of conception still present in gestational sac	Empty gestational sac Normal endometrial stripe	Variable
Treatment	May observe for 24 hours RhoGAM prn*	Observation Bed rest	IVF Rhogam prn	IVF Rhogam prn	Observation Bed rest	IV antibiotics IVF Rhogam prn
Disposition	Discharge with follow-up in 48 hrs. Schedule D&C	Discharge with follow-up in 48 hrs to check doubling of β-hCG	Emergency D&C	Emergency D&C	Discharge with follow-up in 48 hrs. Schedule D&C	Admit to obstetrics and gynecology Emergency D&C

*RhoGAM = Rhô (D) immune globulin. RhoGAM prn is given if mother is Rh−. Dose is 300 μg IM within 72 h of event or procedure
β-*hCG* = Beta human chorionic gonadotropin; *C* + *S* = culture + sensitivity; *D*+*C* = dilatation and curettage; *IV* = intravenous; *IVF* = intravenous fluids; *prn* = as needed.

—blood, which may be either bright red or dark

—bleeding, either external or internal

b. **Physical examination findings** may include:

—signs of blood loss: e.g., orthostatic hypotension, pallor

—signs of fetal distress: e.g., heart rate decelerations

—**vasa previa triad:** membrane rupture, vaginal bleeding, fetal bradycardia

3. **Diagnostic tests**

a. Standard admission laboratory studies: complete blood count (CBC), chemistry panel, prothrombin time (PT), activated partial thromboplastin time (APTT), and urinalysis.

b. Type and crossmatch for 4 units of blood

c. **Fibrinogen, d-dimer,** and **fibrin split products** to look for disseminated intravascular coagulation (associated with abruption)

d. Abdominopelvic ultrasonography to look for:

—fetal position

—fetal heart tones

—free fluid (blood) and clots

4. **Treatment**

a. Immediate consultation with obstetrics and gynecology (ob/gyn) service

b. Vaginal or rectal examination only if consultation with obstetrics will be significantly delayed (> 1 hour)

c. Intravenous hydration

d. Blood transfusion if patient is hemodynamically unstable from blood loss

5. **Disposition**

—All patients are admitted to the ob/gyn service.

C. **Postpartum hemorrhage**

—The most common causes of early (<48 hours after delivery) postpartum hemorrhage are uterine atony and intrapartum traumatic injuries, which may include both vaginal and uterine 3rd-degree tears.

—The most common causes of delayed (>48 hours after delivery) postpartum hemorrhage are retained placenta and endometritis.

1. **Early postpartum hemorrhage**

a. **Clinical features** may include:

—persistent uterine bleeding after delivery

—boggy uterus

—pallor and orthostatic hypotension if blood loss is significant

b. **Diagnostic tests**

—Type and crossmatch in case transfusion becomes necessary

c. **Treatment**

(1) For uterine atony:

—Manual massage

—Oxytocin: 10 units at 20–40 mU/minute

(2) For traumatic injuries:
—Repair of lacerations

d. Disposition

—Patients are admitted to the ob/gyn service for observation.

2. Retained placenta

a. Clinical features

(1) **Symptoms** may include:
—prolonged vaginal bleeding after delivery
—lower abdominal pain

(2) **Physical examination findings** may include:
—cervical bleeding
—minimal cervical discharge
—enlarged or tender uterus
—mild cervical motion and adnexal tenderness

b. Diagnostic tests

(1) Preoperative laboratory studies: CBC, chemistry panel, PT, APTT, and type and crossmatch

(2) Ultrasonography to look for:
—retained placenta (seen as areas of echogenicity in the uterine cavity)
—blood clot
—a thin endometrial stripe. This is a normal finding that indicates that no retained placenta is present.

c. Treatment

—See Disposition section (I C 2 d)

d. Disposition

(1) Patients who are bleeding heavily are admitted to the ob/gyn service for dilatation and curettage (D & C).

(2) If the patient is not bleeding heavily, the consulting obstetrician may consider administering methylergonovine and discharge the patient home with follow-up in 24 hours.

3. Endometritis

—The most commonly involved organisms include *Bacteroides* species (spp), Group B streptococci, *Enterobacteriaceae* spp, and *Chlamydia trachomatis*.

a. Clinical features

(1) **Symptoms** may include:
—fever
—abdominal pain
—vaginal bleeding
—vaginal discharge

(2) **Physical examination findings** may include:
—very tender uterus
—cervical motion and adnexal tenderness
—purulent discharge from cervical os

b. Diagnostic tests

(1) Human chorionic gonadotropin (β-hCG) level to confirm pregnancy

(2) Admission laboratory studies: CBC, chemistry panel, PT, APTT, and urinalysis

(3) Ultrasonography to look for tuboovarian abscess (see section IV C)

c. Treatment

—Broad-spectrum antibiotics: many regimens can be used. One combination commonly used in the ED is cefoxitin 2 g intravenously (IV) + clindamycin 900 mg IV+ gentamycin 2 g loading dose IV

d. Disposition

—Patients with endometritis are admitted to the ob/gyn service.

D. Vaginal bleeding in a non-pregnant patient

1. Causes include:

—dysfunctional uterine bleeding

—fibroids

—endometrial or cervical cancer

—trauma (including traumatic intercourse)

—vulvovaginitis (atrophic, infectious)

2. Clinical presentation

a. Symptoms may include:

—lightheadedness

—weakness

b. Physical examination findings may include:

—orthostatic hypotension

—enlarged uterus

—bleeding from cervical os

—blood in vaginal vault

3. Diagnostic tests

a. β-hCG to determine if patient is pregnant

b. CBC to look for anemia

c. Type and screen (or crossmatch) in case transfusion becomes necessary

d. Cultures for gonorrhea and chlamydia

e. Papanicolaou (Pap) smear

4. Treatment

a. In premenopausal women:

—for severe bleeding: 20 mg IV estrogen administered slowly

—for mild to moderate bleeding: medroxyprogesterone 5 mg orally per day for 10 days

b. In post- or perimenopausal women:

—Administer hormone replacement therapy, but only after a negative result on endometrial biopsy is obtained.

—If the patient is already on hormone replacement therapy, treat as in premenopausal women and send for a repeat biopsy.

5. Disposition

a. Most patients can be discharged home with outpatient follow-up.

b. Patients with evidence of severe bleeding, hypotension, severe anemia (Hct < 20), and active bright red bleeding that does not stop should be admitted to the hospital.

II. Obstetric Emergencies

A. Ectopic pregnancy

—An ectopic pregnancy is a pregnancy located outside the uterus

—A heterotopic pregnancy is one in which there is both an intrauterine pregnancy (IUP) and an ectopic pregnancy. This occurs in only 1 in 30,000 pregnancies in the general population, but is seen in 8 of 100 patients on fertility drugs.

—The most common site of ectopic implantation is the fallopian tube.

—The risk of rupture is greatest at 12–16 weeks.

1. Clinical presentation

a. Symptoms may include:

—amenorrhea

—vaginal bleeding (often preceded by abdominal pain)

—nausea

—fatigue

b. Physical examination findings may include:

—adnexal mass

—tenderness, rebound, or guarding of abdomen

—uterine size normal or smaller than expected

—normal physical examination findings, particularly if the ectopic pregnancy has not ruptured.

2. Risk factors

—Previous ectopic pregnancy

—Pelvic inflammatory disease (PID)

—Sexually transmitted diseases (STDs)

—Previous surgeries, particularly tubal ligation

—Presence of intrauterine device (IUD)

—Use of fertility agents

3. Diagnostic tests

a. β-hCG to confirm pregnancy (Table 16-2)

b. Serum progesterone: a level < 5 ng/ml is highly suggestive of an ectopic pregnancy; a level > 25 ng/ml is highly suggestive of an intrauterine pregnancy.

Table 16-2. β-hCG Levels and Transvaginal Ultrasonography Findings

Finding	Minimum β-hCG level	Weeks gestation
Gestational sac	1500 mIU/ml	4–5 weeks
Yolk sac	7200 mIU/ml	5–6 weeks
Fetal cardiac activity	10,800 mIU/ml	6–7 weeks

β-hCG = beta human chorionic gonadotropin

c. Ultrasonography to look for:
(1) empty uterus
(2) presence of blood in the cul-de-sac
(3) presence of an adnexal mass
(4) presence of echogenic halo around the fallopian tube
(5) presence of fetal heart tones outside the uterus

d. Culdocentesis if ultrasonography is not available: a positive test is aspiration of 0.5 ml of non-clotting blood from the posterior cul-de-sac, and is an indication for surgery. A positive test cannot differentiate between a ruptured ectopic pregnancy and a ruptured corpus luteum cyst. Aspiration of straw-colored fluid is nondiagnostic.

e. Preoperative laboratory studies: CBC, chemistry panel, PT, APTT, LFTs, and blood type and screen.

4. Treatment

a. Airway, breathing, and circulation (ABCs) must be ensured, including IV fluids.

b. Blood transfusion if patient is hemodynamically unstable from blood loss

5. Disposition

a. A patient with a ruptured ectopic pregnancy needs immediate surgery.

b. Patients with non-ruptured ectopic pregnancies are admitted to the ob/gyn service. Definitive treatment may be done operatively or with methotrexate.

c. Stable patients with low suspicion and inconclusive testing may be discharged home with follow-up in 48 hours to check a β-hCG level. The β-hCG rises by at least 66% every 48 hours in early pregnancy. Ectopic pregnancy should be suspected in patients with an abnormally low rise in β-hCG levels.

B. Hyperemesis gravidarum

1. Clinical features

a. Symptoms may include:
—vomiting
—decreased oral intake
—epigastric pain
—heartburn

b. Physical examination findings may include:
—a benign abdominal examination

2. **Diagnostic tests**
   a. β-hCG to confirm pregnancy
   b. Chemistry panel to look for hypokalemia, hyperchloremia, hypernatremia, mild azotemia, and metabolic acidosis
   c. Urinalysis to look for ketones
   d. Ultrasonography to look for hydatidiform mole
3. **Treatment**
   a. Intravenous hydration with dextrose
   b. Antiemetics: metoclopramide 10 mg IV/IM may provide symptomatic relief (Table 16-3)
   c. Patient should be counseled to eat small, frequent meals.
4. **Disposition**
   a. Most patients can be discharged home with outpatient follow-up
   b. Patients who are unable to tolerate oral intake after 6–8 hours in the ED despite IV fluids and antiemetics should be admitted for intravenous hydration.

C. **Preeclampsia and eclampsia**

—Preeclampsia is a syndrome consisting of hypertension (blood pressure >160/110), proteinuria, and peripheral edema.

—Eclampsia is preeclampsia with the addition of central nervous system (CNS) involvement (e.g., coma, seizures)

—Eclampsia also may occur postpartum (uncommon).

—Both occur primarily after the 20th week of pregnancy.

—May be associated with HELLP syndrome (hemolysis, elevated liver enzymes, low platelets)

1. **Clinical features**
   a. **Symptoms** may include:
      —visual disturbances
      —headache
      —oliguria
      —lower extremity swelling
      —altered mental status
      —coma
      —seizures
   b. **Physical examination findings** may include:
      —hypertension
      —nondependent edema of the hands and face
      —brisk reflexes
      —papilledema
2. **Risk factors**
   —Nulliparity (most common)
   —Maternal age <20 or >35 years

Table 16-3. Common ED drugs considered safe in pregnancy (category A, B or generally accepted as safe)

Indication	Drug
Analgesic	Acetaminophen, hydrocodone
Anesthetics and sedatives	Glycopyrrolate, methohexital, propofol
Antibiotics	All cephalosporins, all penicillins, azithromycin, aztreonam, clindamycin, erythromycin (non-estolate preps), fosfomycin, nalidixic acid, spectinomycin
Antifungals	Clotrimazole, miconazole, nystatin
Antidepressants	Bupropion, imipramine, maprotiline
Antidiarrheal	Loperamide
Antiemetics	Chemotherapy-related: dolasetron, granisetron, ondansetron, dronabinol General: metoclopramide
Anti-gout	Probenecid
Antihistamines	Azatadine, chlorpheniramine, clemastine, dimenhydrinate, diphenhydramine, loratadine
Antiplatelet agents	Clopidogrel, dipyridamole, ticlopidine
Antipsychotics	Clozapine
Anti-retroviral agents	Didanosine, nelfinavir, ritonavir, saquinavir
Anti-tuberculosis	Ethambutol, rifabutin
Antiulcer	Aluminum hydroxide, calcium chloride, dicyclomine, magaldrate, sucralfate
Antivirals	Famciclovir, valacyclovir
Anxiolytics	Buspirone, zolpidem
Asthma drugs	Cromolyn sodium, ipratropium, montelukast, nedocromil, terbutaline, zafirlukast
β-blockers	Acebutolol, pindolol
Bladder spasm	Flavoxate
Neurogenic bladder	Oxybutynin
Bladder analgesic	Phenazopyridine
Cholestasis	Ursodiol
Diabetes	Insulin, acarbose, glyburide, metformin, troglitazone
Diuretics	Amiloride, ethacrynic acid, hydrochlorothiazide, metolazone, torsemide, triamterene
Glaucoma	Brimonidine, dipivefrine
H_2-blockers	Cimetidine, famotidine, ranitidine
Laxatives	Bisacodyl, docusate, lactulose, magnesium citrate, milk of magnesia, methylcellulose, psyllium
Muscle relaxant	Cyclobenzaprine
Oncychomycosis	Terbinafine
Ophthalmic antibiotics	Erythromycin, tobramycin
Proton pump inhibitor	Lansoprazole
Scabies	Lindane
Schistosomiasis	Praziquantel
Thrombolytics	Urokinase
Trichomonas spp, *Giardia* spp	Metronidazole (except first trimester)
Thyroid agents	Thyroxine, liotrix, liothyronine
Variceal bleeding	Octreotide
Vertigo	Meclizine

spp = species

—Multiple gestation

—Hydatidiform mole

—Hypertension

—Diabetes mellitus

—Preexisting renal disease

3. **Diagnostic tests**
   a. CBC to look for thrombocytopenia
   b. Peripheral smear to look for hemolysis
   c. LFTs to look for elevated liver enzymes
   d. Urinalysis to look for proteinuria
   e. Fetal heart tones to look for fetal distress
   f. Uric acid level to look for elevation
   g. Preoperative laboratory studies, as necessary

4. **Treatment**

   —Definitive treatment is delivery of the fetus.

   —Preeclampsia may be treated with strict bed rest and observation, with drug therapy initiated only if symptoms become severe or patient progresses to eclampsia

   a. Immediate ob/gyn consultation
   b. For hypertension: **hydralazine** 5–10 mg IV every 15–20 minutes to maintain diastolic blood pressure between 90 and 100 mm Hg
   c. For seizures: **magnesium sulfate** 4–6 g IV over half an hour.

      —Magnesium toxicity is reflected by diminished or absent deep tendon reflexes, bradycardia, and respiratory depression.

      —Antidote is calcium gluconate 1g slow IV push

5. **Disposition**

   —Patients are admitted to the ob/gyn service for further management.

III. Pelvic Pain

A. Pelvic inflammatory disease (PID)

—PID is an ascending infection of the gynecologic tract (including the vagina, fallopian tubes, and ovaries) (Figure 16-1).

—Most cases are caused by *Neisseria gonorrhoeae* and *C. trachomatis*

—PID causes significant morbidity, often resulting in infertility and ectopic pregnancy.

—PID is uncommon in pregnancy beyond 12 weeks.

1. **Clinical features**
   a. **Symptoms** may include:

      —fever

      —general malaise

      —suprapubic pain

—vaginal discharge and bleeding

—pain on ambulation (due to peritoneal irritation)

—right upper quadrant (RUQ) pain, in some patients with Fitz-Hugh-Curtis syndrome (PID + perihepatitis)

b. **Physical examination findings** may include:

—classic triad: **lower abdominal tenderness, cervical motion tenderness,** and **bilateral adnexal tenderness**

—cervical discharge, bleeding, and irritation

—fever

—adnexal mass or asymmetric adnexal tenderness is suggestive of a tubo-ovarian abscess (TOA)

2. **Risk factors**

—Younger age at first sexual contact

—Multiple sexual partners

—Use of IUD

—Prior PID

—Recent intrauterine instrumentation

3. **Diagnostic tests**

a. Complete blood count (CBC) to look for leukocytosis and granulocyte shift

b. Cervical cultures to isolate causative organism

c. Gram stain to look for white blood cells (WBCs)

d. Blood cultures if patient is febrile

e. Ultrasonography if tuboovarian abscess (TOA) is suspected

f. Screening for other STDs

4. **Treatment**

a. Antibiotics: ceftriaxone 125–250 mg IM once and doxycycline 100 mg twice a day for 10–14 days. Azithromycin 1 g orally once may be substituted for doxycycline if patient compliance is a problem.

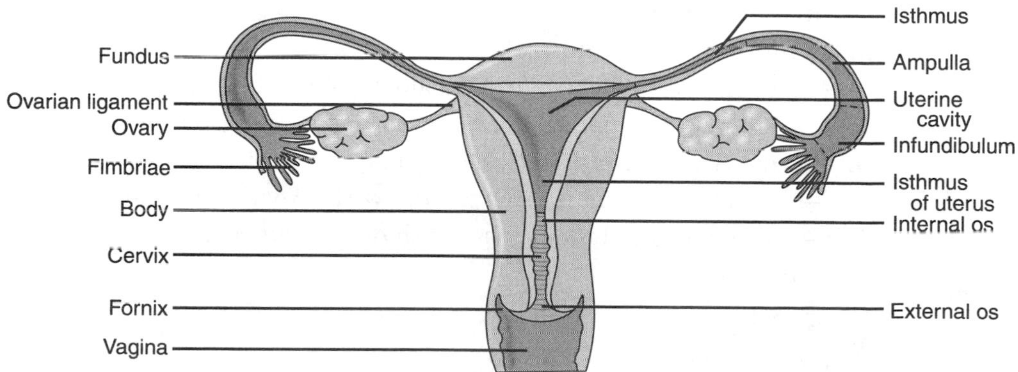

Figure 16-1. Normal anatomy of the female reproductive system. (Redrawn from LifeArt, Emergency Medicine Professional Collection, Lippincott Williams & Wilkins, 1998.)

b. STD counseling

c. Removal of infected foreign body, if present

5. **Disposition**

a. Most patients can be discharged home with outpatient follow-up within 48 hours. HIV testing should be done at follow-up visit.

b. Centers for Disease Control and Prevention (CDC) guidelines for inpatient admission include:

—uncertain diagnosis

—suspected TOA

—fever >39°C (102.2°F)

—failure of outpatient therapy

—pregnancy

—first episode in a nulligravida

—inability to tolerate oral intake

—inability to follow up in 48 hours

—immunosuppression

c. Other considerations for admission include:

—pediatric patient

—presence of infected foreign body

B. Endometriosis

—The diagnosis of endometriosis is not made in the ED.

—Endometriosis should be suspected as a cause of pelvic pain in any young woman with back pain, **dyspareunia,** and irregular or heavy menses.

—ED treatment is supportive with nonsteroidal anti-inflammatory drugs (NSAIDs) for temporary symptomatic relief.

—Disposition involves outpatient referral to a gynecologist so that the patient may be started on hormone therapy or undergo exploratory laparotomy.

C. Hemorrhagic ovarian cyst

1. **Clinical features**

a. **Symptoms** may include:

—sudden onset of sharp lower abdominal pain.

—symptoms of hypotension: e.g., lightheadedness, syncope, weakness

b. **Physical examination findings** may include:

—abnormal vital signs (tachycardia with or without hypotension)

—lower abdominal tenderness with or without rebound

—adnexal mass

2. **Diagnostic tests**

a. β-hCG to look for pregnancy

b. Preoperative laboratory studies: CBC, chemistry panel, PT, APTT, and type and crossmatch

c. Ultrasonography to look for free fluid in the cul-de-sac

3. **Treatment**
   a. IV hydration
   b. Blood transfusion if massive hemorrhage occurs (operative intervention may be needed for massive bleeding)
4. **Disposition**
   a. Most patients can be discharged home with outpatient follow-up.
   b. Any patient with significant bleeding (abnormal vital signs, low hematocrit, large fluid collection by ultrasound) should be admitted to the obstetrics and gynecology service for further management.

D. Ovarian torsion

—An ovary may twist on its vascular pedicle, compromising its blood supply and precipitating ischemia and peritonitis.

—Infarction of the ovary may result without immediate intervention

1. **Risk factors**
   a. **Size of the mass** (the larger the mass, the more likely it is to twist). Presence of cysts or tumors within the ovary increases this risk.
   b. **Length of the pedicle** (a longer pedicle has more mobility)
   c. The **right ovary** is 2 to 3 times more likely to develop torsion than the left one.
2. **Clinical features**
   a. **Symptoms** may include:
      —sudden onset of unilateral colicky pain that radiates from the groin to the flank: "reverse renal colic"
      —nausea and vomiting
      —lower abdominal pain (may be intermittent)
      —history of ovarian cysts
   b. **Physical examination findings** may include:
      —lower abdominal tenderness [generally in the right lower quadrant (RLQ) or left lower quadrant (LLQ)] with rebound
      —cervical motion tenderness
      —tender adnexal mass
3. **Diagnostic tests**
   a. β-hCG to look for pregnancy
   b. Preoperative laboratory studies: CBC, chemistry panel, PT, APTT, and type and screen
   c. Ultrasonography with Doppler to look for:
      —**enlarged cystic ovaries** with small central cystic spaces resulting from hemorrhage. Torsion is unusual with normal-size ovaries
      —Blood flow. A twisted ovary will have **decreased blood flow.**
   d. Kidney, ureter, and bladder (KUB) may be helpful to look for evidence of a large dermoid cyst-e.g., teeth and bones-in the lower abdomen but should not delay ultrasonography or Doppler studies.
4. **Treatment**

   —Treatment is emergency laparotomy.

5. **Disposition**
   a. Patients with suspected ovarian torsion should be admitted to the hospital.
   b. Patients with an adnexal mass but without evidence of torsion may be discharged with outpatient follow-up, although many patients with large masses are admitted for further work-up.

E. Tuboovarian abscess (TOA)

—is an acute infection involving the fallopian tube, ovary, broad ligament, bowel, or omentum, resulting in a pelvic mass.

—usual causes are anaerobes, particularly *Bacteroides* spp.

1. **Clinical features**
   a. **Symptoms** may include:
      —severe pelvic and lower abdominal pain
      —severe back pain
      —rectal pain
   b. **Physical examination findings** may include:
      —an acutely ill-appearing patient
      —fever
      —tachycardia
      —hypotension
      —vaginal discharge, **adnexal tenderness,** and **presence of a mass** revealed on pelvic examination
      —mass revealed on rectal examination
      —abdominal guarding and tenderness
2. **Diagnostic tests**
   a. β-hCG to look for pregnancy
   b. Preoperative laboratory studies: CBC, chemistry panel, PT, APTT, and type and screen
3. **Treatment**
   a. IV hydration
   b. IV antibiotics (e.g., cefoxitin + doxycycline or gentamycin + clindamycin)
   c. Emergency laparotomy if TOA has ruptured
4. **Disposition**
   —Patients with TOA should be admitted to the obstetrics and gynecology service for operative management.

IV. Infections

A. Mastitis

—Inflammation of the breast, usually caused by bacterial infection via damaged nipples.

—Most common causative organism is *S. aureus*.

1. **Clinical features** may include:
   —breast pain
   —erythema of area
   —fever
   —nipple discharge
   —presence of a loculated mass, suggestive of an abscess
2. **Diagnostic tests**
   —No specific diagnostic tests are necessary for a simple mastitis, because the source of the infection is obvious.
   —Other tests may be done if patient has additional complaints.
   —Preoperative laboratory studies should be done if patient has an abscess.
3. **Treatment**
   a. Dicloxacillin 500 mg 4 times a day for 10 days
   b. Cold compresses
   c. Incision and drainage (I & D) for abscesses
   d. Discontinuation of breastfeeding only if an abscess is suspected
4. **Disposition**
   a. Patients with simple mastitis may be discharged home with outpatient follow-up.
   b. Patients with abscesses should be admitted for intravenous antibiotics.

B. Bartholin gland abscess

—Bartholin's glands are paired glands at the introitus whose function is to lubricate the vulva.

—Blockage of the duct leads to the formation of a cyst, and sometimes an abscess.

1. **Clinical features**
   a. **Symptoms** may include:
      —vulvar mass
      —drainage
      —pain
      —difficulty ambulating
   b. **Physical examination findings** may include:
      —fluctuant mass at introitus
2. **Diagnostic tests**
   —No specific diagnostic tests are necessary.
   —Diagnostic aspiration to determine whether there is an abscess (or a cyst) may be performed by introducing an 18-gauge needle into the mass to look for fluid and pus.
3. **Treatment**
   a. For small abscesses (< 2 cm): antibiotics (cephalexin) [250–500 mg

orally 4 times a day for 7 days (adults) or 25–50 mg/kg/day (children)] and warm soaks

b. For large abscesses: incision and drainage or placement of a Word's catheter.

4. Disposition

a. Patients can be discharged home with outpatient follow-up.

b. Patients with recurrent abscesses should be referred for marsupialization.

C. Toxic shock syndrome (TSS)

—is caused by a toxin produced by *Staphylococcus* spp.

—is associated with tampon use, postpartum infections, cutaneous infections, and nasal packing.

1. Clinical features may include:

—fever

—malaise

—hypotension

—diffuse, erythematous macular rash

—nausea, vomiting, diarrhea

—altered mental status

—mucosal injection

2. Diagnostic tests

a. CBC to look for leukocytosis, granulocyte shift, and thrombocytopenia

b. Blood cultures to isolate causative organisms

c. Chemistry panel to look for elevated creatinine kinase (CK), blood urea nitrogen (BUN), and creatinine

d. LFTs to look for elevations

e. Titers for Rocky Mountain spotted fever (RMSF), hepatitis B, leptospirosis, measles, mononucleosis, depending on factors in history

3. Treatment

a. ABCs must be secured.

b. Any source of infection, such as a tampon, should be removed.

c. Antibiotics: nafcillin or oxacillin 1–2 g IV every 4–6 hours (adults) or 50–200 mg/kg/day divided every 4–6 hours (children)

d. Steroids may be considered: methylprednisolone 30 mg/kg

4. Disposition

—Patients with TSS are admitted to the intensive care unit (ICU).

D. Candidiasis

—See Chapter 10 VI A.

—Drugs safe to use in pregnancy for the treatment of candidiasis include clotrimazole, miconazole, and nystatin.

E. Trichomoniasis

—See Chapter 14 IV D.

—Treatment with metronidazole contraindicated in the first trimester. Use clotrimazole 100 mg vaginal suppositories for 7 days instead.

F. Herpes simplex virus (HSV)

— See Chapter 14 IV G.

—Acyclovir is a pregnancy category C drug. Use famciclovir or valacyclovir (both category B) instead.

Review Test

1. For which of the following is outpatient monitoring of β-hCG levels an appropriate treatment?

(A) Inevitable abortion
(B) Threatened abortion
(C) Missed abortion
(D) Incomplete abortion
(E) Septic abortion

Directions: The response options for Items 2–4 are the same. Each item will state the number of options to choose. Choose exactly this number.

Questions 2–4

(A) Previous occurrence
(B) Diabetes mellitus
(C) Presence of intrauterine device (IUD)
(D) Nulliparity
(E) Previous tubal surgery
(F) Multiple gestation
(G) Multiple partners
(H) History of sexually transmitted disease (STD)
(I) Hydatidiform mole

2. Ectopic pregnancy (select 4 risk factors)

3. Preeclampsia (select 5 risk factors)

4. Pelvic inflammatory disease (select 4 risk factors)

Directions: The response options for Items 5–9 are the same. You will be required to select one answer for each item in the set.

Questions 5–9

Match each cause of maternal bleeding to the appropriate statement.

(A) Abruptio placentae
(B) Placenta previa
(C) Vasa previa
(D) Uterine rupture
(E) Uterine atony

5. This factor is the cause of early postpartum hemorrhage.

6. In this condition, bleeding may be internal or external.

7. This cause of maternal bleeding carries the risk of fetal exsanguination as well.

8. Previous cesarean section with the classic vertical incision is a risk factor for this type of maternal bleeding.

9. Bleeding is painless and is secondary to abnormal implantation when this is the cause of maternal bleeding.

Answers and Explanations

1-B. A threatened abortion is characterized by painless vaginal bleeding in a pregnant woman in the first and, sometimes, second trimesters. It is the only one of the conditions listed that has a chance of resulting in a live birth, so it is the only one for which monitoring of β-hCG levels would be necessary. Except for the bleeding, physical examination generally is normal. Inevitable and incomplete abortions require emergent dilatation and curettage (D & C). Missed and septic abortions are treated with a scheduled (vs. emergent) D & C. See Table 16-1 for more information.

2-A, C, E, H. Risk factors for ectopic pregnancy include previous ectopic pregnancy, presence of an intrauterine device (IUD), previous tubal surgery, and a history of sexually transmitted disease (STD).

3-A, B, D, F, I. Risk factors for preeclampsia include preeclampsia in a previous pregnancy, diabetes mellitus, nulliparity, multiple gestation, and hydatidiform mole.

4-A, C, G, H. Risk factors for pelvic inflammatory disease (PID) include previous PID, presence of an intrauterine device (IUD), multiple sexual partners, and a history of sexually transmitted disease.

5-E. Causes of early (<48 hours after delivery) postpartum hemorrhage are uterine atony and intrapartum trauma. Causes of late (>48 hours after delivery) postpartum hemorrhage are endometritis and retained products of conception.

6-A. In abruptio placentae, the bleeding can be external (via vagina) or internal, where it is concealed in the uterus. Unlike the bleeding of placenta previa, this bleeding is associated with severe pain.

7-C. Vasa previa results from fetal vessels taking their origin in placental vessels, so that when the mother's membranes rupture and she bleeds, the fetus bleeds as well. This is why emergency cesarean section is required.

8-D. Uterine rupture is a full-thickness tear of the uterine muscle (myometrium) and occurs more frequently in women who have had a previous cesarean section performed with a classic (vertical) incision versus a Pfannenstiel (low horizontal) incision. Uterine rupture carries high fetal mortality, so emergent cesarean section is required.

9-B. Placenta previa results from premature separation of an abnormally implanted placenta and results in bright red external bleeding that is painless, which distinguishes it clinically from abruptio placenta.

Answers and Explanations

17

Trauma

I. Principles of Trauma [Advanced Trauma Life Support (ATLS) Basics]

A. The initial assessment, or **primary survey,** is a rapid search for and correction of life-threatening problems, which are summarized by the letters **ABCDE:**

1. **Airway**

—Cervical spine injury is assumed; physical examination and airway control are performed with in-line immobilization.

—Patency, secretions, blood, teeth, and jaw or trachea fractures are assessed.

—Suction and modified jaw thrust are used as needed to visualize the field.

—Signs of impending loss of airway (dyspnea, stridor, expanding hematoma, bleeding into airway, dysphagia, hoarseness) are monitored.

—Early intubation may be needed to maintain control of the airway (see Chapter 1 I for methods of airway control).

2. **Breathing**

—Respiratory effort, rate, and chest wall excursion are assessed.

—The chest wall is inspected for signs of penetrating or blunt trauma.

—Breath sounds are checked to ensure they are present and equal.

—The chest is palpated for fractures or subcutaneous emphysema.

—The chest is percussed to listen for hyperresonance or dullness.

—Supplemental O_2 is given as needed.

3. **Circulation**

a. Intravenous (IV) access should be obtained using at least **two large-bore IV catheters.** If damage to the subclavian vessels is suspected, at least one line should be established in the lower extremities.

b. External hemorrhage is best controlled by **direct pressure.**

c. Blind clamping of vessels in an attempt to control bleeding can cause serious damage to surrounding structures and may worsen bleeding.

d. Major vessels should be covered with an occlusive dressing to prevent **air embolus:**

—Air embolus is suspected in a patient who suddenly becomes tachypneic, tachycardic, or hypotensive with a "machinery" murmur.

—Air embolus is managed by placing the patient in the Trendelenburg, left lateral decubitus position in order to trap air in the right ventricle. If the patient's condition does not improve, aspiration of the right ventricle may relieve the embolus.

e. Internal bleeding is best controlled with heavy gauze packing as a temporizing measure until definitive operative intervention can be undertaken.

4. **Disability**

a. A quick **neurologic examination** is performed, including:

—size and reactivity of pupils

—ability to move all four extremities

—presence of reflexes (Table 17-1)

—mental status, assessed using either the AVPU (Alert, responds to Verbal stimuli, responds to Painful stimuli, or Unresponsive) or Glasgow coma scale (Table 17-2; see also Table 17-5 for pediatric patients)

b. A **rectal examination** is performed to assess rectal tone, presence of blood or bony defect, and position of the prostate.

5. **Exposure**

—The patient must be undressed completely to allow a complete physical examination and eliminate the possibility that any injuries could be overlooked.

B. The **secondary survey** consists of:

1. an **AMPLE** history:

—**A**llergies

—**M**edications

—**P**ast history

—**L**ast meal

—**E**vents prior to injury

Table 17-1. Reflexes

Reflex	**Roots**
Biceps	C5, C6
Triceps	C7, C8
Knee jerk	L2–L4
Ankle jerk	S1

Table 17-2. Glasgow Coma Scale

Eyes	Open	Spontaneously	4
		To verbal command	3
		To pain	2
		No response	1
Best motor response	To verbal command	Obeys	6
	To painful stimulus	Localizes pain	5
		Flexion-withdrawal	4
		Decorticate rigidity	3
		Decerebrate rigidity	2
		No response	1
Best verbal response		Oriented and converses	5
		Disoriented and converses	4
		Inappropriate words	3
		Incomprehensible sounds	2
		No response	1
Total			**15**

2. A head-to-toe examination:

—Noncritical injuries are identified and those found on the primary survey are re-examined. This is performed by "log rolling" the patient to maintain spinal immobilization.

3. Following or during the secondary survey, a Foley catheter and nasogastric tube are placed, and radiographs of the cervical spine, chest, and pelvis (trauma series) are obtained.

C. Mechanism of injury

—The mechanism of injury must be determined, because it often guides disposition.

—It may be ascertained by focused history questions. The patient, paramedics, or witnesses may provide information.

—Important clues may be obtained from the following information:

1. **Motor vehicle crashes (MVCs)**

—Speed of vehicle

—Type of collision (frontal, lateral, rear impact, sideswiped)

—Use of seatbelt

—Deployment of air bags

—Status of other passengers

—Position of patient in the car (driver vs. passenger)

—Occurrence of loss of consciousness

—Ability of patient to ambulate at the scene

2. **Falls**

—Height of fall

—Position at impact

—Surface impacted

3. **Gunshot wounds**

—Distance fired from

—Number of shots fired

4. **Stab wounds**

—Length and type of weapon

—Number of wounds inflicted

II. Head Trauma

A. Classification

—Head trauma may be loosely classified as mild, moderate, or severe, based on the Glasgow Coma Scale (GCS). Although these definitions are somewhat arbitrary, they are helpful in classification:

1. Mild: GCS 13–15
2. Moderate: GCS 9–13
3. Severe: GCS < 9

B. Skull fracture

1. Basilar

—**Symptoms** and **physical examination findings** may evolve over hours, so a high index of suspicion is required.

a. **Clinical features** (Figure 17-1) may include:

—periorbital ecchymoses (raccoon sign)

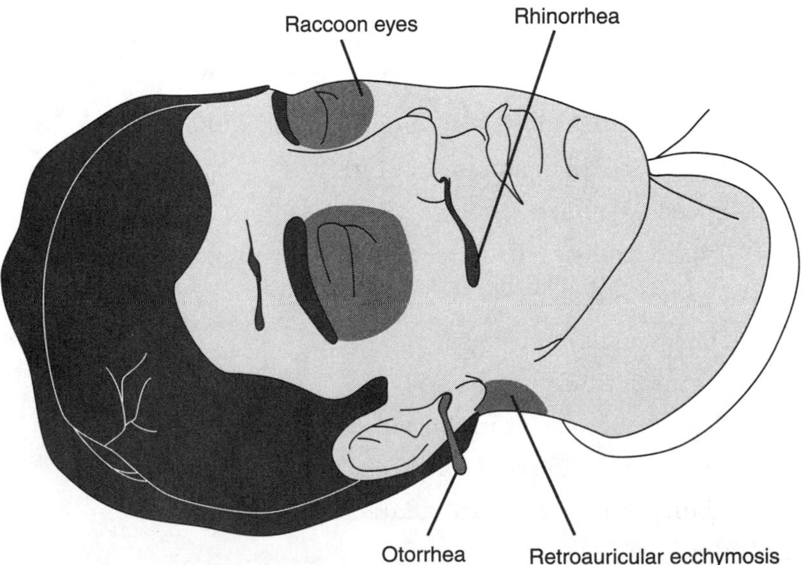

Figure 17-1. Signs of basilar skull fracture. (Redrawn from LifeART Emergency Medicine Professional Collection. Copyright 1998, Lippincott Williams & Wilkins.)

—retroauricular ecchymoses (Battle's sign)
—hemotympanum
—rhinorrhea
—otorrhea
—anosmia
—VIIth nerve palsy
—presence of "step-off" (depression of a skull fragment)

b. Diagnostic tests

—Radiographs of skull to look for fracture (frequently missed)

—Computed tomographic (CT) scan of head with bone windows to look for fracture, intracranial lesions, increased intracranial pressure (ICP), pneumocephalus, and ischemic infarction

—Laboratory studies as needed for admission

c. Treatment

—See section II E for general treatment guidelines.

d. Disposition

—Patients with basilar skull fractures are admitted for observation.

2. Linear and comminuted

—These fractures are more common in children, and may be isolated without underlying brain injury.

—Depressed skull fractures are associated with an increased incidence of intracranial injury, early seizures, and central nervous system (CNS) infection.

a. Clinical features

—Most patients have no significant findings.

—Step-off may be palpable at the fracture line.

—An overlying scalp laceration may be present (open fracture).

b. Diagnostic tests

—As for basilar skull fracture (see section II B 1 b)

c. Treatment

—See section II E.

d. Disposition

—Patients with depressed skull fractures are admitted for observation.

C. Intracranial lesions

1. Contusion

—A contusion results from a direct blow to the skull.

—Injury may occur via the coup or contrecoup mechanism (Figure 17-2).

2. Subarachnoid hemorrhage (see Chapter 6)

3. Subdural hematoma

a. Definition

—A **subdural hematoma** is a hematoma located between the dura mater and the subarachnoid.

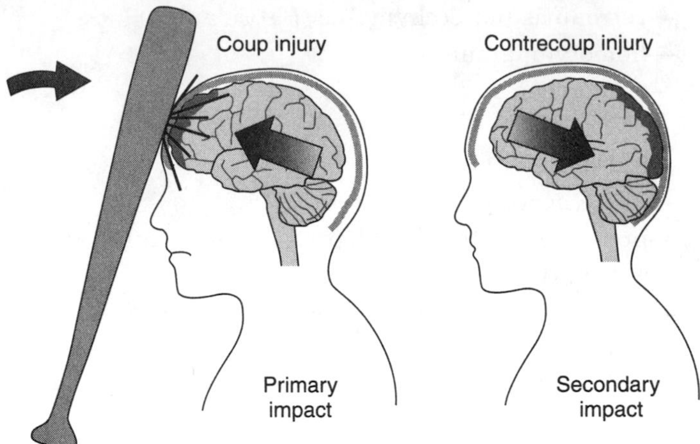

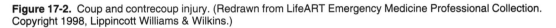

Figure 17-2. Coup and contrecoup injury. (Redrawn from LifeART Emergency Medicine Professional Collection. Copyright 1998, Lippincott Williams & Wilkins.)

b. Cause

—It usually is due to tearing of the bridging veins.

c. Incidence

—These hematomas are relatively common, accounting for one-third of all head injuries.

—Associated brain damage and mortality are higher than for epidural hematomas.

d. Risk factors

—history of falls

—direct head trauma

e. Clinical features may include:

—history of fall or loss of consciousness

—presence of bruise or laceration to the head

—lethargy

—vomiting

—headache

—ipsilateral dilated pupil (late finding, occurs secondary to impending or actual herniation)

f. Diagnostic tests

—CT scan to look for subdural hematoma (Figure 17-3) and skull fracture

—Cervical spine radiographs to look for cervical spine injury

g. Treatment

—Immediate neurosurgical intervention (see section II E)

h. Disposition

—Patients with acute subdural hematomas are admitted to the neurosurgical service.

4. Epidural hematoma

a. Definition

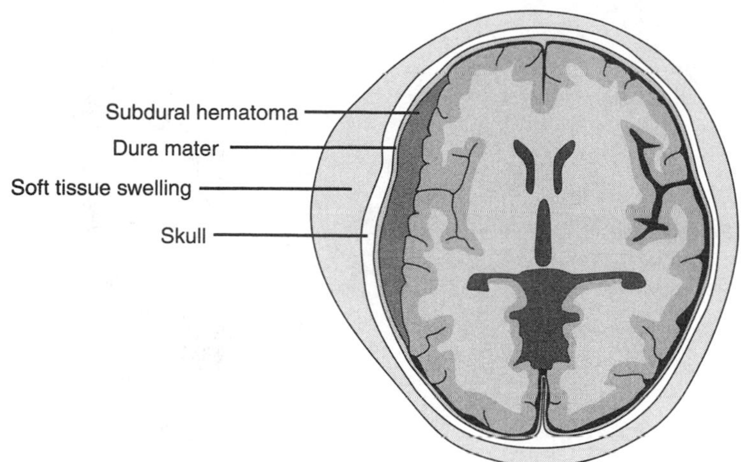

Figure 17-3. Subdural hematoma. (Redrawn from LifeART Emergency Medicine Professional Collection. Copyright 1998, Lippincott Williams & Wilkins.)

—An epidural hematoma is located outside the dura mater but inside the cranium.

—It typically is biconvex or lenticular in shape.

—It usually is located over the temporal region of the brain.

b. Causes

—An epidural hematoma usually is due to a tear of the middle meningeal artery.

—Less commonly, it may be due to a dural sinus.

c. Incidence

—Epidural hematoma is relatively uncommon, accounting for approximately 0.5% of all head injuries.

d. Clinical features may include:

—a patient with direct trauma to the head who loses then regains consciousness with a distinct **"lucid interval"** before becoming comatose. This is the "classic" presentation, seen in less than one-third of cases.

—lethargy

—vomiting

—headache

—ipsilateral dilated pupil (late finding, occurs secondary to impending or actual herniation)

e. Diagnostic tests

—CT scan to look for epidural hematoma (Figure 17-4) and skull fracture

—Cervical spine radiographs to look for cervical spine injury

f. Treatment

—Immediate neurosurgical intervention (see section II E)

g. Disposition

—Patients with acute epidural hematomas are admitted to the neurosurgical service for evacuation of clot.

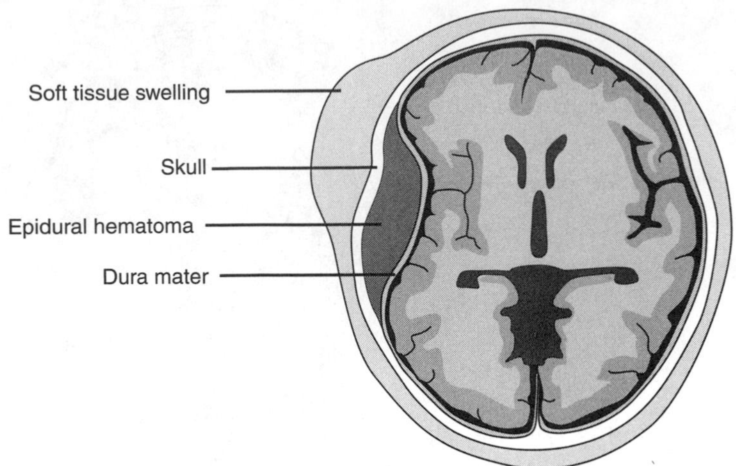

Figure 17-4. Epidural hematoma. (Redrawn from LifeART Emergency Medicine Professional Collection. Copyright 1998, Lippincott Williams & Wilkins.)

D. Diffuse brain injury

—**Diffuse brain injury** results from acceleration and deceleration injuries.

—The underlying mechanisms are thought to involve shearing of the brain at the time of impact, a transient alteration in neurotransmitter use, and temporary changes in cerebral blood flow.

1. Concussion

—**Concussion** is a brief, temporary interruption of neurological function following head trauma.

a. Clinical features may include:

—GCS score of 15 on arrival to the emergency department (ED)

—headache

—dizziness

—vomiting

—tachycardia

—amnesia for the event

b. Diagnostic tests

—Frequent (every 1–2 hours) neurological checks to monitor for presence or progression of neurologic deficits (Figure 17-5 and Table 17-3)

—CT scan of the head is normal.

c. Treatment

—No special treatment is necessary.

—Most patients' symptoms resolve within several weeks.

—A few patients persist with complaints of inability to concentrate, impaired memory, headache, and dizziness (post-concussive syndrome).

d. Disposition

—Disposition is the same as for mild head trauma (see section II F).

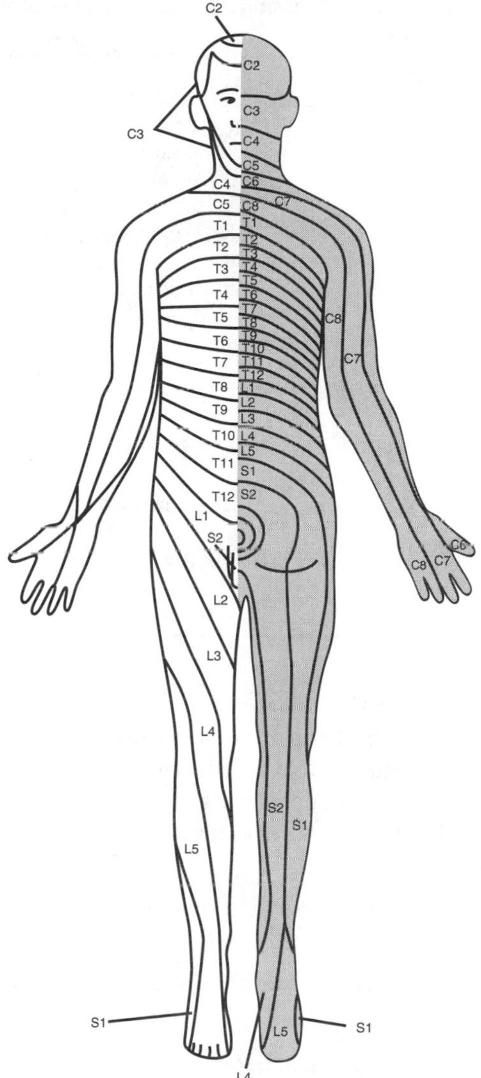

Figure 17-5. Distribution of sensory dermatomes.

2. Diffuse axonal injury (DAI)

a. ATLS definition: prolonged posttraumatic coma that is not due to a mass lesion or ischemic insult. It is difficult to distinguish from hypoxic injury.

b. Risk factors include:

—MVCs

—shaken baby syndrome

c. Clinical features may include:

—posturing (decorticate or decerebrate)

—deep coma

—hypertension

—hyperpyrexia

Table 17-3. Distribution of Selected Motor Innervation

Level	Action
C5	Deltoid
C6	Wrist extensors
C7	Elbow extensors (triceps)
C8	Flexion of middle finger
T1	Finger abductor
L2	Hip flexors
L3	Knee extensors
L4	Ankle dorsiflexion
S1	Ankle plantar flexion
S2–S4	Rectal sphincter

d. Diagnostic tests

—CT scan of the head to look for multiple punctate hemorrhages and nonhemorrhagic foci in the white matter, white-grey junction, and corpus callosum, obscuring of basal cisterns, and effacement of sulci (secondary to cerebral edema)

e. Treatment

—Immediate neurosurgical consult (see section II E)

f. Disposition

—Patients with diffuse axonal injury are admitted to the intensive care unit (ICU).

E. General treatment guidelines

1. **Stabilization** of airway, breathing, and circulation **(ABCs),** including supplemental O_2
2. **Maintenance of systolic blood pressure (SBP) > 90** with intravenous hydration

   —Cerebral perfusion pressure (CPP) = mean arterial pressure (MAP) − intracerebral pressure (ICP)

   —Preventing systemic hypotension prevents a decrease in CPP, thereby reducing hypoxic brain injury.
3. **Treatment of increased ICP** (evidenced by deepening coma, anisocoria, and deteriorating neurological status)

   a. Elevation of the head of the bed

   b. Intubation with sedation

   c. In consultation with the neurosurgical service:

   —Hyperventilation to pCO_2 of 30 mm Hg (effect is immediate, peaks at 6–10 min. Prolonged hyperventilation is not beneficial.)

—20% mannitol solution at 0.25–1.0 mg/kg IV bolus. Peak effect at 1 hour; each bolus lasts 6–8 hours.

—Emergency ventriculostomy for decompression, as needed

4. **Seizure prophylaxis**
   a. Short-term: benzodiazepines (e.g., diazepam or lorazepam 0.1 mg/kg). Children may be particularly susceptible to respiratory depression with benzodiazepines.
   b. Long-term: phenytoin 15 mg/kg IV given over 20 min to prevent hypotension. Dosage for fosphenytoin is the same, but may be given over 7 min.
5. **Antibiotics** for penetrating head injury, including open skull fractures and complicated scalp lacerations
6. **Treatment** of scalp wounds and lacerations may include:

   —copious irrigation

   —closure of scalp wounds with simple interrupted sutures or staples

   —application of pressure dressing to prevent hemorrhage

   —tetanus prophylaxis (see Table 19-5 in Chapter 19)
7. Avoidance of hyper- and hypothermia
8. There is no role for corticosteroids in acute head trauma.

F. Disposition: General guidelines

1. Patients with severe head trauma are admitted to the ICU.
2. Patients with moderate head trauma are admitted to the regular ward or a monitored setting, depending on their neurological status.
3. Patients with mild head trauma who are alert and oriented, are not intoxicated, and have no signs of focal neurological deficit or skull fracture may be released after 6 hours of observation in the ED, provided they have good follow-up and adult supervision at home.
4. Patients who present with mild to moderate head injury that occurred more than 24 hours ago are unlikely to have a lesion that requires operative intervention.

III. Ophthalmologic Trauma (see Chapter 7)

IV. Ear, Nose, and Throat Trauma (see Chapter 8)

V. Maxillofacial and Dental Trauma (see Chapter 9)

VI. Spine Trauma

A. Spinal cord syndromes

1. Anterior cord syndrome

—Anterior cord syndrome is characterized by complete loss of motor and pain and temperature sensation below the level of the lesion.

—Light touch, vibration, and proprioception are intact.

—The prognosis is poor; symptoms are unlikely to resolve.

2. **Posterior cord syndrome**

—Posterior cord syndrome is the opposite of anterior cord syndrome.

—There is complete loss of light touch sensation, vibration, and proprioception below the level of the lesion.

—Motor and pain and temperature sensation are intact.

—The prognosis is poor; symptoms are unlikely to resolve.

3. **Central cord syndrome**

—Central cord syndrome is characterized by variable motor and sensory loss of extremities.

—Upper extremity function loss typically is greater than lower extremity loss.

—Weak handshake is typical.

—Perianal sensation is preserved.

—Urinary retention often is present.

—It is common in elderly patients and in football players following forced hyperextension injury.

—The prognosis for ambulation is good.

4. **Brown-Séquard syndrome** (spinal hemisection) (Figure 17-6)

—Brown-Séquard syndrome is spastic paralysis with vibration and proprioception loss ipsilateral to the lesion (loss is often incomplete).

—Pain and temperature loss are contralateral to the lesion (loss often is incomplete).

—It may occur secondary to penetrating spinal trauma or to an impinging tumor or hematoma.

—The prognosis is good.

5. **Conus medullaris syndrome**

—Conus medullaris syndrome results from injury to the terminal part of the spinal cord.

—It is characterized by loss of reflexes of bowel, bladder, and lower extremities.

—Symmetrical saddle anesthesia

—Sacral sparing (preservation of perianal sensation, rectal tone, or toe flexion) indicates partial injury.

—Pain is uncommon.

6. **Cauda equina syndrome**

—Cauda equina syndrome results from peripheral nerve root compression or injury below L2.

—It is characterized by pain in the distribution of the compressed root.

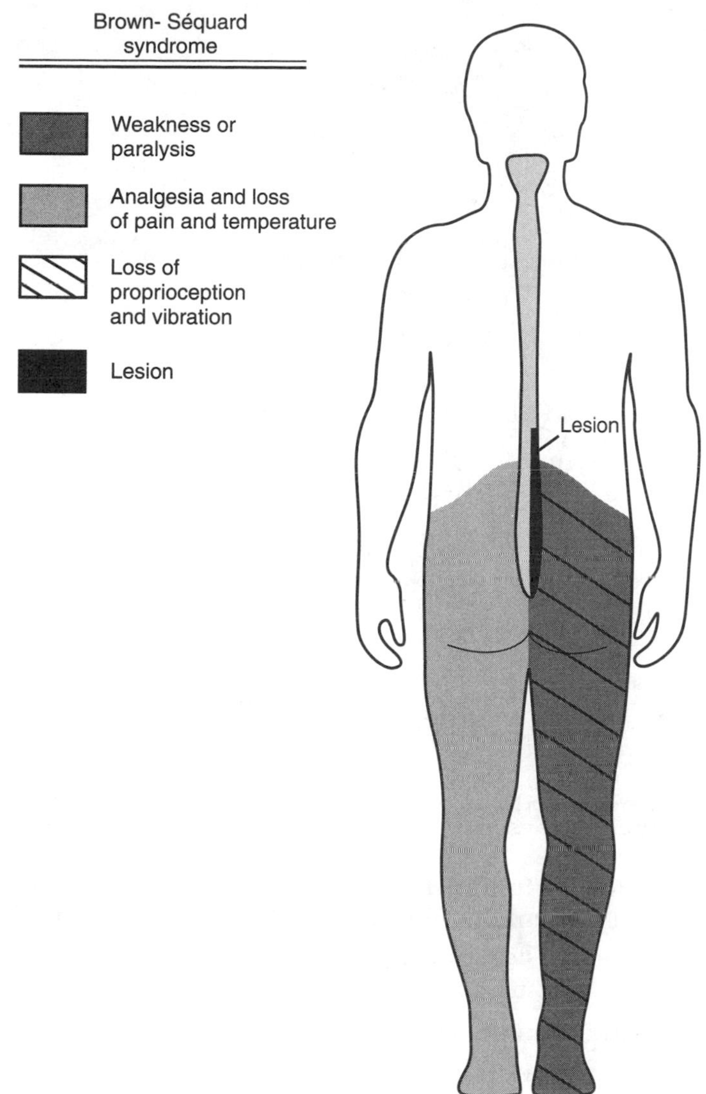

Figure 17-6. Brown-Séquard syndrome. (Redrawn from LifeART Emergency Medicine Professional Collection. Copyright 1998, Lippincott Williams & Williams.)

—Pain is exacerbated with Valsalva maneuver.

—Urinary retention or incontinence is seen due to loss of sphincter function.

—Asymmetric saddle anesthesia

B. Cervical spine injury

1. Anatomy

—The cervical spine can be divided into three columns for purposes of description (Figure 17-7). Disruption of two or more columns results in an unstable injury.

a. Anterior column: the anterior portion of the vertebral bodies, the anterior annulus fibrosis, and the anterior longitudinal ligament

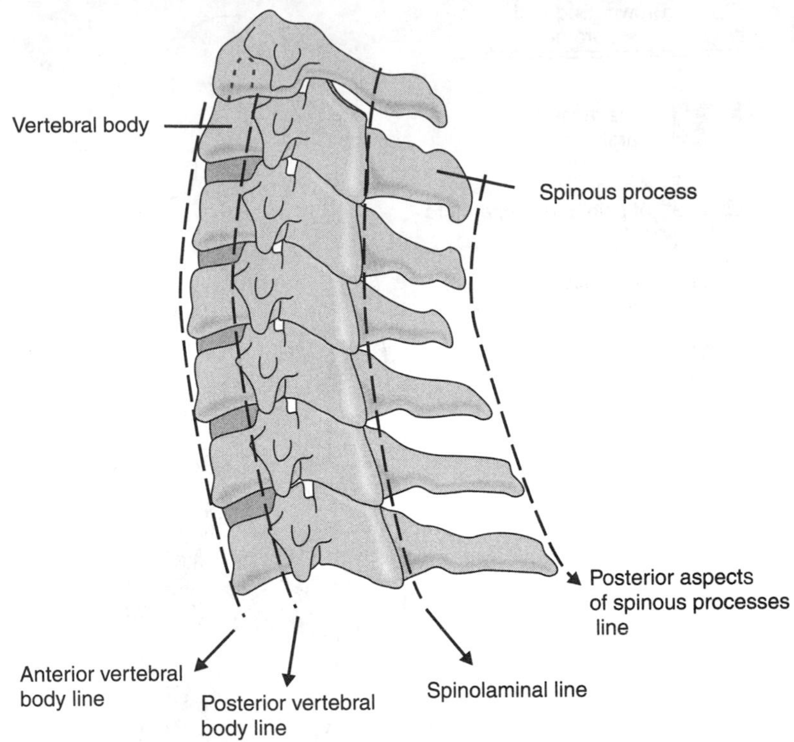

Figure 17-7. Three-column division of the cervical spine. (Modified from Hart RG, Rittenberry TJ, and Uehara DT: *Handbook of Orthopaedic Emergencies.* Philadelphia: Lippincott-Raven Publishers, 1999, p. 377.)

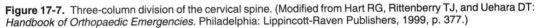

b. **Middle column:** the posterior portion of the vertebral bodies, the posterior annulus fibrosis, and the posterior longitudinal ligament

c. **Posterior column:** the posterior vertebral arch and posterior ligamentous complex

2. **Clinical features** may include:

—pain to palpation of the spine

—loss of natural lordosis

—paraspinal hematoma (seen on radiograph as increased prevertebral thickness)

—deformity

—neurologic deficit

—cerebrospinal fluid (CSF) leak from penetrating spinal trauma (may be obscured by blood)

—**spinal shock:** loss of visceral and peripheral autonomic control with uninhibited parasympathetic impulses

  —flaccid paralysis

  —lack of sweating

—**neurogenic shock:** hemodynamic shock due to loss of vasomotor tone

  —bradycardia

  —hypotension (urine output is preserved; skin is warm, pink, and dry)

  —hypo- or hyperthermia secondary to inability to regulate temperature

—urinary and fecal incontinence

—priapism

—flaccid paralysis (progresses to spastic paralysis if shock does not resolve)

3. **Types of cervical spine injuries**
   a. **Flexion injury**
      (1) **Simple wedge fracture**

      —Anterior column is fractured.

      —Nuchal ligaments and posterior column are intact.

      —Stable

      —Treatment is symptomatic.

      (2) **Flexion teardrop fracture (Figure 17-8)**

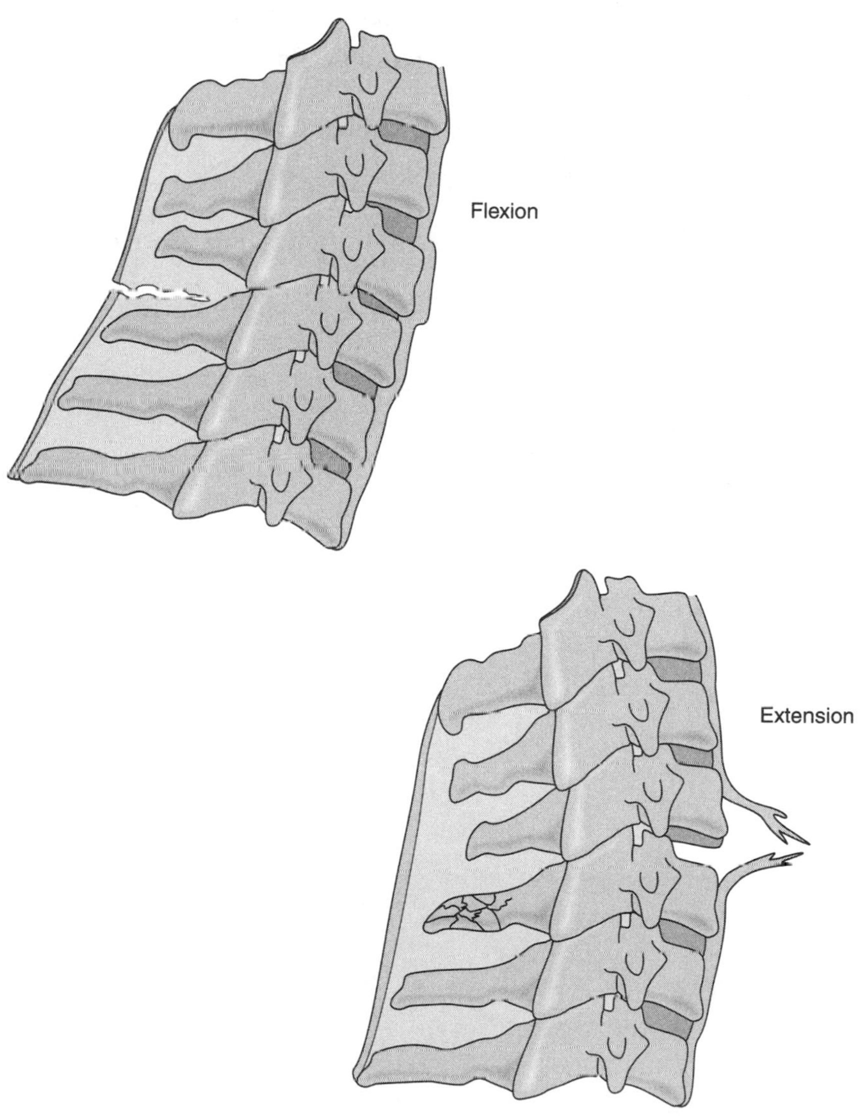

Figure 17-8. Flexion and extension teardrop fractures. (Redrawn from LifeART Emergency Medicine Professional Collection. Copyright 1998, Lippincott Williams & Wilkins.)

—A triangular piece of bone fractures off the anterior vertebral body and is displaced anteriorly.
—Extensive anterior and posterior ligamentous disruption
—Very unstable
—Commonly associated with diving accidents and anterior cord syndrome
—Treatment depends on the severity of the underlying injury.

(3) **Clay shoveler's fracture (Figure 17-9)**
—Avulsion of the base of the spinous process of C6-T1
—Ligaments intact
—Stable injury
—Seen in deceleration injuries and with direct trauma to occiput
—Associated with forceful contracture of muscles attaching to the posterior spinous processes, particularly C7
—Treatment consists of a soft collar and analgesics.

(4) **Subluxation**
—Rupture of ligaments without bony injury
—Described in millimeters of displacement
—Rarely unstable
—Treatment consists of reduction of subluxation.

(5) **Bilateral facet dislocation**
—Disruption of annulus fibrosis with nearly total ligamentous disruption
—Results in anterior displacement of spine above level of injury
—Very unstable

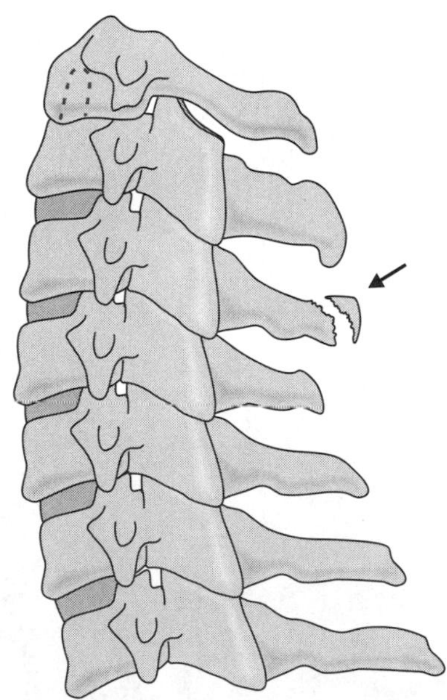

Figure 17-9. Clay shoveler's fracture. (Modified from Hart RG, Rittenberry TJ, and Uehara DT: *Handbook of Orthopaedic Emergencies.* Philadelphia: Lippincott-Raven Publishers, 1999, p. 386.)

—Usually associated with significant neurologic deficit
—Treatment consists of skeletal fixation and traction.

b. Rotation injury

(1) Rotary atlantooccipital dislocation

—Extremely unstable
—Often fatal
—Treatment consists of skeletal fixation and traction.

(2) Rotary atlantoaxial dislocation

—Injury to transverse ligament
—Fatal if dislocation is anterior
—Treatment consists of skeletal fixation and traction.

c. Extension injury

(1) Extension teardrop fracture (see Figure 17-6)

—Same as flexion teardrop fracture, but occurs with hyperextension
—Most common sites are C2, followed by C5-C7
—Ligaments usually are intact.
—Stable with neck in flexion, unstable in extension
—Often associated with central cord syndrome
—Treatment depends on the severity of the underlying injury.

(2) Hangman's fracture (Figure 17-10)

—Bilateral pedicle fracture of C2 with or without dislocation
—Unstable, but cord damage is minimal because spinal canal is widest at this level

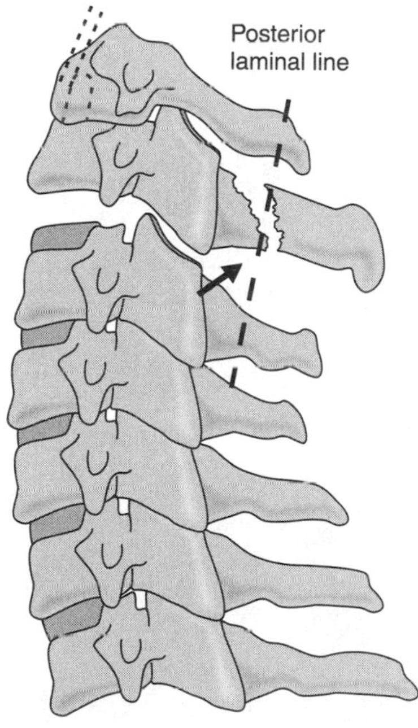

Figure 17-10. Hangman's fracture. (Modified from Hart RG, Rittenberry TJ, and Uehara DT: *Handbook of Orthopaedic Emergencies.* Philadelphia: Lippincott-Raven Publishers, 1999, p. 384.)

—Associated prevertebral swelling may result in respiratory obstruction.

—Associated with high-speed MVCs

—Treatment consists of skeletal fixation.

d. Vertical compression (axial loading) injury

(1) Vertical compression fracture

—Seen in cervical and thoracolumbar spine

—Compression of anterior facets of vertebral body and anterior longitudinal ligament

—If all ligaments are intact, this is a stable fracture.

(2) Jefferson fracture (Figure 17-11)

—Burst fracture of C1, with ring shattered into four or more pieces

—Transverse ligament is disrupted.

—Extremely unstable

—May be associated with retropharyngeal swelling secondary to prevertebral hematoma

—May be missed with plain radiographs if fragments are minimally displaced

—Treatment consists of skeletal fixation.

4. Diagnostic tests

a. Plain radiographs of the cervical spine are indicated for patients with:

—any positive physical examination findings

—altered mental status, including intoxication

—a distracting painful injury

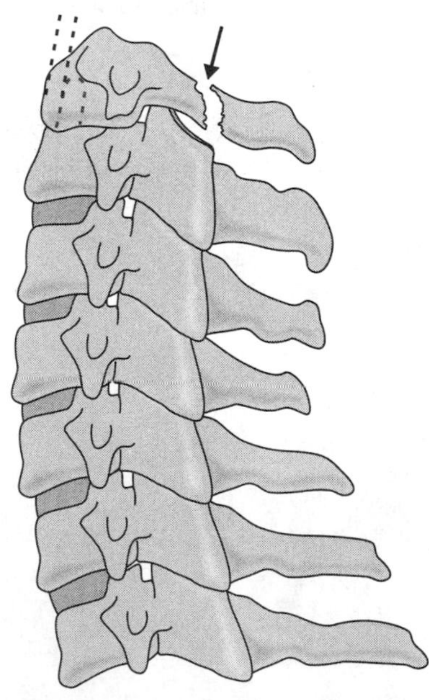

Figure 17-11. Jefferson fracture. (Modified from Hart RG, Rittenberry TJ, and Uehara DT: *Handbook of Orthopaedic Emergencies.* Philadelphia: Lippincott-Raven Publishers, 1999, p. 382.)

(1) **Lateral view**

(a) **Normal findings**

—Anterior and posterior longitudinal ligaments, spinous processes, and laminae from C1-T1 all line up (4 fluid lines, no "bumps").

—Prevertebral soft tissue swelling (Figure 17-12), if present, is < 7 mm at C2 (adults), < 5 mm at C3 (adults), or < 22 mm (adults) and < 14 mm (children) at C6.

—Distances between interspinous processes are consistent.

—No abrupt change in rotation of lateral masses

—Subluxation of < 3.5 mm between any two vertebrae

—Angulation $< 11°$ between any two vertebrae

—No fanning of spinous processes

—Predental space is < 3 mm in adults and < 5 mm in children (see Figure 17-12).

(b) **Abnormal findings**

—Greater swelling is suggestive of a hematoma secondary to a fracture.

—Abrupt change in rotation of lateral masses indicates facet injury.

—Fanning of spinous processes is indicative of posterior ligament injury.

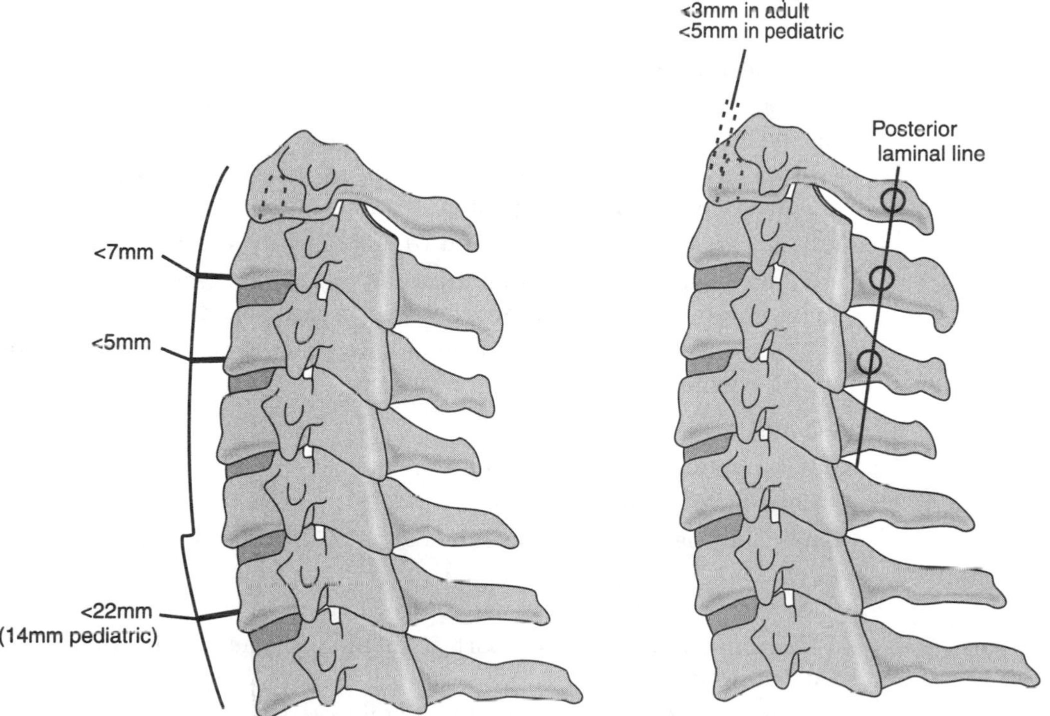

Figure 17-12. Predental and prevertebral spaces. (Modified from Hart RG, Rittenberry TJ, and Uehara DT: *Handbook of Orthopaedic Emergencies.* Philadelphia: Lippincott-Raven Publishers, 1999, p. 378.)

—Predental space > 3 mm in adults and > 5 mm in children is indicative of cruciform ligament injury (see Figure 17-12).

(2) **Open mouth (odontoid) view**

(a) **Normal findings**

—Lateral masses of C1 align with those of C2.

—C1 and C2 interspaces are symmetrical.

(b) **Abnormal findings**

—unequal space on each side of odontoid

(3) **Anteroposterior (AP) view**

(a) **Normal findings**

—Distances between intraspinous processes are symmetrical.

—A given space is no more or less than 50% of the width of the space above it.

(b) **Abnormal findings**

—Abnormal widening indicates an anterior cervical dislocation.

—Abnormal narrowing indicates spinal stenosis, which predisposes to cord injury even in the presence of minor trauma with normally insignificant mechanism.

b. **CT scan of cervical spine** is indicated when:

—Plain films of the cervical spine do not allow adequate visualization (to T1).

—Plain films of the cervical spine are suggestive of an unstable injury.

—Persistent neck pain and decreased range of neck motion are present despite negative plain films.

—Neurologic deficit is present.

—Neurologic deficit in a stable injury is progressing.

c. **Angiography** to look for vascular injury in the presence of penetrating spinal trauma

d. **Endoscopy** to look for injury to pharyngeal viscera and esophagus in the presence of penetrating spinal trauma

e. **MRI** to look for cord compression when clinically suspected

—ED use is limited by availability, long setup and test time, and restriction to patients without metallic foreign objects.

—Difficulties arise in acute trauma situations, where time is of the essence and history often is unknown.

5. **Treatment**

a. **ABCs,** including supplemental oxygen

b. If **neurogenic shock** is present:

—Frequent neurologic checks to document presence and progression of deficits

—Monitoring of vital signs with cardiac monitor

—Blood pressure (BP) support with phenylephrine, dopamine, or dobutamine

—Swan-Ganz catheter for monitoring if pressors used

—External warming for hypothermia

—Atropine for bradycardia

c. **Nasogastric tube to prevent aspiration**

d. **Immobilization** with cervical collar and backboard until cervical spine is clinically or radiographically cleared

e. **Skeletal fixation** for certain specific injuries (see individual injuries) and for *all* injuries involving neurological deficit with Gardner-Wells tongs or halo ring with 4-pin skull fixation

f. **Traction for dislocations** (done in consultation with spine service)
   —5 lbs of traction to start, with weight gradually increased (5 lbs/interspace) at 15-minute intervals
   —Decrease or discontinuation of traction if neurological condition worsens
   —Radiographs post-reduction

g. **High-dose corticosteroids for spinal cord injury** (within 8 hours)
   —methylprednisolone 30 mg/kg IV over 15 minutes, followed by 5.4 mg/kg IV infusion for 23 hours.
   —Note: this approach is controversial in penetrating spinal trauma.

h **Emergent decompression** for progressive neurological deficit secondary to **cord compression**

i. Broad-spectrum **IV antibiotics for penetrating spinal trauma**

j. Aggressive **prevention of decubitus ulcer** formation (can occur within 2 hours) by placing patient in egg-crate or air bed as soon as possible and meticulous nursing care

6. **Disposition**
   —Patients with cervical spine injuries requiring skeletal immobilization or those involving neurological deficit are admitted to trauma service for further management.

C. **Thoracolumbar spine injury**

1. **Background**
   —The thoracic spine requires high-energy force to injure it.
   —When injury does occur, it is significant.
   —The diameter of the spinal cord (in relation to the spinal canal) is widest in the T-spine, so spinal cord injury is more likely there.
   —The thoracolumbar junction (transition zone) is the most mobile part of the spine, and is easily injured.

2. **Clinical features** may include:
   —loss of natural kyphosis (thoracic spine)
   —loss of natural lordosis (lumbar spine)

3. **Types of thoracolumbar spine injuries**

a. **Vertical compression fracture** (see section VI B 3 d 1)
   —This fracture is rare in the thoracic spine, which inherently resists rotation—true axial loading is not possible.
   —When it does occur in the thoracic spine, spinal cord damage is more likely due to the narrowness of the canal at this level.

—In the thoracolumbar spine this fracture is seen most commonly at T12 and L1.

—Vertical height loss of < 50% is treated with orthotics.

b. Burst fracture

(1) Description

—A burst fracture is a vertical compression fracture that results in shattering of a vertebral body.

—The nucleus pulposus of the intervertebral disk is forced into the vertebral body.

—Fracture pieces may impinge on the conus medullaris or cauda equina.

—This fracture is unstable.

(2) Operative treatment is indicated for:

—loss of > 50% of vertical height

—stenosis of canal > 30%

—presence of neurologic deficits

c. Fracture–dislocation (Figure 17-13)

—A fracture–dislocation is characterized by fracture of the posterior elements of the spine with disruption of the posterior ligaments.

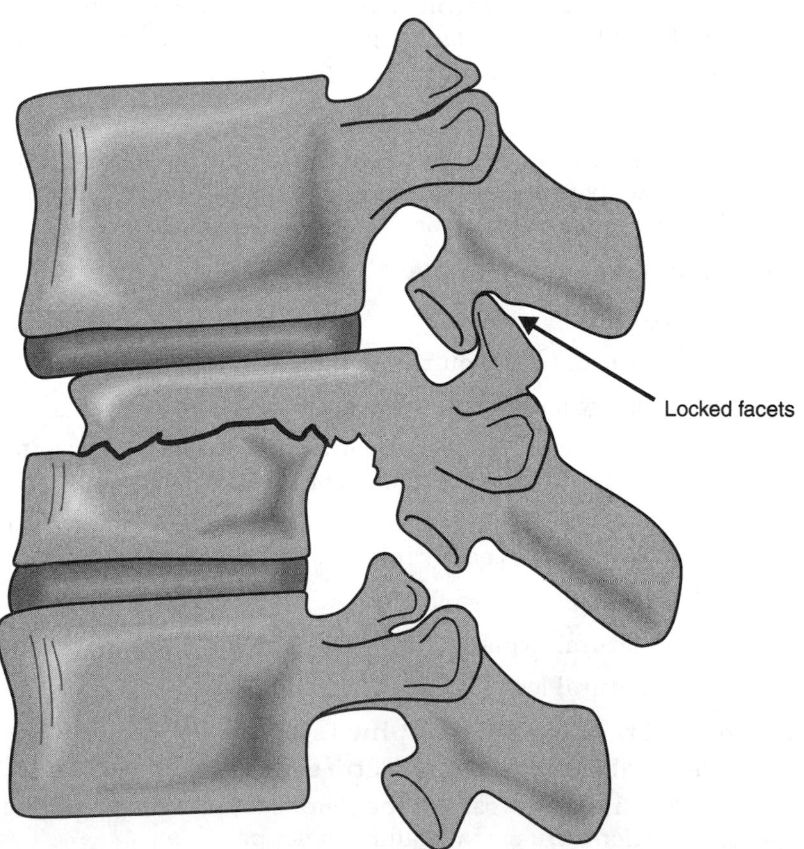

Figure 17-13. Fracture–dislocation of the thoracic spine. (Redrawn from Tintinalli JE, Kelen, GD, Stapezynski JS (eds): *Emergency Medicine: A Comprehensive Review,* 5th ed. New York: McGraw-Hill, 2000, p. 1653.)

—It often is seen in MVC victims with lap-belt-without-shoulder-harness injury

—It is the most unstable thoracolumbar fracture.

—Treatment consists of surgical repair.

d. Chance fracture

—The Chance fracture is a horizontal fracture through the spinous processes, laminae, pedicles, and vertebral bodies, resulting in disruption of the posterior column and compression of the anterior column.

—It occurs in the T12-L2 region.

—It results from flexion and distraction.

—This fracture is unstable.

—It is commonly associated with intraabdominal injury.

—Treatment consists of surgical repair (usually open fixation).

4. Diagnostic tests

a. Thoracolumbar (TL) spine radiographs: AP view

(1) Normal findings include:

—symmetric distance between pedicles

—distance between pedicles that is similar to interpedicular distances one vertebral body above and below

(2) Abnormal findings may include:

—loose fragments of bone (vertebral body)

—loss of vertical height

b. TL spine radiographs: lateral view

(1) Normal findings include:

—alignment of anterior and posterior aspects of the vertebral body and laminae

(2) Abnormal findings include:

—collapse of vertebral height

—loose fragments of bone

—paraspinal hematomas

5. Disposition

—Patients with thoracolumbar spine injuries requiring surgical repair or those involving neurological deficit are admitted for further management.

D. Sacral spine injury

—The sacral spine is rarely injured.

—Sacral spine injury often is associated with pelvic fracture.

1. Clinical features may include:

—sciatica

—perianal anesthesia

—bladder and bowel incontinence

—sexual dysfunction

—impaired motor and sensory function to posterior legs

2. Diagnostic tests

a. Plain films of the sacral spine: may demonstrate pelvic fracture, but do not rule out sacral spine fracture. The sacral spine may be difficult to visualize due to overlying bowel and bladder.

b. CT of sacral spine to look for fracture of sacrum and occult pelvic fracture and sacral hematoma

3. Treatment

—Treatment is supportive.

—Nonsteroidal anti-inflammatory drugs (NSAIDs) are used for analgesia (see Table 11-2 in Chapter 11).

—Opiate analgesia may be necessary in severe cases.

4. Disposition

—Because sacral spine injury rarely is an isolated injury, most patients are admitted to the hospital for further management of their injuries.

E. Coccygeal spine injury

—Coccygeal spine injury usually is the result of a direct blow.

—Severe cases may be associated with rectal tear.

1. Clinical features may include:

—exquisite pain on rectal examination

—pain on sitting down

—pain to palpation of the coccyx

2. Diagnostic tests

a. Radiographs of the coccygeal spine are not helpful.

b. The diagnosis is made clinically, from rectal examination.

3. Treatment

—Treatment is supportive.

a. Analgesia

—NSAIDs (see Table 11-2 in Chapter 11)

—Opiates in severe cases, if necessary

b. Doughnut pillow to minimize mechanical pressure to the coccyx

c. Measures to prevent constipation (prevents painful defecation)

4. Disposition

—Patients may be discharged home with outpatient follow-up.

VII. Neck Trauma

A. Anatomy

1. The sternocleidomastoid muscle divides the neck anatomically into anterior and posterior triangles:

a. Anterior triangle

—Bound by the sternocleidomastoid, the mandible, and the midline of the neck

—Contains the majority of vital structures, including carotid arteries, jugular veins, thyrocervical trunk, larynx, trachea, esophagus, vagus nerve, and sympathetic chain ganglia

b. Posterior triangle

—Bound by the sternocleidomastoid, the clavicle, and the trapezius

—Contains the subclavian vessels, the vertebral arteries, the spinal cord, and the brachial plexus

2. A more clinically useful classification divides the neck into three functional zones (Figure 17-14):

—**Zone I:** extends from the sternal notch to the cricoid cartilage

—**Zone II:** extends from the cricoid cartilage to the angle of the mandible

—**Zone III:** extends superiorly from the angle of the mandible

3. The **platysma** is a superficial muscle that originates on the clavicles and inserts on the mastoids.

—This muscle and its investing fascia play an important role in tamponading internal bleeding and masking outward signs of internal neck injury.

—Violation of this external layer in a penetrating injury is a major clinical indicator in determining the need for future surgical exploration.

B. Mechanisms of injury

1. Penetrating trauma

—**High-velocity injuries** (shotgun or military weapons) carry the potential for more significant damage.

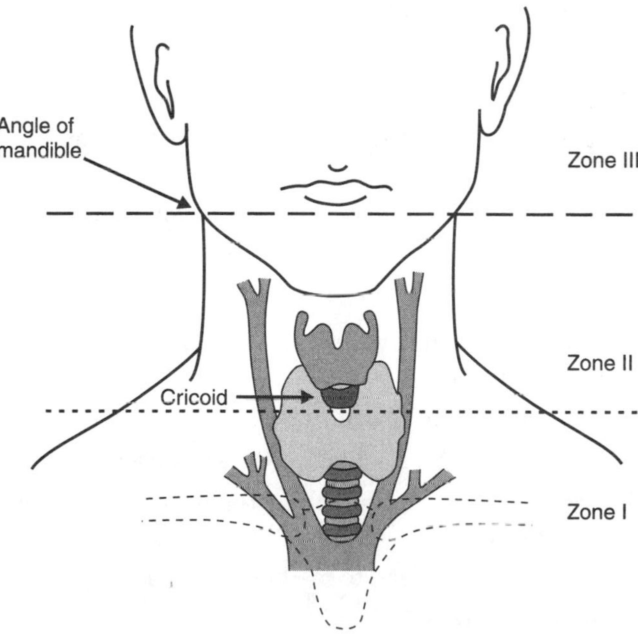

Figure 17-14. Zones of the neck. (Modified from Peitzman, Rhodes, Schwab, and Yealy : *The Trauma Manual.* Philadelphia: Lippincott-Raven Publishers, 1997, p. 151.)

—**Low-velocity injuries** (civilian handguns and stab wounds) are less likely to cause serious injury or death.

—Most injuries in penetrating trauma are vascular.

—Laryngotracheal and pharyngoesophageal injuries are less common.

—CNS and cervical spine injuries are less common than with blunt trauma but must be considered.

2. Blunt trauma

—Injuries to the airway are more common with blunt trauma, which occurs via a number of mechanisms:

a. **Hyperextension** with subsequent direct trauma to the anterior neck (e.g., steering wheel injuries)

b. **Deceleration** with associated shearing neck injuries (e.g., restrained passengers)

c. **Direct trauma** to the anterior neck (e.g., assault with fists or other objects); "clothesline" injuries (e.g., motorcycle and snowmobile riders)

d. **Strangulation**

C. Classification of injury

—Four major organ systems may be involved in penetrating and blunt neck trauma.

1. **Vascular injuries** may be characterized by:

—exsanguination secondary to hemorrhage from an injured vessel

—internal bleeding with hematoma formation

—distortion of neck anatomy and upper airway obstruction

—disruption of cerebral perfusion secondary to carotid artery injury

—dissection with intimal flap

—air embolus

2. **Laryngotracheal injuries** may present as:

—direct blunt trauma to larynx and trachea and associated cartilaginous structures

—fractures, vocal cord disruption, and recurrent laryngeal nerve injury

—deceleration trauma with shearing injuries

—transection of the trachea at its junction with the cricoid cartilage

—penetrating wound with massive subcutaneous emphysema and hematoma formation

3. **Pharyngoesophageal injuries**

—Pharyngoesophageal injuries often are missed during acute evaluation.

—The fascial plane that envelops the esophagus is continuous with the mediastinum.

—These injuries may lead to mediastinitis and sepsis, with high mortality.

4. **Neurologic injuries**

—Neurologic injuries may occur via direct trauma or secondary to hypoperfusion.

—They are seen in cervical spine or other spinal cord injuries.

—Injuries to peripheral nervous structures (e.g., brachial plexus, sympathetic chain ganglia, vagus nerve) must be evaluated.

D. Clinical features may include:

—shoulder drop

—mediastinal crunch

—hoarseness

E. Diagnostic studies

1. **Cervical spine radiographs** to assess bony structures, soft tissue air, and swelling
2. **Chest radiograph** to look for pneumothorax, hemothorax, and mediastinal air
3. **Bronchoscopy/esophagoscopy** using fiberoptic endoscopy to obtain direct visualization of aerodigestive tracts. This should be performed with the patient under sedation to minimize trauma.
4. **Angiography** to look for major vascular injuries and define the area that will require surgical exploration
5. **CT scan** to look for injury to the glottis and supporting cartilaginous structures. Sensitive test, but time-consuming, CT scan is appropriate for evaluation only in stable patients.

F. Treatment

—There is significant controversy and a lack of consensus on how to manage patients presenting to the ED with penetrating and blunt neck trauma.

1. General considerations

—Blind nasotracheal intubation is difficult in the setting of distorted airway anatomy and may rupture a hematoma during insertion; it is, therefore, a poor choice in neck trauma.

—Because the apices of the lungs are in close proximity to structures within the neck, pneumothorax and hemothorax are not uncommon in the setting of neck trauma.

—The signs of a tension pneumothorax must be noted: unilateral decreased breath sounds, jugular venous distention (JVD), and tracheal deviation to the opposite side.

—Treatment is with needle decompression followed by tube thoracostomy (see Chapter 3 III D).

—If damage to the subclavian vessels is suspected, consideration is given to placing at least one IV line in a lower extremity.

2. For penetrating trauma

a. Surgical consultation is necessary for all wounds that penetrate the platysma. (Wounds should be explored in the ED only to determine whether the platysma has been violated; further exploration is inappropriate.)

b. Emergent angiograms are needed for all zone I and III injuries.

c. The role of prophylactic antibiotics is controversial. However, because high morbidity is associated with soilage of tissues from digestive tract injuries, antibiotics routinely are administered.

d. Zone II injuries (where signs and symptoms of injury are more readily apparent) often are managed conservatively.

3. Blunt trauma

—Detecting injury to internal structures after blunt trauma is a diagnostic challenge. A high index of suspicion must be maintained even with minimal outward signs of injury.

—Injuries are poorly localized and not "zone-specific" as with penetrating trauma; therefore, diagnostic studies should be used to define injury whenever clinically suspected.

—Possibility of a closed head injury must be considered in all patients with blunt trauma to the anterior neck.

G. Disposition

—All patients with a significant mechanism of injury should be admitted for 24 hours of observation.

VIII. Chest Trauma

A. Rib fracture

—Mechanisms include MVC, falls, and sports injuries.

—Complications include atelectasis and pneumonia.

1. Clinical features may include:

—point tenderness

—crepitus

—pain on inspiration and movement

—**cough** with or without hemoptysis

2. Diagnostic tests

a. Plain radiographs to look for fractures, pneumothorax, hemothorax, and subcutaneous emphysema

b. Pulse oximetry to look for hypoxia

c. Electrocardiogram (ECG) to look for arrhythmia associated with potential myocardial injury

3. Treatment

a. Supplemental O_2

b. Analgesia (e.g., intercostal nerve block, epidural)

c. Incentive spirometry to prevent atelectasis

d. Pulmonary toilet

e. CT scan of the abdomen for lower rib (9–12) fractures to look for underlying intraabdominal injury

4. Disposition

a. Patients with multiple fractures should be admitted to a monitored setting to optimize pain control and pulmonary toilet and to rule out associated myocardial and pulmonary injuries.

b. Patients with isolated rib fractures who are hemodynamically stable with no other traumatic injuries or comorbidities may be discharged home with outpatient follow-up in one week.

B. Sternal fracture

—The most common cause is steering wheel injury secondary to MVC.

—Sternal fracture itself is not of great concern, but the potential for associated injuries, such as myocardial or pulmonary contusion, cardiac tamponade, and cardiac or diaphragmatic and aortic rupture, is significant.

1. Clinical features may include:

—bruise to chest

—step-off or crepitus over sternum

—pain on inspiration or pressure

—severe chest pain

2. Diagnostic tests

a. **Lateral view chest radiograph** to look for fracture (usually missed on AP view)

b. **ECG** to look for arrhythmia associated with potential myocardial injury

c. **Echocardiogram** if ECG is suspicious for myocardial contusion to look for wall motion abnormalities

d. **CT scan** of sternoclavicular joint if joint disruption is suspected

3. Treatment

—Most uncomplicated sternal fractures can be treated supportively with analgesia and observation.

—Sternal fracture may result in a flail segment (see section VIII D).

4. Disposition

—Patients should be admitted to a monitored setting to rule out associated myocardial and pulmonary injuries.

C. Clavicle fracture

1. Clinical features may include:

—deformity

—hematoma

—ecchymosis

—pain

2. Diagnostic tests

a. Plain radiographs of the clavicle to look for fractures of the lateral and middle thirds of the clavicle

b. Chest radiograph to look for hemothorax from injury to the subclavian vessels

c. CT scan to look for fractures and underlying great vessel injury of the medial third of the clavicle

3. **Treatment**
   a. Immobilization with arm sling for 4–6 weeks
   b. Analgesia with NSAIDs
   c. Surgical reduction for lateral displacement > 1 cm

4. **Disposition**
   a. Patients with isolated clavicle fractures that do not require surgery may be discharged home with outpatient follow-up in one week and referral for physical therapy.
   b. Patients with significant mechanism or other traumatic injuries should be evaluated for pneumothorax, hemothorax, and fractures of ipsilateral humerus and scapula. Admission to a monitored setting should be considered for these patients.

D. Flail chest

—Flail chest is defined as fracture of three or more consecutive ribs at two or more points such that a segment of chest wall is loose, causing chest wall instability.

—Such a fracture results in paradoxical (inward with inspiration and outward with expiration) movement of the flail segment.

—The work of breathing is increased.

—Flail chest is associated with pulmonary contusion.

—This injury carries a high rate of mortality due to associated parenchymal injury.

1. **Clinical features** may include:

   —tenderness of chest wall

   —crepitus

   —paradoxical movement of chest wall (may be missed if internal splinting secondary to muscle spasm is present)

2. **Diagnostic tests**
   a. **Chest radiograph** to look for multiple rib fractures, hemothorax, pneumothorax, and subcutaneous emphysema
   b. **Pulse oximetry** to look for hypoxia
   c. **ECG** to look for arrhythmias

3. **Treatment**
   a. **Airway**
      (1) Intubation is indicated for:
         —presence of three or more injuries
         —fracture of eight or more ribs
         —closed head trauma
         —shock
         —age >65 years

—PaO_2 <60 mm Hg
—deterioration of pulmonary status

(2) Continuous positive airway pressure (CPAP) is a viable alternative for patients who are awake and cooperative.

b. Analgesia via:
—**epidural anesthesia** (choice method)
—intercostal nerve blocks
—It is not practical with multiple rib fractures.
—Note risk of pneumothorax, especially in intubated patients
—patient-controlled analgesia pump
—opiate analgesia

c. Pulmonary toilet via:
—suctioning
—positioning (flail segment down)
—incentive spirometry
—chest physiotherapy
—bronchoscopy

d. Tube thoracostomy for hemo- or pneumothorax on the flail side

4. Disposition
—Patients are admitted to the ICU.

E. Aortic disruption (see Chapter 2 IV)

F. Myocardial contusion

1. Overview

a. Definition
—Myocardial contusion most commonly occurs following blunt trauma to the chest.
—The diagnosis is very difficult to make.

b. Complications may include:
—myocardial rupture
—cardiac tamponade
—ventricular aneurysm
—thromboembolism
—constrictive pericarditis

2. Clinical features

a. Symptoms may include:
—chest pain
—bruise to chest

b. Physical examination findings may include:
—tachycardia
—crepitus or tenderness of chest wall
—**new murmur** or friction rub on auscultation
—transient decrease in cardiac output: CO = SV × HR, (where CO = cardiac output, SV = stroke volume, and HR = heart rate)

3. Diagnostic tests

a. ECG to look for arrhythmias

(1) The most common arrhythmia is sinus tachycardia.

(2) Other arrhythmias seen include:

—premature atrial contractions (PACs)

—premature ventricular contractions (PVCs)

—right bundle branch block (RBBB)

—atrial fibrillation

b. Echocardiogram to look for hypokinesis and wall motion abnormalities

c. Serial cardiac enzymes to look for myocardial injury

4. Treatment

—Treatment is supportive.

a. Supplemental O_2

b. Analgesia as needed

c. Intravenous fluids (IVF) for decreased cardiac output (CO) as needed

d. Antiarrhythmics as needed

e. Pressors for BP support as needed

f. Treatment of congestive heart failure (CHF) if present (see Chapter 2 VII D)

5. Disposition

a. Asymptomatic patients with no other injuries and normal ECG may be discharged home following 12 hours of observation with outpatient follow-up in 48 hours.

b. Symptomatic patients with nonspecific ECG findings or hemodynamic instability but no other injuries are admitted to a monitored setting for observation.

c. Patients with hypokinesis on echocardiogram, ECG changes suggestive of ischemia or new conduction defect, history of coronary artery disease (CAD) or other comorbidities (including age > 65), hemodynamic instability, or other injuries are admitted to the ICU.

G. Pulmonary contusion

—Pulmonary contusion is interstitial and alveolar injury with edema and hemorrhage but no laceration.

—The contused lung has increased airway resistance and decreased compliance.

—The most common mechanism is blunt trauma to the chest secondary to deceleration injury in motor vehicle accidents.

—Other mechanisms include explosions (injury secondary to high-energy shock waves), high-velocity missile wounds, and falls from heights.

1. Clinical features

a. Symptoms may include:

—**dyspnea**

—chest pain

—bruise to chest
— cough
—**hemoptysis**

b. **Physical examination findings** may include:
—tachypnea
—cyanosis
—**rales** or rhonchi on auscultation
—decreased or absent breath sounds
—tachycardia
—hypotension
—rib fractures

2. **Diagnostic tests**
   a. **Arterial blood gases (ABGs)** and pulse oximetry to look for hypoxemia and increased A-a gradient
   b. **Chest radiograph** to look for localized patchy alveolar infiltrates. These usually develop within minutes and are universally present by 6 hours. Infiltrates begin to resolve in a few days.
   c. **ECG** to look for arrhythmias and associated myocardial contusion
3. **Treatment**
   a. Analgesia
   b. Pulmonary toilet
   c. Tube thoracostomy if hemothorax is present
   d. Steroids and prophylactic antibiotics are not indicated.
4. **Disposition**
   —Patients are admitted to the hospital for observation.

H. **Pericardial tamponade** (See Chapter 2 VI)

I. **Pneumothorax** (See Chapter 3 III)

IX. Abdominal Trauma

A. Clinical features

1. **Symptoms** may include:
   —nausea
   —vomiting
   —dyspnea
   —heartburn
   —abdominal pain
   —abdominal distention
2. **Physical examination findings** may include:
   —ecchymoses over the abdomen
   —presence of open penetrating wounds
   —guarding, rebound, and abdominal tenderness

—decreased bowel sounds

—hypotension

—tachycardia

B. Diagnostic tests

—Studies to look for intraperitoneal bleeding and/or organ injury (Table 17-4)

1. **Ultrasonography** to look for hemoperitoneum (minimum threshold = 500 ml)
2. **Diagnostic peritoneal lavage (DPL)** to look for intraperitoneal bleeding

   a. **Diagnosis**

   (1) Aspiration of gross blood, gastrointestinal (GI) contents, vegetable matter, or bile is a positive test and mandates emergency laparotomy.

   (2) Grossly clear lavage is sent for laboratory analysis.

   (3) Positive DPL findings include:

   —red blood cell count (RBC) > 100,000

   —white blood cell count (WBC) > 500

   —Gram stain positive for bacteria

   b. **Contraindications**

   (1) **Absolute contraindication:**

   —Patient injuries clearly warrant surgical exploration.

   (2) **Relative contraindications** include:

   —previous abdominal operations

   —morbid obesity

   —advanced cirrhosis

   —pre-existing coagulopathy

Table 17-4. Detection of Abdominal Trauma: DPL vs. US vs. CT

	DPL	Ultrasonography	CT
Advantages	Early diagnosis Equipment available at all centers	Early diagnosis Noninvasive Can be repeated to assess patient status at different times	Most sensitive Allows for more specific diagnosis
Disadvantages	Invasive Misses injury to diaphragm and retroperitoneum	Operator-dependent Equipment may not be available at all centers Image may be distorted by bowel gas and subcutaneous air Misses diaphragm, bowel, and some pancreatic injuries	Equipment may not be available at all centers Time-consuming Not appropriate for unstable patients Patients need to be transported out of ED Expensive

Adapted from The American College of Surgeons: *Advanced Trauma Life Support (ATLS) student course manual,* 1997.

CT = computed tomography; *DPL* = diagnostic peritoneal lavage; *ED* = emergency department; *US* = ultrasonography

3. **CT scan** of abdomen to look for injury to GI tract, intraperitoneal organs, and renal pedicle injury
4. Upright **abdominal radiograph** (or left lateral decubitus if patient is unable to sit up) to look for free intraperitoneal air
5. **Chest radiograph** to look for elevations or blurring of hemidiaphragms, hemothorax, abnormal gas shadow, or positioning of nasogastric (NG) tube in the chest. All are indicative of diaphragmatic injury. The left side is injured more commonly than the right.
6. Other helpful tests may include:
   —serial abdominal examinations and **CBC** (every 2–4 hours) to look for falling hematocrit as a sign of ongoing hemorrhage
   —serum amylase to look for elevation in cases of blunt trauma (nonspecific)

C. Treatment

1. IVFs
2. Monitoring of hemodynamic status, warmed blood transfusion as necessary
3. Laparotomy
   a. Indications for laparotomy in blunt trauma include:
      —injury to anterior abdomen with hypotension
      —disruption of anterior abdominal wall
      —peritonitis
      —free air on chest radiograph
      —intraabdominal injury diagnosed by CT scan
      —positive DPL (relative)
   b. Indications for laparotomy in penetrating trauma include:
      —abdomen, flank, or back injury with hypotension
      —abdominal tenderness
      —evisceration
      —CT-diagnosed injury
      —positive DPL

D. Disposition

1. Patients who require emergent laparotomy are taken to the operating room.
2. Patients with unstable hemodynamic status are admitted to the surgical intensive care unit
3. Most other patients are admitted for observation

X. Genitourinary Trauma

A. Pelvic fracture

1. **Clinical features** may include:
   —ecchymoses or lacerations of the flank, scrotum, and perianal area
   —mechanical instability following manual manipulation
   —discrepancy in length of extremities in the absence of extremity fracture

2. **Diagnostic tests**
   a. **Radiographs of the pelvis** to look for fracture. Because the pelvis is a ring, the presence of one fracture usually implies at least one more.
   b. DPL, ultrasonography, or CT scan to look for suspected intraperitoneal bleed
   c. Type and crossmatch and other laboratory studies for admission
   d. Angiography if vascular injury is suspected
3. **Treatment**
   a. IV hydration
   b. **Splinting** of unstable fracture with military anti-shock trousers (MAST) suit or **external fixation**
   c. **Antibiotics** for open fracture
   d. Orthopaedic consultation
4. **Disposition**

   —Patients with pelvic fractures may receive external fixation in the ED or the operating room.

   —Some pelvic fractures require operative repair.

   —All patients are admitted for monitoring of hemodynamic status.

B. **Urethral and bladder disruption**

1. **Clinical features**
   a. **Symptoms** may include:
      —inability to void
      —pain
   b. **Physical examination findings** may include:
      —presence of unstable pelvic fracture
      —blood at urethral meatus
      —scrotal hematoma
      —perineal ecchymoses
      —high-riding prostate
      —abnormal rectal tone
2. **Diagnostic tests**
   a. Retrograde urethrogram to look for urethral tear
   b. Cystogram or CT scan to look for bladder rupture
   c. Urinalysis to look for hematuria (obtained via suprapubic catheter if urethra is disrupted)
3. **Treatment**
   a. Urology consultation
   b. Operative repair of urethral or bladder rupture
4. **Disposition**

   —Patients are admitted to the hospital for repair of their injuries and further management.

XI. Extremity Trauma

A. Overview

1. Types of extremity trauma

a. **Subluxation:** an incomplete disruption in the relationship of two bones that form a joint, with imperfect alignment of joint surfaces

b. **Dislocation:** a disruption in the relationship of two bones that form a joint in which the bones have totally moved out of their normal positions

c. **Fracture:** a break in the bone

(1) **Terms used in descriptions of fractures**

—**Angulation:** direction or amount of rotation in which one bone fragment lies in relation to the other. Expressed in degrees

—**Displacement:** the amount (in mm) by which the ends of the bone are offset. May also be expressed as a percentage of the width of the bone shaft

—**Orientation:** transverse, oblique, spiral, greenstick, torus, and segmental **(Figure 17-15)**

(2) **Types of fractures**

—An **open fracture** has overlying broken skin (may be laceration, puncture, or gross protrusion of bone through skin).

—A **spiral fracture** line curves around the bone in a spiral fashion and is caused by transitional or rotational force. In children, these fractures are suggestive of child abuse.

—**Salter-Harris fractures** involve the epiphyseal growth plate; therefore, by definition, they can occur only in children. The classification is based on the extent of involvement (Figure 17-16).

2. **Complications** of extremity trauma may include:

—fat embolism

—compartment syndrome (see section XI B)

—neurovascular compromise

—rhabdomyolysis (seen with prolonged crush injuries)

—avascular necrosis

—malunion

—nonunion

—osteomyelitis (see Chapter 14 V C)

3. Clinical features

a. **Symptoms** may include:

—inability to move the extremity

—pain

b. **Physical examination findings** may include:

—deformity of the extremity

—shorter length of one extremity compared to the other

—swelling

—crepitus

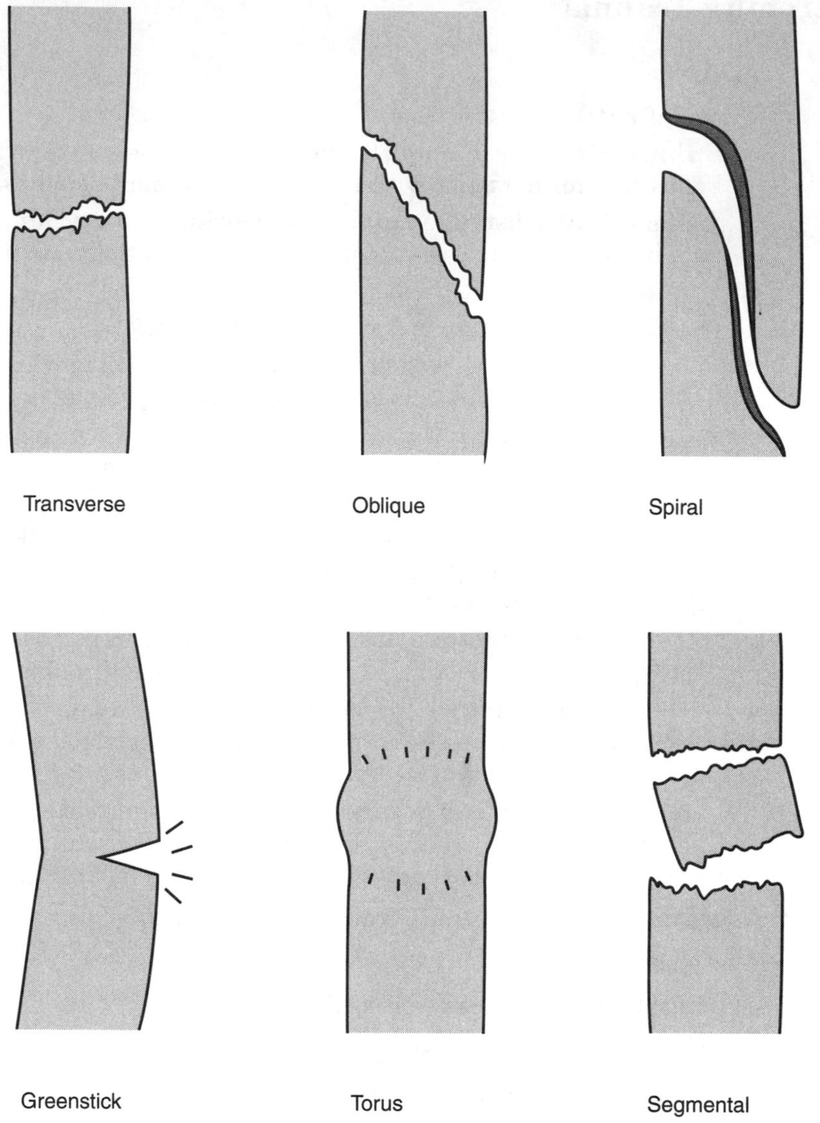

Figure 17-15. Types of fractures.

—laceration or open wound over the extremity
—decreased range of motion
—temperature difference in one extremity compared to the other
—loss of sensation in extremity
—unequal pulses
—abnormal capillary refill
—tenderness to palpation

4. **Diagnostic tests**
   a. Radiographs of extremity: to look for subluxation, dislocation, or fracture
   b. CT scan: may be necessary to further delineate joint plate fracture

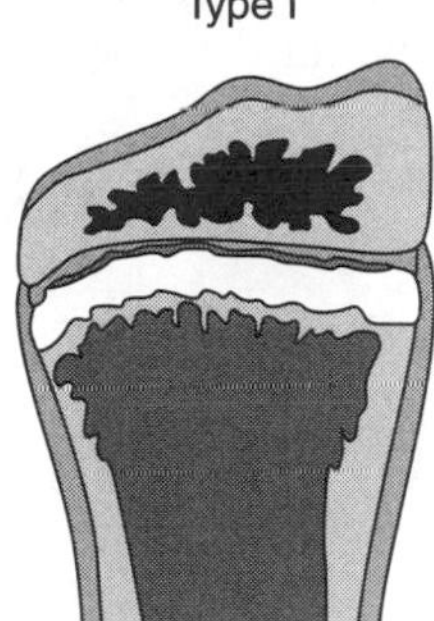

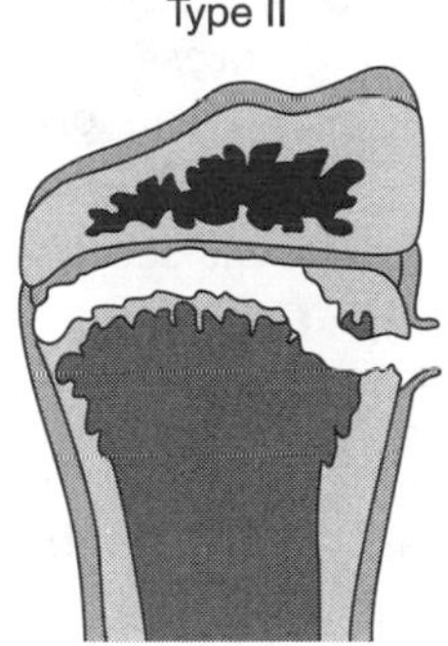

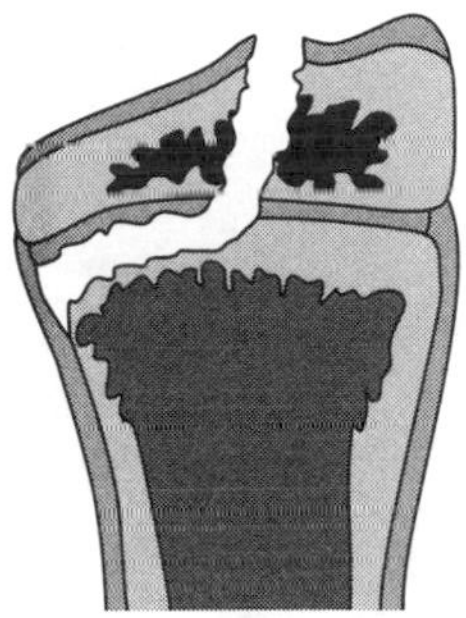

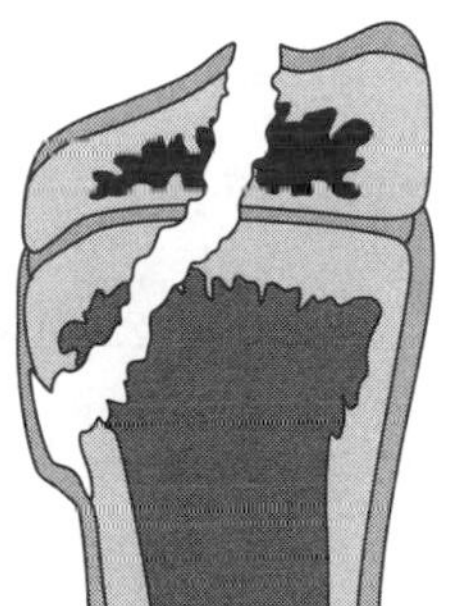

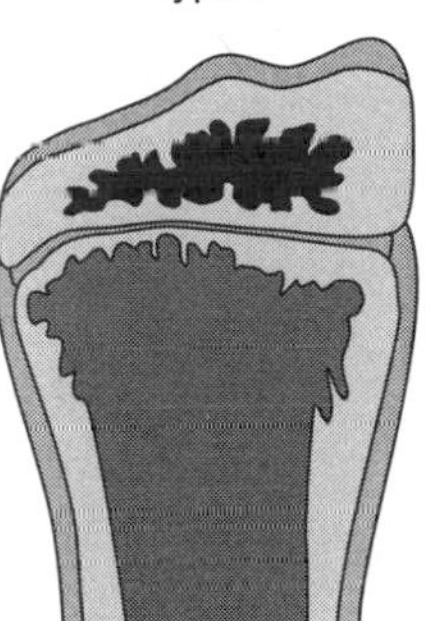

Figure 17-16. Salter-Harris classification of fractures. (Redrawn from LifeART Emergency Medicine Professional Collection. Copyright 1998, Lippincott Williams & Wilkins.)

   c. Further testing such as MRI and angiography: may be ordered by the orthopaedic or vascular surgeon

5. Treatment

   a. For open fractures:

   —thorough irrigation of the wound, with the wound then covered with sterile gauze soaked in saline

   —antibiotics effective against *S. aureus*

   —tetanus prophylaxis (see Table 19-5 in Chapter 19)

   b. Reduction of fracture or dislocation if possible, with IV sedation

   c. Splinting of the injured extremity

6. Disposition

   a. Patients with extremity trauma as part of multiple trauma are admitted to the trauma service.

   b. Patients with isolated extremity trauma are managed per recommendation of the consulting orthopaedic surgeon.

B. Compartment syndrome

1. Overview

   a. Definition

   —Compartment syndrome results when the pressure in a compartment exceeds the arterial perfusion pressure.

—It generally occurs at pressures > 20 mm Hg, but can occur at lower pressures in the setting of prolonged systemic shock where arterial perfusion pressures are low.

—The excess compartment pressure causes muscle and nerve necrosis secondary to ischemia.

b. Compartment syndrome may occur in:

—the hand: associated with crush injury

—the forearm: associated with supracondylar fracture of the humerus

—the thigh: associated with crush injury

—the leg: associated with tibia fracture

—the foot: associated with calcaneus fracture

c. Risk factors

(1) Increase in compartment contents from:

—hemorrhage

—edema

(2) Decrease in compartment size caused by:

—circumferential burns

—constrictive devices (e.g., MAST suit, casts, clothing)

(3) Crush injuries

(4) Patients with altered mental status who cannot report compartment pain

2. Clinical features may include the 6 Ps:

—Pain

—Pale appearance

—Poikilothermic (cold) patient

—Paresthesias are late findings (indicating irreversible damage)

—Pulseless extremity

—Paralysis

3. Diagnostic tests

—Diagnosis is made via measurement of compartment pressure using an 18-gauge needle attached to a manometer or a commercial kit.

4. Treatment

—Treatment is via emergency fasciotomy in the operating room.

5. Disposition

—Patients with compartment syndrome are admitted to the surgical or orthopaedic service, and fasciotomy is performed.

XII. Fractures and Dislocations

A. Overview

1. Clinical findings for all fractures and dislocations may include:

—pain

—deformity

—crepitus

—limited range of motion

—apprehension on the patient's part when the extremity is examined

2. **Radiographic studies**

—**Pre- and postreduction films** should be obtained for all fractures and dislocations unless imminent neurovascular injury is suspected, in which case pre-reduction films may be bypassed in the interest of time.

—Radiographs of the joints above and below a fracture should be obtained to look for additional fractures.

3. **Treatment**

—All **open fractures** require **antibiotics** and **tetanus prophylaxis.**

4. **Disposition**

—Patients with nondisplaced and minimally displaced fractures may be discharged home with orthopaedic follow-up in 1 week.

—Patients with fractures that require early surgical fixation are admitted.

B. Anterior shoulder dislocation

1. **Clinical features** may include:

—**positive sulcus sign:** presence of an indentation between the acromion and the humeral head when the arm is pulled down with the scapula stabilized

—decreased sensation over tip of shoulder: may indicate **axillary nerve damage** and mandates immediate (pre-radiograph) reduction

—accompanying fractures of the glenoid margin (Bankart fracture) or humeral head (**Hill-Sachs fracture**).

2. **Treatment**

—Closed reduction techniques are performed under conscious sedation.

—A cardiac monitor, airway management cart, naloxone, fentanyl, and midazolam are needed for conscious sedation.

a. **Two-person technique**

(1) The patient is positioned supine on a stretcher, and the ipsilateral arm is flexed at the elbow to 90°.

(2) One bedsheet is slung around the patient's torso for the assistant to pull. A second sheet is wrapped around the patient's forearm below the elbow and tied to the ED physician's waist.

(3) The physician and the assistant pull in opposite directions. As the forearm is pulled, gentle rotation is applied to the arm until the dislocation reduces.

b. **Stimson technique**

(1) The patient lies prone on the stretcher, with the arm dangling down with 10–15 lbs of weight attached. Neither the arm nor the weights may touch the floor.

(2) The ED physician gently pushes the humeral head caudally with his or her thumb until the dislocation reduces.

3. **Disposition**

—Patients with anterior shoulder dislocations may be discharged home with an arm sling following successful reduction, with outpatient follow-up in 1 week.

C. Posterior shoulder dislocation

—Posterior shoulder dislocations are less common than anterior dislocations.

—Posterior dislocations are associated with **seizures** and **electrical** and **lightning injuries.**

1. **Clinical features** may include:

—a shoulder that is adducted and internally rotated (arm held in sling position)

—flattening of the anterior shoulder

2. **Treatment**

—Treatment is the same as for anterior dislocations (see XII B 2), except that reduction is in opposite direction.

3. **Disposition**

—Patients with posterior shoulder dislocations may be discharged home with an arm sling following successful reduction, with outpatient follow-up in 1 week.

D. Scapula fracture

—A great amount of force is required to fracture the scapula.

—These fractures usually are seen with high-impact multiple trauma, such as occurs in a motorcycle accident.

—Associated injuries may include rib fractures, pneumothorax, pulmonary contusion, and head or spinal cord injury.

1. **Clinical features** may include:

—tenderness to palpation over the shoulder blade

—swelling, skin abrasions, or open wounds over the back of the shoulder

2. **Treatment**

a. Non- or minimally displaced fractures are treated with a sling, NSAIDs, and early mobilization.

b. Displaced fractures (>2 mm) require open reduction and internal fixation.

3. **Disposition**

—Patients with scapula fractures are admitted for observation due to the high incidence of associated life-threatening injuries.

E. Proximal humerus fracture

—The mechanism most commonly involves fall from a height or onto an outstretched hand

—Pathologic fractures occur often and are secondary to osteoporosis and metastatic disease.

1. **Clinical features**

   a. **Symptoms** and **physical examination findings** may include:

   —a pale forearm and hand: may indicate **axillary artery injury**

   —decreased sensation: may indicate **brachial plexus injury**

   b. Fractures are classified according to the **Neer system,** which divides the proximal humerus into 4 parts: anatomic neck, surgical neck, greater tuberosity, and lesser tuberosity.

   —Neer I: no fragments displaced

   —Neer II: one fragment displaced

   —Neer III: two fragments displaced

   —Neer IV: three fragments displaced

2. **Treatment**

   a. Non- or minimally displaced fractures (fragments are <1 cm off from normal alignment and < 45° angulated) are treated with a sling, NSAIDs, and instructions for pendulum and circumduction exercises.

   b. Most patients with Neer II, III, or IV fractures require surgical intervention.

F. Humerus shaft fracture

1. **Clinical features** may include:

   —**wrist drop:** indicates **radial nerve** damage

2. **Treatment**

   a. **Reduction**

   —Most humeral shaft fractures can be treated with closed reduction.

   —Open reduction may be necessary when there is neurovascular compromise, underlying disease, comminuted injury, or situations of multiple trauma.

   b. **Splint**

   —A sugar-tong splint (one that forms a "U" from elbow to shoulder) is applied, and the arm is held in a sling at 90° of flexion.

G. Elbow dislocation

—Elbow dislocations often occur when an outstretched hand breaks a fall.

—They may be accompanied by brachial artery or median nerve injury.

—Posterior dislocation is more common than anterior dislocation.

1. **Clinical features** include inability to bend the elbow.

2. **Treatment**

   a. **Anesthesia**

   —Closed reduction is performed under conscious sedation.

   —Alternatively, if the injury has occurred within the preceding 6 hours, 10 ml of 1% lidocaine may be injected directly into the hematoma to provide anesthesia.

   b. **Reduction**

   —Reduction is achieved by a slow, steady pull of the forearm in line with the long axis of the humerus.

—The elbow must be checked for full range of motion once reduction is complete.

c. **Splint**

—A posterior splint is applied from wrist to axilla and is worn for 10 days.

3. **Disposition**

—Patients with elbow dislocations may be discharged home following successful reduction, with outpatient follow-up in 1 week.

H. Elbow fractures

—**Radial head fracture** is the most common adult elbow injury.

—**Supracondylar fracture** is the most common elbow injury in **children.**

1. **Clinical features**

a. **Olecranon fracture**

—Inability to extend elbow against resistance

—Possible associated **ulnar nerve** injury

b. **Radial head fracture**

—Pain with pronation and supination

—**Displacement of fat pad** noted on radiograph

c. **Supracondylar fracture**

—Associated **brachial and median nerve** injuries

d. **Intercondylar fractures**

—Rare, seen most commonly in the elderly

—Rarely associated with neurovascular injury

e. **Condylar fractures**

—Medial condyle more frequently involved than lateral condyle

f. **Epicondylar fractures**

—Increased pain with elbow flexion

—Medial condyle more frequently involved than lateral condyle

—May be associated with **ulnar nerve** injury

2. **Treatment**

a. For nondisplaced fractures:

—**RICE** (rest, ice, compression, elevation)

—**NSAIDs** for analgesia

—**Posterior splint**

—**Range of motion exercises** 2–3 weeks post-injury

b. For displaced fractures:

—Open reduction

I. Distal radius fracture

1. **Clinical features**

—Fractures of the distal radius usually result from a fall on an outstretched hand.

— **Colles' fracture** is a distal radius fracture with dorsal angulation.

—**Smith's fracture** is a distal radius fracture with palmar angulation.

—**Galeazzi's fracture** is a distal radius fracture with radioulnar joint dislocation.

2. **Treatment**
   a. Nondisplaced and minimally displaced fractures are treated with closed reduction and immobilization with a posterior or long-arm splint with the elbow in 90° of flexion
   b. Displaced fractures require surgical fixation for definitive repair.
   c. Galeazzi fractures require surgical fixation.

J. Phalanx and metacarpal fracture

—Phalanx fractures are more common in children; metacarpal fractures are more common in adults.

—Extra-articular fractures are more common than intra-articular fractures.

1. **Clinical features** may include:

   —shortened appearance of the involved finger

   —depressed knuckle of the involved finger

2. **Treatment**
   a. Splint or cast for non- or minimally displaced fractures, with the metacarpophalangeal (MCP) joints in flexion and the distal interphalangeal (DIP) and proximal interphalangeal (PIP) joints in extension
   b. NSAIDs
   c. Early mobilization
   d. Non-emergent surgical intervention for displaced and angulated fractures

3. **Disposition**

   —All patients with phalanx or metacarpal fractures are discharged home with outpatient follow-up in 1 week.

K. Thumb fracture

1. **Clinical features**
   a. **Bennett's fracture**

      —The most common type of thumb fracture

      —Oblique fracture at the base of the thumb with proximal displacement resulting in two fragments

   b. **Rolando's fracture**

      —Much less common fracture

      —A comminuted intra-articular fracture at the base of the thumb

2. **Treatment**

   —Non- or minimally displaced fractures are treated with a thumb spica cast for 4 weeks.

   —Displaced (>2 mm) or comminuted fractures require early surgical intervention.

L. Hip dislocation

1. Clinical features

—Numbness of limbs may indicate injury to the **femoral** or **sciatic nerve.**

a. Posterior dislocation

—Hip is adducted, flexed, and internally rotated.

—This type of dislocation usually occurs secondary to direct trauma to flexed knee and hip

—On AP radiograph, the femoral head on the affected side appears smaller than that on the unaffected side.

b. Anterior dislocation

—Hip is abducted, flexed, and externally rotated.

—This dislocation usually is caused by forced abduction and external rotation.

—On AP radiograph, the femoral head on the affected side appears larger than that on the unaffected side.

2. Treatment

a. Hip dislocations usually are treated by closed reduction under conscious sedation within 6 hours of injury, in either the ED or the operating room. Prompt reduction is imperative to prevent the complication of **avascular necrosis** of the femoral head.

b. If conscious sedation is inadequate, closed reduction may be performed under general anesthesia.

c. If closed reduction fails, open surgical reduction is necessary.

3. Disposition

a. Patients who have successful closed reduction and who have no complications may be discharged home with outpatient follow-up in 48 hours.

b. Patients who require open reduction are admitted to the surgical or orthopaedic service.

M. Hip fracture

1. Clinical features may include:

—inability to walk

—pain on weight-bearing

—knee pain (referred)

—limb that is externally rotated, abducted, and shortened when patient is supine

2. Treatment

a. Early open reduction and internal fixation (ORIF)

b. Conservative management with early mobilization may be considered for patients who are nonambulatory prior to injury.

3. Disposition

—Patients with hip fractures are admitted to the orthopaedic service.

N. Femur fracture

—Types include subcapital, intertrochanteric, subtrochanteric, femoral shaft, supracondylar, and condylar fracture.

1. **Clinical features** may include:

—a limb that is externally rotated, abducted, and shortened when the patient is supine

—inability to walk or bear weight on the affected leg

—associated injuries of the hip, tibia, and patella

2. **Treatment**

—Femur fractures require early surgical intervention and monitoring for blood loss, thromboembolism, and compartment syndrome.

O. Knee dislocation

—Knee dislocations are rare overall.

—The most common type is **anterior** dislocation.

—The mechanism involves high-impact force causing extensive damage to ligaments.

—Knee dislocation often is associated with injury to the **popliteal artery,** so angiography should be considered for evaluation.

1. **Clinical features** may include:

—swelling of the popliteal fossa

—absence of distal pulses

—instability of the knee

2. **Treatment**

a. Immediate consultation with orthopaedics
b. Immediate reduction of dislocation
c. Application of long-leg posterior splint with the knee in 15° of flexion
d. Analgesia as needed

P. Patella fracture

—Mechanisms of patella fracture include impact between knee and dashboard in a motor vehicle accident, fall from a height, and direct trauma.

—Transverse fractures are more common than vertical fractures.

1. **Clinical features** may include:

—inability to extend the knee if the extensor mechanism is torn

—pain on knee extension if the extensor mechanism is intact

—hemarthrosis

2. **Treatment**

a. Non- or minimally displaced fractures (<5 mm on AP view, <2 mm on lateral view) with preserved extensor mechanism are treated with a knee immobilizer for 6 weeks with the knee in full extension.
b. Large hemarthroses may be aspirated (contraindicated in sickle cell patients).
c. Open, displaced, or comminuted fractures or fractures associated with subluxation or dislocation require early surgical intervention.

Q. Tibia fracture

1. **Clinical features** may include:
   —pain
   —inability to bear weight
2. **Radiographic findings** may include:
   —fracture on AP and lateral views
   —air in the soft tissue
3. **Treatment**
   a. For nondisplaced fractures: long-leg cast for 12 weeks
   b. For displaced and open fractures and fractures with intraarticular extension: long-leg splint, nothing by mouth, and analgesia while awaiting surgical reduction

R. Tibial plateau fracture

—Tibial plateau fractures may occur secondary to valgus stress or axial loading as a result of skiing accidents, motor vehicle accidents, or falls from a height.

—Lateral condylar fractures are more common than medial condylar fractures.

—Medial condylar fractures have a high incidence of neurovascular complications

1. **Clinical features** may include:
   —inability to bear weight
   —hemarthrosis
   —positive Lachman's test (if anterior tibial spine is fractured)
2. **Treatment**
   a. Initial stabilization: RICE, knee immobilizer, and crutches to avoid weight-bearing
   b. Operative intervention usually is required.
   c. Large hemarthroses may be aspirated (contraindicated in patients with sickle cell disease).
3. **Disposition**
   —Most patients with tibial plateau fractures are admitted for surgical repair.

S. Ankle fracture

1. **Clinical features** may include:
   —disruption of the medial deltoid ligament in **Maisonneuve** fracture, a fracture of the ankle and proximal fibula
   —decreased plantar sensation: may indicate posterior **tibial nerve** injury
2. **Treatment**
   a. Isolated fractures of the ankle (single malleolus without accompanying ligamentous injury) are stable and may be managed with a weight-bearing walking cast for 6 weeks.

b. Bimalleolar fractures and unimalleolar fractures with associated ligamentous injury are unstable and require surgical intervention.

T. Metatarsal fracture

1. Clinical features

—Metatarsal fractures commonly are associated with increased activity or a change in exercise regimen.

2. Treatment

a. Most metatarsal fractures can be managed conservatively with a short-leg walking cast and wooden shoe.

b. Multiple metatarsal fractures and those with > 4 mm displacement may require surgical intervention.

XIII. Pediatric Trauma

—Trauma is the leading cause of death and disability in children.

—MVCs account for about half of these deaths.

—Head injuries are the most common injury.

A. Anatomical and physiological considerations

1. Size

—Children have a greater body surface area–to–mass ratio. The ratio is greatest at birth, then decreases with age.

—Children's heads are proportionally larger than their bodies.

—The organs are in closer proximity in children, so there is a consequently greater risk of multi-organ involvement.

—Children have a smaller body mass, so there is less area to absorb or disperse forces.

2. Skeleton

—The child's skeleton is incompletely calcified and, thus, is more pliable.

—There is less elastic connective tissue and less muscular support.

—The skeletons of children have growth plates and open sutures that close at various ages.

3. Airway

—Children are obligate nasal breathers until about age 6 months.

—The tongue is proportionally larger compared to the mouth.

—The larynx is more cephalad, anterior, and shorter.

—The trachea is smaller in diameter, and there is less tissue support.

—The narrowest portion of the airway is at the cricoid ring, whereas in an adult it is at the vocal cords.

—The large occiput puts the head in flexion.

4. Cardiovascular

—Heart rates (and respiratory rates) are higher.

—Heart rate is the primary means for maintaining cardiac output.

—Stroke volume changes little if at all.

—Children are able to increase systemic vascular resistance very well.

—Blood pressure is maintained until 25%–30% blood loss occurs; therefore, children can decompensate "suddenly."

5. **Neurological**

—Depending on their stage of development, children may not be able to follow commands or to verbalize.

B. Diagnostic tests

1. Diagnostic testing in the pediatric patient is similar to that for adults.
2. **Special radiographic considerations** include the following:
   - **a.** The predental space is wider in children than in adults (see section VI B 4 a 1).
   - **b.** Pseudosubluxation (anterior displacement of one vertebra on another with correct alignment of posterior spinal lines) is commonly seen between C2 and C3.
   - **c.** Children often have spinal cord injury without radiographic abnormality (SCIWORA); therefore, the clinical examination dictates management. If there is tenderness to palpation of the spinal column, fracture is assumed until proven otherwise. The cervical collar should not be removed.
   - **d.** Abuse should be suspected in a child who has fractures that cannot be accounted for by the stated mechanism of injury (see Chapter 20 IX A).

C. Treatment

—Treatment consists of the same ABCDE as in adults (see section I A), with a few special considerations under each category.

1. **Airway**

—An uncuffed endotracheal tube (see Chapter 1 I B 2 a for sizes) is used.

—Cricothyrotomy is not indicated in children younger than 8 years.

2. **Breathing**

—Breath sounds should be auscultated in the axilla, because small chest area makes distinction of right and left breath sounds difficult.

3. **Circulation**
   - **a.** Venous access may be difficult.
   - **b.** The **intraosseous route** is an excellent alternative.
     - **(1) Contraindications** include ipsilateral extremity fracture and obvious infection of ipsilateral extremity.
     - **(2) Complications** include osteomyelitis, fracture, and compartment syndrome.
     - **(3)** Use of this route should be limited to 6 hours.
   - **c. Fluid resuscitation**
     - **(1)** Fluid resuscitation begins with a 20 ml/kg bolus of normal saline or Ringer's lactate.
     - **(2)** The bolus is repeated if the patient's vital signs remain unstable.

(3) If the child still does not respond, 10 ml/kg of packed red blood cells are administered.

(4) If vital signs still are unstable, the child is evaluated for the source of the bleed.

(5) Once the patient is stabilized, maintenance fluids are given at 5 ml/kg.

4. Disability

—Disability is assessed using the modified Glasgow Coma Scale, because many pediatric patients cannot verbalize yet, and most tend to localize pain poorly (Table 17-5).

5. Exposure

—Children are more susceptible to hypothermia, so they should be covered up promptly after they have been examined.

D. Disposition

—Guidelines for disposition are similar to those for adults (see section discussing specific injury).

XIV. Trauma in Pregnancy

A. Pregnant women are managed the same as any adult presenting with trauma, with the ABCDEs, primary survey, and secondary survey.

B. Once initial stabilization is complete, fetal heart monitoring is performed to check for fetal distress. (The patient usually is transferred to the obstetrics service for this.)

C. Special considerations:

Table 17-5. Pediatric Glasgow Coma Scale

	Infant	Child	
Eye opening	Spontaneously	Spontaneously	4
	To speech	To speech	3
	To pain	To pain	2
	No response	No response	1
Best motor response	Spontaneous	Obeys command	6
	Withdraws from touch	Localizes pain	5
	Withdraws from pain	Same	4
	Decorticate	Same	3
	Decerebrate	Same	2
	No response	Same	1
Best verbal response	Coos, babbles, smiles	Oriented	5
	Crying, irritable	Confused	4
	Cries, screams to pain	Inappropriate words	3
	Moans, grunts	Incomprehensible	2
	No response	No response	1
Total			**15**

—By 20 weeks, the gravid uterus is an intraabdominal organ.

—Abruptio placentae and uterine rupture are potential complications of trauma in pregnancy (see Chapter 16 I B 1 a and d).

—RhoGAM must be administered for Rh− patients, especially if fetomaternal hemorrhage is suspected.

—Necessary radiographs are obtained as for the nonpregnant patient, with abdominal and pelvic shielding.

—Pregnant women have a substantial increase in plasma volume and, therefore, can lose relatively large amounts of blood before becoming hemodynamically unstable.

—Pregnant women are maintained in the left lateral decubitus position if possible to minimize the reduction in venous inflow that occurs when the gravid uterus compresses the inferior vena cava.

—**The best chance for the fetus is to resuscitate the mother.**

Review Test

1. A 45-year-old unresponsive man is brought in immobilized on a backboard with a hematoma over his left eye after having fallen off a park bench. His pupils are 4 mm, equal, round, and reactive, but he appears to be posturing with both arms. Which of the following would be your first step in taking care of this patient?

(A) Intubate the patient and get a computed tomographic (CT) scan of his head.
(B) Obtain a CT scan of the head and then intubate.
(C) Give thiamine and 50 g of dextrose.
(D) Check cervical spine and chest radiographs.
(E) Consult with the neurosurgical service.

2. Which of the following would be appropriate placement of a central line in a trauma patient with difficult peripheral access?

(A) Left subclavian vein in a woman with a right lower chest stab wound
(B) Right subclavian vein in a woman with a right upper chest stab wound
(C) Right femoral vein in a man with a gunshot wound to the right leg
(D) Right subclavian vein in a man with a stab wound to the right neck
(E) Left subclavian vein in a man with a left lower chest stab wound

3. The patient with which of the following injuries has the best chance of surviving a thoracotomy done in the emergency department (ED)?

(A) Stab wound to the stomach
(B) Gunshot wound to the chest
(C) Stab wound to the chest
(D) Gunshot wound to the stomach
(E) Blunt trauma to the chest

4. A 33-year-old man presents with a knife stuck in his abdomen after attempting to kill himself. His blood pressure (BP) is 130/70, and his abdomen is nontender on examination except for very localized tenderness around the stab wound site, which is at the level of the umbilicus. Which of the following should be the next step in management of this patient?

(A) Administering local lidocaine and pulling out the knife in the ED
(B) Obtaining a chest radiograph and taking the patient for a computed tomographic (CT) scan
(C) Taking the patient to the operating room to remove the knife
(D) Obtaining a chest radiograph and performing a diagnostic peritoneal lavage
(E) Performing local wound exploration to see whether the knife entered the peritoneum

5. Which of the following statements best describes the optimum management of head trauma in children?

(A) Seizures occurring within minutes of the injury are treated with anticonvulsant therapy.
(B) Vomiting after head trauma in an otherwise normal child requires evaluation by computed tomographic (CT) scan.
(C) The head of the bed should be elevated to 30°, assuming no cervical spine injury.
(D) Skull radiographs are useful in planning the management of head trauma.
(E) D5W should be used in intravenous fluids for children with head trauma.

6. Which of the following studies would be most helpful in diagnosing a penetrating injury to the diaphragm?

(A) Ultrasonography
(B) Computed tomographic (CT) scan
(C) Diagnostic peritoneal lavage
(D) Chest radiograph
(E) Laparoscopy

7. Which of the following statements is correct about the management of stab wounds?

(A) Seventy-five percent of abdominal stab wounds that penetrate the peritoneum injure intraabdominal organs and require surgery.
(B) Liver and spleen injuries are more common with stab wounds, whereas bowel injuries are more common with blunt trauma.
(C) Computed tomography (CT) and ultrasonography will detect small and large bowel injury within several hours of a stab wound injury.
(D) A stab wound between the 3rd and 12th thoracic ribs anteriorly and the 5th and 12th thoracic ribs posteriorly requires a work-up for both chest and peritoneal injuries.
(E) If a patient is coughing or vomiting blood after a stab wound to the abdomen, laparotomy is required.

8. Which of the following statements regarding the resuscitation of pediatric trauma patients is true?

(A) Children are less likely than adults to maintain their blood pressure despite blood loss.
(B) Any intravenous (IV) medication or blood product can be infused by an intraosseus line.
(C) If there is no response to two fluid boluses, further volume expansion should include 20 ml/kg of blood.
(D) Widening of the pulse pressure is an indication of blood loss.
(E) Intraosseus cannulation is the procedure of choice in children older than 6 years after three or four venous attempts have been made.

9. Which of the following statements regarding diagnostic peritoneal lavage (DPL) is correct?

(A) DPL has a high specificity for intraabdominal injury.
(B) Lowering the red blood cell count (RBC) to 20,000 will pick up most diaphragm injuries.
(C) A nasogastric tube and Foley catheter are required before doing a DPL.
(D) If no gross blood comes back on the DPL, a RBC > 50,000 constitutes a positive tap for blunt trauma.
(E) DPL is indicated in the hypotensive patient with an abdominal stab wound.

10. After being slashed with a box cutter, a 35-year-old man has a 3-cm laceration to the right chest at the level of the third intercostal space to the right of the midclavicular line. He is without other complaints, and his vital signs are normal (blood pressure 130/70, heart rate 75, breaths per minute 16). Which of the following statements about the management of this patient is correct?

(A) The patient may be discharged home if the initial and 8-hour chest radiographs are normal.
(B) This patient requires observation for 24 hours to see whether he develops a hemothorax or pneumothorax.
(C) The patient has a potential injury to the heart and requires an echocardiogram.
(D) The patient has an injury to the thoracoabdominal area and requires evaluation for potential injury to the abdomen.
(E) The patient may be discharged home if the initial chest radiograph is normal.

11. Dislocation of which of the following joints is most often associated with an arterial injury?

(A) Elbow
(B) Ankle
(C) Shoulder
(D) Knee
(E) Hip

12. Which of the following statements about flail chest is correct?

(A) Prehospital management involves positioning the patient with the injured side up if possible.
(B) Pain medication should be restricted to prevent further respiratory compromise.
(C) Paradoxical movement of the chest wall is the primary cause of hypoxia.
(D) Intravenous fluids are restricted to prevent fluid overload if the patient is not hypotensive.
(E) Intubation should be used aggressively for patients with hypoxia.

13. Which of the following statements regarding the management of the patient with blunt trauma to the neck is correct?

(A) Orotracheal intubation should not be attempted with suspected laryngotracheal injuries.
(B) Significant laryngotracheal injury is best evaluated by soft tissue lateral radiograph of the neck.
(C) Associated esophageal injuries are common with laryngotracheal injuries.
(D) Life-threatening hemorrhage from blunt neck trauma is common.
(E) Expanding hematoma of the neck requires intervention to secure the airway.

14. A 14-year-old boy complains of lower abdominal pain after straddling the handlebars of his bicycle and then falling to the ground after his bike was struck by a car. Which of the following statements regarding the management of this patient is true?

(A) No immediate study is required to workup microscopic hematuria if he is not in shock or has no significant associated non-genitourinary injuries.
(B) Rectal examination is required before the placement of a Foley catheter.
(C) 100 ml of contrast is instilled into the bladder as part of the cystogram to evaluate gross hematuria.
(D) Indication of extraperitoneal bladder rupture requires surgical exploration.
(E) Straddle injuries typically cause posterior urethral injuries.

15. Which of the following statements regarding head trauma is true?

(A) Subdural hematoma generally has a worse prognosis than epidural hematoma.
(B) Epidural hematomas often are associated with severe underlying injury to the brain.
(C) Seizures occurring within minutes of head trauma indicate a high likelihood of future seizures.
(D) Hyperventilation decreases secondary brain injury by decreasing anoxia.
(E) Epidural hematomas occur more commonly than subdural hematomas in elderly persons.

16. In which patient would performance of diagnostic peritoneal lavage be absolutely contraindicated?

(A) A 37-year-old pregnant woman who is hypotensive after blunt trauma
(B) A 35-year-old man with expanding abdomen after a stab wound to the chest
(C) A 45-year-old obese man who is hypotensive after a rollover car accident
(D) A 65-year-old man with a stab wound to the abdomen with normal blood pressure
(E) A 57-year-old woman with previous surgeries who is hypotensive after falling off a ladder

17. Which of the following statements regarding central cord syndrome is true?

(A) It generally occurs in younger patients.
(B) It results from penetrating injuries.
(C) It occurs with hyperflexion injuries.
(D) It presents with weakness that is worse in the hands than in the arms.
(E) It involves loss of perianal sensation.

18. Which of the following cervical injuries is the most stable?

(A) Clay shoveler's fracture
(B) Flexion teardrop fracture
(C) Jefferson fracture
(D) Hangman's fracture
(E) Bilateral facet dislocation

19. Which of the following statements regarding subdural hematomas is true?

(A) Subdural hematomas are the most common abnormality found on computed tomographic (CT) scan after head injury.
(B) An acute subdural hematoma is symptomatic within 48 hours.
(C) Subdural hematomas often are associated with skull fractures across the middle meningeal artery.
(D) Contrast is not required to detect the presence of subacute or chronic subdural hematoma by CT scan.
(E) Small subdural hematomas require close monitoring, because they often rebleed.

Answers and Explanations

1-C. Although this patient appears to be unresponsive secondary to trauma, his unresponsive state and abnormal neurological findings were due to hypoglycemia. Hypoglycemia caused the patient to lose consciousness, and this in turn caused the patient to fall off the park bench and suffer trauma. He woke up and his neurological findings resolved immediately after he was given one ampule of 50 g dextrose. It is important to check for hypoglycemia in patients with a change in mental status, because it is potentially fatal and easily treatable. Hypoglycemia may present with generalized or focal findings that mimic structural injury. Reversing hypoglycemia may eliminate the need to get radiographs or computed tomographic (CT) scans or to perform intubation. Naloxone is not indicated, because the patient's respiratory rate, large pupils, and apparent structural findings are not consistent with an opiate overdose.

2-E. Venous access should be avoided where possible in veins that may be disrupted by an injury to that area. Placement of subclavian or internal jugular central lines on the same side as a lower chest injury is useful, because the venous access is uninterrupted and possible lung injury from line placement is restricted to the side of the chest that may have been injured in the accident.

3-C. Emergency department (ED) thoracotomy may be helpful to selected trauma patients who have vital signs during those first 5 minutes of arrival in the ED. The patient with an isolated stab wound to the chest has the best chance of surviving an ED thoracotomy. The wound tends to be less extensive than a gunshot wound and is more readily repairable. Isolated injuries to the right ventricle, a systolic BP greater than 50 mm Hg on arrival to the ED, and the presence of cardiac tamponade, are favorable factors for survival. ED thoracotomy is very seldom of benefit to patients with blunt trauma or patients with penetrating injuries to the abdomen or head.

4-C. Penetrating objects such as knives, screwdrivers, or sticks that remain in the patient generally should be removed in the operating room, where minimal damage and maximal control of bleeding can be achieved. If the patient is stable, radiographs may be taken in the emergency department (ED) to help determine the extent of the penetration and resulting damage.

5-C. Elevation of the head of the bed to 30° (assuming no neck injury) is useful in reducing brain swelling. Posttraumatic seizures occur more commonly in children than in adults. Seizures occurring within minutes of the injury are not associated with intracranial injury or subsequent epilepsy, and therefore do not require anticonvulsant therapy. Vomiting after head trauma also is more common in children than in adults, and, by itself (unless persistent), does not require a computed tomographic (CT) scan of the head. Skull radiographs generally are not useful in the diagnosis of head trauma. Normal saline in minimally necessary amounts is preferred over hypotonic intravenous (IV) fluid to decrease swelling of the brain.

6-E. Laparoscopy would be most helpful in diagnosing an injury to the diaphragm. Ultrasound, computed tomographic (CT) scan, and chest radiograph would miss a small hole in the diaphragm unless a piece of bowel or stomach has herniated through it. Diagnostic peritoneal lavage (DPL) can pick up 90% of tears to the diaphragm if the red blood cell count is lowered to 5000. The specificity of this test is low, however, and it will miss injuries to the tendinous portion of the diaphragm, which produces minimal bleeding. Overall, diaphragmatic injuries are still easy to miss in the acute phase.

7-E. Coughing or vomiting blood after abdominal trauma is an automatic indication for laparotomy. Other indications for laparotomy after penetrating trauma include implement in situ, extravasation of bowel or omentum, bleeding from the rectum, and peritoneal findings. Only about 20% of abdominal stab wounds that penetrate the peritoneum injure intraabdominal organs. In view of the low incidence of penetrating abdominal injuries requiring laparotomy, a selective approach has been developed for evaluating whether these injuries require surgery. Penetrating abdominal injuries are likely to injure bowel, stomach, and liver, whereas blunt trauma is more likely to injure solid organs (e.g., spleen and liver) than hollow, viscous organs (e.g, bowel). Computed tomography (CT) and ultrasonography often miss bowel injuries, especially when these tests are done several hours after the injury occurs.

8-B. Any intravenous (IV) medication or blood product may be infused by an intraosseus line. When venous access cannot be obtained in two or three attempts, intraosseus cannulation is the procedure of choice in children younger than 6 years. Initial fluid resuscitation consists of two 20-ml/kg boluses of Ringer's lactate or normal saline. If there is no response to the fluid boluses or vital signs deteriorate after initial improvement, packed red blood cells in boluses of 10 ml/kg should be transfused. Children are able maintain a normal blood pressure despite substantial hypovolemia by significantly increasing their systemic vascular resistance. Tachycardia is the most sensitive indicator of shock in children. Other signs of shock include narrowed pulse pressure, decreased mental status, decreased urine output, prolonged capillary refill, and decreased skin temperature.

9-C. A nasogastric tube and Foley catheter are required before doing a closed diagnostic peritoneal lavage (DPL) in order to decompress the bowel and bladder and decrease the chance of perforating these organs when the DPL needle is placed blindly into the abdomen. Although DPL is a very sensitive test for determining an intraabdominal injury, it has a relatively low specificity and thus may result in substantial nontherapeutic laparotomies. If no gross blood returns when the needle is placed in the abdomen, a red cell count of 100,000 constitutes a positive tap for blunt trauma. A red blood cell count of 5,000 constitutes a positive tap for a diaphragm injury. The only absolute contraindication to a DPL is an obvious abdominal injury requiring laparotomy, such as an abdominal stab wound in a hypotensive patient.

10-A. Studies have shown that pneumothoraces become evident on chest radiograph within 8 hours of penetrating injury. Repeat chest radiographs are warranted at 8 hours to exclude this diagnosis if the initial radiograph is negative for pneumothorax. Because this patient has an isolated stab wound to the right upper chest, which is outside the area of the cardiac silhouette and the thoracoabdominal area, he could be discharged after an 8 hour chest radiograph is normal. The thoracoabdominal area includes the area anteriorly between the 4th rib and the costal margin and posteriorly between the tip of the scapula and the costal margin. It represents the excursion of the diaphragm during inspiration and expiration. Injuries to this area require the exclusion of injuries to both the chest and the abdomen.

11-D. Knee dislocations have a significant risk of arterial injury. Posterior dislocations of the knee are associated with the highest incidence of arterial injury. The initial examination may not reveal a dislocation because of the possibility of spontaneous reduction. This diagnosis should therefore be suspected, and arterial injury should be evaluated when there is severe ligamentous instability of the knee even without radiologic evidence of dislocation. Many centers automatically perform arteriography on patients with knee dislocations.

12-D. The main cause of the hypoxia of flail chest is the underlying lung contusion rather than the paradoxical movement of the unstable chest wall that occurs with breathing. Unnecessary IV fluids should be avoided to minimize the chance of moving fluid into the area of the pulmonary contusion and worsening the paradoxical chest wall motion. The patient may be positioned with the injured side down to help stabilize the chest wall, assuming no injury to the cervical spine is suspected. Pain management is critical with these patients, not only to relieve their severe pain but also to increase the efficiency of their breathing. This may be accomplished with analgesics or intercostal nerve blocks. Patients with flail chest and little underlying pulmonary contusion and associated injuries often can be managed without intubation and mechanical ventilation.

13-E. An expanding hematoma of the neck may quickly close off the airway, and urgent intervention to secure the airway is indicated. Attempting orotracheal intubation is reasonable, but it is important to be prepared to perform a surgical airway if the oral intubation is unsuccessful. Oral intubation should be attempted only if the glottis or vocal cords can be visualized and the tube can be passed gently. Blind intubation by oral or nasal intubation is contraindicated, because it may worsen the already tenuous airway. Additionally, adequate sedation should be used with intubation to avoid causing gagging or coughing that will dislodge a clot, cause massive bleeding, and worsen the airway. Life-threatening hemorrhage and esophageal injuries are not common with laryngotracheal injuries. Laryngotracheal injury is best evaluated by computed tomographic (CT) scan.

14-B. Before placing a Foley catheter in a male trauma patient, it is important to examine the prostate and perineum for a high-riding prostate or perineal hematoma. In addition, the meatus of the penis should be examined for the presence of blood, and the scrotum should be evaluated for ecchymosis, which may indicate an injury to the urethra. Cystograms are used to evaluate potential injuries to the bladder. In the presence of a pelvic ring fracture or gross hematuria, a cystogram is performed using 500 ml of contrast in adults and 5 ml/kg in children to visualize potential injuries to the urinary bladder. The cystogram may be falsely negative unless the appropriate amount of contrast is instilled and adequate bladder pressure is generated. Although microscopic hematuria in stable, adult, blunt trauma patients without major associated injuries does not require immediate work-up, microscopic hematuria in children with trauma requires immediate work-up in the emergency department (ED). It is thought that children have less fat to protect them in falls and thus are at greater risk for potential genitourinary injury. Extraperitoneal bladder ruptures are treated with urethral catheter drainage; no surgery is required. Anterior urethral injuries often result from straddle injuries and kicks to the male genitalia, whereas posterior urethral injuries are associated with pelvic fractures.

15-A. Subdural hematomas are clots that lie between the brain and the dura. Because subdural hematomas are contiguous with the brain, they are more likely to involve injury to the underlying brain than are epidural hematomas. Epidural hematomas are more separated from the brain, lying between the dura and the inner table of the skull. Subdural hematomas are more common than epidural hematomas and are particularly common in patients with brain atrophy, such as elderly or alcoholic patients. Posttraumatic seizures are classified as immediate, early, and late. Immediate seizures have very little morbidity and consequently are not treated unless subsequent seizures or significant findings (e.g., blood) are on the computed tomographic (CT) scan. Hyperventilation decreases the secondary brain injury that results from swelling of the brain by decreasing pCO_2. The drop in pCO_2 causes vasoconstriction, which decreases the brain edema.

16-B. The only absolute contraindication to diagnostic peritoneal lavage (DPL) is an indication for laparotomy or laparoscopy. Indications for laparotomy include penetrating injury to the abdomen with any one of the following: hypotension, expanding abdomen, diffusely tender abdomen (not just at the site of the wound), blood from the rectum, bloody vomiting, evisceration of bowel or omentum, and knife in situ. Relative contraindications to DPL include third-trimester pregnancy, obesity, and previous abdominal surgery. DPL may be done supraumbilically in the first and second trimesters of pregnancy to avoid the enlarged uterus. DPL can be done at a distance from previous surgical scars (e.g., paramedially) using an open technique to avoid adhesions and to provide access to free fluid. It is possible that adhesions from previous surgery may wall off the free fluid, in which case a false-negative reading would be obtained. DPL can be done on the obese patient, but it may be very difficult to cut down through the fat and gain access to the peritoneum.

17-D. Central cord syndrome is the most common of the incomplete spinal cord injuries. It generally is seen in elderly patients with degenerative cervical vertebrae disease with a resulting narrowed spinal canal. The cervical spine is subjected to hyperextension, with the resulting injury to the central portion of the cord causing greater neurological deficit in the upper extremities than in the lower extremities. The hands are more affected than the arms. Treatment usually is nonoperative, and the prognosis is relatively good.

18-A. The clay shoveler's fracture is a fracture of the base of the spinous process of one of the lower cervical vertebrae. Because this flexion-type injury affects only the spinous process, it is not associated with any neurological involvement and is stable. Although it was associated originally with miners shoveling clay, it is now more commonly seen with blows to the back of the neck and sudden deceleration injuries resulting in forced flexion of the neck. The flexion teardrop fracture is a wedge-shaped fracture of the antero-inferior portion of the involved cervical vertebral body. Ligamentous disruption is extensive, and it is very unstable. The Jefferson fracture is a burst fracture of the ring of the first vertebra, resulting from a vertical compression force. It is seen most often on the open-mouth odontoid view with the lateral masses of C1 lying lateral to the articular pillars of C2. This injury is very unstable. The hangman's fracture is a bilateral fracture through the pedicles of C2 that is due to a hyperextension injury. Although the lesion is unstable, cord damage usually is minimal because the size of the spinal canal is greatest at C2, and the bilateral pedicle fractures allow the injury to decompress itself. The associated prevertebral swelling, however, may cause respiratory compromise. Close monitoring is mandatory, and airway intervention may be necessary. Bilateral facet dislocation is a very unstable flexion injury resulting in nearly total ligamentous disruption. On the lateral cervical spine film, there is anterior displacement of more than 50% of the diameter of one vertebral body on the next lower vertebra.

19-E. Up to 40% of subdural hematomas will rebleed. Therefore, patients with even small rim subdural hematomas must be admitted to closely monitored floor beds for observation. Subarachnoid hemorrhage is the most common abnormality seen on computed tomography (CT) after head trauma. Acute subdural hematomas are symptomatic within 24 hours, subacute subdural hematomas are symptomatic in 24 hours to 2 weeks, and chronic subdural hematomas become symptomatic after 2 weeks. Because subacute and chronic subdural hematomas may be isodense to brain parenchyma, they sometimes are difficult to diagnose. Although indirect evidence of the lesion, such as midline shift and ventricular compression, may be seen on a noncontrast head CT scan, contrast will help detect isodense lesions.

18

Toxicology Emergencies

I. Evaluation of the Poisoned Patient

—Evaluation of the poisoned patient consists of thorough diagnostic tests of airway, breathing, and circulation (ABCs), followed by the history and physical examination.

A. Airway. In assessing the airway, evidence of compromise, such as would be suggested by stridor, snoring, loss of the gag reflex, or vomitus in the oropharynx, is looked for.

B. Breathing. The frequency and depth of breathing are noted. Slow, deep breathing may indicate the need for ventilatory support; rapid, shallow breathing may indicate an underlying metabolic acidosis or hypoxemia.

C. Circulation. Blood pressure (BP) and pulse are obtained to assess baseline circulatory status. Bradycardia may indicate cardiotoxicity or parasympathetic overload, whereas tachycardia may be due to cholinergic blockade or central nervous system (CNS) stimulation.

D. History. Because the poisoned patient often presents in a stuporous or at least somewhat altered mental state, obtaining the history may be challenging. It is important to obtain as much information as possible from the paramedics, the patient, the family, and anyone else who was at the scene or who has knowledge of the patient's medical and/or psychiatric history. The objective of the history is to answer the following questions:

1. What poison is involved?
2. How much was taken?
3. By what route was the poison taken (e.g., by mouth, intravenous (IV), skin exposure)?
4. When was it taken relative to evaluation in the emergency department (ED)?
5. What else was taken with it? It is important to remember that the most common co-ingestant in adult poisonings is **ethanol.**

E. Physical examination

1. **Vital signs**

—Any abnormality in vital signs is especially significant in the poisoned patient. Pulse and respiratory rate are determined when the ABCs are checked. It also is important to obtain the temperature and BP. Disturbances in temperature regulation can result from alterations in the CNS (stimulation or depression) and from loss of thermoregulation, often seen with the phenothiazine class of drugs. Hypotension can result from cardiotoxicity, CNS depression, loss of vasomotor tone, and volume depletion (e.g., from diabetes insipidus secondary to lithium, or from diarrhea secondary to organophosphates). Hypertension can result from monoamine oxidase inhibitors (MAOI) overdose, sympathomimetics, and drug withdrawal.

2. Pupillary size

—**Miosis** can be seen in CNS depression, α-adrenergic blockade, and cholinergic stimulation (e.g., opiates, organophosphates, and barbiturates).

—**Mydriasis** can be seen in α-adrenergic stimulation and cholinergic inhibition (e.g., atropine, cocaine, and ethanol).

3. Oral examination

—The odor of the breath is an important diagnostic clue. Table 18-1 lists the odors commonly associated with certain toxins.

—Oral examination also permits examinations for burns, as evidence of caustic ingestions and assessment of mucosal hydration. Increased salivation is associated with organophosphates, strychnine, and arsenic, whereas dry mouth is seen with opiates, anticholinergics, and atropine.

Table 18-1. Odors Associated With Specific Toxins

Odor	Toxin
Acetone	Alcohol, salicylates
Bitter almonds	Cyanide
Carrots	Gemloxin (water hemlock)
Fruity	Ethanol, isopropanol, acetone
Garlic	Arsenic, parathion, organophosphates
Glue	Toluene
Mothballs	Camphor, naphthalene
Pear	Chloral hydrate
Shoe polish	Nitrobenzene
Vinyl	Ethchlorvynol
Wintergreen	Methylsalicylate

4. **Examination of the skin**
   —Track marks provide evidence of IV drug use.
   —Cyanosis refractory to oxygen therapy is suggestive of methemoglobinemia.
   —A red or unusually rosy complexion may be due to cyanide, carbon monoxide, boric acid, or anticholinergic poisoning.
   —Dry skin or lack of sweating is associated with anticholinergic poisoning, whereas moist skin indicates cholinergic or sympathomimetic overdose.
5. **Identification of toxidromes**
   —Knowledge of the cluster of physical findings associated with a particular class of drug can be especially helpful in deciding the course of action. Knowing the type of drug enables the appropriate treatment and antidote to be administered, if available. Table 18-2 lists the common toxidromes.

Table 18-2. Toxidromes

Toxidrome	Examples of toxins	Features
Cholinergics	Organophosphates (insecticides) Carbamates Physostigmine Edrophonium Some mushrooms	Salivation Lacrimation Urination Diarrhea GI upset Emesis
Anticholinergics	Tricyclic antidepressants Belladonna alkaloids Atropine Anti-parkinsonian medications Antihistamines Phenothiazines Scopolamine	Dry mucus membranes Urinary retention Flushed skin Mydriasis Fever
Opioids	Heroin Morphine Meperidine	Coma Respiratory depression Pinpoint pupils (miosis)
Sympathomimetics	Cocaine Amphetamines	Hypertension Tachycardia Hyperpyrexia Mydriasis Anxiety/delirium
Salicylates	Aspirin Many headache and cold medicines	Fever Tachypnea Vomiting Lethargy Tinnitus
Barbiturates	Phenobarbital Secobarbital	Respiratory depression Hypotension Hyperthermia Vesicles or bullae

F. Drugs

1. The "coma cocktail," administered to patients who are unresponsive, consists of **thiamine, dextrose,** and **naloxone.** The cocktail has three components, which commonly reverse many comas. Bedside serum glucose is checked before the cocktail is delivered. Glucose is checked just to make sure coma is not due to non-ketotic hyperosmolar (high sugar) coma. If glucose is high, dextrose should be omitted from the cocktail. The thiamine (100 mg IV) is given before the dextrose (50 g IV push) to prevent **Wernicke-Korsakoff syndrome.** The naloxone (.01 mg/kg) reverses opiate depression, thereby serving as both a therapeutic and diagnostic tool. Several doses of naloxone may be required for patients with a physiological dependence on opioids, or those who have ingested certain synthetic opiate preparations.
2. If the patient is acutely agitated or psychotic, a cocktail of 5–10 mg of **haloperidol** given intramuscularly (IM) and 2–4 mg of **lorazepam** given IM or IV helps to calm the patient so that more definitive therapy may be instituted.
3. **Antidotes**

   —There are antidotes for many of the common poisons encountered in the ED (Table 18-3).

G. Diagnostic tests

1. **Complete blood cell count (CBC):** useful for detecting an infection. Absolute leukocytosis also may be produced by iron, theophylline, and hydrocarbons.
2. **Chemistry panel.** This is especially useful for calculating the anion and osmolal gaps.

   a. The **anion gap (AG) = $[Na^+ - (HCO_3^- + Cl^-)]$.**

   (1) The normal value for an AG is between 8 and 12 mEq/L.

   (2) The presence of an elevated AG means that there is an excess of unmeasured anions, resulting in metabolic acidosis. The differential diagnosis of an elevated AG is summarized by the acronym **CARTMUDPILES:**

   —**C**arbon monoxide (CO), cyanide, caffeine
   —**A**spirin
   —**R**espiratory dysfunction
   —**T**oluene
   —**M**ethanol
   —**U**remia
   —**D**iabetic ketoacidosis (DKA)
   —**P**araldehyde, phenformin
   —**I**ron, isoniazid, ibuprofen
   —**L**ithium, lactic acidosis
   —**E**thanol, ethylene glycol
   —**S**trychnine, starvation, salicylates

   b. The **osmolal gap = [calculated osm] − [measured osm].**

   —**Calculated osm = $2(Na^+)$ + glucose/18 + BUN/2.8**

Table 18-3. Antidotes for Common Toxins

Toxin	Antidote
Acetaminophen	N-acetylcysteine (Mucomyst)
Anticholinesterases, organophosphates	Atropine, pralidoxime
Antimuscarinics, anticholinergics	Physostigmine
Arsenic, mercury, gold	Dimercaprol, D-penicillamine, British Anti-Lewisite (BAL)
α-adrenergic agonists	Phentolamine
β-blockers	Glucagon
Benzodiazepines	Flumazenil
Carbon monoxide	100% oxygen, hyperbaric oxygen
Calcium channel blockers	Calcium gluconate
Copper	Penicillamine
Cyanide	Amyl nitrate + Na-nitrite + thiosulfate
Digitalis	Anti-dig Fab fragments (Digibind)
Heparin	Protamine
Iron salts	Deferoxamine
Isoniazid	Pyridoxine
Lead, arsenic, mercury	CaEDTA
Lead, mercury	Succimer
Methanol, ethylene glycol	Ethanol
Methemoglobinemia	Methylene blue*
Neuromuscular blockers	Neostigmine
Opioids	Naloxone
Organophosphates, carbamates	Atropine, pralidoxime
Tricyclic antidepressants	$NaHCO_3$
t-PA, streptokinase	Aminocaproic acid
Warfarin	Vitamin K

*Contraindicated in glucose 6-phosphate dehydrogenase deficiency. N-acetylcysteine (NAC) is being used investigationally for treatment of methemoglobinemia in GPD deficient patients.

—Normal serum osm = 275–285

—An elevated osmolal gap (> 10 mOsm/L) suggests the presence of low-molecular-weight solutes that were not measured. Common solutes include **ethanol, methanol, ethylene glycol, isopropyl alcohol, mannitol,** and **glycerol.** An elevated gap, therefore, suggests intoxication with one of these solutes. The gap also can be used to make a rough calculation of the amount of solute ingested.

3. **Arterial blood gases (ABGs)** to determine acid–base status. Even the color of the blood—such as the chocolate-colored blood seen in methemoglobinemia—can be helpful.

4. **Abdominal radiograph** to look for radiopaque substances. Some of the common radiopaque substances are summarized by the acronym **CHIPES:**

—**C**hloral hydrate

—**H**eavy metals (arsenic, lead)

—**I**ron, iodide

—**P**henothiazines, psychotropics [tricyclic antidepressants (TCAs)], potassium

—**E**nteric-coated, sustained-release preparations

—**S**alicylates, salts

5. **Electrocardiogram (ECG)** is useful to assess baseline rate and rhythm. Certain drugs have typical toxic patterns on ECG, although these patterns may not be universally present.

   a. **Prolongation of QRS:** TCAs (typical), phenothiazines, calcium channel blockers (CCB)

   b. **Sinus bradycardia/AV block:** β-blockers (BB), CCB, TCAs, digoxin, organophosphates

   c. **Ventricular tachycardia (VT):** cocaine, amphetamines, chloral hydrate, theophylline, digoxin, TCAs

H. Gastrointestinal (GI) decontamination

1. **Syrup of ipecac.** There is very little use for syrup of ipecac. It is definitely contraindicated in caustic ingestions, and unless it will take longer than 1 hour to get from the site of injury to medical assistance, it should not be administered for other ingestions.

2. **Activated charcoal (AC)** is the method of choice for GI decontamination. Some drugs do not adsorb to charcoal, however. These include iron, lithium, hydrocarbons, borates, bromides, mineral acids and alkali, and ethanol. AC in these ingestions is not helpful. Drugs with significant enterohepatic circulation, such as theophylline, digoxin, aspirin, and some β-blockers, require multiple doses of AC (MDAC). Dosage is 1 g/kg.

3. **Gastric lavage (GL)** is helpful for early presentation of ingestions (within 1 hour) and for recovery of pill fragments. It is not as effective in removing the toxin as AC. It is important to remember to use large-bore orogastric tubes (24–32 French in children, 36–42 French in adults) in order to retrieve pill fragments. GL is contraindicated in patients with an unprotected airway, and in ingestions of alkali. Complications include laryngospasm, aspiration pneumonia, and sinus bradycardia.

4. **Whole bowel irrigation** is useful for sustained-release drug preparations, for late presentations, and to aid in massive ingestions in which a significant proportion of the drug may already be in the small bowel. Whole bowel irrigation is accomplished by oral ingestion of a polyethylene glycol electrolyte solution, which decreases transit time via the GI tract without causing electrolyte abnormalities. The dosage is 1.5–2 L/hr (adults), and 25 mg/kg/hr (children). Infusion is continued until the rectal effluent looks the same as the infusate.

5. **Cathartics** are solutions of either saline (MgCitrate, MgSO4, NaSO4) or sorbitol that are administered to promote GI motility and enhance GI transit. They can be given in combination with AC or separately. Although they do reduce GI transit time, they have never been shown to improve morbidity or mortality and therefore are not widely used. They have the additional disadvantages of causing moderate electrolyte disturbances, including hypermagnesemia.

II. Acetaminophen

A. Mechanism of action

—Approximately 10% of acetaminophen (APAP) gets converted in the liver to the toxic metabolite NAPQI, which requires **glutathione** to be metabolized either back to its precursor, or to less toxic compounds. APAP toxicity is thought to occur when glutathione stores drop to < 30%. Glutathione stores are depleted in many situations that put the patient at increased risk for APAP toxicity. These include malnutrition (as seen in patients with AIDS, cancer patients, and chronic alcoholics) and ingestion of drugs that induce the P450 system, including anticonvulsants, isoniazid, and rifampin.

B. Clinical features

—**Table 18-4** describes the stages of APAP toxicity.

C. Diagnostic tests

1. Serum APAP level should be obtained 4 hours post-ingestion, when APAP levels peak. If ingestion time is unknown, draw one level immediately and another one in 2–4 hours.

Table 18-4. Stages of Acetaminophen Toxicity

Stage	Time post-ingestion	Symptoms
1. Initial	0–24 h	Mostly asymptomatic Mild anorexia, nausea, vomiting, diaphoresis
2. Latent	24–48 h	LFTs and PT begin to increase
3. Hepatic	72–96 h	Hepatic dysfunction peaks Hepatic failure signaled by vomiting, metabolic acidosis, jaundice, hypoglycemia, coagulopathy, renal failure, and RUQ pain
4. Recovery	4–14 days	Recovery. Symptoms resolve in 3–5 days LFTs return to normal in 1–3 weeks

LFT = Liver function test; *PT* = prothrombin time; *RUQ* = right upper quadrant.

2. Liver function tests (LFTs), prothrombin time (PT), and bilirubin levels are obtained on initial presentation and several hours afterward to assess extent, if any, of liver damage. Elevated unconjugated bilirubin is suggestive of liver toxicity.
3. Additional baseline tests that are done include CBC, chemistry panel, and a pregnancy test in women of childbearing age.

D. Treatment

1. **AC,** with or without a cathartic.
2. **Antidote. N-acetylcysteine** (NAC) reverses APAP toxicity by replenishing glutathione stores. The nomogram shown in Figure 18-1 helps determine whether treatment with an antidote is necessary. If the APAP level is ≥ 150 mg/ml at 4 hours post-ingestion, it usually is treated.
   a. Indications for antidote
      —APAP levels taken 4 to 12 hours post-ingestion that fall above treatment line on nomogram
      —Single APAP ingestion of > 140 mg/kg with plasma APAP level unavailable at the time
      —Acute liver failure has developed or is imminent.

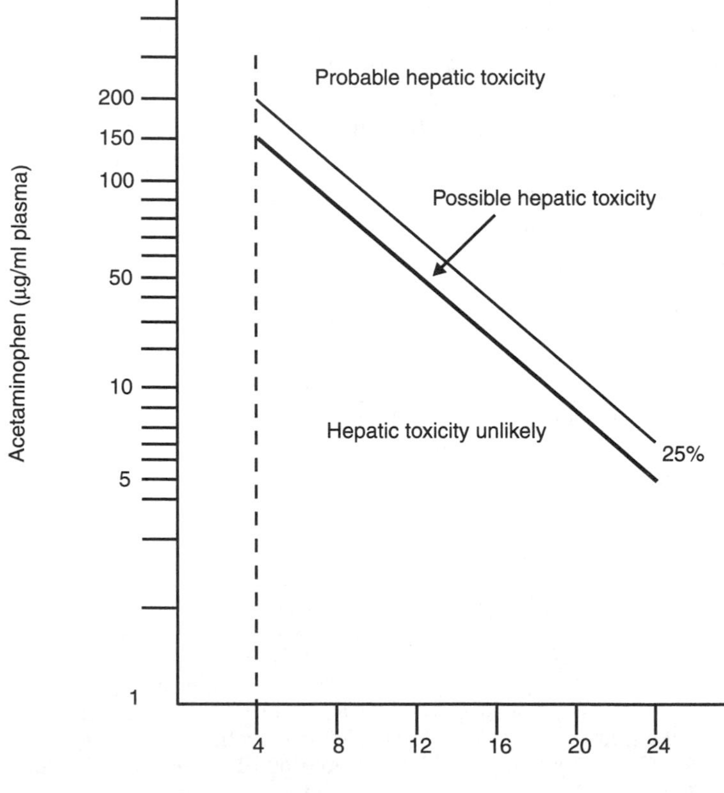

Figure 18-1. Rumack-Matthew nomogram for acetaminophen poisoning. (Reprinted with permission from Rumack BH, Matthew H: *Pediatrics* 55:871, 1975.)

b. **Dosage.** NAC ideally should be given within 8 hours of ingestion, but can be administered up to 48 to 96 hours post-ingestion. Dosage of oral NAC 5% solution is 140 mg/kg initially, followed by 70 mg/kg every 4 hours, for a total of 17 doses. IV NAC is used in other countries, but is only available as an investigational agent in the United States.

3. Blood sugar is monitored. Hypoglycemia is treated with a 10%–20% glucose drip.
4. **Ondansetron** (0.15 mg/kg every 8 hours, 3 times) or **metoclopramide** (1 mg/kg for children; 10 mg for adults) to prevent nausea and improve tolerance to NAC
5. **Vitamin K** for PT more than 1.5 times normal
6. **Fresh frozen plasma (FFP)** for PT more than 3 times normal
7. **Lactulose** enemas (30 ml every 6–8 hr) for encephalopathy
8. **Mannitol** (0.5 g/kg given over 10 minutes) and fluid restriction for cerebral edema that may result from encephalopathy

E. Disposition

1. Patients with negligible APAP levels who present after a known period of time following a single ingestion may be discharged home with outpatient follow-up.
2. Patients with toxic APAP levels, liver damage (per LFTs), who present after an unknown time following ingestion, and who have had multiple ingestions should be admitted to the intensive care unit (ICU).
3. All patients who have ingested substances with suicidal intent should receive psychiatric evaluation.

F. Prognosis. Poor prognostic factors include:

—acidosis with pH < 7.3

—PT > 180 seconds

—Increasing PT between day 3 and 4

—PT > 100 seconds with serum creatinine > 3.4 mg/dl

—Factor V $\leq 10\%$

III. Salicylates

—Salicylates include aspirin, many over-the-counter cold medications, certain prescription pain and migraine relievers, and methyl salicylate.

A. Mechanism of action

1. **Respiratory alkalosis:** Salicylates increase the sensitivity of the medullary respiratory center to pH and pCO_2, resulting in increased alveolar ventilation (hyperventilation).
2. **Emesis and hypokalemia:** Salicylates stimulate the medullary chemoreceptor trigger zone, resulting in vomiting and hypokalemia. Compensation for respiratory alkalosis results in increased renal tubule

permeability and increased excretion of ions, further exacerbating potassium loss.

3. **Hypoglycemia and hyperthermia:** Salicylates disrupt the oxidative phosphorylation pathway, which results in increased heat production and enhanced glycolysis, causing hyperthermia (mild to moderate) and hypoglycemia.
4. **Anion gap metabolic acidosis:** The gap comes from accumulation of unmeasured anions such as ketoacids, lactate, and salicylate. Acidosis stems from three different pathways:
   a. Uncoupling of oxidative phosphorylation results in increased lactate production by tissues.
   b. Inhibition of Krebs' cycle results in accumulation of pyruvate and lactate.
   c. As the buffering capability of the body via urinary excretion of bicarbonate and the Hb-OxyHb system dwindles, metabolic acidosis worsens.
   d. **Pulmonary and/or cerebral edema** are thought to result from increased capillary permeability, although the exact mechanism is unknown. Cigarette smoking and salicylate levels > 40 mg/dl are associated with increased risk of noncardiogenic pulmonary edema.
   e. **GI bleed/hemorrhage:** Salicylates disrupt the coagulation cascade at cyclo-oxygenase, preventing the formation of thromboxane A2, a factor required for platelet aggregation. Although some degree of prolonged bleeding time is associated with even a single dose of aspirin, hemorrhage is a rare complication of salicylate overdose.

B. Clinical features

—**Acute salicylate ingestion** often is associated with suicidal intent but carries a low mortality.

—**Chronic intoxication** usually is seen in very young or very old patients, often due to therapeutic mistakes (overdose). Pulmonary and/or cerebral edema, CNS effects, and hyperventilation are more pronounced and more frequent in chronic intoxication.

—The high mortality (approximately 25%) stems from delay in presentation to the ED, delay in diagnosis (salicylate toxicity is mistaken for other illnesses), and greater systemic acidosis, resulting in higher tissue penetration.

1. **Symptoms** may include:

   —tinnitus or hearing loss (reversible)

   —altered mental status

   —lethargy

   —hallucinations

   —seizures

2. **Physical examination findings** may include:

   —mild to moderate hyperthermia

   —asterixis

   —tachycardia

—tachypnea

—coma

C. Diagnostic tests

1. **Serum salicylate levels** correlate poorly with severity of intoxication. Use of the Done nomogram (Figure 18-2) is severely limited, so the treatment plan must be based on the patient's presentation and the dose ingested.
2. **Chemistry panel** and **serial ABGs** to determine acid–base and electrolyte status and to check for hypoglycemia
3. **LFTs** and **PT** to look for hepatotoxicity
4. **Ferric chloride test** to look for salicylates: 1 ml of urine is mixed with 1 ml of reagent (Trinder reagent, 40 g $HgCl_2$ with 40 g $FeNO_3$ in deionized water and HCl). A purple color indicates positive test for salicylates.

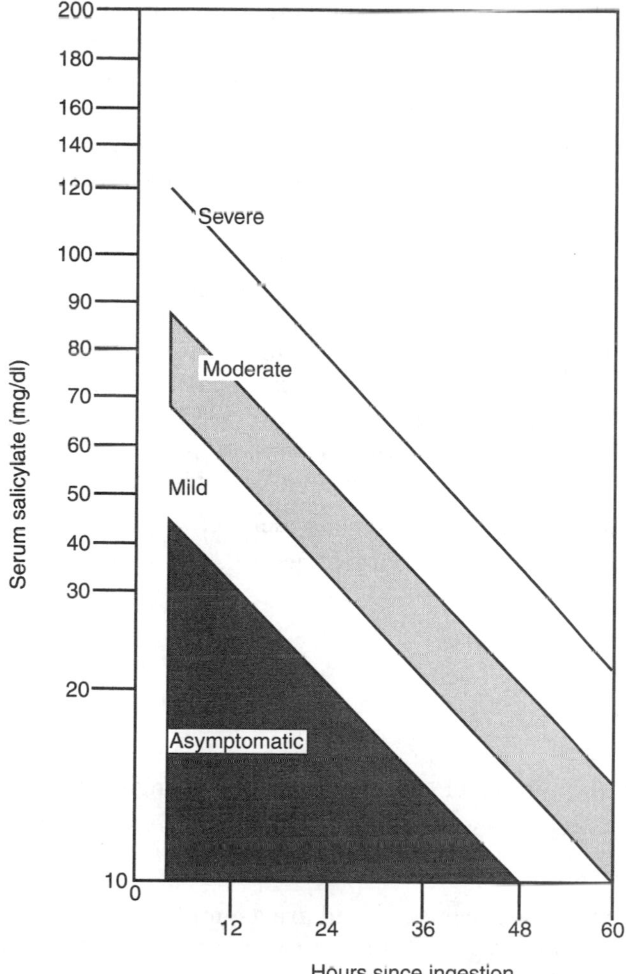

Figure 18-2. Done nomogram for salicylate poisoning. (Reprinted with permission from Done AK: *Pediatrics* 26:00, 1960.)

5. **Urinary pH measurement:** alkaline pH of 7.5–8.0 is desired, to promote renal excretion of salicylate.
6. Pregnancy test for women of childbearing age

D. Treatment

1. **ABCs**
2. **Hydration** with D5NS or D5½NS to maintain a urine output of 3 ml/kg/hr
3. **Electrolyte abnormalities must be corrected.**
   a. Hypokalemia is a particularly bad prognostic factor. It should be corrected with KCl infusions: 40 mEq in 50–250 ml of D5W for 4 to 6 runs.
   b. Hypoglycemia is prevented by adding glucose to IV fluids.
   c. Hypocalcemia can result in tetany. It should be treated with **calcium gluconate.**
4. Seizures are treated with **IV diazepam.**
5. GI decontamination is important. If the patient presents within 24 hours after ingestion or has taken a sustained-release or enteric-coated preparation, then GL is indicated. It is necessary to use a tube large enough in diameter to recover pill fragments.
6. **AC** is given, 1 mg/kg, while results of laboratory studies are awaited. Multiple doses are indicated, because salicylates have large volumes of distribution.
7. **Urine alkalinization** promotes salicylate excretion and should be considered in patients with salicylate levels > 35 mg/dl or when clinical toxicity is evident. It is achieved via administration of **sodium bicarbonate.** Following an IV loading bolus of 1–2 mEq/kg, 3 ampules are added to glucose-containing IV fluids, to run at 1.5 to 2 times maintenance. The aim is to maintain urinary pH at 7.5–8.0. Urinary alkalinization should *not* be undertaken at the expense of causing serum acidosis, however. Serum pH should be maintained at 7.45–7.50.
8. Indications for **hemodialysis** include:
   a. Severe acid–base disturbance
   b. Renal failure
   c. Hepatic failure
   d. Pulmonary edema
   e. Seizures
   f. Coma
   g. Salicylate level > 100 mg/dl in acute ingestions
   h. Salicylate level > 60 mg/dl in chronic ingestions

E. Disposition

1. Patients who receive AC and are asymptomatic after 6 hours of observation (12 hours for sustained-release preparations) may be discharged home with outpatient follow-up.
2. Patients who are symptomatic or have toxic levels should be admitted to the hospital, preferably to the ICU, for further management.

3. All patients who have ingested salicylates with suicidal intent should receive psychiatric evaluation.

IV. β-Blockers

A. Mechanism of action (Fig. 18-3)

—β-blockers (BB) competitively inhibit endogenous catecholamines at the β receptor, preventing activation of adenyl cyclase, the enzyme responsible for converting adenosine monophosphate (AMP) to cyclic AMP (cAMP).

—Table 18-5 lists common β-blockers.

B. Clinical features

1. **Symptoms of toxicity** usually are evident within 2 hours of ingestion and may include:

   —seizures (propranolol)

   —dizziness

   —fatigue

   —mydriasis

2. **Physical examination findings** may include:

   —bradycardia

   —hypotension

   —respiratory depression

   —hypoglycemia

   —bronchospasm (with nonselective agents)

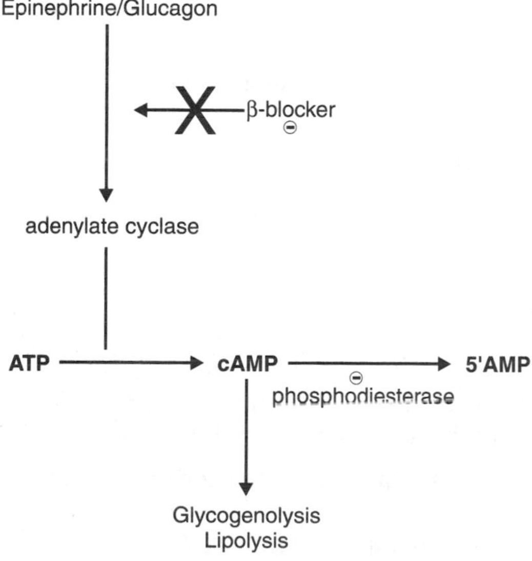

Figure 18-3. β-blocker action

Table 18-5. Common β-Blockers

Nonselective	**β_1 selective**
Labetalol	Acebutol
Nadolol	Atenolol
Penbutolol	Betaxolol
Pindolol	Bisoprolol
Propranolol	Esmolol
Timolol	Metoprolol
Sotalol	Practolol
Carvedilol	

—VT and ventricular fibrillation (VF)

—mild hyperkalemia

C. Diagnostic tests

1. Serum levels correlate poorly with clinical toxicity and therefore are of little use.
2. **ECG** to look for rate and rhythm disturbances
3. **Cardiac enzymes** to look for acute myocardial infarction
4. **ABG** and **chemistry panel** to assess acid–base and electrolyte status

D. Treatment

1. ABCs (IV, oxygen, monitor!)
2. AC for early presentations. MDAC should be considered for all drugs that undergo enterohepatic circulation, including BB.
3. Whole bowel irrigation for sustained-release preparations
4. **Atropine** (0.5 mg adults, 0.02 mg/kg children) for symptomatic bradycardia. Atropine should be given immediately, before endotracheal intubation, to prevent unnecessary vagal stimulation. Atropine can be administered IV or via endotracheal tube (ETT).
5. **Glucagon** for hypoglycemia and bradycardia

   —Adults: 5–10 mg bolus followed by 2–5 mg/hr infusion

   —Children: 0.05–0.10 mg/kg bolus, followed by 0.05–0.10 mg/hr
6. Fluids for hypotension: **Normal saline (NS)** or **Lactated Ringer's (LR)** is infused at 20–40 ml/kg in an effort to expand intravascular volume.
7. If hypotension persists despite fluids, a pressor agent is indicated. Infusions are titrated to BP.

   a. Isoproterenol: 4 μg/min (adults) or 0.05–2.0 μg/min (children)

   b. Dopamine: 5–20 μg/kg/min

   c. Epinephrine: 2–10 μg/min (adults) or 0.05–2.0 μg/min (children)

8. **Amiodarone** is a phosphodiesterase inhibitor that increases cAMP and enhances contractility by increasing Ca^{2+} influx. The loading dose is 0.75 mg/kg; infusion rate is 5 μg/kg/min.

E. Disposition

1. Because BB have a rapid onset of action, an asymptomatic patient at 4 hours post-ingestion (24 hours for sustained-release preparation) can be discharged home with outpatient follow-up.
2. Symptomatic patients should be admitted to the coronary care unit (CCU).

V. Calcium Channel Blockers

A. Mechanism of action

1. Inhibition of slow L-type calcium channels in myocardium results in decreased conduction at the sinoatrial node (SAN) and atrioventricular node (AVN).
2. Inhibition of the fast calcium channels results in decreased myocardial contractility and vasodilation of smooth muscle.

B. Clinical features

1. **Symptoms** may include:

—dizziness

—apnea

—somnolence

—seizures

2. **Physical examination findings** may include:

—metabolic acidosis

—tachycardia

—hypotension

—tetany

C. Diagnostic tests

1. ECG to look for conduction delays and blocks
2. **Cardiac enzymes** to look for acute myocardial infarction
3. **ABG** and **chemistry panel** to assess acid–base and electrolyte status

D. Treatment

—Treatment is the same as for BB (see section IV D). The only difference is the addition of 10–20 ml of a 10% solution of $\mathbf{CaCl_2}$, administered IV, slowly over 10 min, followed by an infusion of 5–10 ml/hr until ECG normalizes and tetany resolves.

E. Disposition

1. Because CCBs have a rapid onset of action, a patient who is asymptomatic at 6 hours post-ingestion (24 hours for sustained-release preparations) can be discharged home.
2. Symptomatic patients should be admitted to the coronary care unit (CCU).

VI. Digitalis

—Digoxin and digitoxin are the most common cardiac glycosides and forms of digitalis. They are compared in Table 18-6. Other cardiac glycosides include oleander, foxglove, and lily of the valley, which also can cause digitalis toxicity. Specifics in this section refer to digoxin, unless stated otherwise.

A. Mechanism of action

—Digoxin inhibits Na^+K^+ATPase. The inhibition increases intracellular Na^+ and Ca^{2+} and extracellular K^+. Digoxin is used in the treatment of congestive heart failure and atrial fibrillation, where it increases the force of myocardial contraction and decreases conduction velocity through the Purkinje tissue.

B. **Risk factors** that increase cardiac sensitivity for digoxin include:

—acute hypoxia

—hypo- or hyperkalemia

—hypercalcemia

—hypomagnesemia

—respiratory alkalosis

—acute myocardial infarction (AMI)

—advanced age

—direct current (DC) cardioversion

C. Clinical features

1. **Symptoms** may include:

—nausea

—vomiting

—malaise

—blurred vision (chronic)

—altered mental status (chronic)

—somnolence (chronic)

2. **Physical examination findings** may include:

—bradycardia

D. Diagnostic tests

1. **Serum digoxin level** 6 hours post-ingestion is drawn to obtain steady-

Table 18-6. Digoxin vs. Digitoxin

	Metabolized by	Half-life	V_D	Enterohepatic circulation	Protein bound
Digoxin	Kidney	30 h	6.0 L/kg	Minimal	25%
Digitoxin	Liver	7 days	0.6 L/kg	Large	95%

V_D = volume of distribution

state level, which correlates with toxicity. A level of > 2 ng/ml is considered toxic. (There is considerable overlap between therapeutic and toxic levels.)

2. **Chemistry panel** to look for:
   a. **Hyperkalemia.** Hyperkalemia often is present in acute toxicity. It is treated with glucose, insulin, and bicarbonate, as necessary. Administration of calcium in the setting of digoxin toxicity may be lethal and is therefore contraindicated.
   b. **Hypomagnesemia.** It is necessary to replace Mg^{2+}, because magnesium has been shown to terminate even refractory VT/VF. Hypermagnesemia may be heralded by loss of deep tendon reflexes, and eventually by respiratory depression.
3. **ECG**
   a. **Acute findings:** AV block and decreased cardiac output. The classic toxic digoxin rhythm is nonparoxysmal tachycardia with 2:1 block. Ventricular dysrhythmias are rare.
   b. **Chronic findings:** premature atrial junctional tachycardia with all grades of AV block, ventricular automaticity, and extrasystoles.
4. **Chest radiograph** to assess patient's volume status. Many patients with congestive heart failure (CHF) easily become fluid overloaded, putting them at risk for pulmonary edema.
5. **Cardiac enzymes** to rule out AMI as one of the causes of increased cardiac sensitivity to digoxin.

E. **Treatment**

1. ABCs, including continuous **cardiac monitoring**
2. Rhythm disturbances must be treated.
   a. Ventricular ectopy and tachydysrhythmias are treated with **lidocaine** (loading dose of 2 mg/kg IV followed by infusion at 1–4 mg/min) or **phenytoin** (loading dose of 10 mg/kg IV followed by infusion at 25–50 mg/min).
   b. Symptomatic bradycardia is treated with **atropine.**
      —Adults: 0.5–1.0 mg every 3–5 min, to a maximum dose of 3 mg
      —Children: 0.01–0.02 mg/kg IV or via ETT if present every 3–5 min, to a maximum dose of 0.04 mg/kg
      —Equipment for transvenous pacing must be ready in case of refractory bradycardia.
3. GI decontamination
   a. GL for early (within 24 hours of ingestion) presentations. Use may be limited, because it produces vagal stimulation, which may be undesirable.
   b. **AC** is appropriate for oral overdose. MDAC should be considered for digitoxin due to its large volume of distribution (V_D).
4. **Antidote** therapy
   —Digoxin-specific Fab fragments are available as an antidote to digoxin poisoning. They prevent digoxin from binding to its receptor.

a. **Indications** include:
—severe, life-threatening dysrhythmias
—symptomatic bradyarrhythmias unresponsive to atropine
—coingestion of other cardiotoxic drugs (BB, CCB)
—serum $K^+ > 5$ mEq/L
—single ingestions of > 10 mg in adults, 4 mg in children
—serum steady-state digoxin level > 10 ng/ml in adults, or > 0.5 ng/ml in children
—cardiac arrest, imminent cardiac arrest, or shock
—rapid clinical deterioration: progressive obtundation, worsening conduction defects, rapidly increasing serum K^+

b. **Disadvantages:** the major disadvantage is cost.

c. **Dosing:** can be given empirically, or calculated as follows:
—If amount ingested is known: # vials Fab = (total body load)/V_D = (amount ingested × 0.8)/0.6 mg/L given IV
—If serum steady-state digoxin level is known: # vials Fab = (serum level) × (weight in kg) given IV
—If neither amount ingested nor serum level is known: 10 vials over 30 minutes for acute ingestions; 4 vials over 30 minutes for chronic ingestions; 20 vials for cardiac arrest

F. Disposition

1. Patients with acute ingestions who presented early, have received AC, and remain asymptomatic 8 hours post-ingestion can be discharged home.
2. All patients with chronic ingestion are admitted to the CCU for monitoring.
3. All patients who have ingested digoxin with suicidal intent are admitted for psychiatric evaluation and cardiac monitoring.

VII. Ethylene Glycol

A. Mechanism of action

—Ethylene glycol is metabolized to glycolaldehyde and then to glycolic acid and glycolyxic acid. Glycolyxic acid can be broken down into six metabolites, the most toxic of which is oxalic acid. Cofactors pyridoxine and thiamine are required to generate the less toxic metabolites.

B. Toxicokinetics

—Volume of distribution = 0.8 L/kg

—Plasma protein binding = 0%

—Elimination half-life = 3–8 hours

—Peak plasma level time = 1–4 hours

—Lethal dose = 1.0–1.5 ml/kg

C. Clinical features

—The patient with acute ethylene glycol intoxication presents much like one with ethanol intoxication. The clinical picture unwinds in three stages (Table 18-7).

D. Diagnostic tests

1. **Serum levels** of methanol, formate, ethylene glycol, and ethanol
2. **Serum osmolarity** and **serum electrolytes** to calculate osmolal gap
3. **ABGs** to assess acid base status
4. **Urinalysis** to look for calcium oxalate crystals and fluorescence to ultraviolet light
5. **ECG** to look for dysrhythmias (rare)
6. **Chest radiograph** to look for pulmonary edema
7. **Computed tomographic (CT) scan** for patients with severe alterations in mental status

E. Treatment

1. **ABCs.** Patent airway must be ensured.
2. GI decontamination: **GL** if patient presents within 1 hour of ingestion
3. **Sodium bicarbonate** for metabolic acidosis with pH < 7.2
4. IV fluids and Foley catheter to promote aggressive diuresis
5. **Pyridoxine** 50 mg IV every 6 hours to aid in detoxification of metabolites
6. **Thiamine** 100 mg IV every 6 hours to aid in detoxification of metabolites
7. Antidote therapy
   a. Indications include:
      —suspicion of ethylene glycol poisoning
      —metabolic acidosis
      —increased osmolal gap
   b. **Fomepizole**
      —Fomepizole is a competitive inhibitor of alcohol dehydrogenase.
      —Loading dose is 15 mg/kg infused over 30 minutes.
   c. **Ethanol**
      —Dosage is 0.8mg/kg followed by an infusion at 130 mg/kg/hr.

Table 18-7. Stages of Ethylene Glycol Intoxication

Stage	Time of onset post-ingestion	Signs and symptoms
1. CNS stage	30 min–12 h	Slurred speech, ataxia, hallucinations, convulsions, coma
2. Cardiopulmonary stage	12–24 h	Hypertension, tachycardia, tachypnea, congestive heart failure
3. Renal stage	24–72 h	Flank pain, oliguria, crystalluria, acute tubular necrosis, acute renal failure

—Serum EtOH levels must be obtained every hour to maintain a **target blood ethanol level of 100–150 mg/dl.**

8. **Hemodialysis** is indicated in the presence of:

—serum ethylene glycol level > 25 mg/dl

—acidosis refractory to bicarbonate therapy

—crystalluria

—renal failure

—pulmonary edema

F. Disposition

—All patients with ethylene glycol ingestions, even if asymptomatic, should be admitted to the ICU, because some of the toxic manifestations may not become evident until as late as 72 hours post-ingestion.

VIII. Methanol

A. Mechanism of action

—Methanol is oxidized to form formaldehyde and then formate, an ophthalmic toxin that produces metabolic acidosis.

B. Toxicokinetics

—Volume of distribution = 0.6 L/kg

—Plasma protein binding = 0%

—Elimination half life = 14–30 hours

—Peak plasma level time = 30–90 minutes

—Lethal dose = 15–30 ml (adults)

C. Clinical features

1. Symptoms and physical examination findings are much like those seen with ethanol intoxication.
2. **Symptoms** may include:

—euphoria

—confusion

—abdominal pain

—nausea

—vomiting

—seizures

—coma

—blurred vision

3. **Physical examination findings** may include:

—decreased visual acuity (“snowstorm effect”)

—slow-reacting pupils, retinal edema, and optic disc hyperemia seen on funduscopic examination

D. **Diagnostic tests**

1. **Serum levels** of methanol, formate, ethylene glycol, and ethanol
2. **Serum osmolarity** and **serum electrolytes** to calculate osmolal gap
3. **ABGs** to assess acid–base status
4. **Urinalysis** to look for myoglobinuria
5. **Visual acuity testing** to evaluate toxicity
6. **ECG** to look for dysrhythmias (rare)
7. **CT scan** for patients with severe alterations in mental status

E. **Treatment**

1. ABCs. Ensure patent airway.
2. GI decontamination: GL if patient presents within 1 hour of ingestion
3. **Sodium bicarbonate** for metabolic acidosis with pH < 7.2. Loading dose is 1–2 mg/kg IV bolus, followed by 3 ampules in 1 L IV fluid, to run at 200–250 ml/hr.
4. **Folic acid** 50 mg IV every 4 hours to aid in detoxification of formate
5. Antidote is **ethanol.**
   a. Loading dose is 0.8 mg/kg, followed by an infusion at 130 mg/kg/hr until **target blood ethanol level** of **100–150 mg/dl** is reached.
   b. Indications include:
      —peak methanol level > 20 mg/dl
      —metabolic acidosis
      —increased osmolal gap
6. **Hemodialysis** is indicated in the presence of:
   —peak methanol level > 50 mg/dl
   —peak formate level > 20 mg/dl
   —acidosis refractory to bicarbonate therapy
   —visual impairment
   —renal failure

F. **Disposition**

—All patients with methanol ingestions, even if asymptomatic, should be admitted to the ICU, because some of the toxic manifestation may not become evident until as late as 72 hours post-ingestion.

IX. Tricyclic Antidepressants

—Tricyclic antidepressants (TCAs) are among the most commonly prescribed drugs in the United States. They are used to treat a variety of conditions, including depression, anxiety, panic disorder, obsessive compulsive disorder, eating disorders, enuresis, attention deficit disorder, chronic pain syndromes, and migraine headache. Their wide use and narrow therapeutic window make them responsible for more intentional drug overdose related deaths than any other prescribed drug.

A. **Mechanism of action**

1. Inhibition of fast Na+ channels
2. K+ channel blockade
3. Antagonism of ACh at muscarinic receptors
4. Inhibition of α-adrenergic receptors
5. Inhibition of GABA receptors
6. Inhibition of amine uptake

B. **Clinical presentation**

1. Na+ channel blockade produces negative inotropy and results in cardiac rhythm disturbances including sinus tachycardia, and wide QRS and PR intervals.
2. K+ channel blockade results in prolongation of the QT interval.
3. GABA receptor antagonism can produce seizures.
4. Antagonism of α-adrenergic receptors causes hypotension with reflex tachycardia.
5. Inhibition of serotonin uptake can result in myoclonus and hyperreflexia.
6. Inhibition of norepinephrine produces sympathomimetic effects and may exacerbate cardiac dysrhythmias.
7. Central antimuscarinic effects include agitation, delirium, hallucinations, slurred speech, ataxia, sedation, and coma.
8. Peripheral effects include dilated pupils, blurred vision, tachycardia, and decreased secretions (opposite of **SLUDGE** acronym—See section XX B later in this chapter).

C. **Diagnostic tests**

1. ECG to look for prolonged PR, QRS, and QT intervals
2. ABGs to assess need for mechanical ventilation
3. Chemistry panel to look for electrolyte abnormalities, especially hypokalemia

D. **Treatment**

1. ABCs. Patent airway must be ensured.
2. GI decontamination. GL may be considered for early presentations; otherwise, AC is used. In most cases 1–2 doses (1 mg/kg) are sufficient.
3. Sodium bicarbonate infusion for all dysrhythmias
4. IV fluids for hypotension
5. Vasopressor infusion (norepinephrine, dopamine) if hypotension is refractory to fluids and bicarbonate
6. Benzodiazepines for seizures
7. Flumazenil and physostigmine are **contraindicated** in the treatment of TCA overdose, because both can induce seizures.

E. **Disposition**

1. Patients in stable clinical condition after 6 hours of cardiac monitoring can be discharged home.

2. Symptomatic patients or patients with cardiac abnormalities should be admitted to the ICU.
3. All patients with suicidal ingestions should receive a psychiatric evaluation.

X. Lithium

—Lithium is the drug of choice for bipolar disorder. It also is used in the treatment of schizoaffective disorder and alcoholism, for prophylaxis against cluster headaches, and for chemotherapy-induced leukopenia.

A. Mechanism of action

—Lithium interferes with hormonal response to cAMP and prevents the reuptake of norepinephrine. It is not known how these mechanisms produce mood stabilization.

B. Toxicokinetics

—Volume of distribution = 0.6 L/kg

—Plasma protein binding = 10%

—Elimination half-life = 25 hours

—Peak plasma level time = 30 minutes to 2 hours; up to 72 hours in overdose

—Bioavailability > 95%

—Toxic dose = 2 mEq/ml, or a single ingestion of 40 mg

C. Clinical features

1. The main systems affected are the CNS and the kidneys.
2. **Symptoms** and **physical examination findings** may include the following, in order of increasing toxicity:

   —vomiting

   —diarrhea

   —polyuria

   —blurred vision

   —weakness

   —drowsiness

   —vertigo

   —increasing confusion

   —slurred speech

   —muscle fasciculation

   —myoclonus

   —urinary and fecal incontinence

   —restlessness

   —stupor

   —coma

   —seizures

D. Diagnostic tests

1. **Serum lithium level:** correlates reasonably well with clinical toxicity
2. **Chemistry panel** to monitor electrolytes and renal function. Some degree of renal insufficiency is common with lithium therapy.
3. **Urinalysis** and **urine electrolytes.** High volumes of dilute urine are expected. Lithium interferes with antidiuretic hormone (ADH) and causes a transient nephrogenic diabetes insipidus.
4. **ECG** to look for cardiac dysrhythmias (rare)
5. **Thyroid function tests (TFTs).** Lithium inhibits thyroid hormone synthesis and metabolites at several stages. Lithium intoxication can worsen preexisting hypothyroidism to the point of myxedema coma.
6. **Pregnancy test** for women of childbearing age. Lithium is mildly teratogenic and is associated with Ebstein's anomaly. It should be discontinued prior to all planned pregnancies, and immediately in the case of an unplanned one.

E. Treatment

1. ABCs
2. GI decontamination. AC is not useful, because lithium does not bind to charcoal. GL should be considered in early presentations. **Whole bowel irrigation** is especially useful for sustained-release preparations.
3. For lithium levels < 2.5 mEq/L, **IV saline** is useful not only for replacing volume and sodium, but also for enhancing lithium elimination. 1–2 L are given over 6 hours. A Foley catheter is placed to monitor input and output.
4. With lithium levels > 2.5 mEq/L, or in the presence of significant neurotoxicity or underlying renal or cardiac disease, **hemodialysis** is the treatment of choice.

F. Disposition

1. Asymptomatic patients with lithium levels < 2.5 mEq/L may be discharged home after 4–6 hours of observation.
2. Symptomatic patients or patients with lithium levels > 2.5 mEq/L should be admitted to the CCU.
3. All patients who have ingested lithium with suicidal intent should receive a psychiatric consult.

XI. Neuroleptics

—The class "neuroleptics" comprises the antipsychotics, including the phenothiazines, butyrophenones, and thioxanthenes. Examples of drugs in this class are haloperidol, thioridazine, chlorpromazine, clozapine, and thiothixene.

A. Mechanism of action

—Neuroleptics exert their effects via inhibition of dopamine uptake.

—Antipsychotic effects are produced by inhibition in the limbic system.

—Inhibition at the basal ganglia results in the movement disorders associated with neuroleptics.

—The antiemetic properties of neuroleptics are due to inhibition of dopamine uptake at the chemoreceptor trigger zone. An exception is the atypical neuroleptic clozapine, which exerts its action via a different subclass of dopamine receptors. It has a lower incidence of tardive dyskinesia but carries a risk of agranulocytosis, requiring weekly monitoring of WBCs.

B. Clinical features

1. The hallmark of neuroleptic overdose is CNS depression, which can range from mild sedation to coma.
2. Other **symptoms** and **physical examination findings** may include:

   —miosis

   —extrapyramidal symptoms (e.g., akathisia, rigidity, dystonia, tremors)

   —seizures
3. Neuroleptic malignant syndrome (NMS) is a life-threatening complication of neuroleptics, characterized by hyperthermia, muscular rigidity, altered mental status, tachycardia, and labile BP.

C. Diagnostic tests

1. Serum drug levels are not useful.
2. **Toxicology screen** to look for coingestants
3. **Chemistry panel, creatinine kinase (CK),** and **urinalysis** to look for electrolyte abnormalities and rhabdomyolysis
4. **ECG** to look for VT/VF, torsades de pointes, and heart block
5. **WBC** count for clozapine ingestions to look for agranulocytosis
6. **CT** can be considered in cases of altered mental status.

D. Treatment

1. **ABCs.** Patent airway must be ensured.
2. GI decontamination. **AC** 1 g/kg is administered orally.
3. **IV fluids** for dehydration and hypotension
4. Vasopressors for hypotension. Choices include high-dose **dopamine** (10–20 (μg/kg/min), **norepinephrine,** and **phenylephrine.**
5. **Benzodiazepines** or **phenytoin** for seizures
6. **Lidocaine** or external pacing for ventricular dysrhythmias
7. **Magnesium sulfate** 2 g IV for torsades de pointes
8. **Diphenhydramine** or **benztropine** for dystonic reactions
   a. Diphenhydramine 25–50 mg every 6 hours (adults) or 5 mg/kg/day (children) IV, IM, or orally
   b. Benztropine 2 mg/day IM or IV
   c. Symptoms resolve in 15–30 minutes. Medication should be continued for 48–72 hours longer in order to prevent further episodes.
9. ED treatment of NMS: ABCs, benzodiazepines to relieve muscular rigidity, cooling measures, and intubation with neuromuscular blockade as necessary

E. Disposition

1. Patients who are asymptomatic 4 hours post-ingestion can be discharged home.
2. Patients with CNS or respiratory depression, seizures, or cardiac dysrhythmias should be admitted to the ICU.
3. Patients with non–life-threatening symptoms should be admitted to a monitored bed.
4. All patients who have ingested neuroleptics with suicidal intent should receive psychiatric evaluation.

XII. Benzodiazepines

A. Mechanism of action

—Benzodiazepines stimulate the inhibitory neurotransmitter γ-aminobutyric acid (GABA), which binds to the $GABA_b$ receptor, opening the chloride channels. The equalization of gradient prevents further nerve impulses from being conducted.

—Many drugs belong to the benzodiazepine group, each of which has a different duration of action and varying sedative, anxiolytic, anticonvulsant, and muscle relaxant properties. Table 18-8 compares some of the more common preparations.

B. Toxicokinetics (see Table 18-8)

C. Clinical features

1. The patient with benzodiazepine overdose presents with signs of CNS depression.
2. **Symptoms** and **physical examination findings** may include:

—drowsiness

—lethargy

—apathy

Table 18-8. Toxicokinetics of Common Benzodiazepines

	Generic name	Trade name	Half-life (h)	V_D (L/kg)	Peak serum concentration (no. hours post-ingestion)	Protein binding (%)
Ultra–short-acting	Midazolam	Versed	2–5	1.1	0.4–1.7	95
	Temazepam	Restoril	0–40	1.4	2–3	97
Short-acting	Alprazolam	Xanax	10–15	0.7–1.0	0.7–1.6	70
	Lorazepam	Ativan	10–25	0.8–1.6	0.5–3.0	92
Long-acting	Diazepam	Valium	15–60	1–2	1–2	98
	Chlordiazepoxide	Librium	5–25	0.3–0.6	1–2	95

V_D = volume of distribution

—ataxia

—short-term memory loss

—hypotonia

—hypotension

—respiratory depression

—coma

D. Diagnostic tests

1. Serum benzodiazepine levels do not necessarily correlate with clinical toxicity and therefore are not useful for management.
2. **Urine toxicology screen** to look for coingestants
3. Bedside glucose testing to look for hypoglycemia
4. **ECG** to look for dysrhythmias (rare)

E. Treatment

—Pure benzodiazepine overdose is almost never fatal. Only supportive treatment is required, because it wears off and resolves in 12–36 hours.

1. **ABCs.** Patent airway must be ensured.
2. **IV fluids** for BP support
3. **AC** for GI decontamination
4. Antidote therapy. **Flumazenil** is a competitive inhibitor of benzodiazepines that binds to the same $GABA_b$ receptor. It reverses all effects of benzodiazepines. Use of flumazenil usually is limited to reversal of benzodiazepine-induced anesthesia (conscious sedation) for minor surgical procedures. The major adverse effect of flumazenil is seizure activity. It is therefore contraindicated in patients in the following categories:
   a. those who are on benzodiazepine therapy for seizure prophylaxis
   b. patients who chronically use or abuse benzodiazepines for their anxiolytic effect
   c. patients who have ingested combinations of benzodiazepines and drugs that are epileptogenic, such as TCAs and antihistamines

F. Disposition

1. Asymptomatic patients who are awake following a pure benzodiazepine overdose can be discharged home.
2. Patients with mixed ingestions, patients with respiratory or CNS depression, and patients who received flumazenil should be admitted.

XIII. Cocaine and Amphetamines

A. Mechanism of action

—The euphoria and "power high" are due to sympathetic nervous system (SNS) stimulation. Cocaine and amphetamines stimulate the release of norepinephrine while blocking its reuptake. The blockade floods synapses with neurotransmitter, causing sustained stimulation of the postsynaptic receptors.

B. Clinical features

1. **Symptoms** may include:
   —mydriasis
   —euphoria
   —agitation
   —paranoia (cocaine)
   —visual hallucinations
   —formication (cocaine)
   —hyperthermia
   —tremor
   —seizures
   —chest pain
   —palpitations
2. **Physical examination findings** may include:
   —tachycardia
   —hypertension
   —tachypnea
   —dyspnea

C. Diagnostic tests

1. **Urine toxicology** screen to confirm drug ingestion and to look for coingestants
2. **Cardiac enzymes** and **ECG:** over 50% of patients who present to the ED with chest pain following cocaine abuse have AMI.
3. **ABG:** to determine acid–base status and to look for A-a gradient if pulmonary pathology is suspected
4. **CBC, chemistry panel, LFTs,** and **coagulation studies** to rule out other causes for presentation, including infection and ethanol withdrawal
5. **Chest radiograph** to look for pneumothorax, pulmonary edema, and pneumonia
6. **Abdominal radiograph** to look for cocaine packets in body packers
7. **Blood cultures** in patients who are septic or who have a new-onset cardiac murmur. IV drug abusers are at increased risk of endocarditis.
8. **Urinalysis** to look for RBC, Hb, rhabdomyolysis
9. **Pregnancy test** in women of childbearing age: cocaine is a known teratogen, and use should be discontinued immediately upon discovering pregnancy.

D. Treatment

—There is no specific treatment for cocaine or amphetamine overdose.

—Treatment is directed at addressing individual manifestations and complications.

—Benzodiazepines are the mainstay of treatment, controlling agitation, seizures, tachycardia, and hypertension. The drug of choice is diazepam. Alternatives to diazepam include lorazepam (0.05 mg/kg IV) and midazolam (0.2 mg/kg IV). Other drugs may be used in addition to benzodiazepines if they are not sufficient on their own.

1. **ABCs.** Supplemental oxygen is given for increased myocardial demand.
2. **Diazepam** 2.5–10 mg IV push every 5 minutes as needed to control anxiety, agitation, tachycardia, hypertension, and hyperthermia
3. **Advanced Cardiac Life Support (ACLS)** protocol for cardiac arrest, myocardial infarction
4. **Phenytoin** 15 mg/kg IV slowly, or diazepam, for seizures. (Dosing for diazepam for children under 5 years of age: 0.05–0.3 g over 3 minutes, maximum dose 5 g; for children over 5 years of age: same dose, maximum dose is 10 g; adults: 10 mg every 15–30 minutes, maximum dose is 30 mg)
5. **Lidocaine** 1 mg/kg loading dose, then 2–4 mg/kg infusion for ventricular dysrhythmias
6. Ice baths, **cool water mist with fanning** to promote evaporative loss for hyperthermia
7. **Nitroprusside** drip 0.5–10 mg/kg/min IV for malignant hypertension
8. For **body packers:** GI decontamination including AC, gastric lavage, and whole-bowel irrigation with cathartics are appropriate. In cases of rupture, emergent abdominal laparotomy is required.
9. Certain drugs should be used with caution or avoided in the treatment of sympathomimetic overdose. These include:
   a. β-blockers—which can potentiate coronary artery vasoconstriction and aggravate bronchospasm
   b. Aspirin—which binds to protein-bound thyroxine and may aggravate missed thyroid storm and hyperthermia
   c. Haloperidol and phenothiazines—which may increase risk of seizures and malignant hyperthermia

E. Disposition

1. Asymptomatic patients may be discharged after 4–6 hours of observation.
2. Patients with evidence of cardiac or neurologic dysfunction (AMI, CVA) should be admitted to the ICU.
3. Symptomatic patients without evidence of cardiac or neurologic dysfunction can be admitted to the regular ward.
4. All patients should be referred to drug counseling and rehabilitation.
5. All patients who have ingested cocaine or amphetamines with suicidal intent should have a psychiatric evaluation.

XIV. Phencyclidine (PCP)

A. Mechanism of action

—PCP acts as a false neurotransmitter, preventing the reuptake of dopamine,

5HT, norepinephrine, and GABA. The psychoactive effect is due to the inability of the brain to translate sensory input into meaningful behavior.

B. Clinical features may include:

—**nystagmus**

—**hypertension**

—normal-sized pupils

—blank stare

—violent agitation

—confusion

—profuse diaphoresis

—cholinergic signs

C. Diagnostic tests

1. **Toxicology screen** to document ingestion and look for mixed ingestions
2. **Urinalysis** and **CK** to look for rhabdomyolysis
3. **Chemistry panel** to look for hypoglycemia and electrolyte abnormalities

D. Treatment

1. Physical and chemical **restraint** for violently agitated patients. **Haloperidol** 5–20 mg IM is used for chemical restraint.
2. **ABCs**
3. Sedation with **benzodiazepines** to control tachycardia, hypertension, anxiety, and seizures
4. **Sodium nitroprusside** for life-threatening hypertension
5. Fluids and urine alkalinization with **sodium bicarbonate** for rhabdomyolysis

E. Disposition

1. Patients with life-threatening symptoms and violent agitation beyond 4 hours should be admitted to the hospital.
2. Patients who are stable and without agitation or psychoses following 4–6 hours of observation can be discharged home.

XV. Lysergic Acid Diethylamide (LSD)

A. Mechanism of action

—Inhibition of 5HT release at the postsynaptic neuron

B. Toxicokinetics

—Half-life: 4 hours

—Onset of action: 30 minutes

—Duration of psychoactive effects: 12 hours

—Drug is marketed in mg quantities, so overdose is rare. Pure LSD intoxication rarely is fatal.

C. Clinical features

1. **Symptoms** may include:
   —euphoria
   —visual hallucinations
   —loss of boundaries between self and the world, making everything fascinating and awe-inspiring
2. **Physical examination findings** may include:
   —mydriasis
   —tachycardia
   —mild hypertension
3. The environment in which the user takes the drug impacts the experience. The same drug taken in a threatening environment can produce an intensely frightening experience (a "bad trip") instead of a "beautiful" one.

D. Diagnostic tests

—No specific diagnostic tests are necessary if the diagnosis is clear. If the diagnosis is unclear, proceed with a general toxicology work-up.

E. Treatment

—The mainstay of treatment involves reassurance and the provision of a relaxing, non-threatening atmosphere. **Benzodiazepines** help in alleviating anxiety.

F. Disposition

1. Most patients calm down after a few hours of observation and can be discharged home.
2. Patients with persistent anxiety, massive ingestions, or mixed ingestions should be admitted.

XVI. Opioids

—The opioids are a group of drugs that are widely used therapeutically for analgesia and anesthesia but unfortunately also have high abuse potential. Examples of drugs in this group include heroin, methadone, codeine, morphine, meperidine, fentanyl, and propoxyphene.

A. Mechanism of action

—Opioids bind competitively to opioid (mu, kappa, delta) receptors to produce decreased affective pain perception by reducing neurotransmitter release, mimicking endorphins.

B. Toxicokinetics

—See Table 18-9 for toxicokinetics of common opioids.

C. Clinical features may include:

Table 18-9. Toxicokinetics of Common Opioids

Drug	Duration of action
Weak analgesic agonist	
Pentazocrine	2 h
Codeine	4 h
Strong analgesic agonist	
Fentanyl	30 min
Meperidine	2 h
Morphine	4 h
Heroin	4 h
Methadone	6–8 h
Antagonist	
Naloxone	< 5 min

—**miosis** (note: meperidine may cause pupillary dilatation secondary to its antimuscarinic activity).

—**respiratory depression**

—**coma**

—euphoria

—nausea

—vomiting

—pruritus

—seizures (meperidine and propoxyphene)

—noncardiogenic pulmonary edema (NCPE)(heroin)

—cardiac dysrhythmias (propoxyphene)

D. Diagnostic tests

1. Serum drug levels are not useful for immediate management.
2. **ABGs** to assess need for mechanical ventilation
3. **ECG** for suspected propoxyphene ingestion
4. **Chest radiograph** for suspected heroin ingestion
5. Pregnancy test for all women of childbearing age. Many opioids are teratogenic.

E. Treatment

1. **ABCs.** Patent airway must be ensured. **100% oxygen** may be administered.
2. Antidote therapy: **Naloxone** (both diagnostic and therapeutic)
   —In adults: 0.4 mg test dose for diagnosis, then 2 mg every 3 minutes to a total of 10 mg until patient is awake
   —In children: 0.01 mg/kg, repeated as necessary to a maximum of 0.2 mg/kg

3. Loop diuretics for NCPE
4. Antiarrhythmics for dysrhythmias. Class Ia drugs (e.g., quinidine, procainamide) should be avoided.

F. **Disposition**

1. Known heroin abusers who respond to naloxone and remain without respiratory depression for 6 hours can be discharged home.
2. Patients with long-acting ingestion (methadone) should be admitted.
3. Patients who sustained hypoxia secondary to opioid overdose should be admitted for 24 hours of observation.
4. All patients should receive referral for drug counseling and rehabilitation.
5. All patients who have ingested opioids with suicidal intent require psychiatric evaluation.

XVII. Iron Toxicity

A. **Mechanism of action**

—Iron toxicity is the condition of free iron present in the circulation. This occurs after 100% of transferrin becomes saturated and results in tissue penetration of iron.

B. **Clinical features**

—Clinical features can range from mild GI upset to severe cardiovascular collapse, depending on the amount ingested. Mild symptoms occur with ingestions of 20 mg/kg or less. Moderate symptoms are associated with ingestions of 20–60 mg/kg, and severe toxicity is seen with ingestions exceeding 60 mg/kg. Table 18-10 summarizes the stages of acute iron poisoning. Note that not all stages occur in all patients.

C. **Diagnostic tests**

1. **Serum iron levels.** The first level should be drawn 3–5 hours post-ingestion, or immediately if time of ingestion is unknown. A second level is drawn 6–8 hours post-ingestion to account for sustained-release preparations. A serum level of < 350 μg/dl indicates minimal toxicity, whereas a level > 500 μg/dl is potentially fatal. Because iron is rapidly metabolized, serum levels can be deceptively low, even as the patient is going into shock.
2. **CBC** to look for leukocytosis. A white cell count $> 15{,}000$ in the presence of hyperglycemia suggests high serum iron levels, and warrants antidote therapy.
3. **ABGs** to assess need for mechanical ventilation
4. **Chemistry panel** to look for hyperglycemia and electrolyte imbalances
5. **PT/APTT** and **LFTs** to look for liver dysfunction
6. **Abdominal radiograph:** iron is radiopaque unless it is completely dis-

Table 18-10. Stages of Iron Toxicity

Stage	Time after ingestion	Signs and symptoms
I. Initial	0–6 h	Tachycardia, tachypnea, metabolic acidosis, hypotension, nausea, vomiting, diarrhea, seizures, lethargy, coma
II. Pseudo-recovery	6–24 h	Patient appears clinically stable
III. Recurrent	12–48 h	Anion gap metabolic acidosis, hyperglycemia, cyanosis, pulmonary edema, hypotension, cardiovascular collapse, leukocytosis, gastrointestinal bleeding, lethargy, seizures, coma
IV. Hepatic	2–5 days	Rare. Acute hepatic failure, coagulopathy, hypoglycemia
V. Late	2–7 wk	Uncommon. Small bowel obstruction, gastrointestinal scarring, stricture formation

solved. Radiographs are useful to assess the amount of the ingestion and the effectiveness of GI decontamination.

7. **Type and crossmatch** for cases of severe toxicity where transfusion may become necessary

D. Treatment

1. **ABCs**
2. GI decontamination
   —AC is useless because iron does not adsorb to charcoal.
   —**GL** with NS is indicated. It is necessary to use a tube with a diameter large enough to retrieve pill fragments.
   —**Whole bowel irrigation** is helpful when abdominal radiograph reveals iron tablets retained in the stomach or small bowel.
3. Antidote therapy: **Deferoxamine mesylate** should be administered to all symptomatic patients, without waiting for serum levels. If patients are asymptomatic, a deferoxamine "challenge" of 50 mg/kg IM or 10 mg/kg IV over 1 hour is administered. If the urine turns a "vin rosé" color (reddish brown) or changes color at all, the test is considered positive, and antidote therapy should be administered to the patient despite being asymptomatic. Dosages are:
   a. IV: 15 mg/kg/hr. Hypotension and rash should be checked for.
   b. IM: 40–90 mg/kg up to a maximum of 6 g/day. Injections should be administered 4–12 hours apart.
   c. Antidote therapy should be continued until the urine is clear and the patient becomes asymptomatic.
4. **Exchange transfusion** for severely symptomatic patients and for those with serum iron levels > 1000 μg/dl
5. **Hemodialysis** for patients who develop shock or coma

E. Disposition

1. Patients with serum iron levels < 300 mg/dl, who remain asymptomatic 6 hours post-ingestion can be discharged home.
2. Patients with severe toxicity should be admitted to the ICU.

XVIII. Carbon Monoxide

A. Mechanism of action

—Carbon monoxide (CO) competes with oxygen for hemoglobin (Hb) with 250 times the affinity of oxygen, resulting in hypoxia to all tissues. Historical clues that may point to CO poisoning include confined space fires, presentation of several household members who are sick at the same time, history of a car engine left on, malfunctioning furnaces, and cold weather.

B. Toxicokinetics

1. Elimination: 100% via lungs
2. Half-life

   —320 minutes on room air

   —82 minutes on 100% oxygen via non-rebreather mask

   —23 minutes on 3.0 atmospheres of hyperbaric oxygen (HBO)

C. Clinical features

1. **Symptoms,** in order of severity, may include:

   —headache

   —nausea

   —vomiting

   —malaise

   —chest pain

   —weakness

   —apathy

2. **Physical examination findings,** in order of severity, may include:

   —cherry red skin

   —abnormal reflexes

   —altered mental status (may be subtle)

   —hypotension

D. Diagnostic tests

1. **Carboxyhemoglobin** (CoHb) **level** makes the diagnosis.
2. **ABGs** to look for low O_2 saturation. Pulse oximetry in the setting of CO poisoning will reveal a falsely normal O_2 saturation.
3. **ECG** and cardiac enzymes to look for myocardial damage
4. **Head CT** to look for white matter changes (poor prognosis) and to rule out other causes of altered mental status

5. **Chemistry profile** to look for metabolic acidosis
6. **Methylated hemoglobin** and **cyanide** levels may be checked, based on clinical suspicion.

E. **Treatment**

1. **ABCs.** Oxygen is the cornerstone of therapy. Oxygenation with a 100% non-rebreather mask should be done.
2. **HBO therapy**
   a. Indications include:
   —asymptomatic patients with CoHb levels > 20%
   —symptomatic patients (e.g., neurologic impairment, ischemia/chest pain, nausea, vomiting, headache)
   —pregnant patients
   —patients who experienced loss of consciousness (syncope)
   b. **Risks and complications** include:
   —barotrauma in closed spaces (including sinus, middle ear, and stomach)
   —O_2 toxicity (convulsions, pulmonary edema)

F. **Disposition**

1. Patients who are asymptomatic and have a normal ECG can be discharged after 4–6 hours of observation.
2. All patients with chest pain, ECG changes, or altered mental status should be admitted.

XIX. Anticholinergics

A. Mechanism of action

—Anticholinergic drugs such as atropine, scopolamine, benztropine, and diphenhydramine inhibit muscarinic cholinergic receptors at parasympathetic end-organs. Muscarinic receptors regulate sweat, salivary, and mucosal gland activity and are present in the smooth muscle of the eye, the GI tract, and the urinary bladder.

—Excessive stimulation of these receptors results in the cholinergic syndrome discussed in section XIX B.

—Cholinergic receptors in the myocardium regulate AVN conduction.

B. Clinical features

1. The clinical features of a patient with anticholinergic poisoning can be summarized with the following expression: **mad** as a hatter, **dry** as a bone, **red** as a beet, **blind** as a bat, and **hot** as Hades.
2. **Symptoms** may include:
   —absence of sweating
   —flushed skin
   —fever

—**altered mental status**

—hallucinations

3. **Physical examination findings** may include:

—**mydriasis**

—**dry mucous membranes**

—decreased bowel sounds

—bladder distention

C. **Diagnostic tests**

1. Serum drug levels are not useful. Because many over-the-counter preparations of anticholinergics include APAP or aspirin, however, APAP and salicylate levels may reveal a mixed poisoning.
2. ECG to look for dysrhythmias (rare). Usually only sinus tachycardia is seen.
3. ABGs to look for signs of respiratory compromise (rare)
4. CBC and chemistry panel as part of general work-up

D. **Treatment**

1. ABCs. Patent airway must be ensured.
2. **Benzodiazepines** for agitation
3. **Cooling measures** and **antipyretics** for hyperthermia
4. GI decontamination: **MDAC** is indicated.
5. Antidote therapy: **Physostigmine** is an anticholinesterase inhibitor that can reverse both the peripheral and central effects of anticholinergic drugs. Use of physostigmine should be limited to patients with seizures, severe hallucinations, or delirium.
   a. Dosage is 1–2 mg for adults and 0.5 mg for children infused IV slowly. Dose can be repeated if needed (rare).
   b. Contraindications

   —Significant conduction abnormalities on ECG

   —Evidence or suspicion of TCA or other cardiotoxic drug ingestion

E. **Disposition**

1. Patients who have received AC and have been symptom-free for 6 hours in the ED can be discharged home with outpatient follow-up.
2. Patients with moderate to severe symptoms, or those who required physostigmine, should be admitted to a monitored bed.
3. Psychiatric evaluation for all suicidal ingestions

XX. Organophosphates

—Organophosphates are a class of compounds commonly found in pesticides and weapons of mass destruction such as nerve gas.

A. **Mechanism of action**

1. **Competitive inhibition of acetylcholinesterase** (ACE) results in prolongation of the actions of acetylcholine (ACh).

2. ACh acts at three different types of receptors:
   a. **Nicotinic:** sympathetic, parasympathetic, skeletal muscle
   b. **Cholinergic:** postganglionic sympathetic (e.g., sweat glands)
   c. **Muscarinic:** parasympathetic

B. Clinical features

1. The clinical features of a patient with cholinergic poisoning are summarized in the acronym **SLUDGE** (salivation, lacrimation, **u**rination, **d**iarrhea, **G**I upset, **e**mesis).
2. Other symptoms and physical examination findings may include:

   —**rhinorrhea**

   —**excess bronchial secretions**

   —**miosis**

   —**involuntary twitches**

   —**muscle fasciculations**

   —rancid breath and vomitus

C. Diagnostic tests

1. RBC **cholinesterase levels** represent "true" levels of activity, whereas plasma levels represent "pseudo" levels and are not as accurate. Unfortunately, tests are not readily available for either level in many hospitals. If available, serial levels should be obtained to assess toxicity.
2. **ABG** to assess respiratory status
3. **ECG** to look for dysrhythmias (rare)
4. CBC, chemistry panel, and LFTs as part of the general work-up

D. Treatment

1. **ABCs.** Suctioning of secretions and maintaining the airway are especially important.
2. **Dermal decontamination.** The patient's clothing must be removed and the exposed skin flushed thoroughly with water. This is extremely important to reduce chances of health care worker poisoning.
3. **GI decontamination:** may be of limited benefit because of the rapid absorption of organophosphates and carbamates. May be more appropriate in the pre-hospital setting.
4. **Atropine:** given until control of secretions is achieved. Dosage is 2–5 mg IV push every 5 minutes for adults and 0.05 mg/kg in children. Atropine effect produces tachycardia and mydriasis, and works only on muscarinic receptors.
5. **Pralidoxime:** reverses effects at both nicotinic and muscarinic receptors. Dosage is 1 g IV in adults, 20–40 mg/kg IV in children (maximum dose is 1 g for both adults and children). Dose can be repeated in 1 hour and then again every 6–8 hours over a 48-hour period until signs and symptoms resolve. Best if administered within first 24 hours.
6. **Benzodiazepines** for seizures

E. Disposition

1. Patients with minimal exposure who remain asymptomatic 6–8 hours post-ingestion can be discharged home.
2. Symptomatic patients and those who received antidote therapy should be admitted to the ICU. Full recovery generally occurs within 10 days.

XXI. Carbamates

A. Mechanism of action

—Carbamates are another class of anticholinesterase inhibitors. Their major difference from organophosphates is their **short duration of action** and **reversible (transient) inhibition of cholinesterase,** resulting in lesser toxicity than organophosphates.

B. Clinical features

—are the same as for organophosphates (see section XX)

—Pralidoxime is not administered for pure carbamate poisoning, because patients are not sick enough to need it (risk vs. benefit ratio).

C. Diagnostic tests

—are the same as those for organophosphates (see section XX C)

D. Treatment

—is the same as that for organophosphates (see section XX D)

—The only exception is that the use of pralidoxime in pure carbamate poisoning is controversial, and thus not usually given. However, it is not withheld in cases where mixed or uncertain ingestions are suspected.

E. Disposition

—Due to the short duration of action of carbamates, patients are rarely symptomatic beyond 6–8 hours, and most can be discharged home safely.

XXII. Corrosive Ingestions

—Corrosive ingestions include strong acids such as HCl, H_2SO_4, and H_3N, and strong alkalis such as NaOH and KOH.

A. Mechanism of action

—Acids exert their effect via a **coagulation necrosis,** which has a slow penetration.

—Alkalis exert their effect via a **liquefaction necrosis,** which has a more rapid penetration.

B. Clinical features

1. Acids

—Acute complications of acid ingestion include corrosive gastritis, hemorrhage, and perforation.

—Delayed complications include gastric outlet obstruction and achlorhydria.

—The esophagus is mostly spared in acid ingestions.

2. **Alkalis**

—Esophageal injury is prominent.

—Acute manifestations include perforation and infection.

—Delayed complications include strictures and altered motility.

C. Diagnostic tests

1. **CBC, chemistry panel** for significant ingestions
2. **ABGs** to assess need for mechanical ventilation
3. **Type and crossmatch** for significant blood loss
4. **Chest** and **abdominal radiographs** to look for perforation

D. Treatment

1. For both acid and alkali ingestions:
   - **a.** ABCs. Patent airway must be ensured.
   - **b.** Haloperidol for acute psychosis as needed
   - **c.** Narcotic analgesia as needed
   - **d.** Endoscopy to determine severity of injury
   - **e.** Methylprednisolone, 125 mg IV, for injuries that penetrate the mucosa
   - **f.** Antibiotic coverage of oral flora if infection is anticipated or if steroids are used
2. For acid ingestions:
   - **a.** Emetics, AC, and neutralizing solution are contraindicated.
   - **b.** Ice water GL is indicated.
3. For alkali ingestions:
   - **a.** Ingested foreign body (e.g., alkaline battery) should be removed.
   - **b.** GL is contraindicated.

E. Disposition

1. Patients who are asymptomatic 6 hours post-ingestion may be discharged home.
2. Symptomatic patients should receive endoscopic evaluation, which may require admission.
3. All patients who have ingested acid or alkali substances with suicidal intent should receive psychiatric evaluation.

Review Test

1. A 72-year-old woman has a shoulder dislocation reduced in the emergency department (ED) under a conscious sedation protocol that used midazolam and fentanyl. Ten minutes after successful reduction of the shoulder, the patient is still quite lethargic. You decide to try a dose of flumazenil. Which of the following is the mechanism of action of this drug?

(A) Competitive inhibition of benzodazepines at GABA inhibitory receptors
(B) Competitive inhibition of barbiturates at GABA inhibitory receptors
(C) Non-competitive inhibition of benzodiazepines at GABA stimulatory receptors
(D) Non-competitive inhibition of barbiturates at GABA stimulatory receptors
(E) Up-regulation of benzodiazepine receptor sites

2. In which of the following situations may flumazenil be used?

(A) A patient with a history of seizure disorder treated with benzodiazepines
(B) A patient with a history of anxiety disorder treated with benzodiazepines
(C) A patient with a history of chronic benzodiazepine use/abuse
(D) A patient with a concomitant tricyclic antidepressant ingestion
(E) A patient with a concomitant ethanol ingestion

3. A 25-year-old man is brought to the emergency department (ED) because he was found unconscious. Upon arrival, he is acutely agitated and restless. Physical examination reveals a well-developed male, with fever of 102°F, pulse rate 100 beats per minute (bpm), and blood pressure (BP) of 140/100. His mental status is waxing and waning. His pupils are 2 mm bilaterally, and reactive to light. There is bidirectional nystagmus. He denies any past medical history and admits only to "partying with friends" a few hours earlier. Which of the following agents is the most likely toxin in this scenario?

(A) Cocaine
(B) Crystal methamphetamine
(C) PCP
(D) LSD
(E) Ethanol

4. A 20-year-old college student is brought to the emergency department (ED) by her roommate. The patient had been vomiting since the previous evening, following the university provost's luncheon. She took two 10 mg tablets of prochlorperazine. The vomiting has subsided, but she now presents with sustained spasm of the sternocleidomastoid and trapezius muscles, and is unable to turn her head to the left. Her vital signs are within normal limits. Which of the following is the most appropriate treatment at this time?

(A) Observation for 4–6 hours
(B) Diphenhydramine
(C) Diazepam
(D) Ibuprofen
(E) Dantrolene

5. A 27-year-old man is brought to the emergency department (ED) by his family because he has been agitated and unable to sleep, and insists there are dung beetles crawling under his skin, when in fact there are none. Physical examination reveals mydriasis, a temperature of 101°F, a pulse rate of 120 beats per minute (bpm), and blood pressure (BP) of 150/110. The patient is diaphoretic and appears to be in acute distress. The family states that the patient does have a history of drug abuse. Which of the following drugs is most likely to produce this reaction?

(A) Heroin
(B) Alcohol
(C) Cocaine
(D) Phenobarbital
(E) Diazepam

6. A 37-year-old intoxicated man presents to the emergency department (ED) disoriented and staggering. As you undress him to look for signs of trauma, you notice a bottle of antifreeze in his pocket and suspect ethylene glycol toxicity. Which of the following criteria is necessary before antidote therapy can be instituted?

(A) Serum ethylene glycol level of 25 mg/dl
(B) Presence of pulmonary edema
(C) Impending renal failure
(D) Serum pH < 7.2
(E) None of the above

7. A 72-year-old woman presents to the emergency department (ED) because for the past few hours, she has been experiencing watery eyes, a runny nose, and diarrhea, and states she feels "hot as hell" although it is only 50°F outside. She states she was doing garden work earlier today and may have spilled some garden chemicals on herself. Which of the following is the *most* likely poison in this case?

(A) Organophosphate insecticide
(B) Atropine
(C) Poisonous mushroom from the garden
(D) Tricyclic antidepressant (TCA) overdose
(E) None of the above

8. For which of the following ingestions is activated charcoal useful?

(A) Hydrocarbons
(B) Lithium
(C) Aspirin
(D) Iron
(E) Mineral acid

9. Which of the following drugs is the drug of choice for treating ventricular dysrhythmias in tricyclic antidepressant (TCA) overdose?

(A) Flecainide
(B) Procainamide
(C) Sodium bicarbonate
(D) Flumazenil
(E) Physostigmine

10. Which of the following is an important cofactor administered to detoxify formate in the treatment of methanol poisoning?

(A) Pyridoxine
(B) Folic acid
(C) Vitamin B_{12s}
(D) Thiamine
(E) Vitamin C

11. Which of the following drugs is the mainstay in the treatment of cocaine overdose?

(A) A benzodiazepine such as diazepam
(B) A barbiturate such as phenobarbital
(C) A β-blocker such as propranolol
(D) An antipsychotic such as haloperidol
(E) A tricyclic antidepressant such as imipramine

12. What is the most common coingestant in adult drug overdoses?

(A) A benzodiazepine
(B) An antidepressant
(C) A sympathomimetic
(D) Ethanol
(E) A household cleaner

13. For which one of the following ingestions is abdominal radiograph useful?

(A) Aspirin
(B) Methadone
(C) Meperidine
(D) Acetaminophen
(E) Diazepam

Answers and Explanations

1-A. Flumazenil is a benzodiazepine antidote that works via competitive inhibition of GABA inhibitory receptors. Because of its major adverse effect of producing seizures, its use is limited to situations where the cause of altered mental status, lethargy, or coma is known to be a pure benzodiazepine ingestion, such as iatrogenic administration for conscious sedation protocols or witnessed pediatric ingestions (See section XII A).

2-E. The major adverse effect of flumazenil is seizure activity. It is therefore contraindicated in patients who are on benzodiazepine therapy for seizure prophylaxis, such as phenobarbital, and in those patients who chronically use or abuse benzodiazepines for their anxiolytic effect. Flumazenil also is contraindicated in mixed ingestions of benzodiazepines and drugs that are epileptogenic, such as tricyclic antidepressants and antihistamines. Ethanol is not a known epileptogenic toxin and would therefore not promote seizure activity (See section XII E 4).

3-C. The most consistent clinical finding in phencyclidine (PCP) intoxication is bidirectional nystagmus. The waxing and waning of mental status also is characteristic of PCP overdose. In cocaine and amphetamine overdose, there is an early peak of euphoria and agitation, after which the patient "crashes." Note also that the patient's pupil size is 2 mm. If this were a cocaine or amphetamine overdose, you would expect to see mydriasis. The findings of hyperthermia and tachycardia are common to sympathomimetic and PCP overdose; diaphoresis and significant hypertension are more common with sympathomimetics. In terms of mental status, agitation is common to all choices listed. Whereas cocaine and amphetamine toxicity is associated with paranoia and hallucinations, however, LSD toxicity commonly manifests with the patient reporting a feeling of dissociation and the presence of synesthesias. Ethanol intoxication usually is not associated with extreme agitation, fever, or bidirectional nystagmus (See section XIV B).

4-B. This patient is experiencing an acute dystonic reaction, which is an extrapyramidal side effect associated with the phenothiazine class of drugs, to which prochlorperazine belongs. The reaction is a non–dose-related, idiosyncratic one. Treatment consists of 25–50 mg of intravenous diphenhydramine and/or 2 mg of intramuscular benztropine mesylate, so diphenhydramine is the correct answer. Symptoms should resolve within 15–30 minutes after administration of the drug. To prevent recurrence of symptoms once the medication effect has worn off, the patient should be discharged with oral medication to cover the next 72 hours. Observation will only prolong the patient's suffering and anxiety and is therefore inappropriate, although the symptoms probably will resolve eventually without treatment. Diazepam is an anticonvulsant and muscle relaxant. Although it probably would help with the spasm, it is reserved for seizures associated with phenothiazines, whereas simple dystonic reactions are treated with anticholinergics. Ibuprofen is a nonsteroidal anti-inflammatory agent, which may help with pain relief, but is ineffective in reversing the cholinergic effect. Dantrolene is used to treat malignant hyperthermia, which can be seen with phenothiazine overdose (rarely), but is not present in this case (See section XI D 8).

5-C. Cocaine and amphetamine overdoses typically result in paranoia. Formication, the feeling that bugs are crawling all over one's skin, also is classically associated with cocaine overdose. Physical findings in cocaine overdose are mydriasis, tachycardia, hypertension, and diaphoresis. The patient usually appears anxious. Heroin (opiate), alcohol, diazepam (benzodiazepine), and phenobarbital (barbiturate) are CNS depressants; therefore, overdose of these would result in a comatose patient, not an acutely agitated one (See section XIII A).

6-E. If ethylene glycol ingestion is suspected, antidote treatment with fomepizole or ethanol is instituted right away. It is not necessary to have any other criteria. Target blood ethanol level is 100–150 mg/dl. A serum ethylene glycol level of 25 mg/dl, pulmonary edema, renal failure, and severe acidosis are criteria for hemodialysis (See section VII E 7).

7-A. Given the patient's history, the most likely toxin is an organophosphate or carbamate insecticide. Although there are mushrooms that cause cholinergic toxicity, these would have to be ingested, so that possibility is very unlikely. Atropine ingestion and tricyclic antidepressant (TCA) overdose produce the opposite syndrome of *anti*cholinergic excess and are therefore inappropriate (See section XIX B).

8-C. Activated charcoal (AC) is not useful for substances that will not bind to it, including lithium, iron, bromides, hydrocarbons, borates, and mineral acids and alkali. However, AC is appropriate in any ingestion where it is not otherwise contraindicated (e.g., caustic or corrosive ingestions) (See section I H 2).

9-C. Because tricyclic antidepressants (TCAs) are, themselves, class Ia antiarrhythmics, other class I (a, b, or c) agents such as procainamide (Ia) and flecainide (Ic) would only potentiate the effect, and are, therefore, contraindicated. Flumazenil is a benzodiazepine antagonist. Its use is contraindicated in ingestions involving TCAs, because they can contribute to the epileptogenic potential of flumazenil. Finally, physostigmine is contraindicated in the treatment of anticholinergic symptoms associated with TCA overdose, again due to the potential for inducing seizures. Although other drugs such as lidocaine and bretylium can be used to treat TCA-induced dysrhythmias, sodium bicarbonate remains the drug of choice, and is effective for most ECG abnormalities (See section IX D 3).

10-B. Pyridoxine and thiamine are cofactors administered in the treatment of ethylene glycol poisoning. Vitamin B_{12} is administered in megaloblastic anemia, not for methanol poisoning. Vitamin C is an important cofactor in the production of collagen, but is irrelevant here (See section VIII E 4).

11-A. The drug of choice for cocaine overdose is a benzodiazepine, which counters the anxiety, agitation, hypertension, hyperthermia, and seizures associated with cocaine toxicity. There is no role for the use of barbiturates or tricyclic antidepressants in cocaine overdose. β-blockers and haloperidol can be used, but they are second-line agents to benzodiazepines (See section XIII D 1).

12-D. Ethanol is the most common coingestant in adult drug overdoses. This must be kept in mind, because ethanol may mask or exacerbate toxicity of the other drug(s) ingested (See section I D 5).

13-A. An abdominal radiograph can detect radiopaque pill fragments, so it is useful for detecting aspirin ingestion. Common radiopaque substances seen in overdoses are summarized by the acronym CHIPES: chloral hydrate, heavy metals, iron, isoniazid, psychotropics (TCAs), phenothiazines, potassium, enteric-coated preparations, salicylates, and salts (See section I G 4).

19

Environmental Emergencies

I. Heat Injury

A. Heat stroke

1. Overview

a. Definition

—Heat stroke is defined as heat injury with altered mental status (AMS).

b. Causes may include:

—high ambient or environmental temperature

—increased endogenous heat production

—decreased ability to dissipate heat

c. Prognosis

—Mortality is high because of the potential for multi-organ failure.

d. Risk factors include:

—extremes of age (infants and the elderly)

—medications: anticholinergic agents, sympathomimetic agents, α blockers, calcium channel blockers (CCBs), tricyclic antidepressants (TCAs), monoamine oxidase inhibitors (MAOIs), lysergic acid diethylamide (LSD), salicylates, diuretics, phenothiazines

—cardiovascular disease

—dehydration

—constrictive, impermeable clothing

—skin disorders that do not permit adequate sweating (e.g., eczema, scleroderma)

—hyperthyroidism

—alcoholism

e. Complications include:

—heart failure

—pulmonary edema

—hepatic failure (usually resolves)

—acute tubular necrosis

—coagulation abnormalities resulting in hemorrhages, fibrinolysis, and, occasionally, disseminated intravascular coagulation (DIC)

2. **Clinical features** may include:

—hyperpyrexia

—AMS

—lack of or minimal sweating

—ataxia

—neurological deficits (e.g., posturing, positive Babinski reflex, hemiplegia)

3. **Diagnostic tests**
   a. Electrocardiogram (ECG) to look for arrhythmias
   b. Chemistry panel to look for electrolyte abnormalities
   c. Urinalysis (UA) to look for myoglobin
   d. Complete blood cell count (CBC), chest radiograph, blood and urine cultures to look for sepsis
   e. Activated partial thromboplastin time (APTT), prothrombin time (PT) to look for coagulopathies
   f. Computed tomographic (CT) scan and lumbar puncture as needed to look for cause of AMS

4. **Treatment**
   a. Stabilization of **airway, breathing,** and **circulation (ABCs),** including supplemental oxygen and replacement of intravenous (IV) fluids
   b. Reduction of core temperature via:

      —evaporation: water is sprayed on undressed patient with breeze from fans directed toward him or her [most practical approach to use in the emergency department (ED)]

      —cold water immersion
   c. Monitoring of core temperature with rectal probe, while cooling the patient to 40°C (104°F)
   d. Benzodiazepines to reduce shivering secondary to cooling

5. **Disposition**

—Patients with heat stroke are admitted to the hospital to monitor for complications.

B. Heat cramps

1. **Overview**
   a. **Definition**

      —**Heat cramps** are painful, spasmodic, involuntary contractions of skeletal muscles that most commonly involve the calves, thighs, and shoulders.
   b. **Causes**

      —Causes are the same as those for heatstroke (see I A 1 b).
   c. **Risk factors** include:

      —replacement of sweating losses with plain (hypotonic) water

      —the same risk factors as for heatstroke (see I A 1 d)

d. **Prognosis**

—Heat cramps are painful but usually self-limiting, with low morbidity and a good prognosis.

2. **Clinical features** may include:

—muscle cramps

—pain

—diaphoresis

3. **Diagnostic tests**

a. **Chemistry profile** to look for hyponatremia and hypokalemia

b. ECG to look for U waves (hypokalemia)

4. **Treatment**

a. ABCs and rest in a cool environment

b. **Replacement of fluids** with isotonic solutions such as:

—IV normal saline (NS)

—commercially available electrolyte-balanced drinks

5. **Disposition**

—Most patients with heat cramps may be discharged home after rehydration, with outpatient follow-up in 24 hours.

II. Cold Injury

A. Hypothermia

1. Overview

a. **Definitions**

—**Mild hypothermia:** core temperature 32°C–35°C (89.6°F–95°F)

—**Moderate hypothermia:** core temperature 28°C–32°C (82.4°F–89.6°F)

—**Severe hypothermia:** core temperature lower than 28°C (82.4°F)

b. **Causes** include:

—environmental exposure

—sepsis

—hypothyroidism

—hypoadrenalism

—hypopituitarism

c. **Risk factors** include:

—extremes of age (infants and the elderly)

—alcohol (acute intoxication and Wernicke's encephalopathy)

—drug overdose

—immobility

—neurological disease

—head trauma

—burns over a significant percentage of the body

—severe exfoliative dermatitis

d. **Complications** include:
—ventricular fibrillation
—DIC
—rhabdomyolysis
—acute tubular necrosis

2. **Clinical features**

a. **Symptoms** may include:
—gradually deteriorating mental status: incoordination→confusion→lethargy→coma
—body that is cold to touch
—dysarthria

b. **Physical examination findings** may include:
—rales on pulmonary auscultation secondary to bronchorrhea
—increased urinary output secondary to cold diuresis
—fixed and dilated pupils with coma
—from mild to severe hypothermia:
—tachycardia→bradycardia
—tachypnea→bradypnea
—hypertension→hypotension
—hyperreflexia→areflexia

3. **Diagnostic tests**

a. **ECG** to look for J (Osborne) wave (Figure 19-1)
—The typical arrhythmia sequence is: sinus bradycardia, atrial fibrillation, ventricular fibrillation, asystole

b. **Chest radiograph** to look for aspiration pneumonia

c. Arterial blood gases (ABG) to determine acid-base status

d. CBC to look for leukocytosis

e. Chemistry panel to look for electrolyte abnormalities

f. UA, urine and blood cultures for sepsis workup as indicated

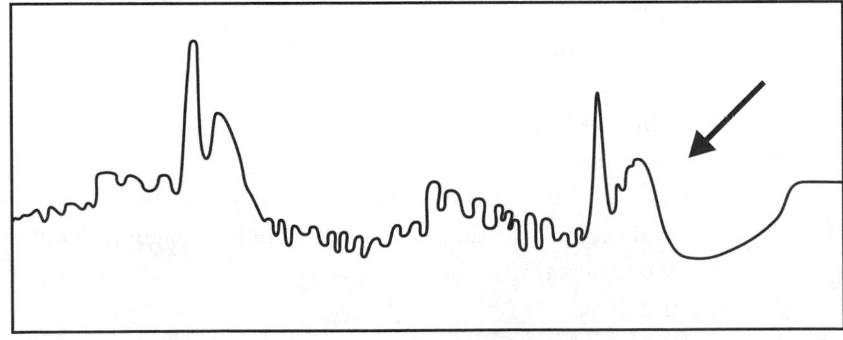

Figure 19-1. ECG demonstrating the J (Osborne) wave seen in hypothermia. (Reprinted with permission from Tintinalli JE, Kelen GD, Stapczynski JS (eds): *Emergency Medicine: A Comprehensive Study Guide,* 5th ed. New York: McGraw Hill, Co, Inc., 2000)

4. Treatment

a. ABCs, including supplemental oxygen

—*Note:* Gentle physical handling of the hypothermic patient is imperative to prevent ventricular fibrillation, because the myocardium is easily irritated in this situation.

b. Passive re-warming via:

—removal of wet clothing

—light covering with a dry bedsheet

c. Active internal (core) re-warming via:

—administration of warm, humidified air using face mask or endotracheal tube (ETT) to prevent further heat loss

—administration of warmed IV fluids via short tubing

—closed circuit pleural or peritoneal lavage with warmed NS

—extracorporeal warming circuit device for severe hypothermia

—*Note:* Gastric lavage is not recommended because it provides little heat transfer and carries the risk of aspiration and vomiting.

d. Active external (surface) re-warming via:

—heating blanket and heating pads

—heat packs to groin and axilla

—warm water immersion

—*Note:* Disadvantages to this method include peripheral vasodilation, resulting in further core temperature drop (after-drop). This can result in relative hypotension and hypovolemia (aftershock), leading to venous pooling, acidosis, and hypoxia.

e. Naloxone, thiamine, glucose cocktail as necessary to address mental status

f. Broad-spectrum antibiotics for suspected sepsis

g. Steroids for suspected adrenal suppression or myxedema coma

5. Disposition

a. Patients with mild hypothermia secondary to environmental exposure who are asymptomatic after re-warming may be discharged home with outpatient follow-up.

b. Most other patients require hospital admission to look for the underlying cause of the hypothermia and further management.

B. Frostbite

1. Overview

a. Definition

—Frostbite is a contact cold injury.

—It is seen most commonly in the face, ears, nose, hands, feet, penis, and scrotum.

b. Causes include:

—inadequate clothing

—constrictive clothing

—wet clothing

c. **Risk factors** include:
—diabetes mellitus
—peripheral vascular disease
—entrapment
—vascular injury
—hypovolemia
—Raynaud's disease

d. **Complications** include:
—hyperhidrosis
—cold intolerance
—arthritis
—amputation

2. **Clinical features**

a. **Symptoms** may include:
—throbbing shooting pain
—numbness
—tingling
—joint pain

b. **Physical examination findings** may include:
—blisters (clear or hemorrhagic)
—edema
—eschars (developing over a few days)

3. **Diagnostic tests**

a. No special diagnostic tests are necessary to make the diagnosis of frostbite.

b. Tests that may be considered on an individual basis include:
—radiographs of the affected extremity for suspected fractures
—CBC, chemistry panel, chest radiograph, and urine and blood cultures if underlying sepsis is suspected
—bone scan for suspected osteomyelitis

4. **Treatment**

a. Removal of wet, constrictive clothing
b. Active re-warming of the frostbitten part via immersion in circulating clean water at 41°C
c. Elevation of the extremity
d. Débridement of tense blisters
e. Topical therapy: may include silver sulfadiazine, bacitracin, aloe, or dry sterile dressings
f. Ibuprofen 12 mg/kg every 24 hours for 3 days to combat arachidonic acid cascade effects
g. IV analgesia (e.g., morphine) titrated to pain
h. Tetanus prophylaxis (see Table 19-5)
i. Antibiotic prophylaxis as needed

5. **Disposition**

a. Most patients with frostbite are admitted to the hospital for further management.

b. Patients with minimal superficial injury may be discharged home with an aloe vera cream, ibuprofen, instructions not to smoke (because smoking decreases circulation to peripheral veins), and outpatient follow-up in 24 hours.

III. Lightning Injury

A. Overview

1. Definition

a. Injury may occur secondary to the high energy of lightning.

b. Three mechanisms of injury are possible:

—Lightning can strike the victim directly.

—Lightning can strike a nearby object and ricochet over onto the victim.

—Lightning can strike the ground and spread up into the victim where his or her body is touching the ground.

c. The energy content of a lightning bolt can exceed 100 million volts.

2. **Complications** include:

—cardiopulmonary arrest

—seizure

—coma

B. **Clinical features** may include:

—**cutaneous fern-like streak burns**

—loss of consciousness

—AMS

—confusion

—**cardiac arrhythmias**

—tympanic membrane rupture

C. Diagnostic tests

a. **ECG** to look for arrhythmias—asystole and ventricular fibrillation

b. Cardiac enzymes to look for evidence of myocardial injury

c. Baseline CBC, chemistry profile, and coagulation studies

d. UA to look for myoglobin (renal involvement is rare)

e. **Cervical spine radiographs** in cases of suspected trauma (e.g., fall after being struck by lightning)

f. Radiographs of any extremity that appears deformed (fractures after a fall are common)

g. Chest radiograph to look for evidence of aspiration, pulmonary edema, or trauma

h. CT scan of the head if head trauma or AMS is present

D. Treatment

a. ABCs

—*Note:* death from lightning injuries is usually immediate or not at all, making it one of the few situations where efforts are concentrated on those who appear dead.

b. Advanced cardiac life support (ACLS) protocol for cardiac arrhythmias (see Chapter 1)

c. Anticonvulsants for seizures

d. Local wound care

e. Tetanus prophylaxis (see Table 19-5)

E. Disposition

—Patients are admitted to the hospital for monitoring of cardiovascular and neurologic status.

IV. Near Drowning

A. Overview

1. Definition

—Drowning is death from suffocation secondary to submersion.

—Near drowning is survival of suffocation secondary to submersion.

2. Mechanism (Figure 19-2)

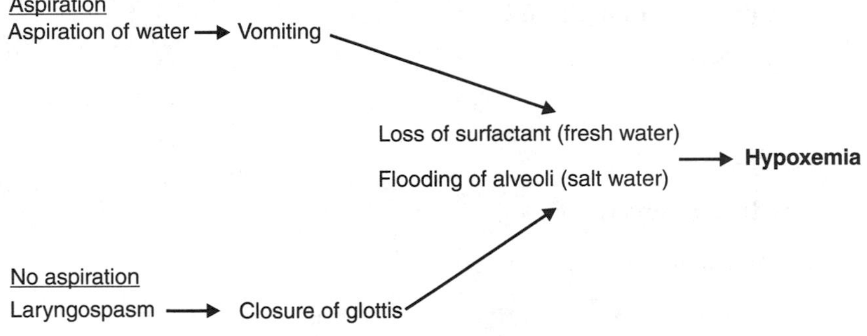

Figure 19-2. Mechanism of near drowning.

3. Risk factors include:

—alcohol or drug abuse

—cervical spine trauma

—seizures

—hypothermia

—inability to swim

4. Complications may include:

—pulmonary edema

—brain damage

—acute tubular necrosis

5. **Prognosis** depends on a number of variables, including:

   —length of time submerged

   —temperature of the water

   —whether loss of consciousness occurred

   —necessity for pre-hospital cardiopulmonary resuscitation (CPR)

   —necessity for cardiac medications in the ED

   —presence of neurological deficits

   —patient's age and underlying health problems

B. Clinical features may include:

—dyspnea

—cyanosis

—tachypnea

—wheezing, rales or rhonchi, on auscultation

—AMS

C. Diagnostic tests

1. ABG to look for hypoxemia
2. Chemistry panel to look for metabolic acidosis and hypoglycemia
3. CBC to look for leukocytosis, hemoconcentration, or hemolysis (usually is normal)
4. UA to look for proteinuria, hemoglobinuria, or myoglobinuria
5. ECG to look for arrhythmias
6. Chest radiograph to look for pulmonary edema or perihilar infiltrates (may also be normal)
7. Cervical spine radiographs to look for injury
8. Toxicology screen to look for potential causes of AMS

D. Treatment

1. ABCs, including supplemental oxygen
2. Early intubation, if necessary
3. Treatment of hypothermia if present (see section II A 4)
4. Nasogastric tube for stomach decompression
5. Albuterol nebulizers for bronchospasm
6. Steroids and antibiotics not indicated

E. Disposition

1. Most patients with any degree of persistent hypoxemia are admitted to the hospital for monitoring of complications.
2. Patients who are asymptomatic, fully conscious, and not hypoxemic may

be discharged home after a 6-hour observation period, with outpatient follow-up in 24 hours.

V. High-Altitude Illness

A. Overview

1. Definition and cause

—High-altitude illness results from acute hypoxia, usually secondary to rapid ascent to a high altitude by an unacclimatized individual.

2. Risk factors include:

—pulmonary disease (secondary to difficulty increasing vital capacity)

—overexertion

—alcohol or drug abuse

—dehydration

—lack of carbohydrates

3. Complications include:

—high-altitude cerebral edema (HACE)

—high-altitude pulmonary edema (HAPE)

B. Clinical features

1. Symptoms may include:

—headache

—anorexia

—nausea

—vomiting

—weakness

—irritability

—with HACE: AMS, seizures, coma

—with HAPE: cough, dyspnea

2. Physical examination findings may include:

—with HACE: ataxia, facial edema

—with HAPE: rales, tachypnea, tachycardia

C. Diagnostic tests

1. Diagnostic tests often are unnecessary, because the nature of the illness usually is obvious from the history. They also usually are not available at the time the patient presents, which is at altitude.

2. Helpful tests may include:

—Pulse oximetry or ABG to look for hypoxia

—Chest radiograph to look for pulmonary edema

—CT scan of the head to look for cerebral edema and other causes of AMS

—Carbon monoxide (CO) level if CO poisoning suspected

D. Treatment

1. For mild high altitude illness sickness:
   a. The patient should remain at present altitude until acclimatization occurs, then ascend at a slower rate.
   b. Acetazolamide for prophylaxis produces a bicarbonate diuresis, which results in a metabolic acidosis, which in turn causes hyperventilation.
   c. NSAIDs for headache
   d. Antiemetic [e.g., 10 mg prochlorperazine or metoclopramide given orally, IM, or IV] for nausea
   e. Low flow (0.5L/min) oxygen, particularly at night
2. For HACE and HAPE:
   a. **Immediate descent**
   b. 100% oxygen
   c. Dexamethasone 4 mg orally/IM/IV every 6 hours to reduce edema
   d. Hyperbaric oxygen (HBO) at descent as needed; HBO also may be provided at altitude via a Gamow bag.

E. Disposition

1. Asymptomatic patients and those who return to baseline following oxygen therapy may be discharged with outpatient follow-up.
2. Symptomatic patients and those with cerebral or pulmonary edema, altered mental status, or concurrent comorbidities are admitted to the hospital for further management.

VI. Diving Injuries

A. Overview (Table 19-1)

—Diving injuries can occur during any phase of the dive.

B. Clinical features of various diving injuries include:

1. **Squeeze**

   —disorientation (secondary to inner ear imbalance)

   —nausea

   —vertigo

   —tinnitus (inner ear)

   —nystagmus (inner ear)

   —ruptured tympanic membrane (TM)
2. **Nitrogen narcosis**

   —altered mental status
3. **Reverse squeeze**

   —same as for squeeze, plus:

   —tooth pain

   —stomach distention
4. **Pulmonary overpressurization syndrome (POPS)**

Table 19-1. Types of Diving Injuries

Type of injury	Phase of dive	Cause	Risk factors
Squeeze	Descent	Compression of a gas in an enclosed space secondary to an increase in ambient pressure	Upper respiratory tract infection, Sinusitis, Nasal polyps
Nitrogen narcosis	During dive	Elevation of partial pressure of nitrogen	
Reverse squeeze	Ascent	Expansion of a gas in an enclosed space secondary to a decrease in ambient pressure	Upper respiratory tract infection
POPS	Ascent	Expansion of compressed air in diving equipment	
AGE	Within 10 min of ascent	Entry of gas bubbles into systemic circulation via ruptured pulmonary veins	
DCS	Usually beyond 10 min after ascent	Release of inert gas into body tissues	Advanced age, obesity, dehydration, alcohol or drug abuse

AGE = acute gas embolism; *DCS* = decompression sickness; *POPS* = pulmonary overpressurization syndrome.

—mediastinal and subcutaneous emphysema

5. Acute gas embolism (AGE)

—syncope within 10 minutes of ascending

6. Decompression sickness (DCS)

—DCS type I: joint pains, skin itching

—DCS type II: neurologic symptoms

C. Treatment

1. 100% oxygen
2. Ascent if still underwater
3. Decongestants and elevation of the head of the bed for ear and sinus squeeze or reverse squeeze
4. Antibiotics for ruptured tympanic membrane
5. Nasogastric tube decompression for stomach reverse squeeze
6. HBO for AGE and DCS. Higher pressures (5–6 atmospheres) often are used for AGE, as compared to the standard 3 atmospheres used for DCS.

D. Disposition

1. Patients who are asymptomatic after 6 hours of observation in the ED may be discharged home with outpatient follow-up.
2. Patients who remain symptomatic after oxygen therapy or those with AMS or other complications should be admitted for further management.

VII. Burns

A. Overview

1. Definitions

—**First-degree burns:** involve epidermis only

—**Second-degree burns:** involve epidermis and varying levels of dermis

—**Third-degree burns:** involve all layers of skin including blood vessels and nerve endings

2. Risk factors include:

—extremes of age (infants and the elderly)

—child abuse

—AMS secondary to alcohol or drug overdose

—immobility

—neurological disease

—head trauma

3. Complications

a. Thermal burn complications include:

—renal failure
—sepsis
—hypothermia
—hypovolemic shock
—contractures

b. Electrical burn complications include:

—cardiopulmonary arrest
—rhabdomyolysis
—delayed hemorrhage from the labial artery in children with oral electrical burns

B. Clinical features

1. Signs of **burns to skin,** by degree, include:

—first-degree: painful, dry, erythematous, no blisters

—second-degree: painful, edematous, with blisters

—third-degree: painless, dry, edematous, insensate, charred areas

—*Note:* **Third-degree burns commonly are interspersed within islands of second-degree burns** and vice versa, meaning that a given area of third-degree burn may not be totally anesthetic. This is important to note for pain management.

2. Estimating the **percentage of total body surface area (TBSA) burned:**

—rule of nines (Figure 19-3)

—palm of patient's hand is equal to approximately 1% of the TBSA

3. Signs of **smoke inhalation injury** include:

—soot in the naso- and oropharynx

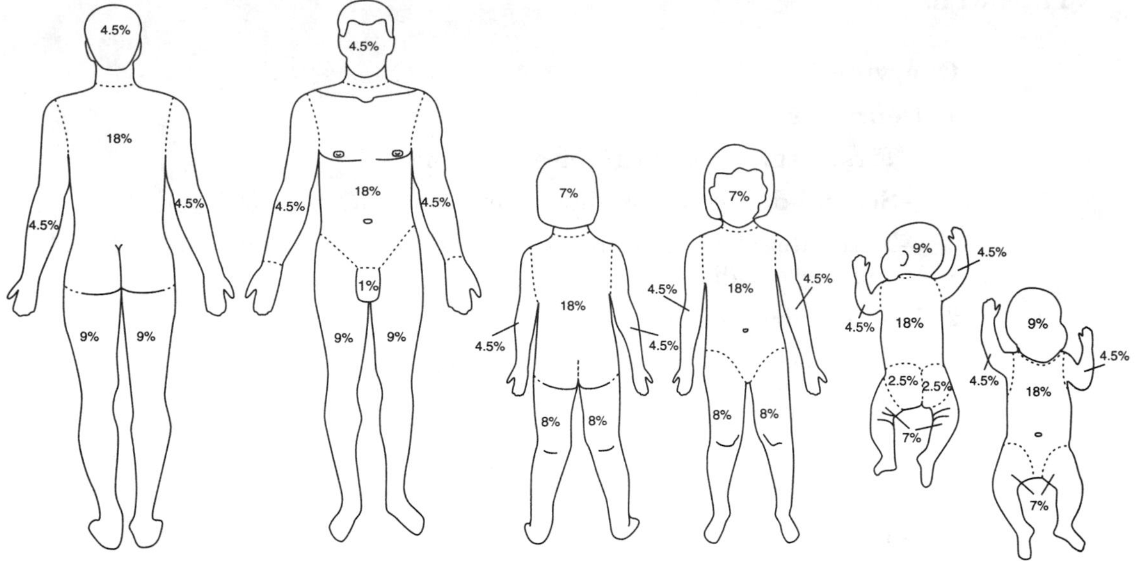

Figure 19-3. The "rule of nines" for adults (*left*), children (*center*), and infants (*right*). (Modified from LifeART Emergency Medicine Professional Collection. Copyright 1998, Lippincott Williams & Wilkins.)

—burnt nose hairs

—dyspnea

—*Note:* Significant smoke inhalation injury can occur in the absence of any signs.

4. Electrical burns

—Alternating current (AC) is more dangerous than direct current (DC) because it causes tetanic muscle contraction and pulls the victim in, preventing him or her from releasing hold; DC usually throws the victim away.

—Observable skin damage does not correlate with extent of underlying tissue destruction.

C. Diagnostic tests

1. **Carboxyhemoglobin level** to assess severity of CO poisoning, particularly for smoke inhalation injuries. See Chapter 18 XVIII E for treatment of CO poisoning.
2. Chemistry panel to look for electrolyte abnormalities and elevated creatine kinase (CK), particularly for electrical burns
3. ECG to look for arrhythmias (the most common arrhythmias in electrical burns are sinus tachycardia and premature ventricular contractions)
4. UA to look for myoglobin (electrical burns)

D. Treatment

1. Airway, Breathing, Circulation, Disability, and Exposure (ABCDE) are checked as for trauma patients (see Chapter 17 I), with supplemental **humidified oxygen.**

2. **Early intubation**
3. IV hydration via two large-bore peripheral lines; output is monitored with a Foley catheter. Urine must be alkalinized if myoglobinemia is present.
   —The Parkland formula for fluid resuscitation is total volume given over first 24 hours = **4 ml** (for adults) or **3 ml** (for children) × **weight (kg)** × **TBSA burned**
   —One half of this volume is given over the first 8 hours from the time of the burn and the remaining one half over the next 16 hours.
4. Parenteral analgesia as needed (e.g., morphine)
5. All affected areas of the body are cleaned with a mild antiseptic solution, and all affected mucous membranes are irrigated with NS.
6. For first- and second-degree burns:
   —**Bacitracin ointment** may be applied to affected parts of the face, and **silver sulfadiazine** cream may be applied to affected parts of the body.
   —Burns are wrapped in sterile gauze.
   —Blisters are left intact. If blisters have already ruptured, dead tissue is débrided.
7. For circumferential and torso burns, **escharotomy** is done to prevent compartment syndrome and distal neurovascular impairment.
8. Third-degree burns require eventual skin grafting, but this is not done in the ED.
9. If burns cross a joint, the joint is immobilized in extension to prevent contractures.
10. Tetanus prophylaxis (see Table 19-5)
11. Hypothermia prevention
12. Nasogastric tube to relieve paralytic ileus, seen in patients with > 20% TBSA
13. Prophylactic antibiotics are not indicated in the ED.

E. Disposition

1. Patients with first-degree and minimal second-degree burns may be discharged home after burns are dressed and fluid status is stabilized, with outpatient follow-up in 24 hours.
2. Patients in the following categories should be considered for hospital admission or transfer to a burn center:
   —Children or elderly patients with burns to > 10% TBSA
   —Adults with second-degree burns to > 20% TBSA or third-degree burns to > 10% TBSA
   —Patients with burns to the face, hands, feet, or perineum
   —Patients with burns associated with inhalational injury
   —Patients with electrical burns

VIII. Wound Care

A. Overview

1. Definition

— A wound is defined as violation of intact skin or mucosa.

2. Causes include:

—shear

—tension

—crush

3. Risk factors for infection

a. **Host factors** include:

(1) immunocompromised states

—diabetes mellitus

—malignancy

—peripheral vascular disease

—HIV

—alcoholism

—malnutrition

(2) drugs

—steroids

—chemotherapeutic agents

(3) other

—obesity

—advanced age

—smoking

b. **Wound factors** include:

—presence of devitalized tissue in margins of the wound

—location (extremity wounds are more prone to infection than scalp or face wounds)

—human bites

—grossly contaminated wounds (especially with pus, feces, vaginal secretions, or saliva)

—deep wounds (full-thickness)

—wounds secondary to burns or frostbite

—stellate (vs. linear) wounds

c. **Repair** and **technical factors** include:

—excessive suture tension

—use of natural (vs. synthetic) suture material

—poor hemostasis

—inadequate cleansing and prepping of wound

4. Complications include:

—infection

—scarring

—contractures

B. Wound preparation

—Few agree on the perfect method of wound preparation. Some general guidelines include:

1. Thorough, **copious pressure irrigation** of the wound. One excellent method employs a 30- to 60-ml syringe with an 18-gauge needle or catheter. This generates about 5 to 8 psi of pressure and is adequate for most wounds. Excessive pressure can result in increased inflammation and destruction of wound edges.
2. **Exploration** (under local anesthesia if necessary) to look for foreign objects, damage to tendon or nerve, or any evidence of joint involvement. Injection of methylene blue into a joint to look for seepage is useful to look for joint disruption.
3. **Débridement** of any grossly necrotic tissue
4. Preparation of the skin surrounding the wound with povidone-iodine, with care taken not to get it into the wound edges, because it is toxic. Direct contact with wound edges delays healing.
5. Clipping rather than shaving of hair around the wound. One exception is the hair of the eyebrow, which should not be tampered with.
6. Draping of the area to create a sterile surgical field

C. Types of anesthesia

—There are two main types of anesthesia, **intradermal** and **topical**. Intradermal administration provides better anesthesia, but the initial injection causes great fear for many patients, especially children.

1. Intradermal injectable local anesthetics included procaine, lidocaine, mepivacaine, and bupivacaine (Table 19-2)
2. **Topical anesthetics**

   —Topical anesthetics provoke less anxiety, but are adequate only for small, superficial lacerations of the face and extremities. They also may be used as a preparation for intradermal injection. Choices include:

   a. TAC (tetracaine 0.5%, epinephrine 1:2000, and cocaine 11.8%). Contraindicated in mucous membranes.

   b. EMLA ointment (50:50 lidocaine 2.5% and prilocaine 2.5%)

Table 19-2. Injectable Local Anesthetics

	Onset of Action	Duration (hr)	Maximum dose Without Epinephrine (mg/kg)	With Epinephrine (mg/kg)
Procaine	Slow	1.0–1.5	7	9
Lidocaine	Fast	1.5–4.0	4.5	7
Mepivacaine	Fast	2.0–4.0	7	8
Bupivacaine	Moderate	3.0–10.0	2	3

c. Ethyl chloride 25% + dichlorotetrafluoroethane 5% refrigerant spray

d. Benzocaine 5% spray, ointment, gel, or cream (good for mucous membranes)

D. Sutures

—The two main types of suture materials are **absorbable** and **nonabsorbable** (Table 19-3).

a. The main advantage of **absorbable sutures** is that they do not need to be removed. They are particularly helpful in infants and children who fear removal, in patients who are noncompliant or will have difficulty returning for follow-up, in patients who are prone to keloids,

Table 19-3. Suture Types

	Composition	Brand name	Advantages	Disadvantages
Absorbable	Plain gut		Rapidly absorbed, good for oral mucosal lacerations	Poor tensile strength
	Chromic gut		Causes less infection than plain gut	Delayed absorption due to chromium
	Synthetic braided Polyglycolic acid Polyglactin	 Dexon Vicryl	Less reactive than gut, good tensile strength	
	Synthetic monofilament polyglyconate polydiaxonone	 Maxon PDS II	Best tensile strength	Low reactivity
Non-absorbable	Monofilament nylon	Ethilon Dermalon	Relatively nonreactive, excellent tensile strength, low coefficient of friction	Knots have tendency to unravel if not tied correctly
	Polypropylene	Proline	Stronger than nylon	Greater memory than nylon so more difficult to work with
	Polybutester	Novofil	Strongest monofilament, best knot security, expands with wound edema and resumes shape	
	Silk		Best knot security	High risk of infection
	Cotton		Excellent knot security	High risk of infection

and in wounds that will be covered by a cast or otherwise will be inaccessible.

b. Nonabsorbable sutures are used for percutaneous closure. The main advantage of nonabsorbable sutures is that they have a decreased tendency to cause infection, because the material is relatively inert. Suture size and timing of suture removal depend on the location of the wound (Table 19-4).

E. Suture alternatives

1. Staples

—Staples are particularly suitable for sharp, linear lacerations of the scalp, trunk, and extremities, and for wounds that need to be closed temporarily before the patient is taken to the operating room.

a. Advantages

—fast

—offer the best resistance to infection

b. Disadvantages

—Cannot be used in areas that will undergo CT or MR imaging

—offer less control in approximating wound edges, and the resulting scar may be cosmetically unappealing

2. Tape

—Tape is particularly suitable for closure of wounds to the forehead, face, malar eminence, and thorax.

a. Advantages

—fast

—painless and requires no anesthesia

—good cosmetic result

—good alternative for patients with very thin, fragile skin (e.g., elderly or steroid-dependent patients)

b. Disadvantages

—limited use

Table 19-4. Suture Size and Timetable for Removal

Location of Wound	Size of Suture	Days to Removal
Scalp	2-0, 3-0	7–10
Face	6-0	3–5
Torso	4-0, 5-0	7–10
Arm	4-0, 5-0	7–10
Hand	5-0, 6-0	7–14
Leg and foot	4-0, 5-0	7–10
Joint surfaces	3-0, 4-0	10–14+

—does not stick well to surfaces exposed to secretions, such as axilla and groin

—is not good for wounds subject to anything but minimal tension

3. Adhesive glue (cyanoacrylate)

—Adhesive glue is particularly suitable for young children with superficial lacerations.

a. Advantages

—fast

—painless, requires no anesthesia

—antimicrobial properties

b. Disadvantages

—Glue polymerizes quickly (about 30 seconds), so there is no time for revising wound approximation.

—Some patients may be allergic to the glue.

—Glue is impractical for large, deep lacerations.

F. After-closure care

1. Dressings

—Most wounds are dressed with an antimicrobial ointment (e.g., bacitracin) and sterile gauze.

—If the wound crosses over a joint, the joint is immobilized.

—For wounds with potential to bleed into closed space and wounds involving ear cartilage, a compression dressing (elastic wrap) is applied.

2. Tetanus prophylaxis (Table 19-5)

3. Antibiotic prophylaxis for:

—immunocompromised patients

—human bite wounds

—grossly contaminated wounds

—late-presenting wounds (> 12 hr)

Table 19-5. Tetanus Prophylaxis

No. Td shots in past 10 yrs	For clean wounds		For all other wounds	
	Td*	TIG	Td*	TIG
Unknown or < 3	Yes	No	Yes	Yes
3 or more	No	No	No	No
Last shot > 10 yrs ago	Yes	No	Yes	Yes

TIG = tetanus immune globulin. Dose is 250–500 U IM. *Td* = tetanus and diphtheria toxoid adsorbed. Dose is 0.5 ml IM.

*If patients are < 7 years old, administer DTP (diptheria-tetanus-pertussis) or DT (diphtheria-tetanus only, when pertussis is contraindicated) vaccine

G. Disposition

1. Patients with simple wounds who do not require admission for any associated injuries can be discharged home with outpatient follow-up for suture removal, usually within a week (see Table 19-4).
2. Patients with wounds with a high potential for infection should have follow-up within 48 hours for a wound check.

IX. Bites and Stings

A. Overview

1. Definition

—More than 2 million animal bites and stings are treated each year in the United States.

—Animal bites include injury from pets, domestic animals, and wild animals; human bites; and envenomations from poisonous reptiles, insects, and marine life.

2. **Complications** may include:

—direct trauma to tissues

—infection

—poison-induced toxic reactions

—exposure to rabies

B. Dog bites

—Dog bites account for 60% to 90% of bite wounds treated in the ED.

—Most of the estimated 1 to 3 million dog bites in the United States each year are from pets, not strays, and occur in the home.

—In developing countries, strays in public places inflict most dog bites.

1. Clinical features and mechanism of injury

—The jaws of a dog can exert up to 200 psi, enough pressure to crush bone.

—The teeth are not sharp, so **crush** and **tearing** injuries often result.

—Injury is to the extremities 50% to 80% of the time.

—In children younger than 2 years, dog bites can perforate the cranium, causing brain injury and meningitis.

2. Bacteriology

—The organisms that most commonly infect dog bites include *Staphylococcus aureus, Streptococcus* spp., *Pseudomonas* spp., *Pasteurella multocida,* and ***Capnocytophaga canimorsus.***

3. Diagnostic tests

a. CT scan or skull films to look for fracture or evidence of skull perforation in any child younger than 2 years
b. Radiographs of the injured area to look for fracture, foreign object, or evidence of joint disruption

c. Neurovascular examination to look for any evidence of vascular or neurologic compromise

4. **Treatment**

a. Local wound care (see section VIII B)

b. Dog bites to the hand or those involving extensive crush injury are not closed primarily.

c. Antibiotics

(1) Antibiotics to cover *S. aureus* and *Streptococcus* spp. are indicated for:

—bites of the hand or lower extremity

—full-thickness bites

—bites requiring extensive débridement

—puncture wounds

—wounds involving tendon, joint, ligament, or bony fractures

(2) Antibiotics should be considered in immunocompromised patients.

(3) First-line choices include dicloxacillin or cephalexin.

(4) Second-line choices for penicillin-allergic patients are erythromycin and trimethoprim-sulfamethoxazole.

d. Tetanus prophylaxis (see Table 19-5)

e. Rabies prophylaxis usually is not required (see Table 14-1 in Chapter 14).

f. Orthopaedic or plastic surgery consultation for any tendon or bony disruption

5. **Disposition**

a. Most patients can be discharged home with outpatient follow-up in 48 hours.

b. Patients with signs of systemic infection, tendon involvement, or evidence of gangrenous tissue should be admitted for IV antibiotics.

C. **Cat bites**

—Cat bites account for 5% to 18% of bite wounds treated in the ED.

—The victim most often is the cat's owner.

1. **Clinical features and mechanism of injury**

a. **Symptoms** and **physical examination findings** of infected cat bites may include:

—erythema

—edema

—tenderness

—localized warmth

b. Most bites occur in the hand.

c. Cats have long, pointy teeth that most often produce puncture wounds. Tendons, joints, and bone can be punctured, introducing bacteria to these deep structures.

d. Patients rarely present until infection becomes evident.

2. **Bacteriology**

—***P. multocida*** is the usual pathogen and can cause overwhelming sepsis within 24 hours.

—Other possible infective organisms include *Actinobacter* spp., *Bacteroides* spp., *Streptococcus* spp., *Staphylococcus* spp., *Neisseria* spp., *Propionibacterium* spp., *Enterobacter spp.*, and *Fusobacterium nucleatum.*

3. Diagnostic tests

a. CBC, chemistry panel, and blood cultures if signs of infection are present

b. Radiographs of the injured area to look for fracture, foreign object, or evidence of joint disruption

c. Neurovascular examination to look for any evidence of vascular or neurologic compromise

4. Treatment

a. Local wound care (see section VIII B)

b. Prophylactic antibiotics are indicated for all cat bite wounds. Coverage of *P. multocida* is necessary.

—First-choice antibiotics are cefuroxime or amoxicillin-clavulanate.

—Second-choice antibiotics are azithromycin or trimethoprim-sulfamethoxazole.

c. Tetanus prophylaxis (see Table 19-5)

d. Rabies prophylaxis usually is not required (see Table 14-1 in Chapter 14).

5. Disposition

a. Most patients can be discharged home with outpatient follow-up in 48 hours.

b. Patients who present with signs of infection within 24 hours of the bite are more likely to have infection with *P. multocida* than with other organisms. These patients should be admitted for IV antibiotics.

c. Immunocompromised patients should be considered for admission for IV antibiotics.

D. Rodent bites

—The usual victims are laboratory workers or young children living in rodent-infested housing (these children usually are bitten while they sleep).

1. Clinical features and mechanism of injury

—Small puncture wounds

2. Bacteriology

—The incidence of infection is 2% to 10%.

—*Streptobacillus moniliformis* can cause clinically significant infection.

—Rats can transmit leptospirosis and plague.

3. Diagnostic tests

—Tests rarely are needed because of the nature of the injury.

4. Treatment

a. Local wound care (see section VIII B)

b. Prophylactic antibiotics are not recommended. Antibiotic choices for active infection include amoxicillin-clavulanate and doxycycline.

c. Suturing of these small wounds generally is not recommended.

d. Tetanus prophylaxis (see Table 19-5)

e. Most rat and squirrel bites do not require rabies prophylaxis. Prophylaxis is indicated for bites by groundhogs, raccoons, and skunks (see Table 14-1 in Chapter 14).

5. Disposition

—Most patients can be discharged home with outpatient follow-up in 48 hours.

E. Ferret bites

—More than 1 million pet ferrets are in the United States.

—Infants are the most likely to be attacked, possibly because they are of similar size to the ferret's instinctual prey.

1. Clinical features and **mechanism of injury**

—**Symptoms** and **physical examination findings** may include multiple bites and extensive cosmetic damage.

—Ferrets are bred to hunt rabbits. They attack by inflicting as many as 200 bites to the neck and face of their prey.

—Ferret attacks are notorious for being unstoppable even in the presence of an adult.

2. Bacteriology

—Little is known about the bacteriology of ferret wounds, but infection with *Mycobacterium bovis* has been reported.

3. Diagnostic tests

a. Radiographs of the injured area to look for fracture, foreign object, or evidence of joint disruption

b. Neurovascular examination to look for any evidence of vascular or neurologic compromise

4. Treatment

a. Victims first should be treated for life-threatening trauma, with attention given to ensuring that wounds do not compromise the airway and that life-threatening hemorrhage is controlled. Once the possibility of life-threatening injury is excluded, attention can be turned to the wounds themselves.

b. Local wound care (see section VIII B)

c. Prophylactic antibiotics are not indicated.

d. Puncture wounds are not sutured.

e. Tetanus prophylaxis (see Table 19-5)

f. **Rabies prophylaxis is indicated** (see Table 14-1 in Chapter 14).

5. Disposition

a. Most patients can be discharged home with outpatient follow-up in 48 hours.

b. Hospital admission should be considered for severe injuries.

F. Primate bites

—Monkey bites are not seen often in EDs in the United States, but they have unique features that require discussion.

—The usual victims in the United States are laboratory workers or other primate handlers.

1. **Clinical features and mechanism of injury**

   —**Symptoms** and **physical examination findings** may include scratches or bites inflicted by monkeys.

   —Scratches from monkey cages also are of concern.

2. **Bacteriology**

   a. The organisms that most commonly infect primate bites are *P. multocida* and *Eikenella corrodens*.

   b. The risk of transmission of *Herpesvirus simiae* is of great concern. *Herpesvirus simiae:*

   —is similar to human herpesvirus

   —has a 70% case fatality rate in humans

   —is found in Old World (Asian) macaque monkeys

   —can be shed from asymptomatic animals

   c. **Symptoms** and **physical examination** of *Herpesvirus simiae* include:

   —vesicles

   —ascending neuropathy and anesthesia at the site of injury

   —encephalitis that can lead to coma and death

3. **Diagnostic tests**

   a. Wound culture

   b. Serum titer for herpes virus

   c. Veterinary evaluation of the offending animal

4. **Treatment**

   a. The wound site is scrubbed immediately with soap and water at the scene. *Herpesvirus simiae* is thought to enter cells within 5 minutes. Wounds should be scrubbed for 20 minutes. If fluids have entered the eye, the eyes should be irrigated copiously with saline.

   b. Acyclovir

   —Acyclovir treatment is potentially life-saving if symptoms of *H. simiae* are present.

   —Acyclovir prophylaxis is not indicated unless the bite is felt to be from a high-risk animal.

   —Acyclovir prophylaxis may be considered in more moderate risk cases if initial wound care is deemed to have been inadequate.

   c. Patients should be advised to avoid activities involving exchange of body fluids for 4 weeks following exposure. They then should be tested for presence of the virus before resuming such activities.

5. **Disposition**

   a. Patients without serious trauma or evidence of infection may be discharged home but should have close outpatient follow-up for 4 weeks.

   b. Patients with evidence of *H. simiae* infection are admitted to the hospital.

G. Human bites

—Human bites may account for as many as 23% of the bite wounds seen in the ED.

1. Clinical features

—Human bites to the hand (commonly referred to as closed-fist injury [CFI] for their tendency to occur as one combatant's fist strikes another's mouth) have a high rate of infection.

—Any wound in the vicinity of the metacarpophalangeal joint should be considered a CFI until proven otherwise.

—Complications include tenosynovitis, septic arthritis, and osteomyelitis.

—Human bite wounds to locations other than the hand are not particularly prone to infection.

2. Bacteriology

—The organisms that most commonly infect human bite wounds are *Streptococcus* spp. and *S. aureus.*

—***E. corrodens,*** a facultative anaerobe, is cultured up to 30% of the time and is thought to be responsible for the severity of infections in CFIs.

—Other bacteria known to cause infection include *Corynebacterium* spp. and *Peptostreptococcus* spp.

3. Diagnostic tests

a. Radiographs of the injured area to look for fracture, foreign object, or evidence of joint disruption

b. Neurovascular examination to determine presence of vascular, tendinous, or neurologic compromise

4. Treatment

a. Local wound care (see section VIII B)

b. Prophylactic antibiotics are indicated for all human bites to the hand.

—The first line choice for prophylaxis is amoxacillin-clavulanate.

—For penicillin-allergic patients, clindamycin plus either ciprofloxacin or trimethoprim-sulfamethoxazole may be used.

c. CFIs are not sutured.

d. Human bites elsewhere on the body also receive antibiotic prophylaxis and are left open.

e. Tetanus prophylaxis (see Table 19-5)

f. Rabies prophylaxis is not indicated.

5. Disposition

a. Most patients can be discharged home with outpatient follow-up in 48 hours.

b. Hospital admission should be considered for:

—wounds older than 24 hours

—established infection

—bone injury

—penetration of joint space or tendon sheath

—foreign object in wound

—unreliable patient unlikely to make follow-up visit or take antibiotics

—diabetic or other immunosuppressed patients

H. Venomous snake bites

1. Overview

a. Snakes

(1) Snakes use their venom to subdue and help digest prey and, occasionally, for self-defense.

(2) Only four types of venomous snakes are found in the United States:

—Three of these snakes are in the family known as pit vipers (Crotalidae).

—The fourth is the coral snake (Elapidae).

(3) Poisonous and nonpoisonous snakes can be categorized quickly by a review of distinguishing physical features (Table 19-6).

b. Pit vipers

—Copperheads, water moccasins, and rattlesnakes are pit vipers.

—Bites from these species account for 98% of venomous snakebites in the United States.

—These snakes have a characteristic pit, a heat-sensing organ, between the eye and nostril on each side of the head.

c. Coral snakes

—Coral snakes are small, with a characteristic red, yellow, and black banding pattern. Many other species mimic the coloration of this snake but not with the same band sequence; hence the saying "Red and yellow kill a fellow; red on black venom lack."

2. Clinical features

—**Symptoms** and **physical examination findings** vary, depending on the type of snake bite.

—Victims of snake bites often suffer from overwhelming fear as well, which by itself can cause fainting, lethargy, vomiting, or tachycardia.

a. Pit viper bites

(1) Characteristics

—Pit vipers can control the amount of venom they inject when biting.

—Some bites may result in no envenomation (usually with older and larger snakes).

—Hematologic and local necrosis symptoms predominate. (*Ex-*

Table 19-6. Characteristics of Poisonous vs. Nonpoisonous Snakes

Poisonous	Non-Poisonous
Triangle-shaped head	Rounded head
Elliptical pupil	Round pupil
Pit between eye and nostril	No pit
Fangs	No fangs

ception: The venom of the Mojave rattlesnake causes a prevalence of neurologic symptoms.)

—Edema can be extensive.

(2) Complications

—allergic reaction

—compartment syndromes

—pulmonary edema

—shock

b. Coral snake bites

(1) Symptoms and physical examination findings may not be present until 6 to 12 hours after the bite. They may include:

—tremors

—salivation

—diplopia

—dysarthria

—dyspnea

—seizures

—minimal local symptoms

(2) Complications include death secondary to respiratory paralysis.

3. Diagnostic tests

—Coagulation profile with fibrin split products to look for DIC

—CBC

—Chest radiograph to look for pulmonary edema

—Other tests such as chemistry panel, LFTs, ECG, and UA as needed

4. Grading systems

a. For pit viper bites

(1) Grade 0

—no evidence of envenomation

—fang marks

—minimal pain

—less than 1 inch edema

(2) Grade I

—mild

—1- to 5-inch edema and erythema in first 12 hours

(3) Grade II

—moderate

—fang marks, pain, 6- to 12-inch edema and erythema in the first 12 hours

—occasional systemic symptoms

(4) Grade III

—severe

—fang marks, pain, edema, and erythema > 12 inches in 24 hours

—systemic symptoms, including coagulation defects

(5) Grade IV

—very severe envenomation

—rapid progression to altered mental status, shock, edema, erythema, ipsilateral ecchymosis, blebs, and coagulation defects

b. For coral snake bites

(1) Grade 0

—no envenomation

—fang scratches or punctures

—minimal local swelling

—no systemic symptoms in 24 hours

(2) Grade I

—moderate

—fang scratches or punctures

—minimal local swelling

—systemic symptoms present, but no respiratory paralysis

(3) Grade II

—severe

—respiratory paralysis occurring within 36 hours

5. Treatment

a. Pre-hospital care

—The patient is reassured.

—The area of the bite is immobilized with a splint and maintained below the level of the heart.

—Use of the Sawyer extractor to suck out venom may be helpful.

—Application of ice over the wound is discouraged, because it worsens tissue damage.

—The biting snake should be brought with the victim to the hospital for positive identification, but only if this can be done safely.

b. ED care

(1) The local poison control center is contacted for advice for all snake bites.

(2) ABCs

(3) Tetanus prophylaxis (see Table 19-5)

(4) For severe envenomation, the only proven therapy is IV antivenin.

(a) Pit viper antivenin

—The current preparation is a blood serum preparation of antibodies from horses exposed to the venom of many different snake species. Sheep-derived antivenin is currently being tested.

—It is given for crotalid envenomations of grades II (5 vials), III (5–10 vials) and IV (10 20 vials).

—It is given in a 1:10 dilution, with subsequent doses given every 8–12 hours if swelling progresses. The antivenin is rolled, not shaken, to mix it.

(b) Coral snake antivenin

—Three vials are given for all definite bites, regardless of presence of symptoms, which can be delayed.

—If signs of envenomation are present, additional antivenin is given.

(c) Exotic snake antivenin

—Exotic snake identification often is a problem.

—Antivenin often is not available, and local expertise often is limited.

—Zoos that keep exotic snakes sometimes carry antivenin for the animals in their collection and are a potential resource.

(5) Treatment of serum sickness

—Patients who receive more than 10 vials of antivenin usually develop serum sickness 1 week later.

—This can be treated with diphenhydramine, tapering dose steroids, and IV cimetidine.

(6) Prophylactic antibiotics are controversial.

(7) Treatment of Gila monster bite

—The Gila monster is detached from the bite victim.

—Any teeth that remain in the bite are removed.

—Local wound care is given.

6. Disposition

a. Patients with nonvenomous snake or crotalid bites with no evidence of envenomation at 4–6 hours may be discharged home with outpatient follow-up in 48 hours.

b. Patients with crotalid snake bites with only minimal local edema, no laboratory abnormalities, and no progression after 12 hours in the ED also may be discharged home with outpatient follow-up in 48 hours.

c. Patients with exotic snake, coral snake, or Mojave rattlesnake bites are at risk for developing profound neurologic and respiratory compromise (onset can be delayed longer than 24 hours). These patients should be admitted to the hospital to a monitored setting in case intubation and respiratory support become necessary.

I. Hymenoptera bites (bees, wasps, hornets, yellow jackets and ants)

—Venom varies among species. It is a mix of proteins, enzymes, amino acids, carbohydrates, and low-molecular-weight substances such as bradykinin, serotonin, dopamine, histamine, and acetylcholine.

1. Clinical features may include:

—immediate pain at the site followed by local swelling and redness

—local burning, itching, and the development of pustules (fire ant sting)

—anaphylaxis in susceptible individuals

—stingers with venom sacks embedded in the skin

2. Diagnostic tests

—No special diagnostic tests are necessary.

3. Treatment

a. ABCs, with particular attention to any manifestations of anaphylaxis (see Chapter 11 II A 4 for treatment of anaphylaxis)

b. Removal of any stingers present in skin: a scalpel is scraped parallel to the skin and the stinger lifted up with the knife blade. Care should be taken not to squeeze the exposed venom sack.

c. Oral antihistamines and ice applied to the wound site can reduce local discomfort.

4. Disposition

a. Most patients can be discharged home with outpatient follow-up in 48 hours and referral to an allergist for possible desensitization.

b. Patients with severe symptoms that have resolved should be discharged home with a prescription for an epinephrine syringe and instructions for self-administration should they be stung again.

c. Patients with anaphylaxis are admitted for monitoring. (see ch. 11)

J. Scorpion and spider bites

1. Overview

a. Scorpions produce a predominantly neurotoxic venom that acts by altering sodium channels in neurons.

b. None of the many North American tarantula species are toxic.

c. Two species of spider known for their toxicity are native to the United States: the black widow spider (*Latrodectus mactans*) and the brown recluse spider (*Loxosceles reclusa*).

—The toxin of the black widow spider opens ionic channels, causing a depletion of acetylcholine in the presynaptic terminal.

—The toxin of the brown recluse spider causes hemolytic effects as well as local vasoconstriction and systemic allergic reaction.

2. Clinical features

a. Characteristics of **scorpion bite** include:

—severe pain at the wound site occurring immediately after sting

—hyperesthesia, local weakness, and numbness

—muscle spasms (may be confused with seizures)

—restlessness and anxiety

—vomiting

—dysphagia

—dysarthria

—syncope

—hyperthermia

—respiratory arrest

b. Characteristics of **black widow spider bite** include:

—local erythema

—cramping sensation spreading from the bite site to gradually include the whole body

—headache, dizziness, weakness

—nausea, dyspepsia, vomiting, **abdominal rigidity**

—ptosis

—dysarthria

—conjunctivitis

—profuse diaphoresis

—hypertension

—respiratory arrest and cardiogenic shock (more common in children)

—Symptoms may mimic pancreatitis, appendicitis, or peptic ulcer disease.

—In adults symptoms start to diminish after 3–4 hours and resolve by 2–3 days.

c. Characteristics of **brown recluse spider bite** include:

—local pain and burning (variable)

—fever, chills

—weakness

—vomiting

—petechiae

—jaundice

—rash: vasoconstriction around the bite site within 2–4 hours. The vasoconstricted area becomes necrotic, and the necrotic area slowly spreads to more dependent tissues.

3. Diagnostic tests

a. CBC to look for hemolysis and **thrombocytopenia**

b. Chemistry panel and LFTs to look for **renal failure**

c. Coagulation profile and fibrin split products to look for DIC

d. Chest radiograph to look for pulmonary edema

e. ECG to look for arrhythmias (black widow spider bites may produce a digitalis effect)

4. Treatment

a. General

—Tetanus prophylaxis (see Table 19-5)

—Local wound care (see section VIII B)

b. Scorpion bites

—Antivenin for all stings that present with central nervous system or skeletal neuromuscular dysfunction

c. Black widow bites

(1) Control of hypertension with nitroprusside

(2) Benzodiazepines for muscle relaxation

(3) Antivenin

—Recommended for children, elderly persons, pregnant women, patients with severe toxicity, and those otherwise felt to be unable to withstand the stress of envenomation

—Dose is 1 vial in 50 l NS over 15 minutes.

d. Brown recluse

(1) No antivenin is available in the United States (available in Brazil).

(2) Necrotic areas can develop into extensive scars requiring later surgery.

(3) Dapsone may be helpful in treating local inflammation; however, adverse effects include methemoglobinemia and hemolysis.

(4) Analgesia as needed

(5) Dialysis for acute renal failure

5. Disposition

a. All patients with scorpion stings should be observed for 24 hours. If exotic species are involved, specific recommendations for that species should be sought for disposition decisions.

b. Patients with spider bites who show no signs of toxicity after 6 hours may be discharged home with outpatient follow-up in 48 hours.

c. All patients with spider bites and signs of toxicity require hospital admission.

K. Venomous marine animals

1. Overview

—Marine envenomations can be broken down into 3 general categories:

a. Bites: injury from the mouthparts of offending organisms

b. Stings: injury resulting from specialized skin-piercing delivery devices

c. Nematocysts: injury from specialized venom sacks found in coelenterates

2. Clinical features

a. Bites. Venomous biting animals include:

(1) Octopus

—The venom is a vasodilator with neurotoxic elements.

—A particularly dangerous octopus is the small, blue-ringed octopus, which secretes **tetrodotoxin,** a potent paralytic that blocks sodium fast channels. The blue-ringed octopus is found in Australia.

(2) Seasnake

—Venom contains potent neurotoxins as well as hemotoxins and cardiotoxins.

b. Stings may be inflicted by a variety of bony fish and invertebrates:

(1) Sea urchin

—Sting is inflicted by long spines that usually break off in the wound.

—Little systemic toxicity is seen.

—One Pacific variety causes facial nerve paralysis.

(2) Cone shells

—A long proboscis punctures the skin of persons handling the shells.

—Cone shells are found in the Pacific region.

—Venom produces curare-like neurotoxic effects.

(3) Scorpion fish

—Venom is primarily neurotoxic and heat labile.

(4) Stingrays

—Injury results from piercing of the victim by the spiny tail that the stingray raises defensively when it is in danger of being stepped on in shallow water.

—The venom is cardiotoxic, neurotoxic, and heat labile.

(5) Catfish

—Catfish fins are supported by barbed spines that are coated with toxin.

—Catfish sting is associated with a high incidence of infection.

(6) Weeverfish

—Spines are coated with toxin and are so sharp they can puncture shoe soles.

c. Nematocysts

(1) Jellyfish

—Stings can produce a range of symptoms that range from mild skin irritation to life-threatening systemic toxicity.

—Toxin is delivered by a hard tube that is propelled forward by tactile stimulus.

(2) Box jellyfish (sea wasp, *Chironex fleckeri*)

—Toxin is musculotoxic and causes vasopermeability, resulting in almost instant cardiac and respiratory arrest.

(3) Portuguese man o' war (*Physalia physalis*)

—Toxin promotes vasodilatation, histamine release, and hemolysis.

(4) Sea nettle (*Chrysaora quinquecirrha*)

—Toxin is not lethal to humans.

—It causes painful urticaria.

(5) Fire coral (*Millepora* spp.)

—Sting is accompanied by instant pain.

—Wheals can take a week to resolve.

3. Diagnostic tests

a. Soft tissue radiographs to look for foreign body if it cannot be excluded by physical examination

b. Other (e.g., laboratory) tests as necessary

4. Treatment

a. Local wound care (see section VIII B)

b. Prophylactic antibiotics for venomous marine animal bites

c. Venomous marine animal bites are not sutured.

d. Tetanus prophylaxis (see Table 19-5)

e. Rabies prophylaxis is not indicated.

f. Patients who have been injured by blue-ringed octopus or cone shells may need respiratory support.

g. Specific therapies

(1) Jellyfish

—Deactivation of stingers and removal of any undischarged nematocysts

—Deactivation may be accomplished with acetic acid, isopropyl alcohol, or meat tenderizer (contains papain).

(2) Sea snake

—Victim is kept quiet.

—Bitten extremity is immobilized.

—Antivenin: indicated in the first 24 to 36 hours after envenomation, but available only in Australia. It is thought that polyvalent tiger snake venom may be an acceptable alternative.

(3) **Sea urchin, scorpion fish, stingrays, catfish, and weeverfish**

—Immersion of body part in hot water

—Removal of all spines from the wound

(4) **Sea nettle**

—Deactivation (as for jellyfish)

—Removal of undischarged nematocysts

(5) **Fire coral**

—Application of acetic acid

—Steroid therapy: may be needed for persistent urticaria

5. Disposition

a. Most patients can be discharged home with outpatient follow-up in 24 hours. Patients should return for frequent wound checks, because stings often do not heal well and are prone to infection.

b. Patients with neurotoxic envenomations should be admitted to the hospital.

X. Occupational Exposure to HIV and Hepatitis

A. Clinical features

—Any exposure resulting in a break in the skin (e.g., needlestick) or mucous membrane exposure to a potentially infectious material [i.e., blood, urine, cerebrospinal fluid (CSF), semen, vaginal secretions and saliva] carries the risk of infection with HIV and hepatitis.

—Upon exposure, the health care worker immediately should clean the wound with soap and water or irrigate involved mucous membrane and then immediately report to his or her supervisor for postexposure prophylaxis.

B. Diagnostic tests

1. The following laboratory tests should be done on the exposed health care worker for documentation purposes:

a. HIV test

b. Hepatitis B and C antibody

c. CBC

d. Chemistry panel

e. LFTs

2. Samples for the following laboratory tests should be obtained from the source patient:

a. HIV test (requires consent from the patient before the specimen is sent to the lab)

b. Hepatitis B serum antigen

c. Hepatitis C antibody

C. Treatment

1. HIV prophylaxis

—Prophylaxis is best started as soon as possible, preferably within 2 hours of exposure and no later than 36 hours postexposure. Postexposure prophylaxis is given for 4 weeks.

a. **Zidovudine** 300 mg every 12 hours, *and*
b. **Lamivudine** 150 mg every 12 hours, *and*
c. **Indinavir** 800 mg every 8 hours on an empty stomach *or* **Nelfinavir** 1250 mg every 12 hours with food
d. *Note:* Combivir, 1 tablet every 12 hours, may be substituted for both zidovudine and lamivudine.

2. **Hepatitis B prophylaxis**

—Most medical students and personnel are vaccinated against hepatitis B, so reimmunization is not necessary. If immune status is in doubt, titers are drawn to verify.

—In exposed health care workers who have not received hepatitis B prophylaxis, 1 mg/ml of **Recombivax** (Hepatitis B inactivated virus vaccine) is administered, followed by the second dose in 2 months, and the third dose in 6 months.

D. Disposition

—All patients are discharged home with outpatient follow-up and referral for HIV counseling.

Review Test

1. Parents bring in a two-year-old girl after they found her chewing on an electrical cord. Burns to the corners of her mouth are visible, but the rest of the physical examination and work-up is otherwise negative. The parents should be warned about which of the following potential complications in this child?

(A) Renal failure
(B) Cardiopulmonary arrest
(C) Infection
(D) Bleeding
(E) Neurological deficits

2. A 26-year-old man is brought to the emergency department (ED) after collapsing within minutes of completing an underwater dive and returning to the surface at a nearby resort. Which of the following is his most likely diagnosis?

(A) Decompression sickness
(B) Acute gas embolism
(C) Reverse squeeze
(D) Squeeze
(E) Pulmonary overpressurization syndrome

3. A 5-year-old girl presents with a burn to her arm. The area is painful, red, and dry, but has no blisters. The remainder of the physical examination is normal. Which type of burn does this child most likely have?

(A) First-degree burn
(B) Second-degree burn
(C) Third-degree burn
(D) Eschar
(E) It is not possible to tell from the description given.

4. Which of the following features is associated with poisonous snakes?

(A) Round pupil
(B) Presence of fangs
(C) Absence of a pit between eye and nostril
(D) Round head
(E) All of the above

5. Which of the following bites may be sutured at presentation (primary closure)?

(A) Jellyfish bite (sting) to the foot
(B) Dog bite to the face
(C) Ferret bite to the head
(D) Human bite to the hand
(E) Sea nettle bite (sting) to the ankle

Directions: The response options for Items 6–9 are the same. You will be required to select one answer for each item in the set.

Questions 6–9

For each environmental injury, select the characteristic ECG finding.

(A) J (Osborne) wave
(B) Premature ventricular contractions
(C) Asystole
(D) Digitalis effect

6. Lightning injury

7. Hypothermia

8. Black widow spider bite

9. Electrical burn

Directions: The response options for Items 10–13 are the same. You will be required to select one answer for each item in the set.

Questions 10–13

Match each type of bite to the bacteria that is most likely to cause infection in that bite.

(A) *Pasteurella multocida*
(B) *Capnocytophaga canimorsus*
(C) *Eikenella corrodens*
(D) *Streptobacillus moniliformis*

10. Dog

11. Cat

12. Rodent

13. Human

Answers and Explanations

1-D. Oral electrical burns have a tendency to present with delayed (1–2 weeks later) bleeding from the labial artery. Parents should be warned about this complication at the time of discharge. Usually the bleeding can be controlled with pressure, and further treatment is not necessary. Electrical injuries can present with renal failure and cardiopulmonary arrest, but these are early rather than late complications. Neurological deficits are also possible, but they are unlikely in this child, who had local injury. Infection is not a usual sequela of electrical burns; rather, it is seen with thermal burns.

2-B. The classic presentation of an acute gas embolism (AGE) is syncope within 10 minutes of ascending from a dive. AGE is caused by gas bubbles entering the systemic circulation from ruptured pulmonary veins. Decompression sickness follows later. Reverse squeeze and pulmonary overpressurization syndrome also occur during ascent, but are not characterized by syncope. Squeeze occurs during descent, not ascent.

3-A. This child's burn fits the description of a typical first-degree burn. Second-degree burns usually present with blisters. Complete third-degree burns usually are painless. Eschars are associated with third-degree burns.

4-B. The presence of fangs is associated with poisonous snakes. All the other features listed—round pupil, absence of a pit between eye and nostril, and a round head—are associated with non-poisonous snakes. See Table 19-6.

5-B. Dog bites to the face have a low risk of infection (between 1% and 5%) and therefore can be closed primarily. Dog bites to the hand or those involving crush injury are not closed primarily. Ferret bites are puncture wounds, and these are not closed. Human bites to the fist are described as closed fist injury. They are not closed primarily either, because of the potential complications of tenosynovitis, septic arthritis, and osteomyelitis. Similarly, marine venomous animal bites are not sutured because of high risk of infection.

6-C, 7-A, 8-D, 9-B. Certain environmental problems have characteristic, although not pathognomonic, ECG findings that may be useful in leading to the correct diagnosis, especially when no history is available.

10-B, 11-A, 12-D, 13-C. Although various bacteria can be found in many different bites (e.g., *P. multocida* in cat, dog, and primate bites), certain bacteria are more typically seen with certain types of bites. It is useful to know which bacteria are commonly seen with specific types of bites when choosing antibiotics.

20

Pediatric Emergencies

I. Neonatal Disorders

A. Fever in the neonate

1. Clinical features

a. Symptoms may include:

—decreased feeding
—decreased urination
—increased sleeping
—lack of social smile
—inconsolable or irritable or floppy infant

b. Physical examination findings may include:

—fever > 38°C (100.4°F)
—tachycardia
—tachypnea
—cyanotic or pale infant
—dry mucous membranes
—meningeal signs (may or may not be present, difficult to assess)

2. Diagnostic tests

a. Work-up for **sepsis** consists of:

—complete blood cell count (CBC) to look for leukocytosis (Table 20-1)
—blood and catheterized urine cultures to look for causative organism
—urinalysis to look for leukocytes and bacteria
—chest radiograph to look for infiltrates
—lumbar puncture to look for bacteria and chemistry of cerebrospinal fluid (CSF) (see Chapter 6 II C)

b. Diagnostic test results suggestive of sepsis include:

—serum white blood cell count (WBC) > 15,000/mm^3
—urine WBC > 10 per high-power field (hpf)
CSF with WBC > 8/mm^3 or positive Gram stain
—chest radiograph demonstrating an infiltrate

Table 20-1. Normal CBC Values in Children

Age	WBC (× /10³ μl)	Hgb (g/dL)	Hct (%)	Plt (× 10³ /μl)
0–3 days	9–35	15–20	45–61	250–450
1–2 weeks	5–20	12.5–18.5	39–57	250–450
1–6 months	6–17.5	10–13	29–42	**300–700**
7–24 months	6–17	10.5–13	33–38	**250–600**
2–5 years	5.5–15.5	11.5–13	34–39	250–550
5–8 years	5–14.5	11.5–14.5	35–42	250–550
13–18 years	4.5–13	12–15.2	36–47	150–450

CBC = complete blood cell count; *Hct* = hematocrit; *Hgb* = hemoglobin; *Plt* = platelets; *WBC* = white blood cell count.

3. Treatment

a. Antibiotics

—One common regimen is ampicillin 25–50 mg/kg given intrvenously (IV) every 6 hours and ceftriaxone 25–50 mg/kg IV every 12 hours

b. Acetaminophen 10–15 mg/kg every 6 hours (maximum dose, 2.6 g/day) or **ibuprofen** 10 mg/kg every 6 hours (maximum dose, 40 mg/kg/day) for fever reduction and analgesia

4. Disposition

a. Infants with suspected meningitis, pneumonia, or urinary tract infection, or infants younger than 2 months with fever of unknown origin should be admitted for IV antibiotics.

b. Infants > 1 month of age who do not appear acutely ill and have reliable parents or caregivers may be discharged home on ceftriaxone with outpatient follow-up in 24 hours.

B. Jaundice

—Neonatal jaundice may be either physiologic or pathologic.

—**Physiologic jaundice** is the type that most commonly affects newborns

—**Pathologic jaundice** may result in kernicterus, the deposition of bilirubin in the brain, with serious neurologic sequelae.

1. Clinical features

a. Physiologic jaundice

(1) Description

—**Physiologic jaundice** peaks on days 3 to 5 of life.

—Yellowing of the skin and sclera progresses in a caudal fashion.

—This type of jaundice corresponds to normal rise of bilirubin from 0.5 mg/dL at birth to 5 mg/dL on days 3 to 5.

—The level declines to normal by 2 weeks of age.

(2) **Incidence**

—The rate of rise and peak value are higher in **Asian, Native American,** and **Inuit** infants.

(3) **Special circumstances**

—Premature infants have exaggerated physiologic jaundice.

—**Breast milk jaundice** occurs in breast-fed infants due to an unidentified factor that increases uptake of unconjugated bilirubin from the gut, and results in prolonged hyperbilirubinemia through weeks 6 to 9.

b. **Pathologic jaundice**

(1) **Causes**

—The most common cause of pathologic jaundice in the newborn is **hemolytic disease.**

—**Breast-feeding jaundice** occurs in infants fed insufficiently in the first week of life, and is analogous to starvation jaundice in the adult. It is distinct from **breast milk jaundice,** which occurs in the 3rd week of life.

(2) **Early manifestations** may include:

—lethargy

—opisthotonus

—seizures

—high-pitched cry

—dark urine

—light stools

—vomiting

—poor feeding

—fever

—death

(3) **Late manifestations** may include:

—choreoathetoid cerebral palsy

—high-frequency hearing loss

—upward gaze palsy

—motor deficit

—decreased intelligence

(4) **Laboratory findings**

—Pathologic jaundice should be considered in infants with jaundice presenting in the first 24 hours of life or with bilirubin levels > 10 mg/dl.

—Conjugated direct serum bilirubin > 2 mg/dl or 10% of total serum bilirubin suggests hepatobiliary disease or a general metabolic disorder.

—Bilirubin crosses the blood–brain barrier at levels of about 25 mg/dL in the normal newborn, 10–20 mg/dL in the premature infant.

2. Pathophysiology

—Bilirubin production, transport and metabolism in the newborn is different from that of adults:

a. Red blood cells (RBCs), the primary source for hemoglobin, have a life span of only 70–90 days

b. Albumin in newborns has a reduced binding affinity for bilirubin.

c. Hepatic uptake of bilirubin is reduced.

d. Hepatic conjugation of bilirubin is deficient.

e. Uptake of unconjugated bilirubin from the gut is greater, especially in infants fed breast milk.

3. Diagnostic tests

a. **Chemistry panel** to look for direct and total bilirubin levels

b. **ABO, Rh blood typing,** and **direct Coombs** test in the mother and neonate if not previously done

c. **CBC, reticulocyte count,** and **peripheral smear** to look for schistocytes, helmet cells, target cells, and other RBC forms that represent hemolytic anemias

d. **Glucose-6-phosphate dehydrogenase (G6PD) assay** to look for this inherited form of hemolytic anemia in Asian or Mediterranean infants

e. Urinalysis to look for reducing substances and WBCs

f. Thyroid function tests to look for hypothyroidism as a cause for the lethargy

g. Diagnostic procedures such as lumbar punctures usually are done only if the infant has signs of sepsis.

4. Treatment

—The goal of treatment of neonatal hyperbilirubinemia is prevention of neurologic injury (Table 20-2).

a. **Phototherapy:** makes bilirubin water-soluble, allowing it to be excreted by the liver and kidneys instead of through the gut

b. **Exchange transfusion:** reserved for patients with bilirubin levels above that at which kernicterus is likely to occur: 25–30 μg/dL in the term infant, 10–20 μg/dL in the premature infant

c. **Treatment of the underlying condition** in patients with direct hyperbilirubinemia (e.g., hepatobiliary disease, metabolic disorder)

5. Disposition

a. Hospital admission should be considered for patients with the following indications:

—suspected kernicterus or encephalopathy

—presentation in first 24 hours of life

—history of prematurity

—suspected large pool of recirculating bilirubin (e.g., from cephalohematoma)

—extensive caudal progression of jaundice

—exchange transfusion required

—suspected low likelihood of follow-up

Table 20-2. Hyperbilirubinemia in Infants

Bilirubin	< 10 μg/dL	10–15 μg/dL	15–25 μg/dL	25–30 μg/dL
Preterm infants < 1500 g at birth	Phototherapy	Phototherapy, consider exchange transfusion	Exchange transfusion	
Preterm infants > 1500 g at birth transfusion	Observe	Phototherapy	Phototherapy; exchange transfusion	Exchange consider
Healthy term infant > 9 wks or < 9 wks and not breast-fed	Observe	Consider phototherapy	Phototherapy	Exchange transfusion
Breast-fed infant 5d–2 wk	Breast-feeding jaundice: increase frequency of feedings to 12 feedings in 24 hours		Feeding changes; consider photo-therapy	Consider other causes, exchange transfusion
Breast-fed infant 3–9 weeks	Observe	Breast milk jaundice: supplement breast milk with formula or halt breast milk feeding for 24–48 hours	Feeding changes; consider phototherapy	Consider other causes, exchange transfusion

Note: Infants at risk for rapidly rising serum bilirubin or increased deposition of bilirubin in the brain include those with Apgar <7, hypoxia, acidosis, hypothermia, hypoalbuminemia, hypoglycemia, and sepsis. These patients require conservative management.

b. Healthy patients with breast-feeding or breast milk jaundice are discharged home with outpatient follow-up and appropriate feeding recommendations.

II. Seizures

—Seizures in the infant or child have many similarities to seizures in adults (see Chapter 6 VIII)

—Disorders exclusive to the pediatric population include **neonatal seizures; febrile seizures;** and one disorder sometimes mistaken for seizures, **breath-holding** spells.

—Neonatal movements confused with seizures include tremulousness or jitteriness and movements associated with the rapid eye movement (REM) phase of sleep.

—Paroxysmal conditions that may mimic seizure activity include syncope, narcolepsy, night terrors, complicated migraine, breath-holding, and Tet spells (Table 20-3).

A. Neonatal seizures

1. Clinical features

—Neonatal seizures occur in the first month of life.

—Most neonatal seizures are generalized tonic-clonic.

Table 20-3. Paroxysmal Conditions Mimicking Seizure Activity

Condition	Hallmark	State of consciousness	Treatment
Breathholding spell	Apnea following anger, frustration, or fright	Briefly unconscious, then return to normal	Reassurance given to parents
Complicated migraine	Neurologic symptoms followed by headache	Loss of consciousness (rare)	NSAIDs, rarely anticonvulsants
"Tet" spell	Transient worsening of congenitally poor pulmonary perfusion	Possible loss of consciousness	Volume infusion, oxygen, surgical repair of congenital heart disease
Syncope	Poor cerebral perfusion	Loss of consciousness	Varied
Narcolepsy	Irresistible urge to sleep	Asleep, easily aroused	Amphetamines
Night terrors	Child awakes, terrified, tachycardic, diaphoretic. The child does not remember the event.	Awake, but may appear to be hallucinating	Psychological intervention only if episodes are persistent
Pseudoseizure	Presence of secondary gain	May appear to be postictal	Reassurance given to parents

NSAIDs = nonsteroidal anti-inflammatory drugs;

2. **Causes** include:
   —hypoxia
   —intracranial hemorrhage
   —hypoglycemia
   —hypocalcemia
   —infection
   —congenital or developmental abnormalities
   —drug withdrawal
   —hyperbilirubinemia
   —vitamin B deficiency
3. **Diagnostic tests**
   a. CBC to look for leukocytosis
   b. **Chemistry panel** to look for hypoglycemia, hypocalcemia, hyperbilirubinemia, and other electrolyte abnormalities
   c. **Toxicology screen** to look for ethanol (EtOh) and drugs of abuse
   d. **Computed tomographic (CT) scan of head** to look for intracranial bleed
   e. Lumbar puncture to look for meningitis or bleed
   f. **Serum anticonvulsant levels** if patient is on any such medications

4. **Treatment**
   a. Stabilization of airway, breathing, circulation (ABCs), including supplemental oxygen
   b. Glucose: 0.5–1.0 g/kg of 10% solution bolus or 5 mg/kg/minute infusion
   c. Anticonvulsant: phenobarbital or phenytoin 18 mg/kg IV no faster than 1 mg/kg/minute
   d. Correction of any electrolyte abnormalities
   e. For patients on isoniazid (INH) or for seizures refractory to anticonvulsants, pyridoxine in a dose equivalent to amount of INH ingested (if known), or an empiric dose of 50–100 mg IV, not to exceed 70 mg/kg.
   f. Treatment of underlying disorder, if known
5. **Disposition**
   —Patients are admitted to the hospital for completion of work-up.

B. Febrile seizures

1. **Clinical features**
   a. **Description**
      —Febrile seizures are tonic-clonic, accompanied by fever.
      —Duration ranges from 30 seconds to 15 minutes.
   b. **Incidence**
      —Febrile seizures occur in children aged 3 months to 6 years.
      —They occur in 3% to 4% of children.
      —About half of children will have a second episode.
      —The incidence of epilepsy is 10% in children with febrile seizures whose parents have epilepsy.
   c. **Prognosis**
      —The consequences of single or recurrent febrile seizures are minimal.
2. **Diagnostic tests**
   a. No special diagnostic tests are necessary for simple febrile seizures.
   b. If the diagnosis is unclear, the following tests may be useful:
      —CBC to look for leukocytosis
      —blood and urine cultures to look for occult bacteremia
      —chest radiograph to look for infiltrates
      —lumbar puncture to look for meningitis if patient is ill-appearing or <1 year of age with documented source of infection
      —electroencephalogram (EEG) is not indicated for first-time febrile seizure.
   c. The diagnosis of febrile seizure can be made only after other causes have been ruled out.
3. **Treatment**
   a. Anticonvulsant therapy is given only to patients with:
      —family history of epilepsy
      —prolonged initial seizure
      —developmental or neurologic abnormality

b. Parents of patients without risk factors just listed should be offered reassurance regarding their child's excellent prognosis.

4. **Disposition**

a. Most patients with febrile seizures can be discharged home with outpatient follow-up after a 4-hour period of observation in the emergency department (ED).

b. Patients in whom the diagnosis is unclear should be admitted for further work-up.

C. **Breath-holding spells**

1. **Clinical features** may include:

—child aged 6 months to 4 years

—severe crying in response to anger or frustration, fear, or pain, and subsequent development of apnea

—loss of consciousness

—jerky movements reminiscent of seizure activity or rigid back and limbs

—spells that are either "cyanotic" or "pallid," depending on changes in skin color

—pallid spells that are precipitated by extreme fright

2. **Diagnosis**

—No specific diagnostic tests are necessary unless the diagnosis is unclear (see section II B 2 b)

3. **Treatment**

—Parents should be offered reassurance.

4. **Disposition**

—Patients can be discharged home with outpatient follow-up in 1 week.

III. Tooth Eruption in Infants

A. **Clinical features**

1. **Overview**

a. Teeth usually begin to erupt between 6 and 9 months of age.

b. The first teeth to erupt usually are the mandibular incisors.

c. Teeth erupt in the following order:

—mandibular central incisors
—mandibular lateral incisors
—maxillary central incisors
—maxillary lateral incisors
—mandibular 1st molars
—maxillary 1st molars
—mandibular 2nd molars
—maxillary 2nd molars

2. **Symptoms** may include:
   —fever
   —diarrhea
   —dehydration
   —skin rash
3. **Physical examination findings** may include:
   —cranky but consolable infant
   —increased salivation

B. Diagnostic tests

—Laboratory testing or radiological imaging is necessary only in the following circumstances:

1. Systemic symptoms present for > 24 hours: possible upper respiratory tract infection
2. Increased salivation accompanied by stridor: possibility of partial airway obstruction
3. Abnormal tooth eruption pattern: refer to pedodontist, consider alveolar bone films

C. Treatment

—Treatment consists of supportive care.

1. Increased fluid intake
2. Acetaminophen or ibuprofen for analgesia and fever reduction
3. Topical benzocaine gel or ice rings to gingiva to reduce pain and irritation
4. Reassurance to parents that symptoms will subside once teeth erupt

D. Disposition

—Patients can be discharged home with outpatient follow-up.

IV. Heart Disease in Children

A. Overview

1. Definition

—Pediatric heart disease is classified as congenital or acquired.

—Although congenital heart disease (CHD) is rare (affecting 7 per 1000 live births), it is the most common form of life-threatening anatomic abnormality.

—Congenital heart disease usually is sporadic, but has also been linked to multiple genetic and environmental factors, including **trisomy 21** (Down syndrome), **Turner syndrome,** maternal **rubella** infection, alcohol, and prescription and illicit drug use.

2. Causes

—Heart disease in children often is identified at birth or through investigation of a murmur heard on a well-child examination.

—Acquired heart disease in children most often is the result of an infectious agent (Table 20-4).

—Emergency presentations of heart disease include **shock, congestive heart failure,** and **cyanosis**. The emergency physician must be able to identify and stabilize life-threatening heart disease in children; in most cases, a pediatric cardiologist will handle definitive diagnosis and therapy.

B. Fetal and neonatal circulation

1. In utero, fetal blood is oxygenated by the placenta, returns to the right heart via the hepatic ductus venosus, and bypasses the pulmonary circulation at two sites: the **foramen ovale,** which connects right atrium to left atrium, and the **ductus arteriosus,** which connects the pulmonary artery to the descending aorta. The right ventricle effectively pumps blood to the placenta and lower body, and the left ventricle pumps blood to the upper body.
2. At birth, pulmonary vascular resistance drops, and left-sided pressures become greater than right-sided pressures, closing the foramen ovale by way of a flap valve. Closure of the ductus arteriosus is mediated by inhibition of prostaglandins and usually is completed in the first few hours of life, but may be prolonged in preterm infants or those with ductus-dependent congenital heart disease.

C. The infant with cardiogenic shock

1. Overview

—Shock, or systemic hypoperfusion, has many different causes, including hypovolemia, sepsis, and pump failure.

—Cardiogenic shock in the infant most often is due to left heart obstructive disease **(aortic stenosis** and **coarctation of the aorta), myocarditis,** or a congenital **arrhythmia**.

Table 20-4. Inflammatory Heart Disease in Infants and Children

Disease	Distinguishing Features	Complications
Myocarditis	Affects child of any age; symptoms of shock and congestive heart failure; may have increased CPK-MB	End-stage cardiomyopathy; sudden death
Pericarditis	Affects older children; pleuritic or positional chest pain; may see pulsus paradoxus	Can cause tamponade; diuresis is contraindicated
Endocarditis	Associated with congenital heart disease, usually aortic stenosis and tetralogy of fallot; unexplained fever	Embolization of vegetations; valvular insufficiency
Rheumatic fever	2–3 weeks post–group A streptococcal infection; arthritis often precedes carditis	Mitral valve insufficiency
Kawasaki disease	Affects younger children; high fever, characteristic rash, oral changes; arthritis	Coronary aneurysm; myocardial infarction

CPK-MB = creatinine phosphokinase MB fraction

2. Clinical features

a. Shock in infants **from any cause** may be manifested by:

—pallor
—poor peripheral pulses
—poor capillary refill
—dyspnea
—poor feeding
—tachycardia

b. Shock in infants **in association with specific disorders**

(1) Factors associated with infantile **aortic stenosis** include:

—male sex
—dramatic onset
—ventricular arrhythmias
—loud systolic murmur

(2) Factors associated with **coarctation of the aorta** include:

—male sex
—dramatic onset
—Turner syndrome
—cool lower extremities
—pressure gradient and pulse difference between upper and lower extremities
—systolic ejection murmur at base radiating to back

(3) Factors that may be associated with **myocarditis** include:

—fever
—tachycardia
—low-voltage electrocardiogram (ECG)
—history of recent viral illness
—evidence of congestive heart failure

(4) Common infantile **arrhythmias** include:

—**supraventricular tachycardia:** narrow complex tachycardia at rate of 220–350 beats/min
—**complete heart block:** dissociation of atrial and ventricular impulses, seen with maternal lupus
—**ventricular tachycardias,** usually seen with myocarditis or cardiomyopathy

3. Pathophysiology

a. Neonates with **left heart obstructive disease** rely on a **patent ductus arteriosus** to supply the systemic circulation. These patients rapidly decompensate when the ductus closes.

b. Aortic stenosis is characterized by narrowing of the left ventricular outflow tract at or near the level of the aortic valve. Severe cases may be associated with hypoplasia of the mitral valve, left ventricle, and ascending aorta (**hypoplastic left heart syndrome**).

c. Coarctation of the aorta is characterized by the abnormal persistence of the posterior aortic shelf. In utero, this shelf directs flow from the ductus toward the placenta. In the infant with coarctation, this shelf blocks flow from the ascending to descending aorta.

d. Infants with myocarditis or arrhythmias have no obstruction to systemic flow, but rather have diminished cardiac output due to:
—poor ventricular filling (supraventricular tachycardia)
—reduced heart rate (complete heart block, bradycardia)
—myocardial hypokinesis (myocarditis)

4. **Diagnostic tests**

a. **Laboratory tests**
—**Arterial blood gas** to look for metabolic acidosis
—CBC to look for anemia
—Chemistry panel to look for electrolyte abnormalities
—Blood cultures to look for infection (endocarditis)

b. **Imaging studies**
—**ECG** to look for tachycardia, A-V dissociation, left ventricular hypertrophy (aortic stenosis), right ventricular hypertrophy (coarctation)
—**Chest radiograph** to look for cardiomegaly
—**Echocardiogram** to look for valvular defects (best screening test for infants in cardiogenic shock)

5. **Treatment**

a. ABCs

b. **For left heart obstructive disease:**
—Prostaglandin therapy should be considered for infants less than 1 week old (after confirmation of diagnosis by ECG) to maintain patent ductus arteriosus until definitive therapy is achieved. Initial dose is 0.1 μg/kg/min.
—Inpatient management may include cardiac catheterization, balloon angioplasty across the coarctation or aortic valve, and surgical repair.

c. **For converting supraventricular tachycardia:**
—Vagal maneuvers
—Adenosine (0.1 mg/kg) IV push
—Digoxin (total digitalizing dose 30–35 μg/kg IV, half given initially, one fourth given at 8 hours and one fourth at 16 hours): will convert some patients after several hours
—Direct current cardioversion if patient becomes unstable (0.5–1.0 J/kg)

d. **For myocarditis:**
—Emergency department treatment is supportive.

6. **Disposition**
—All infants with evidence of shock should be admitted to the hospital for further management.

D. The infant with congestive heart failure

1. **Clinical features**
—Congestive heart failure in the infant, a well-compensated form of low cardiac output, most commonly is due to congenital heart disease char-

acterized by left-to-right shunts, including large **ventriculoseptal defect** (VSD), large **patent ductus arteriosus** (PDA), and **complete atrioventricular canal** (CAVC) **(Table 20-5.)**

—The most common of these is the VSD.

a. **Symptoms** may include:
   —easy tiring
   —poor feeding
   —poor weight gain
   —generalized or peripheral edema

b. **Physical examination findings** may include:
   —dyspnea
   —tachypnea
   —diaphoresis
   —pulmonary edema
   —hepatomegaly
   —**jugular venous distention** (seen less commonly in the infant than in older children or adults)
   —**murmur:** may be harsh systolic murmur, fixed split S2 (in ASD), or infrascapular machinery murmur (in PDA)

2. **Pathophysiology**

a. The **VSD** is characterized by an abnormal hole in the interventricular septum. It may occur alone, in multiples, or as part of more severe disease (e.g., tetralogy of Fallot). Blood shunts from the left to the right ventricle across the defect when there is no associated pulmonary obstruction

b. **Atrial septal defects (ASD)** rarely cause severe disease in the infant but may cause symptoms in the older child or adult. The undiscovered ASD, or **patent foramen ovale,** has been linked to paradoxical emboli in the adult

c. **ASDs,** including **complete AV canal,** are characterized by deficiency of the atrial septum, the ventricular septum, and the mitral and tricuspid valves. A single AV valve with six leaflets often is present, and pulmonary and systemic flow is intermixed.

d. The **PDA** may persist past the perinatal period, most often in preterm infants or infants with left heart obstructive disease. Large **PDAs** in

Table 20-5. Cyanotic vs. Non-cyanotic Heart Disease

Non-cyanotic: left-to-right shunt	Ventricular septal defect Atrial septal defect Coarctation of the aorta Patent ductus arteriosus
Cyanotic: right-to-left shunt	Total anomalous pulmonary venous circulation Hypoplastic left heart Truncus arteriosus Tetralogy of Fallot Transposition of the great vessels

the otherwise structurally normal heart permit shunting of flow from the aorta to the pulmonary artery.

e. Surgical shunts sometimes are created to supply the pulmonary circulation with flow in **pulmonary stenosis** or **pulmonary atresia** before definitive repair. The **Blalock-Taussig** shunt is an anastomosis of the right subclavian artery to the right pulmonary artery.

f. Each of these malformations features abnormal left-to-right flow of blood across the defect. The pulmonary vasculature is forced to sustain greater than systemic flow, resulting in **pulmonary venous congestion,** endothelial damage, medial hypertrophy and **pulmonary hypertension**

g. As pulmonary pressures rise, the right ventricle hypertrophies to overcome the load. When obstruction to right ventricular outflow exceeds that of the left ventricular outflow, direction of flow across the shunt is reversed. This event is known as **Eisenmenger's syndrome**. The development of pulmonary hypertension carries a very poor prognosis.

3. Diagnostic tests

a. **ECG** to look for left, right, or biventricular hypertrophy

b. **Chest radiograph** to look for cardiomegaly and pulmonary venous congestion

c. **Pulse oximetry** to assess O_2 saturation and measure any improvement on administration of supplemental O_2

4. Treatment

a. ABCs, including supplemental oxygen. (Tertiary care centers may provide extracorporeal membrane oxygenation [ECMO] for the infant who oxygenates poorly with mechanical ventilation.)

b. Diuretics as needed

c. Inotropic agents as needed

d. **Nitric oxide:** improves pulmonary hypertension in some cases

5. Disposition

—All infants with congestive heart failure should be admitted to the hospital for definitive diagnosis and treatment.

E. The child with cyanosis

1. Overview

a. Cyanosis in the infant or child may result from poor ventilation secondary to airway obstruction, poor perfusion, or shunting of deoxygenated blood to the systemic circulation (as seen with many CHDs).

b. **Methemoglobinemia** may mimic cyanosis.

c. **Congenital lesions**

—The most common congenital cyanotic lesion in children is **tetralogy of Fallot.**

—The most common congenital cyanotic lesion seen in the first few days of life is transposition of the great arteries.

d. **Complications** may include:

—convulsions

—cerebrovascular accident
—death

2. **Clinical features** may include:
—dyspnea on exertion
—clubbing
—hemoptysis
—systolic ejection murmur
—hypercyanotic **"Tet" spell:** worsening cyanosis, limpness, and syncope

3. **Pathophysiology**

a. **Tetralogy of Fallot** involves anterior displacement of the infundibular interventricular septum and is characterized by:
—pulmonary stenosis or right ventricular outflow tract obstruction.
—ventricular septal defect
—aorta that overrides or "straddles" the VSD
—right ventricular hypertrophy

b. **Pulmonary stenosis** may occur alone at or near the level of the pulmonary valve. If the stenosis is severe enough that right ventricular hypertrophy develops, deoxygenated blood may shunt across a **patent foramen ovale.**

c. **PDA** may provide flow to the pulmonary arteries in severe pulmonary stenosis.

d. **Total anomalous pulmonary venous connection (TAPVC)** is characterized by the return of pulmonary veins (carrying newly oxygenated blood) to the right-sided circulation, usually to the right atrium, coronary sinus, or superior vena cava.

e. Infants with **truncus arteriosus** have a persistent single great vessel, from which both the left and right pulmonary arteries and the aortic arch arise. Truncus arteriosus is accompanied by a **VSD,** permitting mixing of circulations at the level of the ventricles and in the single great vessel.

4. **Diagnostic tests**

a. **Laboratory studies**
—CBC to look for polycythemia
—Arterial blood gas to look for acidosis and oxygen saturation level. In cases that cannot be distinguished on the basis of characteristic physical findings or chest film, pulmonary causes of cyanosis may be ruled out by the infant or child's response to oxygen (Table 20-6).

b. **Imaging studies**
—ECG to look for right ventricular hypertrophy
—Chest radiograph to look for **boot-shaped heart (coeur-en-sabot)** seen in tetralogy of Fallot
—Definitive diagnosis is made by echocardiography and cardiac catheterization.

5. **Treatment**

a. ABCs

Table 20-6. Response of Cyanosis to Supplemental Oxygen

Cause of cyanosis	Response
Pulmonary parenchymal disease	Cyanosis resolves
Hypoventilation	Partial improvement
Arterial/venous mixing	Minimal improvement
Decreased pulmonary perfusion	No change

—Some forms of cyanosis respond to oxygen, whereas others do not, depending on the etiology (see Table 20-6).

—Supplemental oxygen should *not* be given, however, because it can hasten closure of a PDA.

b. Intravenous hydration to maintain systemic blood pressure

c. Peripheral vasoconstrictors for blood pressure as needed

d. For "tet" spells:

—morphine, 0.2 mg/kg/dose IM or IV

—propranolol, 0.05 to 0.1 mg/kg IV

6. Disposition

—All patients with cyanosis should be admitted to the hospital for definitive diagnosis and treatment.

V. Respiratory Disorders

A. Small airways obstruction

1. Overview

a. Bronchiolitis

—**Bronchiolitis** is an acute disease of infancy, characterized by inflammation and obstruction of the small airways, often with a reactive, bronchospastic component.

—From 80% to 90% of cases of bronchiolitis are thought to be due to **respiratory syncytial virus** (RSV).

—Mortality from bronchiolitis is about 1%.

—Bronchiolitis shares many features with **asthma**. The diagnosis of bronchiolitis due to RSV requiring hospitalization in the first year of life is associated with a 23% chance of development of childhood asthma.

b. Asthma

—**Asthma** is a chronic disease in children > 2 years of age.

—It is characterized by inflammation and obstruction of small airways and alveoli in response to infectious and environmental triggers. (See Chapter 3 VIII for further discussion.)

2. Clinical features

a. Bronchiolitis

—Age < 2 years

—History of nasal congestion and cough for 3 to 5 days
—Tachypnea
—Wheezing and fine rales on examination
—Poor feeding and cyanosis if severe

b. **Asthma**
—Any age
—Cough, wheezing, or dyspnea
—Tachypnea
—History of prior bronchiolitis or asthma attack
—Positive family history of asthma or eczema
—Variable history of allergen exposure

c. Factors associated with **worsening small airways disease** may include:
—O_2 saturation less than 95%
—use of accessory muscles for respiration (retractions of sternocleidomastoid, subcostal, and intercostal muscles)
—nasal flaring
—grunting
—head bobbing
—poor hydration status
—cyanosis
—decreased breath sounds
—peak flow less than 50% baseline (in older children)
—inability to speak full sentences without pause (in older children)

3. **Pathophysiology**

a. **Bronchiolitis**
—RSV causes infiltration of peribronchial tissues with lymphocytes, and necrosis of respiratory endothelium.
—The regenerated endothelium lacks effective mucociliary function, prolonging obstruction of the small airways.

b. **Asthma**
—Allergens bind to mast cells, causing degranulation and release of histamine, leukotrienes, prostaglandins, and platelet activating factor.
—These factors cause bronchoconstriction, increased microvascular permeability, and a cellular inflammatory response.

4. **Diagnostic tests**

a. **Peak flow:** peak flow values are useful both in assessing severity of asthma attack and in guiding treatment decisions. Serial measurements allow assessment of ED interventions (i.e., is the patient getting better?) These simple noninvasive tests should be performed in all patients who present with asthma (Table 20-7).

b. **CBC** to look for leukocytosis and eosinophilia. *Note:* prior administration of corticosteroids or epinephrine may produce an artificial leukocytosis. A high eosinophil count points to other causes of wheezing, e.g., aspergillosis and Loeffler's pneumonia.

Table 20-7. Average Peak Flow Values in Children

Height (inches)	Peak flow (L/min)
43	145
44	160
46	185
48	215
50	240
52	265
54	295

c. **Chest radiograph** to look for infiltrates and foreign bodies. Findings that may be present in asthma include increased anteroposterior (AP) diameter, flattening of the diaphragms, and scattered atelectasis from mucous plugs. Not required for routine presentations of asthma.

d. **Nasal culture** to look for **RSV**

e. **ECG** to look for right axis deviation (RAD), clockwise rotation, and right bundle branch block (RBBB). Abnormal p-waves and nonspecific ST changes also may be seen. ECG is not diagnostic and is not required in the ED.

5. **Treatment**

a. **Bronchiolitis**

—**ABCs,** including supplemental **oxygen** and **hydration**

—**Ribavirin:** an antiviral agent used in the treatment of RSV and influenza A and B infections in immunocompromised children, including premature infants, and those with bronchopulmonary dysplasia and congenital heart disease. Dose is 6 g in 300 ml of sterile water given 12–18 hours per day as an aerosol for up to 7 days.

b. **Asthma**

(1) **Racemic epinephrine** given over 15 min every 1–4 hours. Dosages, by body weight, are:

—weight $<$10 kg: 2 ml of 1:8 dilution

—weight 10–15 kg: 2 ml of 1:6 dilution

—weight 15–20: 2 ml of 1:4 dilution

—weight $>$ 20 kg: 2 ml of 1:3 dilution

(2) **Albuterol nebulizer** (0.05% solution)

—age $<$ 12 years: 1.25–2.5 mg every 15–30 min as needed

—age $\geq$ 12 years: 2.5–5.0 mg every 15–30 min as needed

(3) **Ipratropium nebulizer** (0.02% solution) every 15–30 minutes, as needed

(4) **Prednisone** 1–2 mg/kg orally for 3–5 days

6. **Disposition**

a. Patients with good hydration, feeding, and oxygenation, and good response to therapy may be discharged home with outpatient follow-up.

b. Patients with poor oxygenation, respiratory fatigue, or poor response to therapy after 1 hour should be admitted to the hospital for further management.

c. Hospital admission is considered for patients with the following conditions or characteristics:
—age < 3 months
—history of prematurity
—congenital heart disease
—bronchopulmonary dysplasia
—cystic fibrosis
—immunosuppression

B. Upper airway obstruction

—The **most common causes** of upper airway obstruction are croup (laryngotracheobronchitis), epiglottitis, bacterial tracheitis, and foreign bodies.

—**Less common causes** of upper airway obstruction include diphtheria, abscess, trauma, and congenital causes.

1. Croup

a. Overview

—**Croup** is the most common type of upper airway obstruction.

—It is a viral infection, characterized by laryngeal, tracheal and epiglottic edema.

—The most common agent associated with croup is **parainfluenza virus,** but RSV and influenza virus also have been implicated.

—Spasmodic croup is sometimes distinguished from viral croup; it is thought to be an allergic reaction, although treatment is the same for both types.

b. Clinical features may include:
—seasonal increase in fall and winter
—worsening at night and early morning
—patient age between 3 months and 3 years
—a preceding upper respiratory illness
—inspiratory or expiratory stridor
—hoarse voice
—"barking seal" cough
—inspiratory or expiratory stridor
—high fever (present in most cases)
—no dysphagia

c. Diagnostic tests

—The diagnosis of croup often is clear from the history and physical examination findings.

(1) CBC to look for leukocytosis (see Table 20-1)
(2) **Lateral view of the soft tissue of the neck** to look for a **"thumb sign,"** or a widened epiglottis or a foreign body
(3) Chest radiograph to look for distal airway trapping secondary to a foreign body
(4) Blood cultures to identify causative organism

d. Treatment

—Airway must be secured—approximately 2% of children with croup require intubation

—For mild croup: **humidified mist**

—For moderate–severe croup: **nebulized racemic epinephrine** (0.5 ml in 3.5 ml normal saline) and IM **dexamethasone** (0.6 mg/kg)

—Acetaminophen or ibuprofen for analgesia and fever reduction

e. **Disposition**

—Patients who have improved with treatment in the ED may be discharged home with outpatient follow-up after a 4-hour observation period, with follow-up in 48 hours.

—Patients with respiratory fatigue, cyanosis, suspicion of epiglottitis, or failure to improve within 4 hours should be admitted to the hospital.

2. **Epiglottitis** (See Chapter 8 VIII for further discussion)

a. **Overview**

—**Epiglottitis** is a bacterial infection of the epiglottis caused by *Haemophilus influenzae*

—It causes **life-threatening airway obstruction.**

—Due to routine immunization against *H. influenzae,* epiglottitis in children has become less common.

—Children of any age may be affected

b. **Clinical features**

(1) **Symptoms** may include:

—no cough

—high fever

—muffled voice

—drooling

—dysphagia

(2) **Physical examination findings** may include:

—**toxic-appearing** patient

—**"cherry red"** epiglottis

—patient who prefers to sit up or lean in "tripod" position

c. **Diagnostic tests**

—Patients suspected of having epiglottitis should not be examined using a tongue blade, because any provocation may result in airway obstruction.

—Diagnostic tests are deferred if epiglottitis is suspected; these patients must go to the operating room (OR) immediately.

—Other diagnostic tests as for croup (see section V B 1 c)

d. **Treatment**

—Airway is secured using direct laryngoscopy under general anesthesia (in the OR)

—Dexamethasone 10 mg IV in a single dose (optional)

—**Antibiotics:** cefuroxime or cefotaxime 50 mg/kg every 8 hours IV, or ceftriaxone 50–75 mg/kg IV every 24 hours

—Humidified air or oxygen

—Acetaminophen or ibuprofen for analgesia and fever reduction

—*H. influenzae* b vaccine in unimmunized children < 5 years old

e. Disposition

—Same as for croup (see section V B 1 e)

3. Bacterial tracheitis

—Bacterial tracheitis is a rare infection of the upper airway, most often caused by *S. aureus*.

—It should be suspected when any patient diagnosed with croup fails to respond to therapy or deteriorates abruptly.

a. Clinical features may include:

—an earlier diagnosis of croup

—high fever (to 40.8° C[105.6°F])

—inspiratory stridor

—no dysphagia

—toxic-appearing patient

—brassy cough

—thick, purulent secretions

b. Diagnostic tests

—Same as for croup (see section V B 1 c)

c. Treatment

(1) Airway is secured

(2) Antibiotics against *S. aureus:*

—Nafcillin or oxacillin 50 mg/kg every 6 hours IV plus cefuroxime or cefotaxime 50 mg/kg IV every 8 hours for 14 days

—For penicillin-allergic patients: clindamycin 3–13 mg/kg every 8 hours IV plus chloramphenicol 3–6 mg/kg every 6 hours IV for 14 days

d. Disposition

—Same as for croup (see section V B 1 e)

4. Foreign body in the respiratory tract

—Inspiration of a foreign body should be considered in any toddler or pre-school-aged child.

—This injury is most common in children younger than 4 years old or older, mentally challenged children.

a. Clinical features may include:

—cough

—hemoptysis

—history of a choking episode

—dyspnea

—inspiratory stridor (if level is extrathoracic)

—expiratory stridor (if level is intrathoracic)

b. Diagnostic tests

—Same as for croup (see section V B 1 c)

c. Treatment

—Consultation with otorhinolaryngologist or pulmonary specialist for removal

d. Disposition

—Same as for croup (see section V B 1 e)

C. Cystic fibrosis

1. Overview

a. Definition

—Cystic fibrosis is an **autosomal recessive** disorder characterized by abnormal mucus production. It results in chronic pulmonary disease and impaired pancreatic, biliary, and intestinal function.

—The gene is carried by one in 25 Caucasians, and almost never occurs in other populations.

—Pulmonary infection with ***Pseudomonas*** spp. is pathognomonic for cystic fibrosis.

—Infants and children with cystic fibrosis suffer from chronic **bronchiolitis,** due to recurrent obstruction of bronchioles with mucus. Bronchiectasis, or permanent bronchial dilatation and pulmonary hypertension, often results.

b. Complications may include:

—pneumothorax

—hemoptysis

—cor pulmonale

—respiratory failure

—rectal prolapse

—intestinal obstruction

2. Clinical features

a. Symptoms may include:

—failure to thrive

—chronic cough

—hemoptysis

—foul-smelling sputum and stool

—meconium ileus

—chronic abdominal pain

b. Physical examination findings may include:

—dyspnea

—tachypnea

—barrel chest

—clubbing

—hilar lymphadenopathy

3. Diagnostic tests

a. Laboratory studies

—CBC to look for leukocytosis (see Table 20-1)

—Chemistry panel to look for metabolic alkalosis, hyponatremia, hypokalemia, and hypochloremia

—ABG if hypoxemia is suspected

—**Sweat chloride test** (quantitative pilocarpine iontophoretic sweat test) to look for Na or Cl level >60 mEq/L to make definitive diagnosis (this test is not done in the ED)

—Gram stain and sputum culture and sensitivity to look for gram-positive *S. aureus* and *Pseudomonas* spp.

b. **Chest radiograph** to look for infiltrates, hyperaeration, cystic bronchiectasis, or pneumothorax

4. **Treatment**

a. ABCs, including supplemental oxygen

b. Antibiotics to cover *S. aureus* and *Pseudomonas* spp.

c. Bronchodilators as needed

d. Maintenance therapy includes:

—**vigorous pulmonary toilet**

—antibiotic therapy (**intermittent inhaled tobramycin**) to combat *S. aureus* and *P. aeruginosa*

—**aerosolized recombinant human DNase** to lyse DNA released from neutrophils in clogged airways, reducing sputum viscosity

5. **Disposition**

—Most patients with exacerbation of cystic fibrosis and all patients with pulmonary complications should be admitted to the hospital.

VI. Gastrointestinal Disorders

A. Pyloric stenosis

1. **Clinical features**

—The mean age at diagnosis is 4 weeks.

—Pyloric stenosis is more common in boys than in girls, by a ratio of 4:1.

a. **Symptoms** may include:

—**projectile, non-bilious vomiting**

—dehydration

—malnourished infant (or infant not gaining weight)

b. **Physical examination findings** include a small olive-shaped mass palpable in the right upper quadrant.

2. **Diagnostic tests**

a. **Laboratory studies**

—**Chemistry panel** to look for hypochloremic, hypokalemic metabolic acidosis

—Other standard admission laboratory tests as needed

b. **Imaging studies**

—**Abdominal radiograph** to look for air-filled stomach with no air distally

—Ultrasonography of abdomen to look for hypertrophied pylorus

—Barium swallow to look for "string sign," of narrow, elongated pyloric channel

3. Treatment

a. Nothing by mouth

b. Nasogastric tube to suction

c. IV hydration

d. Consultation with surgery department

4. Disposition

—Patients are admitted to the surgical service.

B. Intussusception

1. Overview

a. Definition

—Intussusception is the telescoping of the proximal into the distal bowel.

—It is the **most common cause of acute obstruction** in infants.

—The most common site is **ileocecal.**

—It can advance as far as the rectum.

b. Pathophysiology

—Intussusception often begins at the site of an abnormality in the gut, such as an enlarged Peyer's patch, a Meckel's diverticulum, a polyp, or a tumor.

—Intussusception impedes venous return at the site, causing swelling, with resulting poor arterial perfusion and a high risk of perforation.

2. Clinical features

a. Symptoms may include:

—severe, crampy abdominal pain

—vomiting

—currant jelly stools (late finding)

—drawing up of legs or assuming a squatting position

b. Physical examination findings may include:

—palpation of a **sausage-shaped mass** in the right upper or lower quadrant

—guaiac-positive stool

3. Diagnostic tests

a. Laboratory studies

—Admission laboratory studies, as needed: CBC, chemistry panel, PT, APTT, type and screen, urinalysis

b. Imaging studies

(1) Abdominal radiograph to look for air-fluid levels and soft tissue mass at site of intussusception (most often a normal bowel gas pattern is seen in intussusception, however)

(2) Air or **saline enema**

—To look for a **coiled-spring** appearance of the head of the intussusception (this is the diagnostic gold standard)

—Can be therapeutic: the hydrostatic force of an enema will reduce most cases of intussusception

(3) Ultrasonography to look for intestinal mass

4. **Treatment**

   a. **General**

   —Nothing by mouth

   —Nasogastric tube to suction

   —Intravenous hydration

   —Consultation with surgery department

   b. **If perforation is suspected:**

   —Enema not given

   —IV antibiotics to cover both gram-negative and gram-positive organisms: ampicillin 50 mg/kg every 6 hours plus gentamicin 2.5 mg/kg every 8 hours

5. **Disposition**

   —Patients are admitted to the surgical service.

C. Congenital duodenal obstruction

—Children with congenital duodenal obstruction often have multiple congenital anomalies.

—30% have trisomy 21 (Down syndrome).

—20% have congenital heart disease.

1. **Clinical features** may include:

   —**bilious vomiting after feedings**

   —history of passing meconium

2. **Diagnostic tests**

   a. Abdominal radiograph to look for **double bubble** sign. Air is seen in the stomach and duodenum, but little or none is seen beyond the level of the ampulla of Vater

   b. Barium enema to differentiate duodenal atresia from intestinal malrotation

   c. Laboratory studies for admission, as needed: CBC, chemistry panel, PT, APTT, type and screen, urinalysis

3. **Treatment**

   a. Nothing by mouth

   b. Nasogastric tube to suction

   c. Intravenous hydration

   d. Consultation with the surgery department

4. **Disposition**

   —Patients are admitted to the surgical service.

D. Meckel's diverticulum

1. **Overview**

   a. **Definition**

   —Meckel's diverticulum is a congenital anomaly of the small bowel that usually is found 60 to 100 cm proximal to the ileocecal valve.

   —It may contain ectopic gastrointestinal mucosa.

b. **Incidence**

—Most patients are younger than 2 years of age.

c. **Complications** may include:

—intestinal obstruction from **intussusception** or **volvulus** at the site of the diverticulum

—**gastrointestinal hemorrhage** (Table 20-8)

—**perforation** and **diverticulitis,** usually due to ectopic gastric tissue–secreting acid

2. **Clinical features**

—Most patients are asymptomatic

a. **Symptoms** may include:

—hemorrhage of copious bright red blood per rectum

—abdominal pain and tenderness near the umbilicus

—perforation and diverticulitis

—symptoms that mimic those of **appendicitis** (see Chapter 4)

—toxic-appearing child

b. **Physical examination findings** may include:

—normal findings on examination

—guaiac-positive stool

—cellulitis of the umbilicus

3. **Diagnostic tests**

a. **Laboratory studies**

—Admission laboratory studies, as needed: CBC, chemistry panel, PT, APTT, type and screen, urinalysis.

b. **Imaging studies**

—Nuclear scan using technetium TC 99m to look for uptake in the ectopic gastric mucosa. Cimetidine (30 mg/kg IV) administered before the scan improves retention.

—Barium studies are not helpful

4. **Treatment**

a. Nothing by mouth

Table 20-8. Causes of Lower GI Bleeding in Children < 1 year: "MASSIVE" Acronym

Meckel's diverticulum
Anal fissure, milk allergy
Intu**SS**usception
Infectious colitis
Volvulus
Necrotizing **E**nterocolitis

b. IV hydration

c. IV antibiotics to cover both gram-negative and gram-positive organisms, e.g,, ampicillin 50 mg/kg every 6 hours plus gentamicin 2.5 mg/kg every 8 hours

d. Consultation with surgery department

5. Disposition

—Patients are admitted to the surgical service.

E. Volvulus

1. Overview

a. Definition

—Volvulus is the abnormal twisting of intestine, resulting in partial or complete obstruction.

—It is more common in the neonatal period.

b. Causes

—Volvulus most often is due to congenital **malrotation** of the midgut and **meconium ileus,** which is seen in **cystic fibrosis.**

c. Complications may include:

—impaired local perfusion

—gangrene (about 30% of children with volvulus due to malrotation die from gangrene)

—perforation

2. Clinical features

a. Symptoms may include:

—bright red blood per rectum

—intermittent abdominal pain after meals

—**bilious vomiting**

—weight loss

b. Physical examination findings may include:

—abdominal mass or distention

—signs of peritonitis or acute abdomen

3. Diagnostic tests

a. Laboratory studies

—Admission laboratory studies, as needed: CBC, chemistry panel, PT, APTT, type and screen, urinalysis

b. Imaging studies

—Abdominal radiograph to look for **double bubble sign** (similar to duodenal atresia) or **free air**

—**Barium enema** to look for **bird's beak** sign, or sharp tapering of the barium-filled bowel at the site of volvulus

—If volvulus is due to **meconium ileus,** barium enema will show **microcolon** with meconium flecks.

4. Treatment

a. Nothing by mouth

b. Nasogastric tube to suction

c. IV hydration

d. Consultation with surgery department

5. **Disposition**

—Patients are admitted to the surgical service.

F. Hirschsprung's disease (aganglionic megacolon)

1. **Overview**

a. **Definition**

—Hirschsprung's disease is characterized by an absence of ganglion cells from the anus proximally.

—10% of cases involve the distal rectum.

—65% of cases involve the rectum to the sigmoid colon.

—10% of cases involve the rectum to the proximal colon.

—15% of cases extend through the entire colon and involve the small bowel.

b. **Incidence**

—Hirschsprung's disease is more common in boys than in girls.

c. **Complications**

—Untreated patients may progress to enterocolitis and death

2. **Clinical features** may include:

—scant (or no) meconium after birth

—history of chronic constipation since birth

—subsequent intermittent constipation or **foul-smelling diarrhea**

—worsening abdominal distention

—vomiting

—poor feeding

—small-caliber stools

3. **Diagnosis**

a. **Laboratory studies**

—Admission laboratory studies: CBC, chemistry panel, PT, APTT, type and screen, urinalysis as needed

—**Rectal biopsy** to look for lack of ganglion cells in Meissner's plexus (this test is not done in the ED)

b. **Imaging studies**

—Abdominal radiograph to look for dilated loops of bowel

—Barium enema to look for narrow distal bowel and a dilated proximal bowel

4. **Treatment**

a. Saline enemas

b. Stool softeners

c. Manual disimpaction as needed

d. Definitive surgical repair when patient weighs at least 9 kg (infants may require a preliminary colostomy)

5. Disposition

—Patients are admitted to the surgical service.

G. Necrotizing enterocolitis

1. Overview

a. Definition

—Necrotizing enterocolitis (NEC) is necrosis of the neonatal intestinal mucosa with risk of progression to full-thickness perforation.

—Most patients who develop NEC are inpatients in the NICU or nursery, but some present as outpatients.

b. Causes

—NEC is associated with the overgrowth of *Clostridium difficile* and other bacteria in susceptible patients.

c. Incidence

—80% of cases are in premature infants.

—Full-term babies with NEC usually present in the first week of life.

d. Complications

—Perforation occurs in 20% of cases.

2. Clinical features may include:

—abdominal distention

—blood in stools

—lethargy

—apneic episodes

—increasing amounts of residual tube feeds

—bilious vomiting

3. Diagnostic tests

a. Laboratory studies

—Blood cultures to identify causative organism

—Admission laboratory studies as needed: CBC, chemistry panel, PT, APTT, type and screen, urinalysis

b. Imaging studies

—Abdominal radiograph to look for bowel distention (early), pneumatosis (late), and peritoneal free air (late)

4. Treatment

a. Nothing by mouth

b. Nasogastric tube to suction

c. IV hydration

d. Hyperalimentation

e. Supplemental oxygen as needed

f. Antibiotics: broad-spectrum, including coverage for *C. difficile* (e.g., metronidazole, vancomycin, or bacitracin)

g. Consultation with surgery department

5. Disposition

—Patients are admitted to the neonatal intensive care unit.

VII. Viral Exanthems and Infections

A. Measles

1. Clinical features

a. Symptoms may include:

—fever

—malaise

—cough

b. Physical examination findings may include:

—conjunctivitis

—coryza

—day 3: **Koplik's spots** on buccal mucosa

—day 5: erythematous macular rash that appears on face and neck, spreads to trunk. The rash coalesces, turns coppery brown, and may desquamate (Table 20-9).

2. Complications include:

—laryngotracheitis

—bronchitis or pneumonia

—otitis media

—myocarditis

—pericarditis

—appendicitis

—subacute sclerosing panencephalitis: may occur many years following an infection; mortality is 15%

3. Diagnostic tests

—Diagnosis is best made by recognition of the characteristic rash.

—Measles can be distinguished from rubella by the toxic appearance and high spiking fever of children with measles.

4. Treatment

—Measles runs a self-limited course. Treatment is supportive.

5. Disposition

a. Children with complications of measles should be admitted to the hospital.

b. All other children may be discharged home with outpatient follow-up in 1 week.

B. Rubella

1. Overview

a. Definition

—Rubella is a TORCH (Table 20-10) virus (TORCH = **t**oxoplasmosis, **o**ther, **r**ubella, **c**ytomegalovirus, **h**erpesvirus)

Table 20-9. Causes of Erythematous Maculopapular rash

Disease	Agent	Clinical Features
Chicken pox	Varicella zoster virus	Erythematous vesicles on face and trunk, progressing to crusted lesions
Drug rash	Variable	Generalized rash commonly associated with ampicillin use in infectious mononucleosis
Erythema infectiosum	Parvovirus B19	"Slapped cheek" rash followed by maculopapular rash on trunk and extremities. May look lacey.
Herpangina	Cocksackievirus A4	Bright red macules on face, with vesicle formation, ulcerative lesions on palate and mouth
Infectious mononucleosis	Epstein-Barr virus	Pink maculopapular rash on trunk and limbs, petechial hemorrhages on palate, cervical lymphadenopathy
Kawasaki disease (mucocutaneous lymph node syndrome)	Agent unknown	High fever lasting 5 or more days, conjunctivitis, oral changes (strawberry tongue), extremity changes, rash
Measles	Paramyxovirus	High spiking fever, cough, conjunctivitis, coryza followed by rash on face and neck progressing downward
Rocky Mountain spotted fever	*Rickettsia rickettsii*	Maculopapular to hemorrhagic lesions spreading from wrists and hands to trunk
Roseola	Herpes-6 virus	Young child with high fever; pink maculopapular rash appears on trunk after fever drops in 2–4 days
Rubella	Togavirus	Low-grade fever, cough, conjunctivitis, rash on face and neck
Scarlet fever	*Streptococcus pyogenes*	Generalized punctate erythema (gooseteeth or sandpaper texture) on trunk and limbs, circumoral pallor, strawberry tongue
Stevens-Johnson syndrome	Sulfa drugs, penicillins, cefaclor, phenytoin	Erythema multiforme rash
Toxic shock syndrome	*Staphylococcus aureus*	High fever, headache, vomiting and diarrhea, rash, hypotensive shock

Table 20-10. Findings in Newborns Congenitally Infected With a TORCH Agent

Agent	Findings
Toxoplasma	Hydrocephalus, calcifications, chorioretinitis, elevated CSF protein
Other (cocksackievirus, varicella, syphilis, others)	Cocksackievirus: CNS findings Syphilis: mucocutaneous lesions (snuffles), osteochondritis, periostitis Varicella: microcephaly, cutaneous scars, limb or digit abnormalities
Rubella	Microcephaly, cataracts, cloudy cornea, congenital heart disease, "blueberry muffin" skin, deafness
Cytomegalovirus	Microcephaly, inguinal hernias, thrombocytopenia, petechiae, pneumonitis
Herpesvirus	Cutaneous vesicles, fever, lethargy, hepatosplenomegaly, encephalitis, keratoconjunctivitis

CNS = central nervous system; *CSF* = cerebrospinal fluid; *TORCH* = **T**oxoplasma, **O**ther, **R**ubella, **C**ytomegalovirus, **H**erpesvirus.

b. **Epidemiology**

—Rubella occurs in epidemics every 6–9 years in unimmunized children or adolescents in whom immunity may have faded.

—Recent outbreaks have occurred in college students.

c. **Complications** may include:

—encephalitis

—thrombocytopenia

—arthritis or arthralgias

—congenital anomalies (deafness, eye defects, mental retardation, and cardiac malformations) in children born to mothers who contracted rubella during pregnancy

2. **Clinical features**

a. **Symptoms** may include:

—prodrome of fever, malaise, and cough

—conjunctivitis

b. **Physical examination findings** may include:

—erythematous maculopapular rash appearing on the face and spreading downward

—low-grade fever

—tender posterior cervical lymphadenopathy

3. **Diagnostic tests**

—No specific diagnostic tests are necessary.

—**CBC** may be done to look for **leukopenia** and thrombocytopenia

—Any adolescent or adult woman with suspected or known pregnancy should have rubella confirmed by titer.

4. Treatment

—Treatment is supportive.

5. Disposition

a. Patients with suspected complications of rubella should be admitted to the hospital.

b. All other patients can be discharged home with outpatient follow-up.

c. Care should be taken that patient's contacts do not include unimmunized pregnant women.

C. Roseola (exanthem subitum)

—Roseola is caused by herpesvirus-6.

—It usually is seen in children younger than 2 years old.

1. Clinical features

a. Symptoms may include:

—rapid onset of high fever followed by rash

—febrile seizure

b. Physical examination findings may include:

—generalized nonpruritic erythematous macular rash that appears upon defervescence (usually on day 2–3). This rash is most prominent on buttocks, back, and trunk.

—a child who is otherwise well: no pharyngitis, conjunctivitis, or hepatomegaly

2. Diagnostic tests

—Diagnosis is made by the characteristic appearance of the rash following defervescence. It sometimes is misdiagnosed as a drug rash when antibiotics are given to combat the fever-producing infection.

—No specific diagnostic tests are necessary.

3. Treatment

—Treatment is supportive.

4. Disposition

—Patients can be discharged home with outpatient follow-up.

D. Kawasaki disease (mucocutaneous lymph node syndrome)

1. Overview

a. Definition

—Kawasaki disease causes a vasculitis of small and medium-sized arteries, most notably the coronary arteries.

b. Causes

—The exact etiological agent is unknown.

—It is associated with HLA B5 in Caucasians, and HLA BW22 J2 in Asians.

c. Complications. Approximately 1%-2% of children with Kawasaki disease die from cardiac complications. Possible complications include:

—**coronary aneurysm**
—myocardial infarction
—pericarditis
—hydrops of gallbladder
—hemolytic-uremic syndrome
—abdominal aortic aneurysm
—cerebrovascular accident
—renal or peripheral artery aneurysm

2. **Clinical features**
   a. **Acute phase**
      —**fever** for 5 or more days
      —bilateral conjunctivitis
      —oropharyngeal edema
      —dry, cracked lips
      —**strawberry tongue**
      —erythematous, edematous hands or feet with or without desquamation
      —erythematous maculopapular rash
      —cervical lymphadenopathy
      —abdominal pain and vomiting secondary to biliary obstruction
   b. **Subacute phase**
      —irritability
      —arthritis
      —arthralgias
      —myocarditis
      —more prominent desquamation
   c. **Convalescent phase**
      —gradual resolution of symptoms
3. **Diagnostic tests**
   a. Diagnosis is made when the child has a high fever and four of the remaining five conditions (bilateral conjunctivitis, oral changes, extremity changes, rash, and cervical lymphadenopathy) in the absence of another diagnosis.
   b. **Laboratory tests** that may be useful include:
      —erythrocyte sedimentation rate (ESR) to look for elevation
      —CBC to look for leukocytosis and thrombocytosis
      —serum immunoglobulin levels to look for elevated IgE level (this test is not done in the ED)
      —chemistry panel to look for elevated bilirubin
      —blood and throat cultures to identify causative organisms
   c. **Imaging studies**
      —ECG to look for arrhythmias
      —Chest radiograph to look for cardiomegaly and infiltrates
      —Echocardiogram to look for valvular abnormalities and cardiomyopathy

4. Treatment

a. Aspirin: 20–30 mg/kg 3 times a day. (Aspirin is thought to be associated with Reye syndrome [see section VII F] and normally is not given to children, but in this case the benefit outweighs the risk.)

b. IV IgG (inpatient)

5. Disposition

a. Children presenting in the acute phase should be admitted to the hospital for IV IgG.

b. Children presenting in the subacute or convalescent phase should be evaluated for development of cardiac complications, but may be discharged home with outpatient follow-up biweekly.

E. Erythema infectiosum (fifth disease)

1. Overview

a. Causes

— Erythema infectiosum (fifth disease) is caused by parvovirus B19.

b. Complications

(1) Parvovirus B19 infection in pregnant women can cause fetal death.

(2) Transient aplastic crisis (TAC) in patients with hereditary hemolytic anemias or immunodeficiency, including:

—sickle cell disease

—hereditary spherocytosis

—alpha-thalassemia

—autoimmune hemolytic anemia

—G6PD deficiency

—acute lymphocytic anemia

—congenital immunodeficiency

—HIV infection

2. Clinical features may include:

—characteristic **"slapped cheek"** rash that progresses to erythematous maculopapular rash on trunk and extremities.

—rash that appears lace-like after a few days

—arthralgias

—arthritis (most often in hands, wrists, and knees)

—lymphadenopathy

3. Diagnostic tests

—No specific diagnostic tests are necessary, but diagnosis may be confirmed by IgM-antibody assay.

4. Treatment

—Treatment is supportive.

—Patients who develop TAC may require blood transfusion.

5. Disposition

—Most patients can be discharged home with outpatient follow-up.

F. Reye syndrome

1. Overview

a. Definition

—Reye syndrome is a rare disease seen in children with a history of a febrile illness (especially varicella or influenza A) and concurrent **aspirin** use.

b. Prognosis

—Most children do not progress to stages IV and V and recover without sequelae.

—Cerebral edema and high ammonia levels are associated with a poor prognosis.

c. Complications may include:

—permanent neurologic deficit

—cerebral edema

—seizures

—respiratory failure

2. Clinical features

a. Symptoms and **physical examination findings** are characterized by a progressive deterioration in mental status and neurologic function.

b. This deterioration may be grouped into 5 clinical stages:

—Stage I: sleepiness, lethargy, vomiting

—Stage II: altered mental status (confusion, combativeness, delirium), hyperreflexia, hyperpnea

—Stage III: obtundation, seizures, decorticate rigidity, intact pupillary reflex, loss of oculocephalic reflex

—Stage IV: coma, decerebrate posturing, fixed pupils

—Stage V: coma, flaccid paralysis, isoelectric EEG, respiratory arrest

3. Diagnostic tests

a. LFTs to look for elevations of AST and ALT

b. Chemistry panel to look for hypoglycemia and metabolic acidosis

c. ABG to look for respiratory alkalosis

d. PT to look for prolongation

e. Lumbar puncture: will reveal increased intracranial pressure without pleocytosis

f. Ammonia level to look for elevation

4. Treatment

a. Treatment is supportive.

b. Treatment may include:

—ABCs, with mechanical ventilation as needed

—10–15% glucose IV to prevent hypoglycemia

—vitamin K for prolonged PT

—environment with minimal stimulation

—dialysis for very high ammonia levels

—treatment of increased intracranial pressure

5. Disposition

—Patients require admission to the intensive care unit.

VIII. Orthopaedic Disorders

A. Legg-Calvé-Perthes disease

—Legg-Calvé-Perthes disease is an idiopathic aseptic necrosis of the femoral capital epiphysis, which becomes avascular, is resorbed, and is revascularized.

—It occurs most commonly between the ages of 4 and 10 years.

—The condition **usually** is **unilateral.**

—It is more common in males.

1. Clinical presentation

a. Symptoms may include:

—pain in the hip joint

—groin pain

—knee pain

—gradual onset

—slow progression

b. Physical examination findings may include:

—disturbance of gait

—limping

—decreased range of motion, especially abduction and inward rotation

—atrophy of thigh muscles

2. Diagnostic tests

—Radiographs to look for flattening and, later, fragmentation of the femoral head, which contains areas of lucency and sclerosis.

3. Treatment

a. Containment of the femoral head in the acetabulum with mobile traction and slings

b. Prolonged bed rest

c. Abduction plaster casts and splints

d. Subtrochanteric osteotomy with internal fixation

4. Disposition

—Patients are managed according to consultation with the orthopaedics department.

B. Slipped capital femoral epiphysis

—Slipped capital femoral epiphysis is the abrupt or gradual displacement of the proximal femoral epiphysis on the femoral neck.

—It often is seen in overweight teenagers, usually boys.

—Onset usually is insidious.

—It commonly occurs during a growth spurt.

—Early diagnosis is vital, because treatment becomes more difficult in the more advanced stages.

—Associated endocrinopathy may be present.

1. **Clinical presentation**
   a. **Symptoms** may include:
      —hip stiffness that improves with rest
      —**limping**
      —hip pain that radiates down the anteromedial thigh to the knee
      —apparent loss of height
   b. **Physical examination findings** may include:
      — external rotation on flexion of the affected hip
      —limited flexion, abduction, and internal rotation
      —affected limb 1–3 cm shorter than the contralateral one
2. **Diagnostic tests**
   —Radiographs of the affected hip to look for widening of the epiphyseal plate or displacement of the femoral head:
   a. AP view to look for posterior displacement
   b. Lateral view to look for medial displacement
3. **Treatment**
   a. Cessation of weight bearing
   b. Corrective surgery
4. **Disposition**
   —Patients can be discharged home but need either orthopaedic consultation in the ED or prompt outpatient referral to confirm the diagnosis and evaluate the need for corrective surgery.

C. Ewing sarcoma

—Ewing sarcoma is an undifferentiated sarcoma of uncertain origin that arises primarily in the long bones

—It is seen primarily in adolescents.

—It is more common in males.

—It is rare in African-Americans.

1. **Clinical presentation** may include:
   —pain
   —fever
   —localized swelling
2. **Diagnostic tests**
   a. CBC to look for leukocytosis

b. ESR to look for elevation

c. **Radiographs** to look for destructive lesion, periosteal elevation, and soft tissue mass

3. **Treatment**

a. Surgery

b. Chemotherapy

c. Consultation with oncology and orthopaedic services

4. **Disposition**

—Patients are managed per recommendations of consultation with oncology and orthopaedics.

D. Osteogenic sarcoma

1. **Overview**

a. **Definition**

—Osteogenic sarcoma is a malignant tumor of the bone-producing mesenchyme.

—It is the most common primary malignant bone tumor seen in pediatric patients.

—Half of all cases occur in proximity to the knee joint.

b. **Incidence**

—It is seen mainly in adolescents.

—It is twice as common in males.

c. **Complications**

—Metastases are primarily to the lungs.

2. **Clinical presentation** may include:

—pain

—deformity of extremity

—swelling

3. **Diagnostic tests**

a. Radiographs of the extremity to look for:

—Codman's triangle (a cuff of periosteal new bone formation at the margin of the soft tissue mass)

—characteristic radial "sunburst" as the tumor breaks through the cortex and new bone spicules are produced

b. Chest radiograph to look for metastases

c. MRI to look for soft tissue involvement

4. **Treatment**

a. Surgery: limb may or may not be salvaged

b. Chemotherapy

c. Consultation with oncology and orthopaedics

5. **Disposition**

—Patients are managed according to consult recommendation.

E. Osgood-Schlatter disease

1. Overview

a. Definition

—Osgood-Schlatter disease is believed to result from trauma from excessive traction by the patella tendon on its immature epiphyseal insertion.

—It is characterized by painful enlargement of the tibial tubercle.

—It often is **bilateral**.

b. Epidemiology

—It is related to vigorous physical activity (e.g., running, jumping).

—It occurs between the ages of 10 and 15 years.

—It is more common in boys.

2. Clinical presentation may include:

—pain (more common with prolonged knee flexion)

—swelling

—tenderness over the tibial tubercle at the patellar tendon insertion

—stable patellofemoral joint

3. Diagnostic tests

—Lateral radiographs of the knee to look for fragmentation of the tibial tubercle and possible ossicles in the tendon

4. Treatment

—Resolution usually is spontaneous after a course of weeks or months.

a. RICE
b. Immobilization with casting
c. Crutches for ambulation, with progression from non-weight-bearing to gradual weight-bearing
d. NSAIDs for analgesia (see Table 11-1 in Chapter 11)
e. Avoidance of excessive sport and exercise
f. Surgical removal of loose bodies considered if pain persists

5. Disposition

—Patients can be discharged home with referral to an orthopaedist or sports medicine specialist.

IX. Psychosocial Emergencies of Children

A. Child maltreatment

—The term **child maltreatment** encompasses physical abuse and nonaccidental trauma, emotional abuse, sexual abuse, and neglect.

—Most states require reporting of child maltreatment by health care professionals.

—Child maltreatment most often occurs when the physical, financial, or emotional resources of the child's caretakers are stretched.

1. **Clinical features**
   a. Characteristics of the **patient** or **victim** often include:
      —age < 4 years
      —premature birth
      —developmental delay (Table 20-11)
      —twin or member of other multiple gestation
      —signs of low self-esteem, poor school performance, suicidal ideation, or antisocial personality traits (in older children)
   b. Characteristics of the **abuser** may include:
      —abuse as a child
      —low self-esteem
      —financial instability
      —emotional instability
      —authoritarian personality
   c. **History** and **physical examination findings** may include:
      —young child who was alone at the time of injury
      —mechanism of injury that is inconsistent with physical findings or abilities of the child
      —caretaker delay in seeking care for patient
      —many injuries in different stages of healing
      —immunization record that is grossly incomplete for age (Table 20-12)
2. **Diagnostic tests**
   a. The health care professional is **not required to diagnose** child maltreatment; a reasonable suspicion is all that is needed to mobilize social work resources and report to state authorities.

Table 20-11. Developmental Milestones

Age	Motor skills	Language/social skills
1 mo	Raises head	Responsive smile, regards face
2–4 mo	Rolls over Grasps rattle	Spontaneous and social smile, coos Laughs
6 mo	Sits without support Passes cube hand to hand	Imitates speech sounds Resists toy pull
12 mo	Stands alone well Neat finger-thumb grasp	Drinks from cup Says "Dada" or "Mama"
18 mo	Walks up steps Scribbles	Combines words Uses spoon
2 y	Jumps in place Draws vertical line	Uses plurals Plays interactive games, 2-word sentences
4 y	Hops on one foot Draws a human figure	Recognizes colors Dresses without supervision
6 y	Walks backward	Defines words

Table 20-12. Recommended Childhood Immunization Schedule

Vaccine	Birth	2 mo	4 mo	6 mo	12–15 mo	4–6 y	11–12 y
MMR					1st	2nd	
Hepatitis B	1st	2nd		3rd			
DTaP		1st	2nd	3rd	4th		
Td							1st
Hib		1st	2nd	3rd	4th		
Varicella					1st		2nd
Polio		1st IPV	2nd IPV	3rd OPV	4th OPV		

DTaP = diphtheria-tetanus-pertussis; *Hib* = *Haemophilus* influenzae, type b; *IPV* = inactivated polio vaccine; *MMR* = measles-mumps-rubella; *OPV* = oral polio vaccine; *Td* = tetanus.

b. Depending on the nature of maltreatment or injury, the following studies may be helpful:

—radiographic studies to look for fractures in different stages of healing

—CBC to look for infection

—PT, APTT, and bleeding time to look for bleeding diathesis

—oral, genital, and rectal cultures for *Chlamydia* species and *Neisseria gonorrhoeae*

—rape kit if sexual abuse is suspected

3. Treatment

a. Treatment of any acute injuries with splints, casts, wound care as needed

b. Treatment of any infections or electrolyte abnormalities

c. Consultation with social worker

d. Consultation with psychiatrist

4. Disposition

—Patients are admitted to the hospital.

B. Sudden infant death syndrome (SIDS)

1. Overview

—In sudden infant death syndrome (SIDS) a child aged 1 month to 1 year is found dead in his or her crib, or has a "near miss" episode.

—The peak age is 2–4 months.

—SIDS occurs most commonly in the fall and winter months.

2. Clinical features may include:

—a history of a recent upper respiratory infection

—sleeping in the prone position: associated with a higher risk of SIDS

—passive smoke inhalation and sleeping in the parents' bed: also have been associated with a higher risk of SIDS

3. Diagnostic tests

—SIDS is a diagnosis of exclusion, properly made when a postmortem examination of an infant shows no clear cause of death.

—A careful history and autopsy lead to a diagnosis in many cases initially suspected to be SIDS.

—Infants who have a near miss should be examined for signs of physical abuse such as **shaken baby syndrome,** as well as disorders such as seizure, sepsis, and congenital abnormalities.

4. **Treatment**

—A child who arrives or is pronounced dead in the ED places difficult demands on both parents and providers.

—Parents should be allowed to see and hold the child.

—Grief counselors and clergy should be made available.

—The case must be reported to the medical examiner.

5. **Disposition**

   a. Children who have had a near-miss episodes of SIDS should be hospitalized for work-up.
   b. **Apnea monitor** and alarm may be given to selected patients for outpatient use, although the effectiveness of this method is not clear.
   c. Children should be placed on their backs (supine) to sleep.

Review Test

Questions 1 and 2

A physician in a community hospital is called to the nursery to evaluate a 3-day-old premature infant boy who weighed 1200 g at birth. The nurse practitioner believes that the infant has had a seizure. When examined, the patient is found to be afebrile, lethargic, and jaundiced. Hematocrit is 31, blood type is O+, and serum bilirubin is 18.6.

1. Which of the following management options is most appropriate?

(A) Observation
(B) Complete sepsis work-up
(C) Repeat bilirubin
(D) Phototherapy
(E) Exchange transfusion

2. Which of the following is most likely to provide the answer to the cause of the abnormality in this infant?

(A) G6PD assay
(B) History of seizures in the mother
(C) Blood type of the mother
(D) Blood cultures
(E) White blood cell count (WBC)

Questions 3 and 4

A 15-month-old girl is brought in by her mother because of "convulsions." The mother describes recent cough and nasal discharge in the child, but no other symptoms. The child has no history of prematurity or developmental delay. She is not jaundiced. The child's father developed epilepsy as an adult, and the mother wonders if it is contagious. Physical examination shows a fearful child who cries when examined, temperature of 38.6°C (101.5°F), and occasional wheezes on auscultation of chest. Urinalysis, complete blood cell count (CBC), and chest film are normal.

3. Which of the following tests are required to make the diagnosis?

(A) Blood cultures, lumbar puncture
(B) Lumbar puncture, electroencephalogram (EEG)
(C) EEG, brain auditory evoked response (BAER)
(D) Blood cultures, serum bilirubin
(E) Serum bilirubin, BAER

4. The mother wants to know if the child will have more seizures. Which of the following responses is correct?

(A) Probably not; only 3%–4% of children will have these seizures
(B) Maybe; about 10% of children have recurrent seizures after a febrile seizure
(C) Probably; more than 50% of children like her will have recurrent seizures
(D) Not sure; the child needs evaluation by a pediatric neurologist
(E) Not sure; it depends what kind of seizures the patient's father has.

Questions 5 and 6

A 6-month-old infant is brought to the emergency department for a "bad cold." The father says the child has had a runny nose and cough, and hasn't been feeding well for 4 days. On examination, the child appears well and has no stridor, but has fine crackles in both lung fields. Respiratory rate is 56. Oxygen saturation is 95%.

5. Which of the following diagnoses is most likely to be correct?

(A) Croup
(B) Bronchiolitis
(C) Congestive heart failure
(D) Erythema infectiosum
(E) Congenital syphilis

6. The father says the infant was 8 weeks premature and had some kind of lung trouble. Which of the following management strategies is most appropriate for this child?

(A) Outpatient supportive care
(B) Outpatient apnea monitoring
(C) Admission for administration of ribavirin
(D) Admission for cardiac work-up
(E) Admission for contact isolation

7. A 6-year-old child is brought in by ambulance for difficulty breathing. The child is sitting forward, drooling, and can only speak single words in a muffled voice before gasping for breath. A history of admission for asthma is elicited. Physical examination reveals fever to 103.1°F, respiratory rate 48, oxygen saturation 91%, and inspiratory stridor, but otherwise good breath sounds and no wheezes, rales, or rhonchi. After oxygen is administered, which of the following is the appropriate next step?

(A) Administration of mist
(B) Administration of nebulized racemic epinephrine
(C) Administration of intramuscular dexamethasone
(D) Lateral radiograph of the neck
(E) Laryngoscopy and intubation in operating room

Questions 8 and 9

A 3-month-old infant presents to the emergency department with shortness of breath. On physical examination, she is found to have generalized edema, crackles on auscultation of the lungs, and hepatomegaly.

8. Which of the following congenital cardiac anomalies is most likely to account for this presentation?

(A) Ventriculoseptal defect
(B) Aortic stenosis
(C) Tricuspid atresia
(D) Transposition of the great arteries
(E) Total anomalous pulmonary venous connection

9. Which of the following complications of this infant's abnormality is irreversible?

(A) Pulmonary edema
(B) Peripheral edema
(C) Failure to thrive
(D) Pulmonary hypertension
(E) Left to right shunt

10. Which of the following is true of slipped capital femoral epiphysis?

(A) Usually seen in young children
(B) Seen in girls more often than boys
(C) Onset is usually abrupt
(D) Can occur during a growth spurt
(E) Affected leg is internally rotated

Directions: The response options for items 11–15 are the same. You will be required to select one answer for each item in the set.

Questions 11–15. Match each clinical disorder with the appropriate diagnostic test.

(A) Barium enema
(B) Ultrasonography
(C) Plain film of abdomen
(D) Technetium Tc 99m scan
(E) Rectal biopsy

11. Pyloric stenosis

12. Hirschsprung's disease

13. Meckel's diverticulum

14. Intussusception

15. Necrotizing enterocolitis

Answers and Explanations

1-E. This infant requires exchange transfusion, because he has hyperbilirubinemia in the pathologic range, and has demonstrated neurologic complications. Although full-term neonates can tolerate bilirubin levels up to 25 μg/dl, premature neonates can develop kernicterus at levels of 10 μg/dL and above, depending on weight. Repeat bilirubin and phototherapy would be appropriate management options only if the bilirubin were < 10 μg/dL. A sepsis work-up may be indicated further down the line, but at this time the most appropriate management consists of treating the hyperbilirubinemia to prevent neurological complications.

2-C. Determining the blood type of the infant's mother may explain the abnormality. ABO and Rh incompatibility are major causes of hyperbilirubinemia in the neonate. A glucose-6-phosphate dehydrogenase (G6PD) assay will not reveal any potential cause of hyperbilirubinemia. Although sepsis is an important cause of hyperbilirubinemia, it is less common, so blood cultures and white blood cell count would not be the first choices.

3-A. This child most likely had a febrile seizure. Because a first-time febrile seizure is a diagnosis of exclusion, other causes of seizure must be ruled out, including sepsis and meningitis. Blood cultures and lumbar puncture will reveal or rule out sepsis and meningitis. Brain auditory evoked response is a test used to detect kernicterus in infants. Hyperbilirubinemia also can cause seizures, but patients with bilirubin levels high enough to cause them usually appear jaundiced.

4-C. Although only 3%–4% of all children will have a febrile seizure, of those who have a first seizure, about half go on to have a second seizure. Of those children who do have a febrile seizure and who have a parent with epilepsy, about 10% go on to have epilepsy.

5-B, 6-C. This child most likely has bronchiolitis. Although the distinction between bronchiolitis and asthma is not always clear, a first episode of wheezing in a child under 2 years of age with a preceding upper respiratory infection is characteristic of bronchiolitis. Infants at high risk for morbidity and mortality from bronchiolitis, including those with a history of prematurity, should be admitted for administration of ribavirin.

7-E. This child has epiglottitis. Characteristic features include forward-leaning position, drooling, muffled voice, high fever, and inspiratory stridor. Epiglottitis is a life-threatening inflammation of the epiglottis. Any perturbation of the child can cause airway compromise. These patients should be intubated in the most controlled setting by the most experienced physician available.

8-A, 9-D. This infant has congestive heart failure, caused by congenital heart disease featuring a left-to-right shunt. Ventriculoseptal defect (VSD) and total anomalous pulmonary venous connection are both left-to-right shunts, but VSD is by far the more common. Pulmonary hypertension, caused by abnormally high pulmonary flow, is irreversible.

10-D. Slipped capital femoral epiphysis is the displacement of the proximal femoral epiphysis on the femoral neck. It can occur during a growth spurt. Onset usually is insidious, not abrupt. The condition usually is seen in overweight male teenagers. The affected leg is externally, not internally, rotated when the hip is flexed. Internal rotation is actually limited. The affected limb may be shorter than the contralateral one.

11-B, 12-E, 13-D, 14-A, 15-C. Pyloric stenosis is best diagnosed by ultrasonography, which will show a hypertrophied pylorus. Barium enema is used for both diagnosis and treatment of intussusception; the head of the intussusception will have a "coiled-spring" appearance. Air insufflation will also often reduce intussusception. A technetium Tc 99m study is useful in cases of Meckel's diverticulum, because abnormal ectopic gastric mucosa in the diverticulum will show uptake of technetium. Rectal biopsy will show a lack of ganglion cells in the Meissner's plexus in patients with Hirschsprung's disease. Pneumatosis cystoides intestinalis, or gas pockets in the intestinal wall, are seen on plain film of the abdomen in patients with necrotizing enterocolitis. Both volvulus and congenital duodenal obstruction may show a double bubble sign on plain film of the abdomen.

Comprehensive Examination

1. Which of the following is a feature of ulcerative colitis?

(A) It is seen more often in men than women.
(B) It is limited to the colon.
(C) Fistulas and strictures are common.
(D) Endoscopy reveals a cobblestone pattern.
(E) Endoscopy reveals skip lesions.

2. Which of the following ophthalmic drugs is a mydriatic?

(A) Phenylephrine
(B) Cyclopentolate
(C) Homatropine
(D) Scopolamine
(E) Polyvinyl alcohol

3. A 40-year-old man comes to the emergency department for evaluation of a fractured tooth. Examination of the tooth reveals a pinkish tinge at the fracture site. Which of the following statements regarding this situation is correct?

(A) The patient has an Ellis II fracture.
(B) The pinkish tinge is exposed dentin.
(C) Calcium hydroxide should be used on the fracture site.
(D) Sharp tooth edges should be filed down.
(E) Dental consult should be obtained emergently.

4. What endotracheal tube sizes is recommended for a 6-year-old child?

(A) 4.0 mm
(B) 4.5 mm
(C) 5.0 mm
(D) 5.5 mm
(E) 6.0 mm

5. In which of the following cases would prostaglandin therapy be appropriate?

(A) Infant with coarctation of the aorta suspected on the basis of pulse differential
(B) Infant with tetralogy of Fallot suspected on the basis of hypercyanotic episode
(C) Infant with patent ductus arteriosus confirmed by echocardiography
(D) Neonate with aortic stenosis confirmed by echocardiography
(E) Neonate with truncus arteriosus confirmed by echocardiography

6. A 22-year-old woman comes in with slurred speech and ataxic gait. She reports that she has not been drinking ethyl alcohol. Her blood work reveals an elevated anion gap and osmolar gap. Urine microscopic examination shows calcium oxalate stones. Which of the following substances has the patient most likely ingested?

(A) Isopropyl alcohol
(B) Ethylene glycol
(C) Methyl alcohol
(D) Oil of wintergreen
(E) Ethyl alcohol

7. After preparation of equipment, what is the next step in rapid sequence intubation?

(A) Preoxygenation
(B) Sedation
(C) Paralysis
(D) Analgesia
(E) Intracranial pressure control

8. A 20-year-old man with sickle cell disease presents with abdominal pain. He is not sure whether this is the abdominal crisis that he experiences regularly because of his sickle cell disease. Which of the following findings would indicate that the pain was of a different etiology than sickle cell disease?

(A) A white blood cell count (WBC) of 15,000 with three bands on differential
(B) A hemoglobin of 10 with a reticulocyte count of 8%
(C) Streaking of the peri-appendiceal fat on CT
(D) Poorly localized abdominal pain
(E) Elevated indirect bilirubin

9. Which of the following findings is associated with adrenal insufficiency?

(A) Hypertension
(B) Pale skin
(C) Bradycardia
(D) Alopecia
(E) Increased hair growth

10. Which of the following conditions can present with hypercalcemia?

(A) Hypoparathyroidism
(B) Hypomagnesemia
(C) Pancreatitis
(D) Multiple transfusions
(E) Chronic lithium use

11. What gas detector is used to check for proper endotracheal tube placement?

(A) Carbon dioxide
(B) Carbon monoxide
(C) Oxygen
(D) Nitrogen
(E) Nitric oxide

12. Which of the following statements regarding subarachnoid hemorrhage (SAH) is correct?

(A) The most common cause of SAH is blood dyscrasia.
(B) CT is 100% sensitive for finding SAH.
(C) Protein C deficiency is considered a risk factor for SAH.
(D) Class I SAH presents with coma and abnormal posturing.
(E) The cerebrospinal fluid (CSF) supernatant may be xanthochromic in SAH.

13. Which of the following is the most common site for entrapment of intraocular foreign bodies?

(A) Orbit
(B) Lens
(C) Anterior segment
(D) Posterior segment
(E) Cornea

14. Which of the following statements regarding anorexia nervosa is correct?

(A) This disorder begins in the fourth decade of life.
(B) It is seen equally in men and women.
(C) There may be a history of laxative abuse.
(D) The treatment of choice is benzodiazepines.
(E) Patients are usually of normal or above normal weight

15. A 30-year-old woman who has been stabbed in the left chest and presents to the emergency department with a blood pressure of 60/palpable. Her neck veins are distended, but breath sounds are equal on both sides. The patient receives 2 liters of Ringer's lactate and one unit of O-negative blood, but the cardiac rhythm becomes bradycardic and her pulse is no longer palpable. Which of the following constitutes the best management of this patient at this time?

(A) External chest compression
(B) Placement of subclavian central line
(C) Administration of atropine
(D) Left thoracotomy
(E) Chest radiograph

16. A rapid sequence intubation is needed on a woman who weighs 50 kilograms. Which of the following doses of fentanyl is indicated?

(A) 100 μg
(B) 150 μg
(C) 200 μg
(D) 250 μg
(E) 300 μg

17. Which of the following medications, when taken in a toxic dose, can lead to noncardiogenic pulmonary edema?

(A) Aspirin
(B) Acetaminophen
(C) Ampicillin
(D) Nifedipine
(E) Diazepam

18. Which of the following antibiotic combinations is the first-line treatment of Ludwig's angina?

(A) Gentamicin and metronidazole
(B) Penicillin and metronidazole
(C) Penicillin and cefazolin
(D) Gentamicin and cefazolin
(E) Gentamicin and penicillin

19. A woman who is 9 weeks pregnant comes to the emergency department with profuse, heavy vaginal bleeding and cramping. Cervical examination reveals an open internal os. Ultrasound findings include an empty gestational sac and a normal endometrial stripe. What is the most likely diagnosis?

(A) Missed abortion
(B) Threatened abortion
(C) Inevitable abortion
(D) Completed abortion
(E) Incomplete abortion

20. In which of the following poisonings is mydriasis usually seen?

(A) Opiates
(B) Phenothiazines
(C) Organophosphates
(D) Barbiturates
(E) Cocaine

21. Which of the following statements regarding lithium intoxication is correct?

(A) It may cause syndrome of inappropriate secretion of antidiuretic hormone (SIADH).
(B) It may cause signs of hyperthyroidism.
(C) It may present as urinary retention.
(D) Activated charcoal is useful in treatment.
(E) Hemodialysis is treatment for significant intoxication.

22. What is the correct compression rate and compression-to-ventilation ratio in adult one-person cardiopulmonary resuscitation (CPR)?

(A) A compression rate of 60–80 per minute and a compression-to-ventilation ratio of 15:2. (15 compressions at 60–80 compressions per minute followed by 2 breaths)
(B) A compression rate of 80–100 and a compression-to-ventilation ratio of 15:2
(C) A compression rate of 60–80 and a compression-to-ventilation ratio of 5:1
(D) A compression rate of 80–100 and a compression-to-ventilation ratio of 5:1
(E) The rate and compression-to-ventilation ratio are dictated by the patient's weight

23. A 10 kilogram child presents to the emergency department in asystole. Which of the following dosages of atropine should be administered?

(A) 0.1 mg
(B) 0.15 mg
(C) 0.2 mg
(D) 0.25 mg
(E) 0.3 mg

24. A patient presents with what appears to be acute cholecystitis. Which of the following would be the best test to confirm the diagnosis?

(A) Radionuclide hepatoiminodiacetic acid (HIDA) scan
(B) Barium swallow
(C) Meglumine diatrizoate (Gastrografin) enema
(D) Serum GGT
(E) Abdominal radiograph

25. Which of the following antibiotics is recommended for outpatient treatment of pyelonephritis?

(A) Erythromycin
(B) Ciprofloxacin
(C) Doxycycline
(D) Cephalexin
(E) Ampicillin

26. Which of the following statements regarding central retinal vein occlusion (CRVO) is correct?

(A) Painless loss of vision occurs over hours or days.
(B) The patient has a perception of flashing light.
(C) The eye exam reveals a pale retina with a central cherry red spot.
(D) It is associated with atrial fibrillation.
(E) Surgical repair is needed within 24 hours.

27. Which of the following statements regarding toxic epidermal necrolysis is correct?

(A) It usually occurs in children under 5 years of age.
(B) The patient usually appears well.
(C) The mucous membranes usually are involved.
(D) Antibiotics are indicated for treatment.
(E) Patients can be discharged from the emergency department with follow-up.

28. Which of the following medications acts most rapidly to treat hyperkalemia?

(A) Calcium
(B) Insulin
(C) Glucose
(D) Albuterol
(E) Kayexalate

29. Which of the following benzodiazepines has the shortest half-life?

(A) Midazolam
(B) Alprazolam
(C) Lorazepam
(D) Diazepam
(E) Chlordiazepoxide

30. Which of the following diseases of the bone is associated with hypercalcemia?

(A) Osteoporosis
(B) Osteomalacia
(C) Paget's disease
(D) Legg-Calvé-Perthes disease
(E) Osgood-Schlatter disease

31. Which of the following is a noncompetitive depolarizing agent?

(A) Etomidate
(B) Pancuronium
(C) Vecuronium
(D) Succinylcholine
(E) Fentanyl

32. Which of the following statements regarding pancreatitis is correct?

(A) Serum amylase is most specific for the diagnosis of pancreatitis.
(B) High dose penicillin can be an etiology for pancreatitis.
(C) The patient should receive aggressive oral rehydration.
(D) CT scan is the imaging study of choice compared to ultrasound.
(E) Morphine is favored over meperidine for analgesia.

33. A urinalysis obtained from a patient with hematuria reveals red blood cell (RBC) casts. Which of the following locations is the probable source of the bleeding?

(A) Urethra
(B) Bladder
(C) Prostate
(D) Ureter
(E) Kidney

34. Which of the following medications is the initial treatment for anaphylactic shock?

(A) Diphenhydramine
(B) Hydroxyzine
(C) Hydrocortisone
(D) Epinephrine
(E) Cimetidine

35. A 25-year-old man presents with a 2-day history of a painless nodule on his left eyelid. He does not complain of any vision changes. The examination reveals a nontender, non-erythematous nodule on his left eyelid with mild conjunctival injection. Which of the following conditions does this patient most likely have?

(A) Chalazion
(B) Hordeolum
(C) Blepharitis
(D) Conjunctivitis
(E) Hyphema

36. Which of the following conditions usually presents as euvolemic hyponatremia?

(A) Pancreatitis
(B) Renal tubular acidosis
(C) Syndrome of inappropriate secretion of antidiuretic hormone (SIADH)
(D) Hepatic cirrhosis
(E) Nephrotic syndrome

37. A 4-month-old infant girl is brought in to the emergency department by ambulance after the father finds the child not breathing in her crib. After a failed resuscitation attempt, the infant is pronounced dead. The father does not know the infant's birth or immunization history, but reveals that the baby had had a "cold," which he blamed on the babysitter's cigarette smoke. At this time, how should the cause of the patient's death be described to the father?

(A) Passive exposure to cigarette smoke
(B) Complications of an upper respiratory infection
(C) Improper sleep positioning
(D) Inadequate immunization
(E) Unknown

38. Which of the following statements regarding circulation and intravenous access is correct?

(A) A palpable radial pulse denotes a systolic blood pressure of 120 mm/Hg.
(B) Normal capillary refill time is 2–3 seconds; 5 seconds is considered abnormal.
(C) Central line placement is often faster than peripheral line placement.
(D) When starting a peripheral intravenous line in an infant, a 12 gauge needle should be used.
(E) External jugular access is one method of central venous access.

39. Which of the following statements regarding aspiration pneumonia is correct?

(A) Patients usually present with a normal chest examination.
(B) Double antibiotic coverage is needed in all cases.
(C) Bronchoscopy and pulmonary toilet provide relief from obstruction.
(D) Cystic fibrosis is considered a risk factor.
(E) It is commonly associated with asthma.

40. A 35-year-old woman presents with severe pain in the mouth. She points to the location where a tooth was extracted the day before. Examination of her mouth reveals a deep, empty hole where the tooth used to be. What is the most appropriate action?

(A) Emergency dental or periodontal consult
(B) Intravenous antibiotics to cover mouth flora
(C) Packing of the socket with petroleum gauze
(D) Drainage of the gingiva above the socket
(E) None of the above

41. Which of the following statements regarding dermatomyositis is correct?

(A) The muscle weakness usually is asymmetrical.
(B) The muscle weakness usually is more distal than proximal.
(C) It is associated with a heliotrope rash.
(D) The anti-nuclear antibody (ANA) test usually is negative.
(E) Treatment consists of multiple-dose aspirin.

42. A 35-year-old man presents to the emergency department after a 4-story fall. His blood pressure is 80/60, heart rate is 120 beats per minute, and respiratory rate is 24 breaths per minute. Two large-bore IVs are started, blood work is sent, and type O blood is ordered. He has equal bilateral breath sounds, tender abdomen, and an unstable pelvis on palpation. Portable chest radiograph-ray reveals a wide mediastinum but no hemothorax or pneumothorax. Pelvis film reveals widening of the symphysis pubis and the sacroiliac joints. Repeat vital signs after 2 liters of Ringer's lactate are unchanged. Which of the following should be the next step in management of this patient?

(A) Placement of Foley catheter
(B) Angiogram to rule out traumatic rupture of the aorta (TRA)
(C) Computed tomographic (CT) scan of abdomen and head
(D) Supraumbilical open diagnostic peritoneal lavage (DPL)
(E) Jude views of pelvis

43. Which of the following statements regarding central venous access is correct?

(A) The right side is preferred over the left for subclavian access.
(B) Internal jugular access carries a higher risk of pneumothorax than the subclavian.
(C) The left side is preferred over the right in internal jugular access.
(D) Femoral access carries the highest risk of infection.
(E) External jugular access is one method of central venous access.

44. A 60-year-old woman presents with periumbilical pain for the last day, which is exacerbated by eating. She also complains of vomiting and diarrhea. Her vital signs are: Temperature=99.6°F; pulse=118 beats per minute and irregularly irregular; blood pressure=160/90; respirations=24 per minute. She does not appear well. Her abdominal exam reveals a mildly tender abdomen without rebound or guarding. Her rectal exam reveals guaiac positive stool. The chest radiograph does not show an infiltrate or free air under the diaphragm. Which of the following conditions is the most likely diagnosis?

(A) Acute appendicitis
(B) Perforated ulcer
(C) Acute abdominal aneurysm
(D) Acute intestinal ischemia
(E) Diverticulosis

45. A patient presents with a Mallory-Weiss syndrome. Which of the following tests would be used to identify the source of bleeding?

(A) Endoscopy
(B) Colonoscopy
(C) Angiogram
(D) Radionuclide scanning
(E) Anoscopy

46. Which of the following statements regarding cluster headaches is correct?

(A) More women are affected than men.
(B) The headache is associated with lacrimation.
(C) An aura may precede the headache.
(D) The pain is considered pulsatile in nature.
(E) The pain is usually bilateral.

47. Which of the following is an autoimmune etiology of oral ulcers?

(A) Pemphigus
(B) Epidermolysis bullosa
(C) Varicella zoster
(D) Mononucleosis
(E) Squamous cell carcinoma

48. Which of the following electrocardiographic (ECG) changes can be seen in a patient with hypokalemia?

(A) Peaked T waves
(B) Loss of P waves
(C) Widened QRS complex
(D) Shortened QT interval
(E) First-degree heart block

49. Over what anatomic location should a Heimlich maneuver be delivered to a child?

(A) The sternum
(B) The xiphoid process
(C) Between the xiphoid and the umbilicus
(D) The umbilicus
(E) Between the umbilicus and the pubic symphysis

50. Which of the following is the most common cause of small bowel obstruction?

(A) Adhesions
(B) Neoplasms
(C) Gallstones
(D) Abscess
(E) Diverticulitis

51. Which of the deciduous (baby) teeth are the first to erupt?

(A) Mandibular central incisors
(B) Mandibular lateral incisors
(C) Maxillary central incisors
(D) Maxillary lateral incisors
(E) Mandibular first molars

52. In what condition would an anion gap metabolic acidosis be expected?

(A) Diabetic ketoacidosis
(B) Adrenal insufficiency
(C) Renal tubular acidosis
(D) Diarrhea
(E) Chronic pyelonephritis

53. Which of the following characteristics is considered a risk factor for attempted suicide?

(A) African-American race
(B) Female gender
(C) Married
(D) Recent job loss
(E) The fourth decade of life

54. A patient who presents with head trauma opens his eyes on command, makes incomprehensible sounds in response to rectal examination but says nothing else, and localizes to painful stimuli. What is his Glasgow Coma Score (GCS) ?

(A) 6
(B) 8
(C) 10
(D) 12
(E) It is not possible to calculate a GCS for this patient

55. What is the correct compression depth when performing cardiopulmonary resuscitation (CPR) on an infant?

(A) 0.5–1.0 inches
(B) 1.0–1.5 inches
(C) 1.5–2.0 inches
(D) 2.0–2.5 inches
(E) 2.5–3.0 inches

56. Which of the following findings would suggest that a pleural effusion is an exudate?

(A) Specific gravity < 3g/dl
(B) Protein pleural fluid (PF):serum ratio < of 0.5
(C) Lactate dehydrogenase (LDH) < 200 IU/ml
(D) LDH PF:serum r0atio of < 0.6
(E) Specific gravity > 1.016

57. Which of the following medications is used in the treatment of toxigenic bacterial diarrhea?

(A) Amoxicillin
(B) Clindamycin
(C) Loperamide
(D) Metronidazole
(E) Vancomycin

58. Which of the following statements regarding the physical examination of the eye is correct?

(A) Both eyes should be checked for visual acuity at the same time.
(B) Pinhole testing usually improves vision in retinal disease.
(C) The green light on the slit lamp is used to check for corneal abrasions.
(D) Neovascularization of scleral vessels is checked with the ophthalmoscope.
(E) Normal intraocular pressure is between 10–23 mmHg.

59. A 12-year-old boy presents with left ear pain and decreased hearing. He appears to have retroauricular swelling and tenderness. Otoscopic examination reveals ear discharge and a bulging, erythematous tympanic membrane. His temperature is 38.8°C (102°F). Which one of the following antibiotics and routes is indicated?

(A) Amoxicillin orally
(B) Cefuroxime intravenously (IV)
(C) Erythromycin orally
(D) Metronidazole IV
(E) Tetracycline orally

60. Which of the following statements regarding sialolithiasis is correct?

(A) The stones usually are composed of uric acid.
(B) The pain is made worse with eating sweet food.
(C) There is usually an absence of swelling.
(D) It is associated with systemic lupus erythematosus and rheumatoid arthritis.
(E) Cefazolin is indicated if infection is suspected.

61. A 19-year-old college student presents to the emergency department with fever, cough, and bilateral conjunctivitis. A characteristic maculopapular rash is noted on her face and neck. A urine pregnancy test is positive. Which of the following congenital abnormalities might be found in her child?

(A) Microcephaly, cataracts, congenital heart disease
(B) Microcephaly, thrombocytopenia, pneumonitis
(C) Mucocutaneous lesions, osteochondritis
(D) Microcephaly, limb or digit abnormalities
(E) Cutaneous vesicles, hepatosplenomegaly

62. What is the first intervention recommended in the treatment of ventricular fibrillation?

(A) Lidocaine
(B) Epinephrine
(C) Bretylium
(D) Procainamide
(E) Defibrillation

63. A 50-year-old man who is suspected of having overdosed on labetalol presents to the emergency department. Which of the following choices of medication and dosage is correct to give in this situation?

(A) Atropine 2 mg intravenous (IV) bolus
(B) Glucagon 5 mg IV bolus
(C) Isoproterenol 1 mg IV bolus
(D) Calcium chloride 1 g IV bolus
(E) Epinephrine 1 mg IV bolus

64. A 25-year-old woman presents with several weeks of fatigue, swollen joints, and low-grade fever. She has a butterfly-shaped rash over the malar area of her face. What is the most likely diagnosis?

(A) Rheumatoid arthritis
(B) Systemic lupus erythematosus
(C) Scleroderma
(D) Sarcoid
(E) Dermatomyositis

65. A 16-year-old boy presents with pain and swelling to the right knee with inability to walk properly. A radiograph of the knee reveals a cuff of periosteal new bone formation at the margin of a soft tissue mass. What is the most likely diagnosis?

(A) Ewing's sarcoma
(B) Osgood-Schlatter disease
(C) Osteogenic sarcoma
(D) Osteomalacia
(E) Septic arthritis

66. A patient presents in the emergency department with paroxysmal supraventricular tachycardia. Which of the following statements regarding the use of carotid massage is correct?

(A) It is to be performed after administration of adenosine.
(B) Pressure is applied for 20 seconds.
(C) There is a higher success rate when massaging both carotids at the same time.
(D) It is contraindicated in patients with carotid bruits.
(E) It slows conduction through decreased sympathetic tone.

67. Which of the following statements regarding mania is correct?

(A) It affects men more often than women.
(B) It usually begins in the fifth decade of life.
(C) It is not associated with hallucinations.
(D) Speech is usually slow and deliberate.
(E) Haloperidol may be useful in the acute state.

68. Which of the following substances is absorbed by activated charcoal?

(A) Aminophylline
(B) Ethyl alcohol
(C) Iron
(D) Lithium
(E) Kerosene

69. Which of the following conditions is associated with claudication of the masseter muscles?

(A) Temporal arteritis
(B) Oral thrush
(C) Amyotrophic lateral sclerosis (ALS)
(D) Hyperthyroidism
(E) Aortic dissection

70. Which of the following statements regarding the use of epinephrine in ventricular fibrillation is correct?

(A) The initial adult dose is 0.5 mg.
(B) The dose should be repeated every 10 minutes.
(C) If intravenous access is unavailable, the medication can be given intramuscularly.
(D) The initial pediatric dose is 0.01 mg/kg.
(E) Subsequent pediatric dosages should be the same as the initial dose.

71. If adenosine and verapamil fail to convert a paroxysmal narrow-complex supraventricular tachycardia, which of the following medications may be indicated?

(A) Epinephrine
(B) Lidocaine
(C) Bretylium
(D) Digoxin
(E) Magnesium

72. A 35-year-old woman, with a history of systemic lupus erythematosus (SLE), presents with sudden onset of pleuritic chest pain and shortness of breath. Her vital signs show a respiratory rate of 40 breaths per minute, pulse of 120 beats per minute and blood pressure of 140/80. She is afebrile. Lung exam and chest radiograph are unremarkable. Her oxygen saturation is 80% and her electrocardiogram (ECG) reveals an $S_1Q_3T_3$ pattern. Which of the following conditions does this patient most likely have?

(A) Pulmonary embolus
(B) Pneumonia
(C) Pneumothorax
(D) Pleuritis
(E) Adult respiratory distress syndrome (ARDS)

73. Which of the following antibiotic regimens would be used for an ill-looking patient with acute cholecystitis?

(A) Clindamycin and metronidazole
(B) Cefazolin and ampicillin
(C) Cefazolin, gentamicin, and metronidazole
(D) Ampicillin and gentamicin
(E) Ceftriaxone, gentamicin, and metronidazole

74. On neurologic examination, a 33-year-old patient presents with the following findings: He uses inappropriate words, his eyes open to painful stimuli, and he localizes pain. Which of the following Glasgow Coma Scale scores would you assign to him?

(A) 6
(B) 7
(C) 8
(D) 9
(E) 10

75. Which of the following organisms is the pathogen responsible for malignant otitis externa?

(A) *Staphylococcus aureus*
(B) *Mycoplasma pneumoniae*
(C) *Pseudomonas aeruginosa*
(D) *Haemophilus influenzae*
(E) *Moraxella catarrhalis*

76. A 30-year-old woman comes in after ingesting an unknown substance. The patient is lethargic, febrile, and tachypneic. An arterial blood gas reveals a pH of 7.22, partial pressure of carbon dioxide (pCO_2)of 30, partial pressure of oxygen (pO_2)of 100, and a bicarbonate level of 16. A fingerstick reveals a blood glucose of 55. Which of the following did the patient most likely take?

(A) Aspirin
(B) Barbiturate
(C) Opioid
(D) Physostigmine
(E) It is not possible to tell from the information given

77. A 10-year-old boy presents with difficulty walking and a painful right hip for 4 days. Physical examination reveals an externally rotated, flexed right hip with limited active range of motion. The radiograph of the hip demonstrates displacement of the femoral head. What is the most likely diagnosis?

(A) Septic arthritis
(B) Legg-Calvé-Perthes disease
(C) Toxic synovitis
(D) Ewing's sarcoma
(E) Slipped capital femoral epiphysis

78. Which of the following causes of hypoxemia presents with an A-a gradient which improves with supplemental oxygen?

(A) Hypoventilation
(B) Reduced fraction of inspired oxygen (FiO_2)
(C) $\dot{V}/\dot{Q}$mismatch
(D) Shunt
(E) Diffusion abnormality

79. Which of the following statements regarding pneumothorax is correct?

(A) It is defined as areas of parenchymal collapse.
(B) Thoracocentesis is the treatment of choice.
(C) Chronic obstructive pulmonary disease (COPD) is a risk factor.
(D) Physical examination reveals hyporesonance of the chest wall.
(E) In tension pneumothorax, the heart sounds are increased.

80. Which of the following statements regarding abdominal aortic aneurysm is correct?

(A) Symptomatic and asymptomatic individuals should be admitted.
(B) An aneurysm of 3 centimeters need immediate surgical repair
(C) A calcified aorta may be seen on abdominal radiograph.
(D) In the acute situation, the patient should be kept hypertensive.
(E) Pulses are usually equal in the upper and lower extremities.

81. Which of the following anticonvulsive medications is usually prescribed to a patient with trigeminal neuralgia?

(A) Carbamazepine
(B) Valproate
(C) Phenytoin
(D) Lorazepam
(E) Phenobarbital

82. A 22-year-old man presents with fever, sore throat, and abdominal pain. He appears well, and on throat examination has a mild exudative pharyngitis. A complete blood cell count (CBC) is done, and atypical lymphocytes are identified on the differential. Which of the following pathogens is the most likely cause of the pharyngitis?

(A) Ebstein-Barr virus
(B) Echovirus
(C) *Streptococcus pyogenes*
(D) *Neisseria gonorrhoeae*
(E) *Bordetella pertussis*

83. A 70-year-old woman with a history of thyroid disease presents to the emergency department with a change in mental status, hypotension, bradycardia, and nystagmus. Which of the following medications may be indicated for treatment?

(A) Thyroxine
(B) Propylthiouracil
(C) Methimazole
(D) Iodine
(E) Propranolol

84. A 25-year-old woman presents to the emergency department with right breast pain. Physical examination detects a small tender, erythematous area on the breast. There is no indication of an abscess. The patient is not allergic to any medications. Which of the following antibiotics is the best choice for treatment?

(A) Penicillin
(B) Doxycycline
(C) Dicloxacillin
(D) Erythromycin
(E) Gentamicin

85. A report on a patient's blood work shows the following: sodium: 140; potassium: 5; chloride: 105; bicarbonate (HCO_3^-):20; blood urea nitrogen (BUN): 28; creatinine: 1.0; glucose: 90. What is the calculated osmolality?

(A) 155
(B) 160
(C) 280
(D) 290
(E) 295

86. Which of the following patients is most likely to have Osgood-Schlatter disease?

(A) A 2-year-old boy
(B) An 8-year-old girl
(C) A 12-year-old boy
(D) A 25-year-old woman
(E) A 40-year-old male

87. Which of the following statements regarding the treatment of pulmonary embolus is correct?

(A) The intravenous (IV) bolus dose of heparin is 50 U/kg.
(B) Therapeutic activated partial thromboplastin time (APTT) desired is 2.5–3.0 times baseline.
(C) Low molecular weight heparins are administered once per day.
(D) Coumadin is started after 10 days of heparin therapy.
(E) Coumadin and heparin are not prescribed simultaneously.

88. Which of the following is the medication of choice for dystonic reactions?

(A) Haloperidol
(B) Clozapine
(C) Benztropine
(D) Diazepam
(E) Dopamine

89. An 18-year-old man is unable to move his hands or legs after falling off a 5-foot fence and landing on his head. His Glasgow Coma Score is 15, and no fracture is noted on the cervical, thoracic, or lumbosacral radiographs. What would be the most appropriate initial management of this patient?

(A) Mannitol 1 g/kg
(B) Cefazolin 1 g
(C) Furosemide 40 mg
(D) Methylprednisolone 30 mg/kg
(E) Naloxone 100 mg

90. Which of the following statements regarding cerebral vascular accident (CVA) or stroke is correct?

(A) Hemorrhagic strokes are more common than ischemic strokes.
(B) Atrial fibrillation is considered an etiology for embolic strokes.
(C) The most common site for a hemorrhagic stroke is the medulla.
(D) Ischemic strokes are best seen on CT one hour after occurrence.
(E) Heparin is contraindicated in ischemic strokes.

91. A 17-year-old boy presents with recent facial trauma. On eye examination, you notice a teardrop-shaped pupil. Slit lamp examination reveals a shallow anterior chamber and hyphema. Which of the following conditions does the patient most likely have?

(A) Corneal abrasion
(B) Corneal laceration
(C) Conjunctival laceration
(D) Iridocyclitis
(E) Corneal ulcer

92. Which of the following statements regarding cavernous sinus thrombosis is correct?

(A) There is an absence of pain in the facial area.
(B) Enophthalmos is found on physical examination.
(C) The patient should be admitted to the intensive care unit (ICU).
(D) *Pseudomonas* spp. is a common infecting agent.
(E) The mortality is approximately 2–5%.

93. Which of the following medications is the treatment of choice for torsades de pointes?

(A) Magnesium
(B) Calcium
(C) Potassium
(D) Sodium bicarbonate
(E) Phosphate

94. Which of the following pneumonia etiologies can be treated with doxycycline?

(A) *Streptococcus pneumoniae*
(B) *Moraxella catarrhalis*
(C) *Pseudomonas aeruginosa*
(D) *Chlamydia pneumoniae*
(E) *Pneumocystis carinii*

95. Which of the following statements regarding hemoptysis is correct?

(A) In most situations, a chest radiograph is noncontributory to the diagnosis.
(B) Hemoptysis with renal disease would suggest nonsteroidal anti-inflammatory drug (NSAID) toxicity.
(C) Massive hemoptysis usually results from hemorrhage from pulmonary arteries.
(D) Clubbing may be associated with bronchogenic carcinoma as a diagnosis.
(E) An echocardiogram may be useful to rule out aortic stenosis as an etiology.

96. Which of the following statements regarding epistaxis is correct?

(A) Protein C deficiency is considered an etiology.
(B) Epistaxis usually is more severe in children than in adults.
(C) Bleeding is more common from the posterior nasal septum.
(D) Epinephrine can be used topically as a vasoconstrictor.
(E) A nasal foreign body is the most common cause in adults.

97. What pathogen causes scarlet fever?

(A) Coxsackie virus, type A 16
(B) Group A beta-hemolytic streptococcus
(C) Herpes zoster virus
(D) *Staphylococcus aureus*
(E) Parvovirus B19

98. A worried mother brings her 5-week-old breast-fed daughter to the emergency department because the infant has looked yellow for 3 weeks. What is the most likely explanation of the infant's condition?

(A) Increased enterohepatic circulation of bilirubin
(B) Increased binding affinity of fetal hemoglobin for oxygen
(C) Increased binding affinity of neonatal albumin for bilirubin
(D) Increased need for free water in formula
(E) Increased deposition of bilirubin pigment in basal ganglia and cerebellum

99. Which of the following medications is considered a muscle relaxant?

(A) Ibuprofen
(B) Indomethacin
(C) Naproxen
(D) Sulindac
(E) Cyclobenzaprine

100. A woman presents to the emergency department 4 days postpartum with fever, severe lower abdominal pain, and vaginal bleeding. On physical examination, there is minimal cervical discharge; however, the uterus is enlarged and tender. What is the most likely diagnosis?

(A) Vaginal atony
(B) Intrapartum trauma
(C) Endometritis
(D) Fibroids
(E) None of the above

101. Which of the following statements regarding tuberculosis is correct?

(A) All persons exposed to tuberculosis will develop the disease.
(B) Diabetes and cancer can make a person susceptible to tuberculosis.
(C) Gram staining of sputum can secure the diagnosis of tuberculosis.
(D) Cavitary lesions in the lower lobes are suggestive of tuberculosis.
(E) Prophylaxis for tuberculosis includes the use of isoniazid for 2 months.

102. A 30-year-old man presents with abdominal pain for one day. The pain started in the middle of the abdomen, but now it is in the right lower quadrant. He is also complaining of nausea and vomiting. His vital signs are: temperature=100.8°F; pulse=110 beats per minute; blood pressure=130/80; respirations=24 per minute. His physical examination reveals involuntary guarding in the right lower quadrant. He has a tender rectal exam with guaiac negative stool. He has a normal genital examination. Which of the following is the most likely diagnosis?

(A) Acute diverticulitis
(B) Testicular torsion
(C) Acute appendicitis
(D) Perforated ulcer
(E) Urolithiasis

103. Which of the following statements regarding urolithiasis is correct?

(A) Hypoparathyroidism can lead to stone formation.
(B) The abdominal radiograph tends to underestimate the size of the stone.
(C) Uric acid stones are associated with very alkaline urine.
(D) Patients who have their pain controlled can be discharged from the emergency department.
(E) The most common type of urinary tract stone is cysteine.

104. Which of the following statements regarding scleritis is correct?

(A) It is a condition that usually does not cause a painful eye.
(B) It is associated with clear discharge.
(C) Cells and flare are found on slit lamp examination.
(D) The most common cause of scleritis is sarcoid.
(E) The patient should be placed on neomycin eye drops.

105. A mother brings her 16-year-old son to the emergency department complaining that he has bad breath. Examination of the child's mouth reveals a gray pseudomembrane covering the gingiva by the anterior incisor area. Which of the following conditions does the boy have?

(A) Herpetic stomatitis
(B) Coxsackie infection
(C) Trench mouth
(D) Dental caries
(E) Kawasaki disease

106. Administration of which of the following drugs would exacerbate the condition of a patient presenting with peptic ulcer disease?

(A) Cimetidine
(B) Indomethacin
(C) Sucralfate
(D) Meglumine diatrizoate (Gastrografin)
(E) Omeprazole

107. Which of the following statements regarding diverticular disease is correct?

(A) It is commonly seen in the third and fourth decade of life.
(B) Diverticula are most frequently seen at the ileocecal valve.
(C) Symptoms include left upper quadrant pain and vomiting.
(D) CT is used to look for free air at the splenic flexure.
(E) The patient may complain of urinary frequency.

108. Which of the following viruses is most commonly associated with corneal ulcers?

(A) Cytomegalovirus
(B) Herpes simplex virus
(C) Epstein-Barr virus
(D) Adenovirus
(E) Coxsackievirus

109. A patient suffers a facial fracture that involves the floor of the orbit, zygomaticomaxillary sutures and the pterygoid processes bilaterally, as well as the nasofrontal suture. Which type of fracture does he have?

(A) LeFort I
(B) LeFort II
(C) LeFort III
(D) LeFort IV
(E) Mixed LeFort fractures

110. What breath odor is characteristic of arsenic poisoning?

(A) Acetone
(B) Carrots
(C) Garlic
(D) Mothballs
(E) Wintergreen

111. Which of the following ingested substances may be seen on abdominal radiograph?

(A) Acetaminophen
(B) Chloral hydrate
(C) Atenolol
(D) Nifedipine
(E) Captopril

112. Which of the following medications is useful for the treatment of cocaine toxicity?

(A) Aspirin
(B) Propranolol
(C) Haloperidol
(D) Chlorpromazine
(E) Lorazepam

113. An elevated serum ammonia level and an altered mental status in a patient with a history of alcohol use would suggest which of the following conditions?

(A) Hepatic encephalopathy
(B) Wernicke's encephalopathy
(C) Acute alcohol intoxication
(D) Acute alcohol withdrawal
(E) Delirium tremens

114. Which of the following pathogens is associated with acute gastroenteritis from eating shellfish?

(A) *Vibrio parahemolyticus*
(B) *Staphylococcus aureus*
(C) *Escherichia coli*
(D) *Clostridium botulinum*
(E) *Giardia lamblia*

115. Which of the following statements regarding gastroesophageal reflux disease is correct?

(A) The pain worsens when sitting up and is relieved by lying down.
(B) Workup can include an acid reflux test and endoscopy.
(C) It is caused by an increase in lower esophageal sphincter pressure.
(D) Estrogen has been identified as a precipitating factor.
(E) It is treated with antibiotics.

116. Which of the following medications would be indicated for treatment of conjunctivitis secondary to the herpes simplex virus?

(A) Ciprofloxacin
(B) Ceftriaxone
(C) Azithromycin
(D) Bacitracin
(E) Trifluorothymidine

117. A 2-year-old boy presents with epistaxis and foul-smelling discharge from the left nostril only. On examination of the nose, a fullness can be felt over the left nostril. What is the most likely cause of the nosebleed?

(A) Foreign body
(B) Henoch-Schönlein purpura
(C) Nasal polyp
(D) Sinusitis
(E) Osler-Rendu-Weber syndrome

118. What is the best transportation medium for an avulsed tooth?

(A) Saliva
(B) Milk
(C) Saline
(D) Water
(E) Dry gauze

119. Which of the following signs is associated with organophosphate poisoning?

(A) Hyperthermia
(B) Dry mouth
(C) Urinary retention
(D) Diarrhea
(E) Mydriasis

120. A patient's blood work comes back with the following results: sodium: 148; potassium: 4.0; chloride: 101; bicarbonate (HCO_3^-): 22; blood urea nitrogen (BUN): 28; creatinine: 1.6; glucose: 180. What is the calculated anion gap?

(A) 19
(B) 21
(C) 23
(D) 25
(E) 29

121. Which of the following statements regarding rheumatoid arthritis is correct?

(A) It occurs most often in persons under 21 years of age.
(B) Joint stiffness worsens as the day goes on.
(C) Rheumatoid factor is positive in about one half of cases.
(D) The erythrocyte sedimentation rate (ESR) is elevated in about one half of cases.
(E) Radiographic evidence includes joint space narrowing.

122. Which of the following statements regarding hepatitis is correct?

(A) Liver function tests are usually 10 times normal in alcoholic hepatitis.
(B) Alanine aminotransferase (ALT) greater than asparagine amino transfer (AST) usually suggests alcoholic hepatitis.
(C) Hepatitis A causes permanent liver damage.
(D) Hepatitis C is transmitted through enteral exposure.
(E) Hepatitis D only occurs concurrently with Hepatitis B.

123. A patient has the following results on a urine test: fractional excretion of sodium (FENa): 0.7, urine osmolality (U_{osm}): 600, and a urine sodium (U_{Na}): 10. Which of the following causes of acute renal failure does the patient most likely have?

(A) Cirrhosis
(B) Rhabdomyolysis
(C) Goodpasture's syndrome
(D) Nephrolithiasis
(E) Multiple myeloma

124. A patient was started two days ago on ofloxacin and phenazopyridine for treatment of a urinary tract infection. She states that though the dysuria has resolved, her urine is now orange. Which of the following is indicated?

(A) Repeat urine culture
(B) Repeat urinalysis
(C) Cystogram
(D) Coagulation profile
(E) Patient reassurance

125. Which of the following breathing patterns would suggest a brain lesion in the medulla?

(A) Hyperventilation
(B) Eupneic
(C) Cheyne-Stokes
(D) Kussmaul
(E) Ataxic

126. Which of the following is a clinical feature of peripheral vertigo?

(A) Gradual onset
(B) Intense symptoms
(C) Intact hearing
(D) Multidirectional nystagmus
(E) Neurologic deficit

127. A 30-year-old woman presents with an acid burn to both eyes. Which of the following interventions should be performed first?

(A) Visual field examination
(B) Eye irrigation
(C) Topical antibiotics
(D) Cycloplegic eyedrops
(E) Fluorescein instillation

128. Which of the following pathogens is the most common cause of pharyngitis in adults?

(A) *Streptococcus pyogenes*
(B) *Haemophilus influenzae*
(C) Coxsackievirus
(D) Adenovirus
(E) Herpesvirus

129. Which of the following antibiotics is most likely to cause pseudomembranous colitis?

(A) Tetracycline
(B) Erythromycin
(C) Doxycycline
(D) Cephalexin
(E) Clindamycin

130. What type of microscopic study can be used to diagnose a fungal infection of the skin?

(A) Tzanck test
(B) KOH preparation
(C) Mineral oil preparation
(D) Gram stain
(E) India ink preparation

131. A woman who is 8 weeks pregnant comes to the emergency department with the complaint of mild vaginal bleeding and lower abdominal pain. Bimanual examination reveals a slightly enlarged uterus and tenderness over the left adnexa. The ultrasound reveals no intrauterine pregnancy (IUP) but does show free fluid behind the uterus. What is the most likely diagnosis?

(A) Ectopic pregnancy
(B) Endometritis
(C) Pelvic inflammatory disease
(D) Endometriosis
(E) Endometrial carcinoma

132. A 25-year-old man comes to the emergency department with altered mental status secondary to an unknown ingestion. A urine sample is obtained, and ferric chloride is added to it. The urine turns purple. Which of the following substances is present in the patient's system?

(A) Acetaminophen
(B) Iron
(C) Salicylate
(D) Tricyclic antidepressant
(E) Lithium

133. A 30-year-old woman presents with headache which she says is worse upon awakening, but gets better as the day progresses. She also complains of blurry vision. On funduscopic exam, papilledema is noted. The patient has a head CT which is normal. A lumbar puncture reveals an opening pressure of 380 mmHg, with no red or white cells. Which of the following conditions does this patient most likely have?

(A) Normal pressure hydrocephalus
(B) Subarachnoid hemorrhage
(C) Pseudotumor cerebri
(D) Atypical migraine
(E) Viral meningitis

134. Which of the following treatments is indicated for a hyphema?

(A) Mydriatic eye drops
(B) Eye patch over both eyes
(C) Aspirin
(D) Keeping the patient lying flat
(E) Prochlorperazine

135. Which of the following statements regarding cellulitis is correct?

(A) The most typical locations are the chest and back.
(B) Diabetes mellitus is considered a risk factor.
(C) The borders of the lesion are sharply demarcated.
(D) Most patients should be admitted for intravenous (IV) antibiotics.
(E) The organism most commonly involved is *Pseudomonas.*

136. What is the most common precipitating event for thyroid storm?

(A) Pulmonary emboli
(B) Sepsis
(C) Toxemia
(D) Diabetes
(E) Emotional stress

137. Which of the following conditions is considered a risk factor for toxemia of pregnancy?

(A) Multiparity
(B) Maternal age in third decade
(C) Liver disease
(D) Multiple gestations
(E) Early menarche

138. Which of the following statements regarding meningitis is correct?

(A) Viral meningitis carries a higher morbidity than bacterial meningitis.
(B) Infants with meningitis are usually found to have sunken fontanelles.
(C) The opening pressure on a lumbar puncture is usually very low on a patient with meningitis.
(D) *Staphylococcus pneumoniae* is a leading cause of meningitis in teenagers and young adults.
(E) Erythromycin is the drug of choice for treating bacterial meningitis.

139. Which of the following drugs has the longest duration of action?

(A) Codeine
(B) Meperidine
(C) Morphine
(D) Heroin
(E) Methadone

140. Which of the following drugs is indicated for an acetaminophen overdose?

(A) Sodium bicarbonate
(B) N-acetylcysteine
(C) Thiamine
(D) Protamine
(E) Physostigmine

141. Which of the following cysts is treated with a Word catheter?

(A) Breast cyst
(B) Sebaceous cyst
(C) Bartholin's cyst
(D) Pilonidal cyst
(E) Thyroglossal cyst

142. What odor of the breath is associated with diabetic ketoacidosis?

(A) Bitter almond
(B) Acetone
(C) Feces
(D) Ethanol
(E) Spearmint

143. Which of the following suture materials should be used to close a simple laceration of the eyelid?

(A) 4.0 nylon
(B) 6.0 nylon
(C) 4.0 silk
(D) 6.0 silk
(E) Any of the above are suitable choices

144. Which of the following medications is indicated for isoniazid-induced seizures?

(A) Thiamine
(B) Niacin
(C) Pyridoxine
(D) Methylene blue
(E) Calcium

Directions: The response options for items 145–149 are the same. You will be required to select one answer for each item in the set.

(A) Tophi
(B) Positive birefringent crystals
(C) Sexually active adult
(D) Pediatric population
(E) Positive anti-nuclear antibody (ANA)

For each of the following findings, select the appropriate joint disorder.

145. Systemic lupus erythematosus (SLE)

146. Nongonococcal bacterial arthritis

147. Gonococcal arthritis

148. Gout

149. Pseudogout

Directions: The response options for Items 150–153 are the same. You will be required to select one answer for each item in the set.

For each of the following ventilator modes, select the statement that best describes it or its use.

(A) Continuous mandatory ventilation (CMV) mode
(B) Assist control (AC) mode
(C) Intermittent mandatory ventilation (IMV) mode
(D) Synchronized intermittent mandatory ventilation (SIMV) mode

150. A disadvantage to the use of this mode is breath stacking

151. At this mode setting, the ventilator delivers at a present rate regardless of patient effort

152. This mode facilitates weaning

153. At this mode setting, the ventilator responds to the patient's efforts. If there are none, the ventilator will cycle at the preset rate

Directions: The response options for Items 154–158 are the same. You will be required to select one answer for each item in the set.

For each of the following rhythms, select the statement that best describes its etiology, presentation, or treatment.

(A) Ventricular fibrillation
(B) Asystole
(C) Pulseless electrical activity
(D) Paroxysmal supraventricular tachycardia
(E) Wide complex tachycardia

154. This rhythm can be caused by tension pneumothorax and cardiac tamponade.

155. Magnesium is administered for suspected hypomagnesemic states.

156. There is absolutely no ventricular activity.

157. Verapamil may be indicated for this rhythm.

158. In a stable patient, lidocaine is initially used.

Directions: The response options for items 159–163 are the same. You will be required to select one answer for each item in the set.

(A) Painful, scattered vesicles and pustules
(B) Honey-colored, crusty vesiculopapular rash
(C) Sharply demarcated, painful, erythematous area
(D) Comedones, papules, cysts and scars
(E) Sharply demarcated plaques with silvery scale

For each of the following dermatological emergencies, select the best description of its physical findings.

159. Erysipelas

160. Acne

161. Psoriasis

162. Herpes

163. Impetigo

Questions 164–167

Match each type of bite to the bacteria that is most likely to cause infection in that bite.

(A) *Pasteurella multocida*
(B) *Capnocytophaga canimorsus*
(C) *Eikenella corrodens*
(D) *Streptobacillus moniliformis*

164. Dog

165. Cat

166. Rodent

167. Human

Directions: The response options for Items 168–171 are the same. You will be required to select one answer for each item in the set.

For each of the following medications for asthma, select the statement that best describes its mechanism of action.

(A) Albuterol
(B) Ipratropium
(C) Prednisone
(D) Zafirlukast

168. Acts by blocking leukotriene receptors in the airway

169. Controls inflammation

170. Bronchodilatation through sympathetic receptors

171. Bronchodilatation through anticholinergic receptors

Directions: The response options for Items 172–176 are the same. You will be required to select one answer for each item in the set.

For each of the following signs, select the statement that best describes how each is tested or found on physical exam.

(A) Iliopsoas sign
(B) Obturator sign
(C) Rovsing's sign
(D) Cullen's sign
(E) Grey-Turner's sign

172. Ecchymosis of the flank

173. Ecchymosis at the umbilicus

174. Pain in the right lower quadrant (RLQ) when the left lower quadrant (LLQ) is palpated

175. Pain on internal rotation of flexed right thigh

176. Pelvic pain on flexion of right thigh against downward pressure

Directions: The response options for Items 177–181 are the same. You will be required to select one answer for each item in the set.

(A) Phimosis
(B) Priapism
(C) Penile fracture
(D) Testicular torsion
(E) Acute epididymitis

For each of the following male genitourinary problems, select the statement that best describes its etiology, presentation, or treatment.

177. Can be secondary to benign prostatic hypertrophy

178. A dorsal slit may be indicated for treatment

179. Involves absence of the cremasteric reflex

180. Sudden onset of penile pain associated with a clicking sound

181. Often associated with patients in sickle cell crisis

Directions: The response options for Items 182–185 are the same. You will be required to select one answer for each item in the set.

(A) Multiple sclerosis
(B) Myasthenia gravis
(C) Guillain-Barré
(D) Bell's palsy

For each of the above neurologic conditions, select the statement that best describes its etiology or presentation.

182. Idiopathic seventh cranial nerve paralysis or paresis.

183. Presents as ascending symmetric limb weakness.

184. Physical findings include optic neuritis and intranuclear opthalmoplegia.

185. Repetitive muscle stimulation produces fatigue.

Directions: The response options for items 186–190 are the same. You will be required to select one answer for each item in the set.

For each of the following eye conditions, select the best description of the physical findings.

(A) Acute iritis
(B) Corneal abrasion
(C) Acute glaucoma
(D) Retrobulbar hemorrhage
(E) Orbital blow-out fracture

186. Enophthalmos and subcutaneous emphysema

187. Steamy cornea and high intraocular pressure

188. Cells and flare in the anterior chamber and small pupil

189. Central artery occlusion on funduscopic examination

190. Uptake of fluorescein on slit lamp examination

Directions: The response options for items 191–195 are the same. You will be required to select one answer for each item in the set.

(A) Vitamin K
(B) Methylene blue
(C) Pyridoxine
(D) Deferoxamine
(E) Amyl nitrate

For each of the following toxicities, select the appropriate antidote.

191. Methemoglobinemia

192. Iron salts excess

193. Cyanide poisoning

194. Isoniazid overdose

195. Warfarin overdose

Directions: The response options for items 196–200 are the same. You will be required to select one answer for each item in the set.

(A) Coronary aneurysm
(B) Disseminated intravascular coagulation
(C) Subacute sclerosing panencephalitis
(D) Transient aplastic crisis
(E) Bronchiectasis

Match each disease with the associated complication.

196. Cystic fibrosis

197. Erythema infectiosum

198. Measles

199. Kawasaki disease

200. Rocky Mountain spotted fever

Answers and Explanations

1–B. Complications of ulcerative colitis include rectal prolapse, massive hemorrhage, and toxic megacolon. Ulcerative colitis is found in women more often than men. On the other hand, Crohn's disease is found in men more often than in women and involves the entire gastrointestinal tract. Fistulas, strictures and abscess are more common in Crohn's disease than in ulcerative colitis. Cobblestoning and skip lesions are endoscopic findings of Crohn's disease.

2–A. Phenylephrine is a mydriatic (a drug that will cause pupillary dilatation) that can be used for eye examinations. Cyclopentolate, homatropine and scopolamine are cycloplegics (drugs that will inhibit pupillary dilatation) that are used for conditions such as corneal abrasions or ulcers. Polyvinyl alcohol is artificial tears, and is used as a conjunctival moisturizer for decreased tear production.

3–E. The patient has an Ellis III, not II, fracture. The pinkish tinge seen on physical examination is pulp. Filing of sharp edges and application of calcium hydroxide are used in adults for the other Ellis fractures (I and II, respectively), but not for Ellis III fractures. The dentist should be consulted as soon as possible for a possible pulpectomy.

4–D. The formula to calculate the tube size in a child is (age in years/4) + 4, so 6/4+4=5.5 mm (of the internal diameter of tube). Note this formula is only applicable in children over 2 years of age. The size of the child's pinkie finger can also be used as a gauge for proper tube size. Pediatric tubes do not have cuffs at the end, for the narrowest part of a child's airway is at the cricoid cartilage.

5–D. Prostaglandin therapy prevents closure of a patent ductus arteriosus, and is useful in neonates with ductus-dependent left heart obstructive disease, including aortic stenosis and coarctation of the aorta. It should be administered only after confirmation of the diagnosis by echocardiography.

6–B. A byproduct of ethylene glycol breakdown is oxalate. Just a small amount of oxalate in the urine can combine with calcium to form calcium oxalate stones. Isopropyl alcohol causes ketosis without acidosis; therefore, no anion gap is present. Methyl alcohol and oil of wintergreen do not produce calcium oxalate crystals.

7–A. Before any medications are given, the patient must be preoxygenated with 100% oxygen by mask. The patient should also be on a monitor and measurement of oxygen saturation through pulse oximetry should be done. Proceed only when the oxygen saturation is above 95%. Once the patient has been preoxygenated, administration of medications for intracranial pressure control, sedation, and paralysis can take place.

8–C. This patient's pain is caused by appendicitis, not sickle cell disease. CT signs of appendicitis include peri-appendiceal fat streaking, narrowing of the lumen of the entry to the appendix, thickening of the appendiceal walls and failure to visualize the appendix with contrast.Patients with sickle cell disease usually have elevated white counts up to 16,000 and higher than normal reticulocyte counts in the face of anemia. Secondary to ongoing hemolysis, a slightly elevated indirect bilirubin may be encountered. The abdominal crisis of sickle cell disease is usually a diffuse abdominal pain without rebound or guarding.

9–D. Adrenal insufficiency is characterized by dehydration, hypotension, tachycardia, changes in mental status, increased pigmentation of the skin and mucous membranes and alopecia. This condition may be idiopathic, or may be due to granulomatous or infectious disease. The treatment of adrenal insufficiency is administration of corticosteroids.

10–E. The most likely cause of clinically evident hypercalcemia is malignancy (e.g., multiple myeloma, lung cancer), but sarcoid, hyperparathyroidism, and lithium use or toxicity also can present with hypercalcemia. Hypoparathyroidism, hypomagnesemia, pancreatitis, and multiple transfusions are causes of *hypo*calcemia.

11–A. End-tidal carbon dioxide detectors can be used to check proper endotracheal tube placement. Other acceptable methods to check tube placement include pulmonary and gastric auscultation, resistance to bagging, condensation in the endotracheal tube, and a chest radiograph. Checking for exhalation of other gases exhaled, such as carbon monoxide, oxygen, nitrogen, and nitric oxide, is not recommended to confirm placement.

12–E. The most common cause of subarachnoid hemorrhage (SAH) is a rupture of a saccular aneurysm. The CT misses SAH in up to 10% of cases. Therefore, when clinical suspicion is high, a lumbar puncture (LP) should be performed. In Class I SAH, there are no neurologic deficits found on exam. The CSF on LP will be grossly bloody and the supernatant will be xanthochromic. Protein C deficiency, which causes a hypercoagulable state, is not considered a risk factor for SAH.

13–D. Clinical features of an intraocular foreign body include decreased visual acuity, hyphema, proptosis, and limitation of extraocular movement. The most likely site of the foreign body is the posterior segment. A CT scan or an ultrasound may be needed to localize the foreign body.

14–C. Anorexia nervosa is a disorder that begins in adolescence and is seen ten times more frequently in women than in men. There may be a history of laxative or diuretic abuse. Treatment is individualized; benzodiazepines are not indicated for anorexia nervosa. Patients are significantly underweight.

15–D. This patient requires an immediate emergency department thoracotomy. On arrival, she clearly had signs of pericardial tamponade: stab wound to the left chest, distended neck veins, and hypotension. A reasonable alternative first step would be pericardiocentesis. The presence of equal bilateral breath sounds makes it unlikely that pneumothorax is the cause of her hypotension. Bradycardia is an ominous finding in the face of trauma and requires immediate surgical attention. Intravenous (IV) atropine and external cardiac compression will not help this patient. She needs immediate decompression of her tamponade. Chest radiograph would demonstrate the tamponade as an enlarged cardiac silhouette but is not necessary to make the diagnosis. Since two large-bore peripheral IV lines are in place, access is adequate and, therefore, placement of a subclavian central line is not necessary.

16–B. Fentanyl is a synthetic opioid that can be used as part of rapid sequence intubation. The recommended dose is 3 μg per kilogram of patient's body weight. Fentanyl, which does not release histamine, has an onset of action from 2–4 minutes.

17–A. Aspirin, as well as opiates, can lead to noncardiogenic pulmonary edema. Diazepam may cause respiratory depression, but not pulmonary edema. Acetaminophen, ampicillin, and nifedipine may have effects on renal, cardiac, or hepatic function.

18–B. Ludwig's angina is an infection of the sublingual, submental, and submandibular spaces. Intravenous antibiotics and hospital admission are indicated for this patient. The usual oral pathogens, which include gram-positive organisms and anaerobes, must be covered. Penicillin and cefazolin provide good coverage against gram-positive bugs. Gentamicin covers gram-negative bugs. Metronidazole is effective against anaerobes. An excellent single drug regimen is clindamycin.

19–C. This patient has an inevitable abortion. With a missed abortion there is no vaginal bleeding and the internal os is closed. A threatened abortion usually presents with minimal vaginal bleeding and a closed internal os. A completed abortion also has minimal vaginal bleeding, although the internal os may be open. The history and physical examination findings most likely represent an inevitable abortion. This abortion would be classified as incomplete if there had been passage of tissue.

20–E. Mydriasis (large pupils) usually is seen in cocaine intoxication. Opiates, phenothiazines, organophosphates, and barbiturates usually cause miosis (small pupils). The exception is meperidine, in the opiate class, which also can produce mydriasis. In all circumstances, the pupils should react, at least minimally.

21–E. Lithium intoxication may cause nephrogenic diabetes insipidus, which would present as hypernatremia. Lithium can worsen preexisting hypothyroidism by inhibiting thyroid hormone synthesis. Signs of lithium intoxication include gastrointestinal (GI) distress, urinary incontinence, and altered mental status. Treatment for severe intoxication is hemodialysis. Since lithium does not adsorb to charcoal, treatment with activated charcoal is not effective.

22–C. The correct compression rate in adults is 60–80 per minute, and the ratio of 5:1 compression-to-ventilation is reserved for two-person cardiopulmonary resuscitation (CPR). In an adult, the depth of compression should be 1.5–2 inches. Adequacy of compressions is monitored through the presence of a carotid or femoral pulse on compressions, however, this is impossible in one-person CPR.

23–C. The pediatric dose of atropine, which is a parasympathetic blocking agent, is 0.02 mg/kg. This dose can be repeated up to a total dose of 0.04 mg/kg with a total minimum dose of 0.1 mg to prevent paroxysmal bradycardia.

24–A. A radionuclide hepatoiminodiacetic acid (HIDA) scan can be performed if the right upper quadrant ultrasound is equivocal or negative in the face of high clinical suspicion. Serum gamma-glutamyl transferase (GGT) is not specific for cholecystitis. The abdominal radiograph may not reveal gallstones. Barium swallows and meglumine diatrizoate (Gastrografin) enema are of no use in securing a diagnosis of cholecystitis.

25–B. Excellent coverage of gram-negative bacteria, which is the usual pathogen involved, is essential to the treatment of pyelonephritis. Of all the antibiotics listed, the floroquinolone ciprofloxacin gives the best gram-negative coverage. Erythromycin, doxycycline, cephalexin, and ampicillin are more effective against gram-positive organisms.

26–A. A central retinal vein occlusion (CRVO) is associated with diabetes, arteriosclerosis, hypertension and coagulopathies. It presents as painless loss of vision over hours to days. Perceptions of flashing light are suggestive of a retinal detachment. The retinal examination reveals dilated tortuous retinal veins with associated hemorrhage. Central retinal arterial occlusion (CRAO) presents with a pale retina, and is associated with endocarditis and atrial fibrillation, conditions that predispose to valve or heart wall thrombus formation. Treatment for CRVO includes lowering of the intraocular pressure, direct ocular massage, and anterior chamber paracentesis.

27–C. Toxic epidermal necrolysis (TEN) is a one of the few true dermatologic emergencies. TEN favors adults, and patients appear very ill upon presentation. Both skin and mucous membrane usually are involved. Antibiotics are not indicated. Patients with TEN should be admitted to the intensive care unit (ICU) for strict temperature control, fluid resuscitation, and monitoring of hemodynamic status.

28–A. All the choices listed in the question are appropriate treatments for hyperkalemia. The medication with the fastest onset, however, is calcium, secondary to its effect on the cell membrane (it interferes with sodium/potassium exchange). It can be given as either calcium chloride or calcium gluconate. Calcium chloride contains three times as much elemental calcium per milliliter as calcium gluconate.

29–A. Midazolam (Versed) has the shortest half-life of the benzodiazepines used in the emergency department. It is very useful in situations in which conscious sedation is indicated (e.g., incision and drainage, joint relocations). The other choices (alprazolam, lorazepam, diazepam, and chlordiazepoxide) are simply other benzodiazepines with longer half-lives.

30–C. Paget's disease is a disorder of bone remodeling. Increased osteoclast activity leads to release of calcium from the bone, which results in hypercalcemia. Other symptoms associated with Paget's disease include stiffness, fatigue, and decreased auditory acuity, as well as those associated with hypercalcemia (e.g., dehydration, gastrointestinal [GI] distress, renal calculi).

31–D. For rapid sequence intubation, succinylcholine is the noncompetitive depolarizing agent of choice. Pancuronium and vecuronium are competitive depolarizing agents. Etomidate is a sedative anesthetic. Fentanyl is a potent opioid analgesic.

32–D. Ultrasonography is an excellent modality for identification of pseudocysts, but CT scan remains the preferred technique for overall evaluation of the pancreas. The patient with acute pancreatitis should take nothing by mouth and all hydration should be done intravenously. Serum amylase is not specific for pancreatitis. Amylase may be elevated in diabetic ketoacidosis, renal failure, parotiditis, bowel obstruction, and certain cancers, to name a few conditions. Serum lipase is more specific for pancreatitis. Penicillin is not known to cause pancreatitis. However, tetracycline and sulfonamides can lead to inflammation of the pancreas. Morphine can cause spasm at the sphincter of Oddi, as well as colonic spasm, which should be avoided in pancreatitis.

33–E. Red blood cell casts can be formed only in the kidney. Therefore, the likely source of the bleeding would be renal. Though blood can come from anywhere in the urinary tract, no casts would be found on microscopic examination of the urethra, bladder, prostate, or ureter.

34–D. If a patient with an allergic reaction presents with hypotension or other signs of inadequate tissue perfusion, the medication of choice is epinephrine, which should be given subcutaneously. The other medications listed—diphenhydramine, hydroxyzine, hydrocortisone, and cimetidine—can be given in addition to epinephrine, but epinephrine must be part of the initial drug protocol.

35–A. A chalazion is a painless nontender nodule found on the eyelid. Treatment consists of application of warm compresses. A hordeolum is an erythematous, tender nodule on the inside or outside of the eye. Blepharitis conjunctivitis and hyphemas are not associated with nodules.

36–C. The syndrome of inappropriate secretion of antidiuretic hormone (SIADH) usually presents as euvolemic hyponatremia. Patients with pancreatitis or renal tubular acidosis usually are hypovolemic. Patients suffering from hepatic cirrhosis or nephrotic syndrome usually are hypervolemic.

37–E. Although passive exposure to cigarette smoke, recent upper respiratory infection, improper sleep positioning, and inadequate immunization all have been linked to sudden infant death syndrome (SIDS), the diagnosis of SIDS cannot be made until an autopsy reveals no other cause.

38–B. Normal capillary refill time is 2–3 seconds. A time greater than 5 seconds is considered delayed, and is usually a sign of hypovolemia. A palpable radial pulse usually denotes a systolic blood pressure of 80 mm/Hg. Peripheral line placement is usually faster than a central line. Peripheral access should be the first choice. The choice of intravenous gauge for an infant should be 22–24 gauge for peripheral insertion. The external jugular is considered a peripheral vein.

39–C. Lung auscultation of a patient with aspiration pneumonia will usually reveal either wheezes, rales, or rhonchi. If you suspect a patient has aspiration pneumonia, antibiotics are indicated only if a superimposed bacterial pneumonia is suspected. Cystic fibrosis is not a recognized risk factor for aspiration pneumonia. However, when patients with cystic fibrosis do aspirate, they are more likely to develop pneumonia due to impaired mucociliary clearance. There is no increased incidence of aspiration pneumonia in patients with asthma. Rather, it is associated with patients who have an impaired gag reflex such as those with drug overdose, and certain stroke victims.

40–C. Osteitis sicca, or dry socket, can cause severe pain, which usually occurs 1 to 3 days after tooth extraction. Analgesia, not antibiotics or drainage, is indicated for this condition. The socket can be packed with petroleum gauze or zinc oxide. Dental or periodontal follow-up should be obtained within 48 hours.

41–C. Dermatomyositis is an autoimmune disease that affects both skin and muscle. The muscle weakness usually is proximal and symmetrical. The anti-nuclear antibody (ANA) usually is positive, and the erythrocyte sedimentation rate (ESR) is elevated. Physical examination findings include the heliotrope rash, a violet lesion in a V-distribution over the chest and neck. The treatment for myositis or dermatomyositis is corticosteroids.

42–D. This patient is unstable and has a number of potential injuries that may be causing his instability. He may be losing blood from intraabdominal, pelvic fracture, or thoracic injuries. The injury that is most likely to prove fatal and that is most readily diagnosable and reparable is an abdominal injury. Because he is unstable, it is not possible to take him for a CT scan to make this diagnosis. A diagnostic peritoneal lavage (DPL) can be done in the trauma bay to diagnose whether there is an abdominal injury. It should be done supra-umbilically to minimize the chances of hitting a pelvic hematoma from his pelvic injury and giving a false-positive result. Ultrasound in experienced hands can substitute for DPL in diagnosing whether the patient has an abdominal injury causing his hypotension Although the history of sudden deceleration and a wide mediastinum make it necessary to rule out traumatic rupture of the aorta (TRA), evaluating this injury takes a back seat to evaluating the abdomen. A serious TRA would already have killed the patient, and an intact TRA can wait until the abdomen is addressed. The patient may need an external fixator for his pelvic fracture; this can be placed either in the emergency department or in the operating room, depending on the results of his DPL. Angiography may be necessary to diagnose and embolize arterial bleeding if the patient remains hypotensive.

43–D. Femoral access carries the highest rate of infection. The left side is preferred over the right side when performing a subclavian line placement; however, if the patient already has a hemopneumothorax, choose the side with the hemopneumothorax. The subclavian carries a higher risk of iatrogenic pneumothorax than the internal jugular. For anatomic reasons, there is a better success rate with internal jugulars inserted on the right rather than the left. Also, there is no risk of injuring the thoracic duct with a right-sided approach.

44–D. Intestinal ischemia should be suspected in an elderly person with abdominal pain when that pain is out of proportion to the physical findings. This condition should especially come to mind when the pulse is irregularly irregular, which may be a sign of atrial fibrillation, a risk factor for intestinal ischemia. Perforated ulcer, appendicitis or acute abdominal aneurysm would be suggested by physical findings, such as localized peritonitis or a pulsatile mass in the abdomen. Diverticulosis usually presents as painless lower gastrointestinal bleeding.

45–A. Mallory-Weiss syndrome occurs due to excessive retching and vomiting, and results in upper gastrointestinal (GI) bleeding, for which endoscopy is used to locate the source. Colonoscopy, angiogram, radionuclide scanning, and anoscopy are all used for localization of lower GI bleeding.

46–B. While migraine headaches affect more women than men, cluster headaches affect men more often than women. While the pain of migraine headaches is usually pulsatile, the pain of cluster headaches is usually unilateral and boring. Cluster headache is associated with lacrimation, ptosis, nasal congestion and rhinorrhea. Migraine headaches are preceded by an aura.

47–A. Pemphigus, along with systemic lupus erythematosus and Behçet's disease, are among those autoimmune conditions that can cause oral ulcers. The ulcers may be painless or painful. Although the other conditions listed also can cause ulcers, they are either hereditary (epidermolysis bullosa), infectious (syphilis and mononucleosis/Epstein Barr virus), or neoplastic (squamous cell carcinoma).

48–E. Hypokalemia may present on an electrocardiogram (ECG) with first- or second-degree atrioventricular (AV) block, premature ventricular contractions, or large U waves (especially in the anterior chest leads). The treatment for hypokalemia is supplemental potassium by intravenous drip. It is necessary to check for magnesium in any situation of hypokalemia. The other choices listed in the question—peaked T waves, loss of P waves, widened QRS complex, and shortened QT interval—are ECG findings for hyperkalemia.

49–C. In both the adult and the child, the landmark for the Heimlich maneuver should be two fingerbreadths below the xiphoid process, and the thrusts should be delivered in an upward pattern. Incorrect placement above, below, or to the side may lead to needless chest or abdominal trauma.

50–A. Adhesions and hernias are the most common cause of small bowel obstruction. Gallstones and abscesses can cause small bowel obstruction, but not as frequent. Neoplasms can cause small and large bowel obstruction. Diverticulitis can be a cause of large bowel obstruction.

51–A. Tooth eruption in infants usually occurs between the sixth and ninth month. The eruption may be accompanied by fever and irritability. The mandibular central incisors erupt first, followed by the mandibular lateral incisors, then the maxillary central incisors, then the maxillary lateral incisors, and then the mandibular first molars.

52–A. Diabetic ketoacidosis classically presents with an anion gap acidosis, due to the unaccounted-for ketones. All the other conditions listed can present with a metabolic acidosis, but in most cases there will not be a gap. Some of the other conditions that can present with an anion gap acidosis include uremia, aspirin ingestion, and carbon monoxide intoxication. See Chapter 18 I G a for more information.

53–D. Risk factors for attempted suicide include Caucasian race; male gender (although women make more suicidal gestures); being single, widowed, or divorced; recent loss of job or family member; and age greater than 65. It is very important when interviewing patients for possible suicide, always to take them seriously, especially when they describe how they would kill themselves (i.e., they have a plan). These patients should be kept on hold in the emergency department until they can be evaluated by a psychiatrist.

54–C. This patient has a Glasgow Coma Scale score of 10—3 points for opening his eyes to command, 5 points for localizing to pain, and 2 points for making incomprehensible sounds. The GCS is useful to grossly categorize the severity of head injury and the need for immediate intervention. (See Figure 17-1.)

55–A. To perform cardiopulmonary resuscitation (CPR) on an infant, the landmark is one finger breaths below the nipple line. The compression depth is 0.5–1.0 inches. The ratio of chest compressions to ventilations should be 5:1, with a compression rate greater than 100 compressions per minute.

56–E. Pleural exudates are usually seen in pulmonary infections and neoplasms. Transudates are associated with congestive heart failure, renal failure, or cirrhosis. Exudates usually have a specific gravity of > 1.016 while in transudates it is < 1.016. Other biochemical differences between exudates and transudates are listed in table 3–2. All the incorrect choices are properties of transudates.

57–C. Loperamide is an anti-diarrheal agent used in the treatment of toxigenic bacterial diarrhea. Since the diarrhea is caused by a pre-formed toxin, there is no role for antibiotics. Amoxicillin, clindamycin, metronidazole, and vancomycin are all antibiotics.

58–E. Normal intraocular pressure is between 10–23 mmHg. It is elevated in conditions such as acute angle closure glaucoma, retrobulbar hemorrhage, and hyphema. It is decreased in conditions such as ruptured globe, traumatic iritis, and intraocular foreign body. When performing the examination of the eye, visual acuity should be checked one eye at a time. The visual acuity does not improve with pinhole testing in retinal or optic nerve disease, but will improve if the patient needs corrective lenses for eyesight. The cobalt blue light of the slit lamp, along with fluorescein dye, are used to look for corneal abrasions. The ophthalmoscope is used to check for neovascularization of *retinal* vessels.

59–B. The child has a mastoiditis. The most frequently implicated organisms include *Streptococcus pneumoniae, Streptococcus pyogenes, Staphylococcus aureus, Haemophilus influenzae,* and *Pseudomonas aeruginosa.* (Infection with *H. influenzae* is less common since the advent of the Hib vaccine.) Although it does not cover *P. aeruginosa,* cefuroxime would be the drug of choice; it must be given intravenously. The other antibiotics listed—amoxicillin, erythromycin, metronidazole, and tetracycline—do not reach adequate blood levels to cover (or do not cover at all) the usual pathogens associated with this condition.

60–E. Sialolithiasis is the obstruction of one of the salivary glands by a stone, which usually is composed of calcium. Pain usually is exacerbated by eating bitter or sour foods. Systemic lupus erythematosus and rheumatoid arthritis are not predisposing factors. Usually there is swelling over the affected gland. If infection is suspected, a medication with good staphylococcal and streptococcal coverage, such as Cefazolin, is indicated.

61–A. This woman has rubella. Rubella is one of the TORCH (*t*oxoplasmosis, *o*ther, *r*ubella, *c*ytomegalovirus, *h*erpesvirus) agents (see Table 20–10), and is associated with microcephaly, cataracts, cloudy cornea, "blueberry muffin" skin, deafness, congenital heart disease, and mental retardation in children born to mothers who contract the disease during pregnancy.

62–E. When faced with a patient in ventricular fibrillation, the initial treatment is defibrillation at 200 Joules (J). If the initial attempt fails, proceed with additional attempts at 300 J, then 360 J. If the patient continues to be pulseless, cardiopulmonary resuscitation (CPR) and cardioresponsive medications such as epinephrine, lidocaine, bretylium, and procainamide are indicated.

63–B. Labetalol is a β-blocker. Although all the medications listed may be useful for the treatment of a β-blocker overdose, the only medication for which the correct dosage is specified is glucagon. In addition, isoproterenol should never be given as an intravenous (IV) bolus, because it can cause the patient to go into ventricular tachycardia or fibrillation. Epinephrine IV is reserved for cardiac arrest situations (and severe anaphylactic shock, at a dose of 0.1–0.3 mg; and even then the risk of ventricular tachycardia or fibrillation is still high).

64–B. Systemic lupus erythematosus (SLE) is an autoimmune condition that affects mostly women in their third to sixth decades of life. Associated with this condition are fatigue, arthralgias, and arthritis. The malar (butterfly) rash is typical of SLE. Lupus cerebritis, a condition that affects the central nervous system, can present with headache, personality changes, and seizures.

65–C. Osteogenic sarcoma is a malignant tumor of bone producing mesenchyme and is the most common malignant pediatric bone tumor. Once diagnosed, surgery and chemotherapy are indicated. If osteogenic sarcoma is suspected, the child should receive a chest radiograph to look for metastases.

66–D. Carotid massage is a vagal maneuver that slows conduction down the atrioventricular (AV) node by increasing parasympathetic tone. It should be applied for only 5–10 seconds, and never bilaterally. Auscultation of carotid bruits is a firm contraindication to this procedure. However, a large proportion of patients with significant carotid stenosis have no bruits. Therefore, absence of bruits does not ensure the safety of the carotid massage maneuver. Usually, vagal maneuvers are performed prior to the administration of any medications.

67–E. Mania is a mood disorder that affects men and women equally. It usually begins in the third decade of life. Mania may be associated with paranoia, delusions, and hallucinations. The patient's speech is usually pressured, with flights of ideas. An antipsychotic such as haloperidol may be useful for treatment.

68–A. Activated charcoal is a very useful substance for gastrointestinal (GI) tract decontamination. However, charcoal does not absorb all substances. The recommended dose for activated charcoal is 1 g/kg. If the patient has active bowel sounds, multiple dosing may be indicated.

69–A. Temporal arteritis is an autoimmune disease that is associated with headache and visual disturbances secondary to vasculitis. The patient may also complain of painful chewing due to vascular involvement of vessels that supply the masseter, temporalis, and tongue muscles. Patients with suspected temporal arteritis should be admitted to the hospital and treated with corticosteroids until the diagnosis is either confirmed or ruled out by a temporal artery biopsy.

70–D. The initial pediatric dose of epinephrine is 0.01 mg/kg, with subsequent dose at 0.1 mg/kg, or 10 times the initial dose. The initial dose for an adult is 1.0 mg. This dose can be repeated every 3–5 minutes. Epinephrine in the arrest situation is not given intramuscularly. However, it can be delivered through the endotracheal tube if intravenous access is not available.

71–D. If adenosine and verapamil fail to convert or control paroxysmal supraventricular tachycardia, other medications that can be used include digoxin, β-blockers, and diltiazem (a calcium-channel blocker). Lidocaine and bretylium are used for ventricular ectopy, and magnesium is used for torsade de pointe; they are not indicated for narrow-complex tachycardia.

72–A. Most cases of pulmonary embolus will not present in as straightforward a fashion as this one. However, pulmonary embolus should always be considered when there is unexplained pleuritic chest pain, tachycardia, or tachypnea . Pneumonia, pneumothorax, and adult respiratory syndrome will have abnormal chest radiographs. Pleuritis is not associated with severe hypoxia. The classic $S_1Q_3T_3$ pattern is seen only about 30% of the time. SLE is a hypercoagulable state that is a risk factor for emboli.

73–C. A toxic-appearing patient with an intraabdominal infection such as cholecystitis requires coverage against gram-positive, gram-negative, and anaerobic organisms. Clindamycin and metronidazole are each effective against anaerobes. Cefazolin (a first generation cephalosporin) and ampicillin are each effective against gram-positive organisms. Gentamicin and ceftriaxone (a third generation cephalosporin) are each effective against gram-negative organisms. Therefore, one drug from each category should be used. A regimen of clindamycin and metronidazole misses gram- negative bugs; cefazolin and ampicillin misses gram-negative and anaerobic bugs; ampicillin and gentamicin misses anaerobic bugs; and a regimen of ceftriaxone, gentamicin, and metronidazole misses gram-positive bugs.

74–E. The Glasgow Coma Scale is used to quickly assess neurologic status. It is based on best eye, motor, and verbal response. Its range is from 3 to 15. Based on the description, the patient's score is 10. His use of inappropriate words gives him a 3 for verbal response; eye-opening to painful stimuli gives him another 2 points, while localization of pain gives him 5 points. See Figure 17-1.

75–C. *P. aeruginosa* ear infections in diabetics or immunocompromised patients can cause malignant otitis externa. This condition warrants intravenous antibiotics and hospital admission. The other choices are etiologies of otitis *media;* they do not lead to malignant otitis externa.

76–A. Aspirin ingestion may present with fever, tachypnea, vomiting, lethargy, and tinnitus. It also is associated with a respiratory alkalosis and an anion gap acidosis. Barbiturate and opiate intoxication usually present with hypoventilation. Cholinergic-intoxicated patients present with the SLUDGE toxidrome: *s*alivation, *l*acrimation, *u*rination, *d*iarrhea, *g*astrointestinal (GI) upset, and *e*mesis.

77–E. A slipped capital femoral epiphysis can present either abruptly or gradually. It usually is seen in boys with growth spurts, and the child will give a history of pain and limping. These children may be discharged (non-weight bearing), but should receive urgent orthopaedic follow-up.

78–C. $\dot{V}/\dot{Q}$ mismatch is the prime cause of hypoxia in conditions such as pulmonary embolus and adult respiratory distress syndrome (ARDS). Hypoventilation and a reduced fraction of inspired oxygen (FiO_2) do not present with an A-a gradient. Shunts and diffusion abnormalities do not improve with supplemental oxygen.

79–C. Pneumothorax is the presence of air in the intrapleural space. Chronic obstructive pulmonary disease (COPD), tuberculosis (TB), and lung cancer are just a few of the risk factors. The physical examination usually reveals decreased breath sounds and hyperresonance of the chest wall on the affected side. Tube thoracostomy is indicated for the evacuation of air from the pleural space. Tension pneumothorax usually presents with dull and shifted heart sounds.

80–C. An abdominal radiograph may be helpful to identify a calcified aorta, a predisposition for an abdominal aortic aneurysm.The symptomatic patient with an abdominal aortic aneurysm is a true emergency; however, asymptomatic patients with incidental findings can be discharged. Aneurysms of greater than 5 centimeters will need surgical repair. If symptomatic and hypertensive, medication should be given to lower the blood pressure to remove the threat of rupture. Physical exam will usually reveal pulse deficits in the upper and lower extremities.

81–A. Trigeminal neuralgia (tic douloreaux) presents with a shooting pain in the V2 or V3 distribution. It can be triggered by such things as chewing, smiling or eating. The pain is intense, unilateral, and lasts several seconds. Carbamazepine (with or without baclofen) may be helpful in preventing reoccurrence. Although all of the other choices listed are also anticonvulsants, they are not used in the treatment of trigeminal neuralgia.

82–A. Infectious mononucleosis, caused by the Ebstein-Barr virus, can present with general malaise, low-grade fever, pharyngitis, skin rash, and hepatosplenomegaly. The complete blood cell count (CBC) usually reveals atypical lymphocytes.

83–A. This patient probably is in a condition known as myxedema coma (although the patient need not be in a coma). The most likely cause of this situation is lack of thyroid hormone. Therefore, thyroxine would be indicated. All the other medications listed in the question—propylthiouracil, methimazole, iodine, and propranolol—are used for treatment of states of thyroid hormone excess.

84–C. The patient is suffering from mastitis. If she appears well and is without fever, the patient can be discharged on oral antibiotics with secure follow-up. A good choice of antibiotic is one that would cover normal skin flora. Of the choices listed, dicloxacillin is the best; however, erythromycin would be an alternate if the patient had a history of allergy to beta-lactam antibiotics. Gentamicin is a poor choice as it is not effective against most skin flora which are gram-positive.

85–E. Osmolality is calculated using the following equation: (2 × sodium) + glucose/18 + blood urea nitrogen (BUN)/2.8. The measured osmolality must be checked versus the calculated osmolality to seek a possible osmolar gap. Osmolar gaps often are seen in alcohol intoxications and ketosis.

86–C. Osgood-Schlatter disease is a painful enlargement of the tibial tubercle. It occurs between the ages of 10 and 15 and is found more commonly in boys. The treatment is rest, ice, elevation, pain medication, and temporary non-weight bearing. Resolution is slow, requiring a period of weeks to months.

87–C. The correct dose of heparin in the treatment of pulmonary embolus is 80U/kg bolus dose, followed by an18/U/kg drip. The activated partial thromboplastin time should be kept at 1.5–2.0 times baseline. Coumadin should be started 2–7 days after heparin therapy, and should be overlapped with heparin because coumadin takes approximately two days before therapeutic levels are reached. Fractionated heparins are given once a day subcutaneously.

88–C. Dystonic reactions (e.g., ophthalmoplegia, torticollis) are caused by the ingestion of neuroleptics such as haloperidol, thioridazine and chlorpromazine. Benztropine or diphenhydramine can reverse a dystonic reaction. Benzodiazepines (such as diazepam) should be avoided as first-line drugs because they reverse dystonia caused by other etiologies as well, (such as tetanus), and may lead a physician into making the wrong diagnosis.

89–D. A loading dose of methylprednisolone is indicated in this patient with neurologic deficits after blunt trauma. The National Acute Spinal Cord Injury Study found that patients with blunt spinal cord injury who were treated within 8 hours of their injury with 30 mg/kg methylprednisolone followed by an infusion of 5.4 mg/kg/hr showed neurological improvement at 6 weeks and 1 year. Mannitol, furosemide, and hyperventilation are not indicated, because there is no evidence of increased intracranial pressure.

90–B. Ischemic strokes make up about 85% of all strokes. Embolic stroke etiologies include atrial fibrillation, recent myocardial infarction, endocarditis, or cardiomyopathy. The most common site for a hemorrhagic stroke is the putamen. Patients will usually have a negative CT one hour into an acute ischemic stroke. Heparin may be used in some ischemic strokes, depending upon the size and progression of the stroke.

91–B. Corneal lacerations due to trauma may present with those elements contained in this patient's eye examination. Corneal abrasions and ulcers will not present with these acute signs. A conjunctival laceration will not involve the anterior chamber or cornea. Iridocyclitis will present with a normal-looking pupil; however, the pupillary be slow to react to light and there may be associated photophobia.

92–C. Cavernous sinus thrombosis is an acute emergency that carries a mortality of approximately 33%, even with appropriate treatment. The patient usually presents with eye and/or facial pain, as well as exophthalmos. Antibiotics of choice include nafcillin, ceftriaxone, ampicillin, or gentamicin, according to the type of infection. It is not necessary to cover *Pseudomonas* spp. in the immunocompetent patient.

93–A. Torsades de pointes is an electrocardiogram (ECG) rhythm that may look like ventricular fibrillation except that there will be alternation between high- and low-amplitude waves. Conditions that can cause torsades de pointes include overdoses with type 1A antiarrhythmic agents (e.g., procainamide or quinidine) or tricyclic antidepressants, as well as electrolyte imbalances. Torsades de pointes is not treated like ventricular fibrillation; magnesium is the drug of choice.

94–D. The treatment of choice for *Chlamydia pneumoniae* pneumonia is either doxycycline or erythromycin. The treatment of choice for *Streptococcus pneumoniae* or *Moraxella catarrhalis* is a β-lactam, such as a penicillin or a cephalosporin. The drug of choice for *Pseudomonas aeruginosa* is a β-lactam with or without an aminogylcoside. The drug of choice for *Pneumocystis carinii* is trimethoprim-sulfamethoxasole.

95–D. When presented with a patient with hemoptysis, a chest radiograph may be useful to look for tuberculosis, pneumonia, carcinoma, and other diseases. In association with renal disease, Goodpasture's syndrome or Wegener's granulomatosis would be suggested etiologies. Hemoptysis is usually due to bleeding from bronchial arteries or capillaries. An echocardiogram would be useful to rule out mitral stenosis as a cause of hemoptysis. Clubbing is seen in bronchogenic carcinoma, bronchiectasis, and chronic hypoxic diseases.

96–D. Epistaxis (or nosebleed) usually is more severe in adults than in children. The source of bleeding is usually from the anterior part of the nasal septum (Kiesselbach's plexus). Protein C deficiency usually causes a hypercoagulable state, and is not associated with nosebleeds. Nasal foreign bodies are much more common in children rather than adults.

97–B. Scarlet fever is caused by an endotoxin released by Group A beta-hemolytic streptococcus. The rash consists of punctate lesions on an erythematous base and feels like sandpaper to the touch. It is associated with fever, sore throat, and other constitutional symptoms. Scarlet fever should be treated with penicillin to avoid the risk of rheumatic fever.

98–A. This infant most likely has breast milk jaundice, a common form of neonatal hyperbilirubinemia that is not pathologic. It results from the normal increased uptake of unconjugated bilirubin from the gut in infants fed breast milk. These infants improve with temporary substitution or alternation of breast milk with formula feeds. Breast-feeding jaundice occurs in younger infants and is due to insufficient calories, similar to starvation jaundice in the adult. These infants require increased feeding. Neonatal albumin has a decreased binding affinity for bilirubin.

99–E. Cyclobenzaprine, a muscle relaxant, can be used for situations in which pain may be due to muscle spasm, or in torticollis. All the other medications listed—ibuprofen, indomethacin, naproxen, and sulindac—are nonsteroidal anti-inflammatory agents (NSAIDs) and do not have a direct effect on muscle relaxation. Muscle relaxants may have a sedative effect, and patients should be aware of the side effects associated with this type of medication.

100–C. Delayed postpartum hemorrhage (more than 48 hours after giving birth) is suspicious for either retained products of conception or endometritis. Bleeding from vaginal atony and intrapartum trauma usually occurs within 48 hours. This patient should be admitted to the hospital for observation and, possibly, intravenous antibiotics.

101–B. The lifetime risk of developing tuberculosis after exposure is only about 10% in the healthy host. Special acid-fast staining is used on sputum to help determine the diagnosis of tuberculosis. Cavitary lesions are usually found in the upper lobes of the lung. Isoniazid prophylaxis should be administered for 6 months. Any of the immunocompromised states, such as HIV infection, diabetes, renal failure, and cancer can increase the risk of developing tuberculosis.

102–C. This patient presents with the typical history and physical exam for acute appendicitis. Acute diverticulitis usually presents with left lower quadrant pain. A normal genital exam virtually excludes testicular torsion. Perforated ulcer usually presents with epigastric pain and localized rebound and guarding to the upper aspect of the abdomen. Urolithiasis presents with flank pain and hematuria.

103–D. Hyperparathyroidism, not hypoparathyroidism, can lead to stone formation (due to increased serum and urinary calcium). Abdominal radiographs tend to overestimate the size of the stone. Uric acid stones, which are radiolucent, occur in an acid environment. Patients who have their pain adequately controlled and able to tolerate oral fluid intake can be discharged safely from the emergency department. Cysteine is the least common type of urinary tract stone; the most common type is calcium oxalate.

104–C. Scleritis usually presents with a gradual onset of boring eye pain. There is no discharge. On slit lamp examination, cells and flare (secondary to anterior chamber inflammation) are appreciated. More likely causes of scleritis are from collagen-vascular disease (such as rheumatoid arthritis and lupus) and less likely from sarcoid and other granulomatous diseases. Antibiotic drops are not indicated for scleritis.

105–C. Acute necrotizing ulcerative gingivitis, or trench mouth, is seen commonly in adolescents and young adults. The treatment is warm saline irrigation and antibiotics, as well as viscous lidocaine for local pain control. None of the other conditions listed presents with a pseudomembrane over the gingiva.

106–B. Indomethacin, a nonsteroidal anti-inflammatory medication may exacerbate pain patients with peptic ulcer disease.Cimetidine (an H_2 blocker), sucralfate (coats mucosal lining), and omeprazole (a Na+-K+ ATPase pump inhibitor) are all used for the treatment of peptic ulcer disease. Meglumine diatrizoate (Gastrografin) is safe to use for a radiographic imaging study.

107–E. Diverticulosis and diverticulitis (an inflammation of a diverticula) are usually seen in the sixth decade of life or older. However, younger patients may have the disease. Diverticula are mostly found in the sigmoid colon. Pain is usually epigastric and/or left lower quadrant pain. The CT is used to identify bowel wall thickening or streaking or inflammation of the pericolonic fat. If the inflammation is near the urinary bladder, urinary urgency and frequency may be elicited from the history.

108–B. Herpes simplex is the viral agent that most commonly causes corneal ulcers. Bacterial ulcers, however, are more common in general, and usually follow minor corneal trauma. Fungal corneal ulcers may be seen in immunocompromised patients.

109–B. The fractures the patient suffered fit the description of a LeFort II fracture. A Lefort I fracture is separation of the lower maxilla (free floating jaw). A LeFort III fracture involves separation of the midface from the rest of the cranium. The LeFort IV fracture does not exist. (See Figure 9-5.)

110–C. A patient with arsenic poisoning may present with altered mental status and breath that smells like garlic. An odor of acetone is associated with alcohol or aspirin. Patients with cyanide intoxication present with breath that smells like bitter almonds. A breath odor of mothballs would suggest camphor; a wintergreen smell is suggestive of methylsalicylate.

111–B. Some ingested substances may appear on radiographs. These include, but are not limited to, chloral hydrate, heavy metals, iron, and potassium. The other substances listed in the question—acetaminophen, atenolol, nifedipine, and captopril—do not show up on radiographs.

112–E. Benzodiazepines such as lorazepam are used in cocaine intoxication to control agitation, tachycardia, hypertension, and hyperpyrexia. Aspirin should be avoided because of the possibility that an underlying thyrotoxicosis may be present. Phenothiazines such as haloperidol and chlorpromazine may increase the risk of seizure. Propranolol would control the hypertension and tachycardia but not the agitation, as it lacks sedative properties.

113–A. An elevated ammonia level is usually suggestive of hepatic encephalopathy. Wernicke's encephalopathy is caused by thiamine deficiency. The altered mental status found in acute alcoholic toxic and withdrawal states is not due to elevated ammonia levels. Delirium tremens is seizure activity associated with acute alcohol withdrawal.

114–A. Tetracycline is the treatment of choice for severe gastroenteritis secondary to *Vibrio parahemolyticus* found in shellfish. *Staphylococcus aureus* is associated with mayonnaise and diary products. *Escherichia coli* is associated with hamburger and poorly-cooked meat. *Clostridium botulinum* is associated with honey or canned foods. *Giardia lamblia* can be found in swimming pools and drinking water.

115–B. The pain of gastroesophageal reflux is usually relieved by sitting and is aggravated by lying down. It is caused by a lowering of lower esophageal sphincter pressure, which can be caused by fatty foods, chocolate, peppermint, and alcohol. Estrogen has not been shown to cause reflux disease; however, progesterone has been linked to reflux disease. Barium studies, endoscopy, and acid reflux tests can be used to determine the diagnosis. Gastroesophageal reflux disease is treated with a proton pump inhibitor such as omeprazole.

116–E. Of the medications listed in the question, trifluorothymidine is the only antiviral medication. All the other choices (ciprofloxacin, ceftriaxone, azithromycin, and bacitracin) are antibiotics, and would not be useful for herpes simplex conjunctivitis. Additional treatment would include artificial tears and cool compresses as well as an urgent ophthalmologic follow-up (within 24 hours).

117–A. In the pediatric population, the presence of a foreign body in the nose should always be suspected when there is a unilateral nose bleed with foul-smelling discharge. Sinusitis and Henoch-Schönlein purpura do not present as nosebleeds. Although nasal polyps and Osler-Rendu-Weber syndrome can present as epistaxis, there is no associated foul-smelling discharge or nasal fullness.

118–A. When a tooth is avulsed, the best transport medium is saliva. If possible, and if there is no concern about the risk of aspiration, the tooth should be transported in the patient's mouth. Milk, saline, and water are alternative media, but they are not as good as saliva. Dry gauze is the worst transport medium for an avulsed tooth.

119–D. Organophosphates (insecticides) and carbamate intoxication usually present with the SLUDGE syndrome: *s*alivation, *l*acrimation, *u*rination, *d*iarrhea, *g*astrointestinal (GI) upset, and *e*mesis. The other choices listed in the question—hyperthermia, dry mouth, urinary retention, and mydriasis—are compatible with anticholinergic intoxication. The treatment for organophosphate intoxication is atropine and pralidoxime.

120–D. The anion gap is calculated using the following equation: sodium—(HCO_3 + chloride). A normal anion gap is between 8 and 12 mEq/L. An elevated anion gap may be seen in situations of increased production of lactate (e.g., sepsis, carbon monoxide intoxication) or ketone (e.g., diabetic ketoacidosis, salicylate intoxication).

121–E. Rheumatoid arthritis first occurs most often between 25 and 50 years of age. The history usually reveals stiffness in the joints on wakening that may get somewhat better during the day. Rheumatoid factor and erythrocyte sedimentation rate (ESR) are elevated in most cases. Radiographic evidence includes periarticular erosions, joint space narrowing, and marginal erosions.

122–E. Hepatitis D, caused by the delta virus, occurs only in associated with Hepatitis B. Hepatitis A, transmitted enterally, does not cause permanent liver damage. In alcoholic hepatitis, the liver function test are usually only 2–3 times normal with asparagine amino transfer (AST) greater than the alanine aminotransferase (ALT) (due to liver mitochondrial damage, where AST is found in greater supply). Hepatitis C is transmitted through parenteral contact.

123–A. The analysis of the urine values reveal an acute renal failure which is prerenal in origin. The only cause of prerenal failure listed amongst the choices is cirrhosis. Other causes of prerenal failure include congestive heart failure, sepsis, and hypovolemic states. Rhabdomyolysis, Goodpasture's syndrome and multiple myeloma will cause renal (or intrinsic) causes of renal failure, where the FENa will be greater than 2.0 and the U_{osm} will be less than 300. Nephrolithiasis will cause a renal failure or the postrenal type, which usually presents with a high U_{Na}, usually greater than 40.

124–E. This patient with a urinary tract infection was placed on phenazopyridine, a urinary tract analgesic that will turn the urine a bright orange. Patients should receive reassurance before treatment that this event will likely occur. A repeat urine culture or urinalysis, cystogram, and coagulation profile are all unnecessary.

125–E. Breathing patterns will at times suggest the etiology of a patient's altered mental status. Ataxic breathing is irregularly irregular in rate and amplitude and can be found in medullary lower brain stem lesions. Cheyne-Stokes breathing is associated with upper brain stem lesions and congestive heart failure (CHF). Kussmaul breathing is associated with diabetic ketoacidosis. Hyperventilations are usually from a toxic-metabolic etiology. Eupneic breathing is normal breathing.

126–B. Peripheral vertigo, usually due to a labyrinthitis, is usually acute in onset, with intense dizziness and vomiting. Hearing loss and tinnitus are common. On examination for nystagmus, it is found to be unidirectional, horizontal, fatigable, and inhibited by ocular fixation. Gradual onset, intact hearing, multidirectional nystagmus, and neurologic deficit are typical findings of central vertigo.

127–B. The first intervention for a patient with acid or alkaline eye burns is copious eye irrigation with normal saline, Ringer's solution, or plain tap water. The irrigation should be continued until a neutral pH is reached. All other treatment is deferred.

128–D. Although all of the agents listed in the question can cause pharyngitis, adenovirus is the most likely agent. It can be associated with fever, exudates, and cervical adenopathy. Treatment is supportive.

129–E. Although most antibiotics have been linked as an etiologic agent of pseudomembranous colitis, clindamycin accounts for by far the most cases. Pseudomembranous colitis can develop from days to weeks after the start or termination of an antibiotic. The treatment for pseudomembranous colitis is either vancomycin or metronidazole.

130–B. Fungal infections of the skin (*candida* and *tinea* species), can be diagnosed by looking at skin scrapings of the affected area that have been treated with potassium hydroxide (KOH). The slide should be gently heated before examination to destroy other cellular elements. The Tzanck smear identifies varicella and herpes. India ink is used to identify cryptococcus.

131–A. A pregnant woman who does not have an intrauterine pregnancy (IUP) on ultrasound and has free fluid behind the uterus should be considered to have an ectopic pregnancy until proven otherwise. The free fluid may signify rupture (although some normal pregnancies do have free fluid). If the ectopic pregnancy is ruptured, the woman needs surgery. If it is not ruptured, treatment options include surgery or methotrexate.

132–C. The ferric chloride test is a qualitative measure for the presence of salicylate. The test is not able to quantify the amount of salicylate in the patient's blood or cerebrospinal fluid (CSF). With a positive ferric chloride test, a serum salicylate level should be sent. Other substances should also be considered, because an altered mental status due to intoxication may be the result of a mixed ingestion.

133–C. Pseudotumor cerebri, usually found in young, obese women, usually presents with the complaint of headache and blurred vision. Physical examination will reveal papilledema and occasionally cranial nerve involvement. Head CT is normal and the lumbar puncture (LP) will have a high opening pressure. Normal pressure hydrocephalus and atypical migraine do not have high opening pressure on LP. Subarachnoid hemorrhage would reveal blood on either the CT or LP. Viral meningitis would present with white cells on the LP.

134–E. The treatment for hyphema (blood in the anterior chamber) includes keeping the head of the bed elevated 30°–45°, administering cycloplegic drops, and the application of a transparent eye shield. Because of the risk of rebleeding, aspirin and aspirin-like medications should be avoided. Vomiting will increase intraocular pressure, therefore, the use of an antiemetic, such as prochlorperazine, is indicated.

135–B. Cellulitis, which usually affects the lower extremities, as well as the upper extremities and the face, presents with a warm, erythematous, and indurated area of skin with margins that are not well demarcated. People who are immunocompromised (e.g., those with human immunodeficiency virus [HIV], diabetes mellitus, or renal insufficiency) are at a higher risk for cellulitis. Most patients, however, can be discharged with an antibiotic that covers *Staphylococcus* and *Streptococcus* species with follow-up in 48 hours.

136–B. Thyroid storm is a complication of thyroid disease that, although seldom seen, can carry a mortality of up to 50% if left untreated. Although all the choices listed in the question can predispose a patient with thyroid disease to become thyrotoxic, by far the leading etiology is sepsis. In addition to treatment of the underlying cause, this patient should be given medications such as propylthiouracil, iodine, propranolol, and corticosteroids. Aspirin should be avoided for treatment of fever, because the aspirin may displace thyroid hormone from its carrier protein, thereby making the hormone active.

137–D. The risk factors for toxemia of pregnancy (preeclampsia and eclampsia) include nulliparity, maternal age less than 20 or greater than 35 years, multiple gestations, hydatidiform mole, hypertension, diabetes mellitus, and pre-existing renal disease. Preeclampsia is a syndrome of hypertension, proteinuria, and peripheral edema. Eclampsia is preeclampsia with central nervous system (CNS) involvement, such as coma or seizures. Eclamptic seizures are treated with magnesium. Age of menarche is not a known risk factor for toxemia of pregnancy.

138–D. Bacterial meningitis carries a much higher mortality and morbidity than viral meningitis. Because of high cerebrospinal fluid (CSF) pressures generated in meningitis, the infant's fontanelles are usually bulging, and a high opening pressure would be found on lumbar puncture. *Streptococcus pneumoniae* and *Neisseria meningitides* are leading causes of bacterial meningitis in adolescents and young adults. *Haemophilus influenzae* meningitis is less common since the advent of the *H. influenzae* type B (Hib) vaccine. The drug of choice would be a broad-spectrum β-lactam, such as a third generation cephalosporin (e.g., ceftriaxone).

139–E. Methadone has a duration of action between 6 and 8 hours. When treating a patient with methadone overdose, multiple doses of naloxone may be needed before methadone is adequately cleared from the system. Most patients with methadone overdose should be admitted to the intensive care unit (ICU) for observation and medical management. The other choices (codeine, meperidine, morphine, and heroin) are other opiates with shorter durations of action.

140–B. N-acetylcysteine (NAC) is the recommended drug of choice for acetaminophen overdose. Ideally, it should be given within 8 hours of ingestion, although it may be useful up to 72 hours after ingestion. NAC is given orally, in multiple doses over 3 days. Sodium bicarbonate is used in the treatment of tricyclic antidepressant overdose. Thiamine is administered to alcoholics to prevent Wernicke's encephalopathy. Protamine reverses heparin toxicity. Physostigmine is used to treat anticholinergic overdose.

141–C. A Bartholin's cyst may be found at the introitus of the vagina. It develops from the Bartholin's glands, the function of which is to lubricate the vulva. The Word catheter is a special catheter with a balloon on the end that is inflated with saline while it is placed in the incised cyst. The catheter should stay in place for several weeks before it is removed, and the patient should have follow-up while the catheter is in place.

142–B. Diabetic ketoacidosis is associated with the fruity odor of acetone. This odor should not be confused with the smell of alcohol on the breath, which would be a disastrous mistake. A bitter almond smell on the breath is associated with cyanide poisoning. A fecal smell is associated with hepatic encephalopathy.

143–B. When closing an eyelid laceration, the smallest suture material, at least 6.0, should be used. Though silk is more comfortable, it carries the risk of a more exaggerated inflammatory response, therefore, nylon is a better choice. Complicated lacerations should be referred to an ophthalmologist.

144–C. Pyridoxine, (vitamin B_6) which is a cofactor in the formation of gamma-aminobutyric acid (GABA), is indicated for isoniazid-induced seizures. Isoniazid inhibits GABA formation. GABA is involved with the inhibition of neurons reaching action potential. Thiamine, (vitamin B_1) is administered to alcoholics to prevent Wernicke's encephalopathy, which usually does not involve seizures. Niacin (vitamin B_3) deficiency causes dementia which again does not usually involve seizures. Methylene blue is used to treat methemoglobinemia. Calcium is used to treat hypocalcemia, which can manifest with seizures.

145–E, 146–D, 147–C, 148–A, 149–B. A positive antinuclear antibody in the face of oligoarthritis is consistent with systemic lupus erythematosus (SLE). Young children with joint effusions may have a septic arthritis due to *Staphylococcus aureus* or gram-negative bacilli. Gonococcal arthritis must be considered in a sexually active adult who presents with migratory, polyarticular joint pain and swelling. The joint swelling of gout may be associated with tophi, which are nodular calcifications that may be seen on the toes, elbows, or ears. Analysis of the synovial fluid aspirated from a patient with pseudogout, or calcium pyrophosphate deposition disease, reveals positively birefringent crystals under polarized light (gout has negatively birefringent crystals). In assessing patients with joint effusions, physicians should not go with the odds; effusions should be aspirated for a definitive diagnosis to be made.

150–153. The answers are **150–C, 151–A, 152–D, 153–B.** Continuous mandatory ventilation (CMV) mode, delivers ventilations at a present rate and tidal volume without any need for patient effort. If the patient is not comatose, it requires neuromuscular paralysis and sedation. In assist control (AC) mode, the ventilator responds to the patients efforts, delivering ventilations at the initiation of a patient's ventilatory attempt. If no attempt, the ventilator will breathe for the patient. Intermittent mandatory ventilation (IMV) mode, may cause breath stacking if the patients ventilations are not timed with the ventilations initiated by the ventilator itself. Synchronized intermittent mandatory ventilation (SIMV) mode prevents breath stacking by synchronizing the patients ventilations with those delivered by the ventilator. This mode also facilitates weaning off the ventilator.

154–158. The answers are: **154–C, 155–A, 156–B, 157–D, 158–E.** Causes of pulseless electrical activity, other than tension pneumothorax and cardiac tamponade, include hypovolemia, hypothermia, massive pulmonary embolism, and certain drug overdoses. Magnesium is indicated for a ventricular fibrillation-like rhythm, torsades de pointes, caused by electrolyte disturbances, certain antiarrhythmics, and tricyclic antidepressant overdoses. There is no ventricular activity in asystole. Supraventricular tachycardia may be treated with vagal maneuvers, adenosine or verapamil. If presented with a stable patient with a wide complex tachycardia, lidocaine is indicated. If the patient is unstable, then cardioversion would be the initial intervention.

159–C, 160–D, 161–E, 162–A, 163–B. Erysipelas, usually caused by *Streptococcus* spp., most commonly occurs in children and elderly people. There may be a prodrome of fever and chills. The key differentiating factor between this and cellulitis is that erysipelas is very painful. Acne, which usually affects adolescents, can affect the face and trunk. Psoriasis is a chronic disease, usually worse in the winter. The plaques usually are found on the extensor surfaces of the body, especially the elbow. Herpetic infections usually are painful. Herpes simplex and herpes zoster (shingles) usually are diagnosed on a clinical basis without the need for special tests, such as a Tzanck smear. Treatment includes the use of acyclovir, valacyclovir, or famciclovir. Impetigo usually is due to a staphylococcal or streptococcal infection that affects the most superficial layer. It usually occurs in children, and the most common location is the face. Antibiotics, such as cephalexin, can be used for treatment.

164–B, 165–A, 166–D, 167–C. Although various bacteria can be found in many different bites (e.g., *P. multocida* in cat, dog, and primate bites), certain bacteria are more typically seen with certain types of bites. It is useful to know which bacteria are commonly seen with specific types of bites when choosing antibiotics.

168–171: The answers are: **168–D, 169–C, 170–A, 171–B.** Zafirlukast is a non-specific inhibitor that blocks leukotriene C_4 (LTC_4), leukotriene D_4 (LTD_4), and leukotriene E_4 (LTE_4), receptors. Leukotrienes cause bronchoconstriction through a number of mechanisms. Prednisone, a steroid, controls the late inflammatory aspect of asthma. Albuterol, as well as other β agonists, works by way of bronchial sympathetic receptors to cause bronchodilatation. Bronchodilatation is also the end result of the administration of ipratropium, but its mechanism of action is through inhibition of anticholingeric receptors.

172–176: The answers are: **172–E, 173–D, 174–C, 175–B, 176–A.** Grey-Turner's and Cullen's signs may be found in hemorrhagic pancreatitis. Rovsing's sign is a sign of peritonitis and can be found in acute appendicitis. The obturator sign (found when there is irritation of the obturator externus muscle) and the iliopsoas sign (when there is irritation of the iliopsoas muscle) may be positive findings in acute appendicitis.

177–181: The answers are: **177–E, 178–A, 179–D, 180–C, 181–B.** Acute epididymitis may be associated with benign prostatic hypertrophy in the elderly. The treatment for phimosis may involve an incision on the foreskin on the dorsal aspect of the penis, called a dorsal slit, as a definitive measure. Testicular torsion, a twisting of the testicle and spermatic cord which results in neurovascular compromise, presents with an absent or decreased cremasteric reflex. Penile fractures, which can occur during sexual intercourse, present as a swollen, painful penis. The patient will usually report a clicking sound on history. Priapism, a prolonged, painful erection, is associated with sickle cell disease, metastatic disease, lymphoma, and spinal shock.

182–185: The answers are: **182–D, 183–C, 184–A, 185–B.** Bell's palsy is an idiopathic seventh cranial nerve paralysis or paresis. It may be associated with hyperacusis, pain behind the mastoid or ear, and impaired taste. Other causes of seventh nerve dysfunction include herpes simplex or herpes zoster infection, Lyme disease, sarcoid, and tumor. Guillain-Barré, an acute demyelinating peripheral neuropathy (the peripheral analog of multiple sclerosis) will usually present with symptoms in the lower extremities that will ascend to the upper extremities and chest muscles. Multiple sclerosis, which is a demyelinating disease of the central nervous system axons, can present with different neurologic disturbances at different times. It is associated with optic neuritis and intranuclear opthalmoplegia. Myasthenia gravis, a disease where antibodies are made to acetylcholine receptors, presents with easy fatigability, especially to the cranial nerves.

186–E, 187–C, 188–A, 189–D, 190–B. Orbital blow-out fractures present with limitation of intraocular movement, orbital edema, subcutaneous emphysema, ptosis, and enophthalmos. Acute glaucoma typically presents with high intraocular pressure and a steamy looking cornea on eye examination. Cells and flare usually signify inflammation in the anterior chamber, as in iritis or anterior uveitis. A patient with a central retinal arterial occlusion usually complains about painless vision loss over several hours to days; a retrobulbar hemorrhage as well as a pale retina may be appreciated. Corneal abrasions are superficial tears in the cornea. The patient will complain of eye pain, and the vision may or may not be affected. On slit-lamp examination, an uptake of fluorescein is visualized with the green light.

191–B, 192–D, 193–E, 194–C, 195–A. Therapy with methylene blue is indicated for methemoglobinemia because it is a substitute for a limiting cofactor in NADPH-dependent hemoglobin reduction. Deferoxamine is a chelating agent used for the treatment of toxic iron ingestions. Amyl nitrate is given in cyanide intoxication to produce methemoglobinemia to provide a competitive substance for cyanide binding. Seizures that do not respond to conventional medications may be due to isoniazid intoxication. Pyridoxine is used to help promote GABA production. Vitamin K is instrumental in the carboxylation of certain coagulation factors that are blocked by the use of warfarin.

196–E, 197–D, 198–C, 199–A, 200–B. Children with cystic fibrosis often develop bronchiectasis after chronic and recurrent episodes of bronchiolitis. Parvovirus, the etiologic agent of erythema infectiosum, can cause a transient aplastic crisis in patients with hemolytic anemia, including sickle cell disease. Subacute sclerosis panencephalitis is an uncommon complication of measles that may appear 10 years after infection. Its incidence has decreased with immunizations. Two percent of children with Kawasaki disease, or mucocutaneous lymph node syndrome, die from complications, particularly coronary aneurysm. Disseminated intravascular coagulation occurs in Rocky Mountain spotted fever with invasion of the endothelium by rickettsial organisms.

Index

References in *italics* indicate figures; those followed by "t" denote tables